atlas of HAND SURGERY

by Robert A. Chase, M.D.

Emile Holman Professor of Surgery, and
Chairman, Department of Surgery,
Stanford University School of Medicine, Stanford, California

W. B. SAUNDERS COMPANY • Philadelphia • London • Toronto

W. B. Saunders Company: West Washington Square
Philadelphia, PA 19105

1 St. Anne's Road
Eastbourne, East Sussex BN21 3UN, England

1 Goldthorne Avenue
Toronto, Ontario M8Z 5T9, Canada

Listed here is the latest translated edition of this book together with the language of the translation and the publisher.

Japanese (*1st Edition*) – Igaku Shoin Ltd., Tokyo, Japan

Atlas of Hand Surgery   ISBN 0-7216-2495-2

© 1973 by W. B. Saunders Company. Copyright under the International Copyright Union. All rights reserved. This book is protected by copyright. No part of it may be reproduced, stored in a retrieval system, or transmitted in any form or by any means, electronic, mechanical, photocopying, recording, or otherwise, without written permission from the publisher. Made in the United States of America. Press of W. B. Saunders Company. Library of Congress catalog card number 72-97907.

Print No: 9   8   7   6

To Ann

Preface

The principles of hand surgery have evolved to some extent from research investigation but in larger part from experience. Therefore, if we are to concern ourselves with the proper application of the principles of hand surgery, we must absorb everything in the milieu which may be relevant. Discussions with a mentor and participation with him in the care of patients are the basis for development of competence.

Experience is partly based on one's own attempts to apply surgical principles, but the attempts of others provide equally important knowledge. The principles themselves continue to be modified and improved upon by innovators in surgery—through experience. Since experience in surgery may be passed on by personal interchange with only a limited number of colleagues, the published word and diagram become very important in establishing the educational milieu alluded to above. The urge to record experiences personally participated in and the compelling desire to make available to colleagues some of the valued return of interchanges with my teachers and fellow students prompted the preparation of this atlas.

The excitement in surgery of the hand arises from the fact that each hand problem is different and requires the sequence of (1) thinking through the problem; (2) conceptualizing a course of action; (3) pursuing that course; and (4) assessing the results. This kind of clinical equivalent of research has generated the principles by which we function as hand surgeons.

The material presented in this atlas is based on case experiences. The case examples chosen exemplify fundamentals which may be applied in new combinations to fit the unique problems of any patient who presents himself with a surgical problem in the hand. I have used principles, notions and prejudices passed on to me by those with whom I have had the closest relationship in surgery of the hand, particularly Willie White, Bill Littler, Erle Peacock, Paul Brand, Don Laub and Harry Buncke. I am grateful to them for the occasional use from their experiences of a case example which perfectly exemplifies a principle.

This atlas is a reality in large part because of the enormous effort of Daisy Stilwell, whose drawings better than words depict principles and techniques which have proved useful in clinical experience. I am grateful for the talented hands, keen intellect and perseverance of my secretary, Mrs. Grace Lee, for her help in preparing the manuscript. Their capable hands have made my task of directing the project an easy one.

ROBERT A. CHASE, M.D.

Contents

General Principles

1	ANATOMY	3
2	RECORDS	21
3	TOURNIQUET	22
4	NERVE BLOCK ANESTHESIA	24
5	SKIN AND SUBCUTANEOUS TISSUE	32
6	ELECTIVE SKIN INCISIONS	35
7	SKIN GRAFTING	40
8	INFECTIONS	56

Fingertip Injuries

9	MINOR SOFT TISSUE LOSS	63
10	EXTENSIVE SOFT TISSUE LOSS	66
11	REPLANTATION OF FINGERTIP AFTER AMPUTATION	68
12	FINGERNAIL INJURIES	70
13	CROSS-FINGER FLAP	71
14	FINGER TO THUMB PEDICLE FLAP	74
15	ISLAND PEDICLE FLAP FOR FINGERTIP LOSS	78
16	ADVANCEMENT FLAP FOR FINGERTIP LOSS	82

Contents

Skin and Soft Tissue Losses

Free Skin Grafts

17	Skin Grafting on the Palm of the Hand	86
18	Free Plantar Skin Graft to Palm	90
19	Skin Grafting on the Dorsum of the Hand	92

Pedicle Flaps

20	Soft Tissue Replacement Using Vascularized Pedicles	96

Local Pedicle Flaps

21	Cross-Finger Flaps	97
22	Local Pedicle Shift	100
23	Secondary Digital Fillet	104
24	Finger Fillet to Resurface the Thumb	110
25	The Fillet Principle in Acute Injury	112
26	Two-Stage Amputation with Cross-Finger Flap	116

Distant Pedicle Flaps

27	Pedicle Soft Tissue from Distant Sites	120
28	The Infraclavicular Flap	126
29	Total Hand Degloving Injury	134
30	The First Web Space	136
31	Proper Use and Care of Pedicle Flaps	142

Amputations

32	Single Digit Amputation	148
33	Index Ray Amputation	151
34	Fifth Ray Amputation	158

35	Salvage of Usable Parts in Severe Hand Injuries.......................... 162
36	Use of Damaged Digits as Composite Transfers............................ 164
37	Use of Amputated Parts as a Source of Free Grafts of Skin and Nerves 166
38	Double Use of a Finger Fated for Amputation 168
39	The Primary Island Pedicle Flap for Salvage After Trauma......... 172
40	Metacarpal Transfer... 182
41	Composite Transfer of a Joint... 190

Vascular Reconstruction

42	Allen's Test.. 196
43	Vascular Reconstruction 198

Nerve Surgery

44	Sensory and Motor Deficits in Acute Median Nerve Injury at the Wrist 202
45	Primary Nerve Repair.. 205
46	Findings and Treatment Late After Median Nerve Injury at the Wrist 208
47	Acute Ulnar Nerve Transection at the Wrist 210
48	Acute Injury of the Motor Branch of the Ulnar Nerve............. 213
49	Digital Nerve Repair... 216
50	Small Superficial Sensory Nerve Branches 218
51	Factors Influencing Care of Nerve Injuries at the Wrist 221
52	Injury of the Ulnar Nerve at the Elbow 222
53	Radial Nerve Paralysis... 226
54	Median Nerve Injury at the Elbow 228

Contents

55	Tests to Sharpen Diagnosis Late After Nerve Injury	229
56	Nerve Gaps	234
57	The Island Pedicle Technique	238
58	Combined Island Pedicle and Nerve Transfer	242

Bone and Joint Reconstruction

59	Fractures in the Hand	246
60	Stiff Proximal Interphalangeal Joints	254
61	Bone Grafting	258
62	Use of Bone Grafts in the Phalanges	266
63	Metacarpal Bone Grafting	270
64	Fusion of Thumb Metacarpophalangeal Joint	276
65	Fusion of Thumb Carpometacarpal Joint	280
66	Fusion of Digital Joints	283
67	Fusion of the Wrist Joint	288

Reconstruction of the Thumb

68	Reconstruction of the Thumb	295
69	Thumb Reconstruction by Pollicization	300
70	Pedicle Flap, Bone Graft, Island Flap Reconstruction of the Thumb	310

Surgery of Rheumatoid Arthritis

71	Wrist Arthroplasty	321
72	Metacarpophalangeal Joint Synovectomy	326
73	Finger Arthroplasty	332

74	Synovectomy of Extensor Tendons at the Wrist	340
75	Rupture of Extensor Tendons	342
76	Resection of the Ulnar Head	344

Tendons, Fascia and Muscles

77	Tendon Injuries	346
78	Flexor Tendon Lacerations	348
79	Flexor Tendon Grafting	356
80	Tendon Graft Donor Sites	361
81	Laceration of the Flexor Pollicis Longus	363
82	Palmar Wrist Laceration	366
83	Extensor Tendon Lacerations	368
84	Digital Extensor Tendon Injuries	370
85	The Extensor Pollicis Longus	372
86	Deformities of the Fingers from Tendon Imbalance	374
87	Dupuytren's Contracture	378
88	Tendon Transfers	396
89	Tendon Transfers for Ulnar Nerve Paralysis	400
90	Tendon Transfers for Median Nerve Paralysis	418
91	Tendon Transfers for Radial Nerve Paralysis	427

Index 433

General Principles

1

Anatomy

The unique functional capacity of the human hand has been extolled by anatomical observers since the dawn of medical history. As a functional puppet it responds to the desires of man; its motor performance is initiated by the contralateral cerebral cortex. The conscious demands relayed to the hand and forearm from the central nervous controlling mechanism are sent as movement commands. At the subconscious levels, such a movement command is broken down, regrouped, coordinated, and sent on as a signal for fixation, graded contraction, or relaxation of a specific muscular unit. The degree of contraction or relaxation is then modified by relayed evidence that the motion created is that desired by the person. The modifying factors arrive centrally from a multiplicity of sensory sources such as the eye, peripheral sensory end organs, and muscle or joint sensory endings. The surgeon planning reconstructive surgery on the upper extremity must be aware not only of the complex anatomy of the hand and arm but also of the physiologic interplay of balanced muscular functions under the influence of complex central nervous coordination. The maintenance of physiologic viability by the central and peripheral circulatory and lymphatic systems must also concern the reconstructive surgeon.

1 — Anatomy

THE SKELETON AND ITS NEUROMUSCULAR APPARATUS

In any anatomic study of the hand and forearm, one thought should be kept in mind as one delves into morphologic detail of each structure—that physiologic hand function knows no such specialization as the dissected mechanical categories into which we fit our fragments of anatomic knowledge. Natural function knows only a summation of actions as expressed in phenomena such as grasp, pinch, push, pull, or release. A study of single muscle or tendon function is an anatomic and not a physiologic study. It is essential to recall that the muscular unit never functions alone but is a cooperative contributor to hand posture, fixation, or motion, by its fixed or varied contraction or relaxation with its antagonists, protagonists and modifiers.

Architecture

The ability of the hand to resist and create powerful gross action, combined with its capacity to perform intricate fine movements in multiple planes, reflects the masterful construction of its supporting architecture. Reducing the hand to its supporting skeleton and its restraining ligaments reveals the architectural basis for its varied function. A study of the range of joint motions in the hand and forearm with all motor elements removed discloses the full range and limitations which the skeleton imposes on hand function.

The hand skeleton is divisible into four elements of descending order of specialization. (**A**)

1. The *thumb* and its *metacarpal* with a wide range of motion at the carpometacarpal joint. Five intrinsic muscles and four extrinsic muscles are specifically influential on thumb positioning and activity.

2. The *index finger* with independence of action within the range of motion allowed by its joints and ligaments. Three intrinsic and four extrinsic muscles allow such digital independence.

3. The *third, fourth, and fifth fingers with metacarpals 4 and 5*. This unit functions as a stabilizing vise to grasp objects for manipulation by the thumb and index finger or in concert with the other hand units in powerful grasp.

4. *The fixed unit of the hand consisting of the second and third metacarpals and the distal carpal row.*

The Fixed Unit of the Hand

The distal row of carpal bones forms a solid architectural arch with the capitate bone as a keystone. The articulations of the distal carpals with one another, the intercarpal ligaments, and the important transverse carpal ligament (flexor retinaculum) maintain a strong, fixed transverse carpal arch. Projecting distally from the central third of this arch are the fixed central metacarpals, the second and third. Littler has called this "the fixed unit of the hand." It forms a fixed transverse arch of carpal bones and a fixed longitudinal arch created by the anatomic convexity of the metacarpals. As a stable foundation this unit creates a supporting base for the three other mobile units. This central beam moves as a unit at the wrist under the influence of the prime wrist extensors (extensor carpi radialis longus and extensor carpi radialis brevis) and the prime wrist flexor, the flexor carpi radialis. These major wrist movers insert on the second and third metacarpals. Thus the fixed central unit is positioned for activity of the adaptive elements of the hand around it. (**B**)

The Adaptive Hand Elements

At the level of the metacarpal heads the transverse arch of the hand becomes mobile, which is possible because the first metacarpal moves through a wide range of motion at the saddle-like carpometacarpal joint, and the fourth and fifth metacarpal heads move for-

General Principles

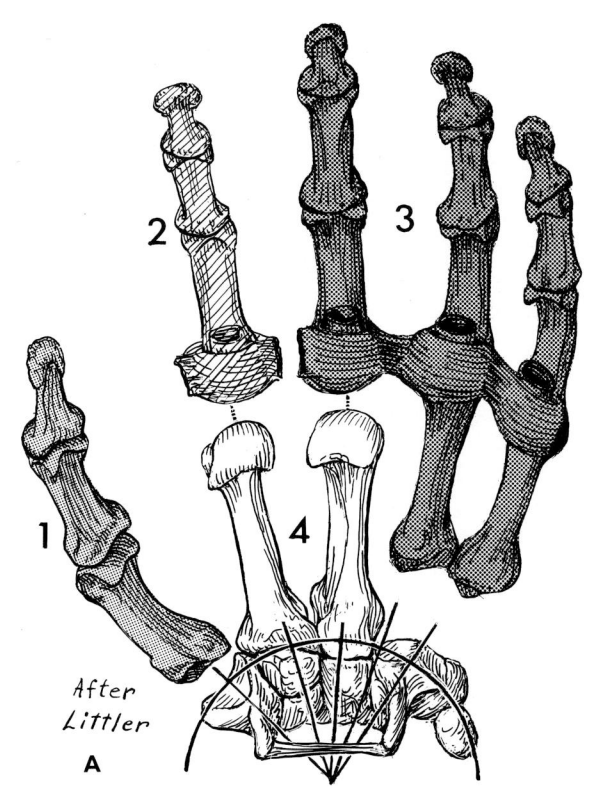

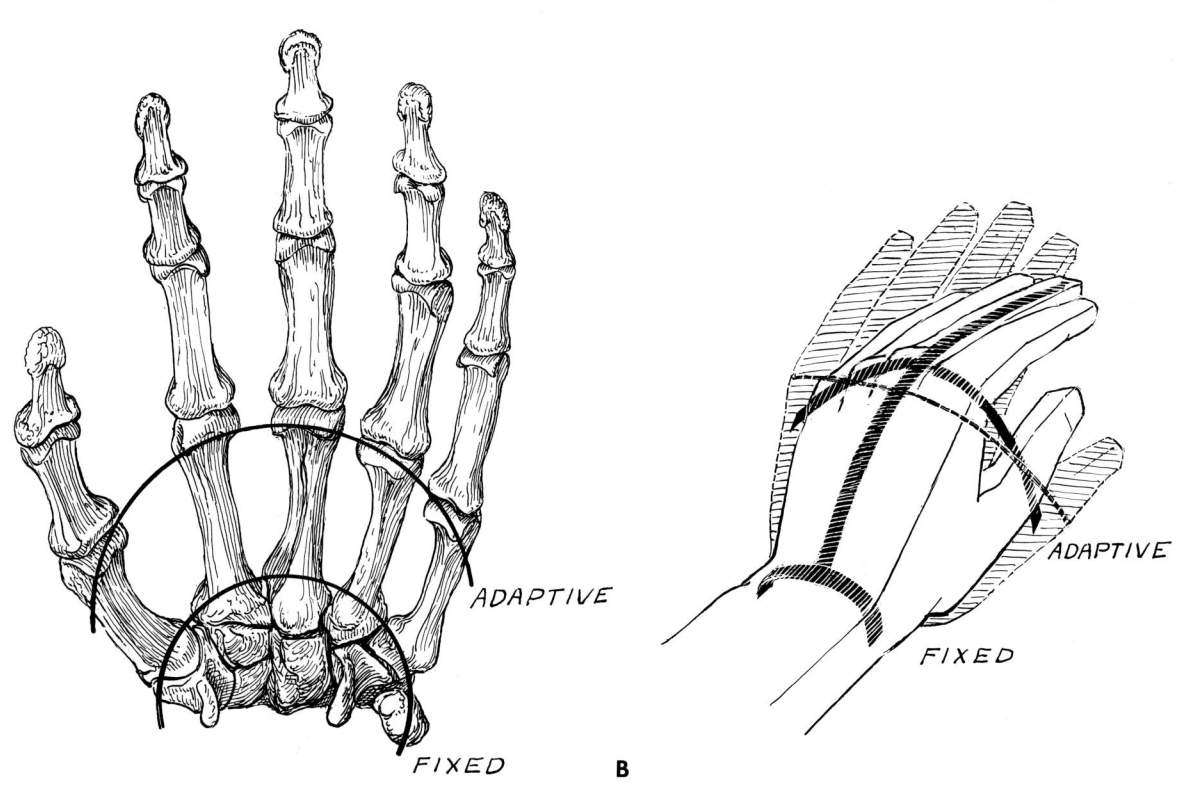

5

ward and back about 15 and 30 degrees, respectively.

The loose capsular ligaments of the thumb carpometacarpal joint with its shallow saddle articulation allow circumduction of the mobile first metacarpal. Its range of motion is checked by these capsular ligaments and by its attachment to the fixed hand axis through the adductor pollicis, the first dorsal interosseous, and the fascia and skin of the first web space. The mobile fourth and fifth metacarpal heads move dorsal and palmar in relation to the central hand axis by limited mobility at the carpometacarpal joints. These metacarpal heads are tethered to the central metacarpals by the intermetacarpal ligaments. The intermetacarpal ligaments unite adjacent metacarpophalangeal volar plates, which are intimate parts of the joint capsules.

When the head of the first metacarpal is palmar abducted by thenar muscles, innervated by the median nerve, and the fourth and fifth metacarpals are palmar abducted by the hypothenar muscles, innervated by the ulnar nerve, a palmar, concave, transverse metacarpal arch is created, approximating a semicircle. The mobile metacarpal heads are pulled dorsally by extrinsic extensor tendons when the thenar and hypothenar muscles relax. It is obvious that a flaccid paralysis of the intrinsic muscles of the hand in median and ulnar nerve palsy will produce a flattened or even reversed transverse metacarpal arch. The active production of a semicircular transverse arch by the thenar and hypothenar muscles creates the proper circumferential arrangement of the metacarpophalangeal joints for convergence of the fingers in flexion. In this position the fingers, flexing at the metacarpophalangeal joints only, converge, forming with the thumb a cone whose apex lies over the anatomic center of the hand. (**C**)

A vertical line dropped from the apex of the cone to the center of its base will strike the third metacarpophalangeal joint. This point at the apex of the transverse metacarpal arch is the anatomic center of the hand. With the fingers fully abducted the tips form radii of equal length from the anatomical center of the hand. The thumb without its distal phalanx is a fifth equal radius. (**D**) The same radius projected proximally falls at the wrist joint.

The Metacarpophalangeal Joints

Lateral activity in the metacarpophalangeal joints in the denuded skeleton with only ligaments intact is limited by the reinlike collateral ligaments. (**E**) These ligaments are loose and redundant while the metacarpophalangeal joints are in extension and hyperextension, allowing maximum medial and lateral deviation. As the metacarpophalangeal joint is flexed, the cam effect of the eccentrically placed ligaments and the epicondylar bowing of the collateral ligaments result in tightening and strict limitation of lateral mobility.

Fingers which have been fixed in extension during periods of healing have had the stage set for collateral ligament shrinkage and locking of the metacarpophalangeal joints in hyperextension.

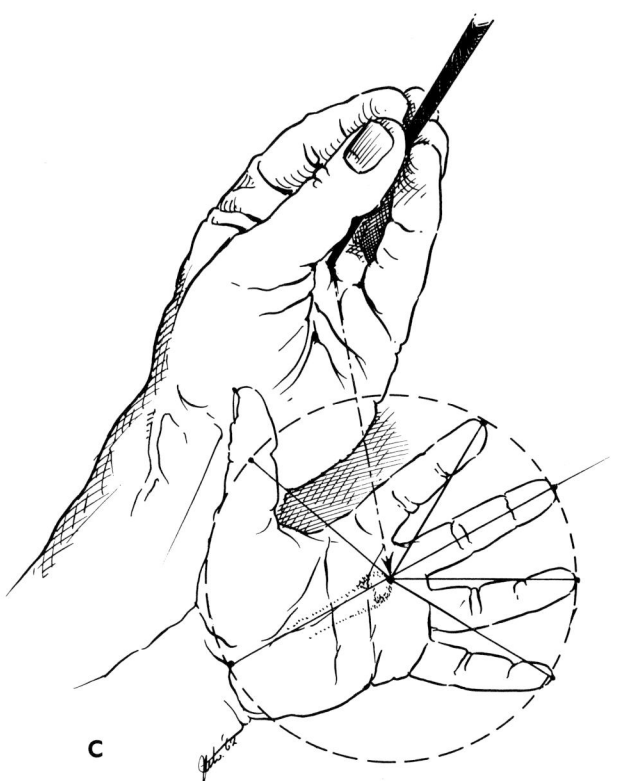
C

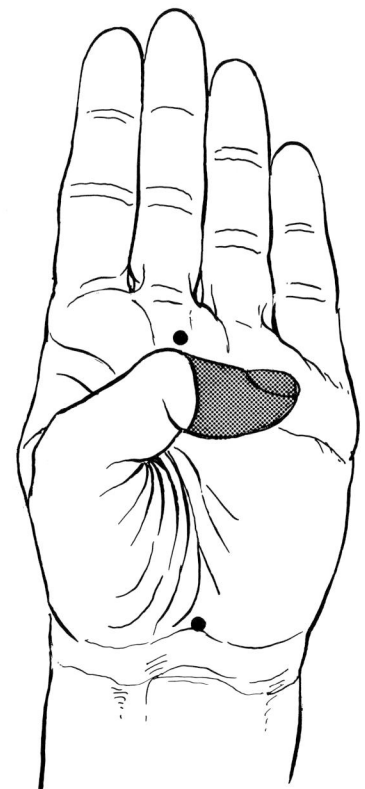
D

General Principles

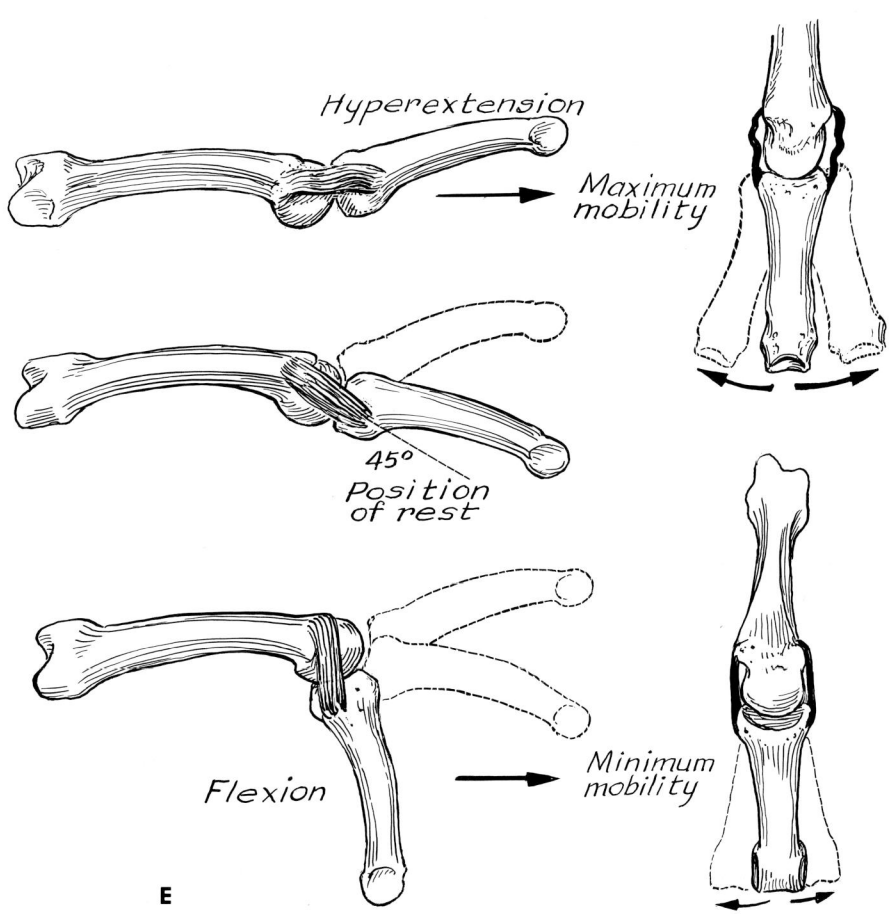

Adapted from Littler, in Converse: Reconstructive Plastic Surgery. Philadelphia, W. B. Saunders Company, 1964, Vol. 4, p. 1620.

The Interphalangeal Joints

The proximal interphalangeal joint can be pushed to 120 degrees of flexion or 30 degrees beyond the right angle, but extension usually cannot be carried beyond 5 degrees of hyperextension because of the ligamentous volar plate, which is an inseparable part of the joint capsule. The medial and lateral collateral ligaments are a part of the capsule. They are radially fixed in a manner which allows no medial or lateral deviation of the joint in any position.

The distal interphalangeal joints of the fingers can be pushed into flexion to about 90 degrees before they are limited by the dorsal joint capsule. The distal interphalangeal joints extend to 30 degrees of hyperextension. There is no lateral mobility in these joints with the collateral ligaments intact. The collateral ligaments of the distal interphalangeal joints are simply thickened medial and lateral portions of the joint capsule.

The proximal interphalangeal joints and the distal interphalangeal joints are hinge joints; any lateral motion is limited in all phases of flexion and extension by radially oriented collateral ligaments which are tight at any angle. The metacarpophalangeal joints, in contrast, allow motion through several axes. The capsule, including the collateral ligaments and volar plate, is quite lax, allowing medial and lateral deviation, flexion, extension, and thereby circumduction and a small degree of distraction. In the absence of other sources of stabilization, upon cutting the collateral ligaments the metacarpophalangeal joint becomes a flail, unstable, mechanism. Nature, fortunately, has created another source of lateral stability—the interosseous muscles. By virtue of the selective variable pull, the interossei normally influence lateral motion in the metacarpophalangeal joint to the extent allowed by the unyielding collateral ligaments. Should the collateral ligaments be sacrificed, the interossei remain the sole source of lateral stability. When intrinsic (ulnar) paralysis exists, if the collateral ligaments are sacrificed, all lateral stability is lost and disastrous ulnar deviation will occur. At the interphalangeal joints lateral stability is again dependent upon the collateral ligaments, but at this level there is no second line of defense. The collateral ligaments of the interphalangeal joints, therefore, cannot be sacrificed without creating a lateral instability correctable only by fusion of the interphalangeal joint or reconstruction of collateral ligaments.

The volar plates of the metacarpophalangeal joints are the sites of insertion of the intermetacarpal ligaments, which limit separation or fanning of the metacarpal heads.* The volar plates also give rise to the vaginal ligament, which creates a tunnel for the flexor tendon. The volar plate is fixed to that portion of the capsule which originates from the proximal phalanx and, therefore, the plate moves with the proximal phalanx in flexion and extension.

The Wrist

The wrist joint is the site for major postural change between the arm beam and the working hand end piece. It has a multiarticulated architecture which creates a potentially wide range of motion in flexion, extension, radial deviation, ulnar deviation, and circumduction. The most extensive range of motion occurs at the radiocarpal joint. The distal radius presents a shallow articular surface which is concave from radial to ulnar extremes as well as in the dorsal to palmar projection. Its articular junction with the distal ulna presents a concave surface in a third plane which allows rotation of the radius around the ulna in supination and pronation. The hand rotates with the distal radius.

The navicular and lunate bones of the proximal carpal row form the convex articular counterparts of the concave distal radius for the major wrist articulation.

All four of the bones in the distal carpal row present articular surfaces for junction with the metacarpals. The distal carpal row forms a solid architectural arch with the central capitate as the keystone. The nature of the articulations of the distal carpals with one another, and of the carpal ligaments and the important transverse carpal ligament (flexor retinaculum), is such that they make up a strong and fixed transverse carpal arch.

Skin Creases

The surgeon must know the relationship of skin creases and the underlying joints to plan precise placement of skin incisions for exposure of joints and their related structures. (**F**)

---

*The attachments of the deep transverse palmar ligament have been specifically noted by Haines (1951) as follows: "The pads, i.e., volar plates of adjacent digits, are attached together by the deep transverse ligaments of the palm, made of ordinary ligamentous tissue.... deep transverse palmar ligament or deep intermetacarpal ligament, the latter a most inappropriate term as the structure is not directly attached to the metacarpal bones."

General Principles

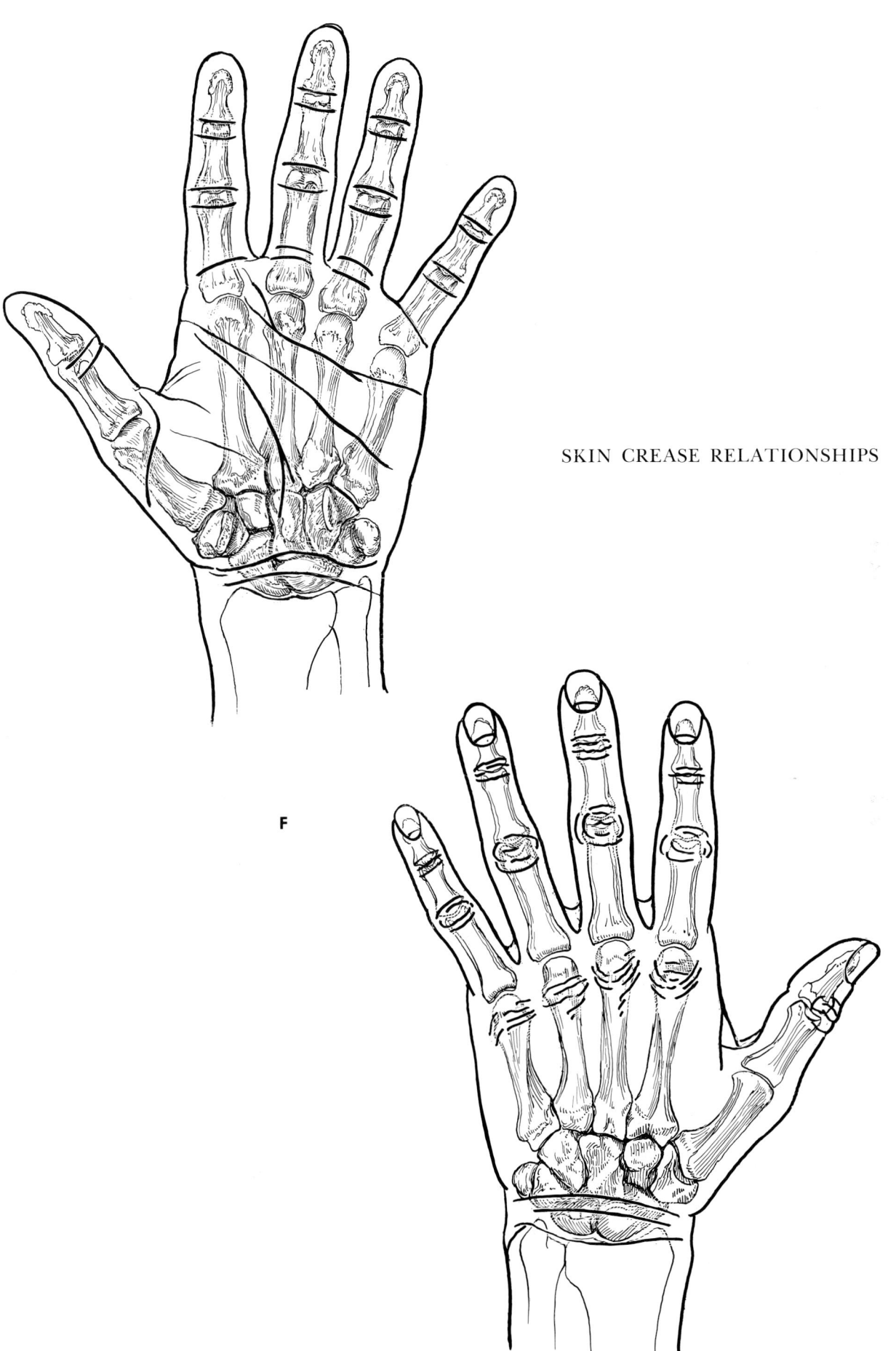

SKIN CREASE RELATIONSHIPS

F

9

DYNAMICS OF HAND FUNCTION

The central backbone of the hand is positioned in extension by the very important extensor carpi radialis brevis and longus. (**A**) Flexion is effected by the flexor carpi radialis. (**B**) All three muscles insert on the central two metacarpals (2 and 3). These key motors are responsible for positioning the hand axis in preparation for operation of the adaptive hand elements around it.

There are numerous other modifying motors to adjust the hand axis in the exact position desired such as the flexor carpi ulnaris and extensor carpi ulnaris which produce ulnar deviation. (**C**)

The fixed unit of the hand is extended from the radius at the radiocarpal joint. The entire complex is a beam attached to the ulna by the distal radioulnar joint, the interosseous membrane and the proximal radioulnar articulation. Rotation around the fixed ulna in supination and pronation is largely under the influence of the median innervated pronator teres and pronator quadratus and the radial innervated supinator. (**D**) The biceps and brachioradialis augment supination.

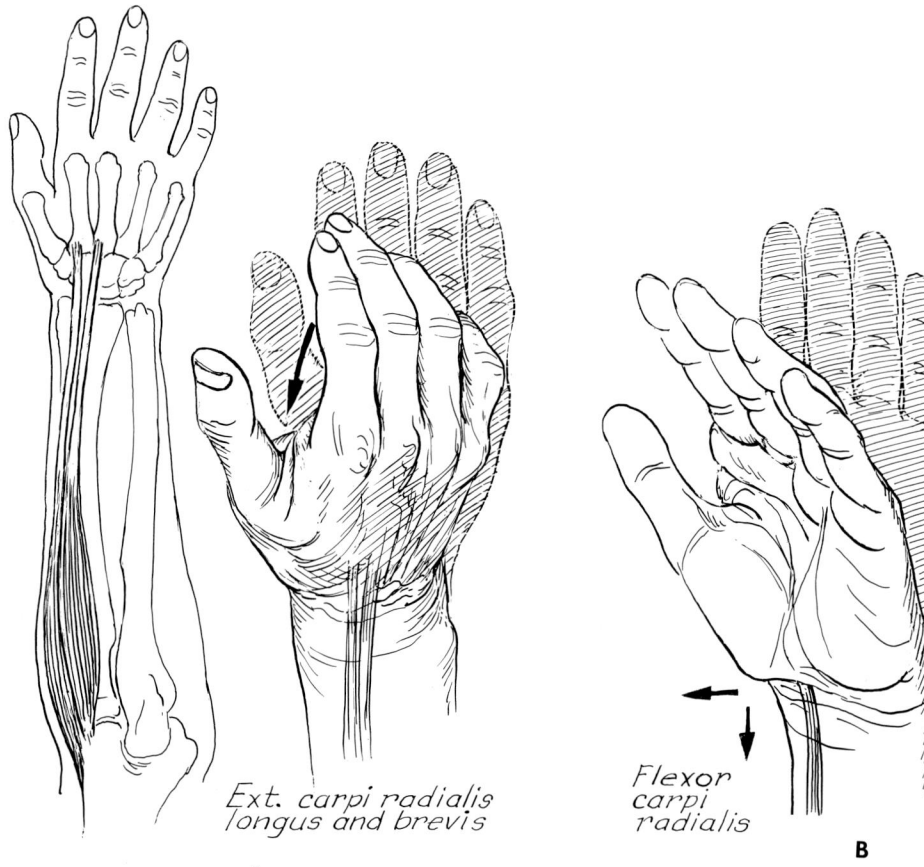

Ext. carpi radialis longus and brevis
A

Flexor carpi radialis
B

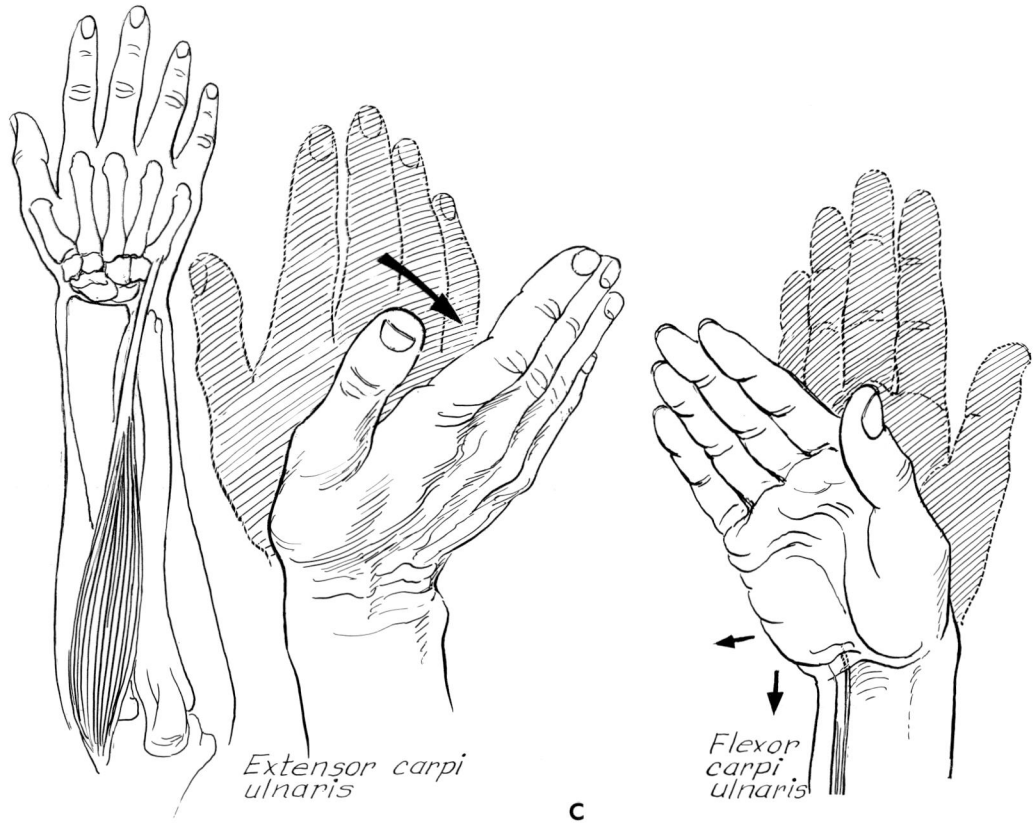

C

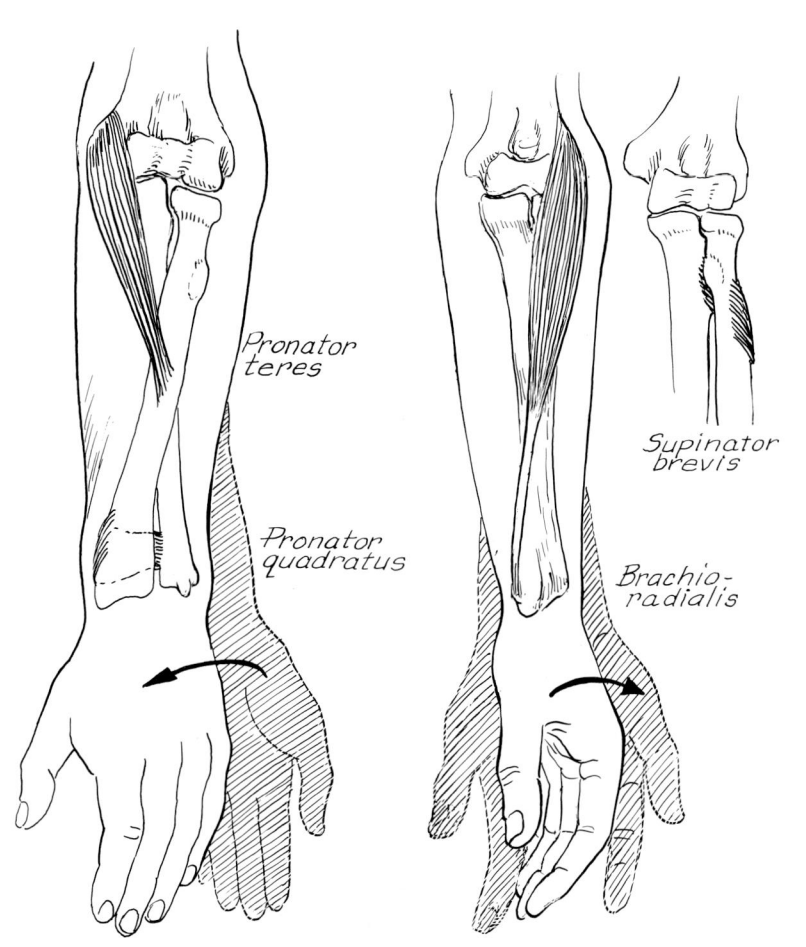

D

1 — Anatomy

Intrinsic Positioning Muscles

With the hand axis or fixed unit in position the metacarpal arch is adjusted primarily by the thenar and the hypothenar muscle groups. The median nerve generally innervates all of the thenar muscles on the radial side of the flexor pollicis longus. These two and one-half muscles (abductor pollicis brevis, opponens pollicis, and superficial head of the flexor pollicis brevis) are positioning muscles which act to bring the first metacarpal into palmar abduction, thus increasing the concavity of the transverse metacarpal arch. (**E**) This, in turn, prepares the thumb for proper pulp-to-pulp opposition with the fingers.

The thumb is steadied in position by contraction of the antagonist to the abductors, the triangular, and very important, thumb adductor. (**F**) Both the adductors and the abductors support flexion of the metacarpophalangeal joint to prevent recurvatum at this joint on pinching which may occur with paralysis of either or both (Froment's sign). With graded relaxation of the abductors, the adductor will dominate and will pull the thumb against the side of the hand.

The ulnar nerve innervates the hypothenar muscle group which serves further to develop the concavity of the transverse metacarpal arch. The opponens digiti minimi exemplifies the action of hypothenar group. (**G**)

General Principles

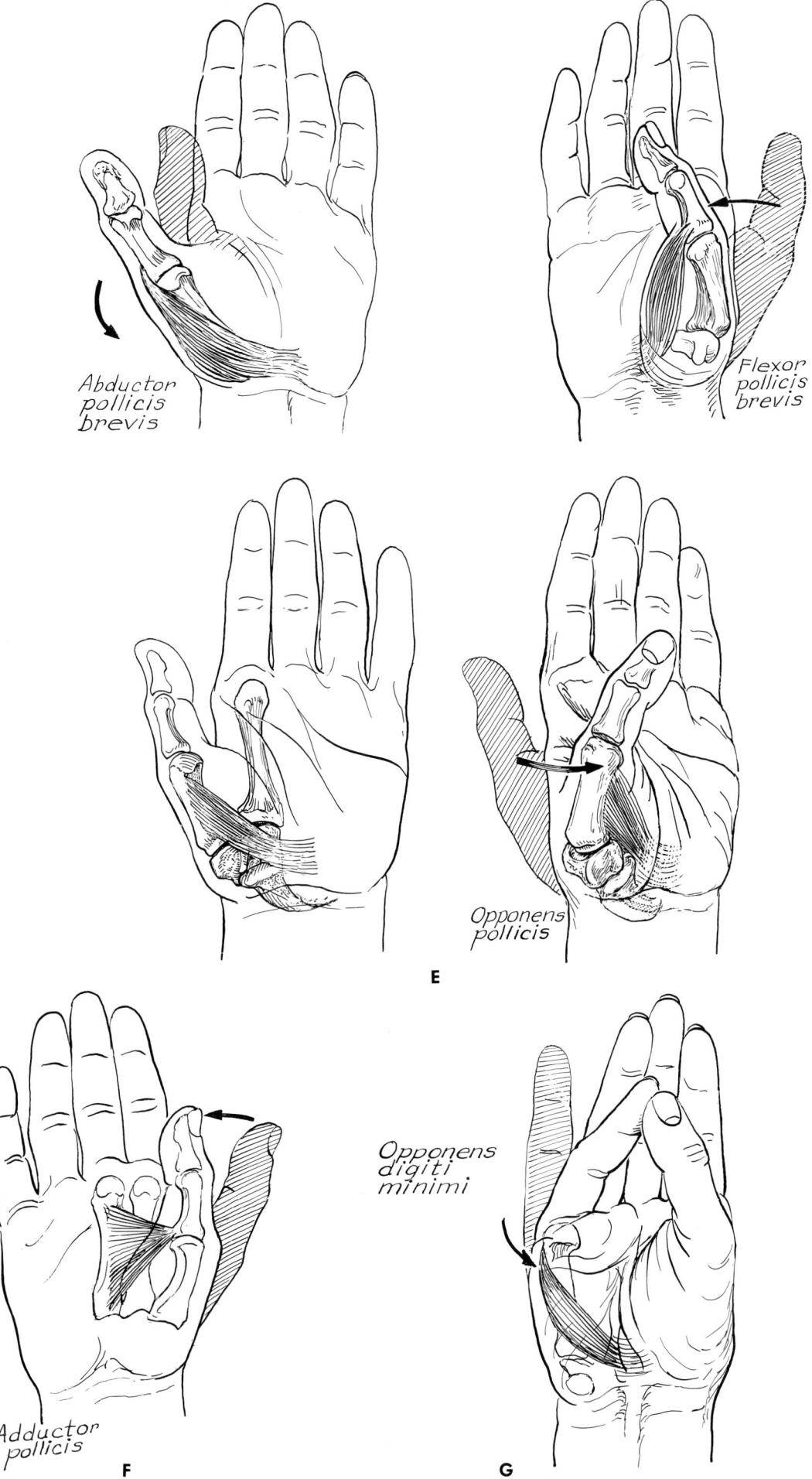

13

1 – Anatomy

Extrinsic Extensors

Extension of the phalanges of the fingers and thumb is dependent both upon long extensors at the metacarpophalangeal joints and upon an interplay between the long extensors and intrinsic muscles at the interphalangeal joints. The extensor digitorum is a series of tendons with a common muscle belly which enters into the central extensor of each of the fingers. (**H**) There are intertendinous bridges between these separate tendons over the dorsum of the hand.

Independent long extensor power is supplied to the index finger through the extensor indicis and to the little finger through the extensor digiti minimi. (**I**) In each case the independent extensor lies on the ulnar side of the long extensor tendon to these two fingers from the extensor digitorum.

Each of the three oblique muscles to the thumb on its extensor surface inserts on one of the thumb bones. The abductor pollicis longus inserts on the metacarpal where it primarily radially abducts the metacarpal, but since it bridges the wrist, it secondarily radially deviates the wrist. (**J**)

The extensor pollicis brevis inserts on the proximal phalanx so it primarily acts as an extensor of the metacarpophalangeal joint but acts at the other joints with the abductor pollicis longus. (**K**)

The extensor pollicis longus inserts on the distal phalanx and is the primary extensor of the interphalangeal joint. (**L**)

Flexion of the phalanges into the palm is a complicated motion representing the sum of actions of the long flexors (profundus and superficialis) and long extensors (extensor digitorum, extensor digiti minimi and extensor indicis), modified and enhanced by the intrinsic muscles (interossei and lumbricals). The long flexors to the fingers are responsible for flexion of the interphalangeal joints and are supplements to active flexion of the metacarpophalangeal joints and the wrist joint.

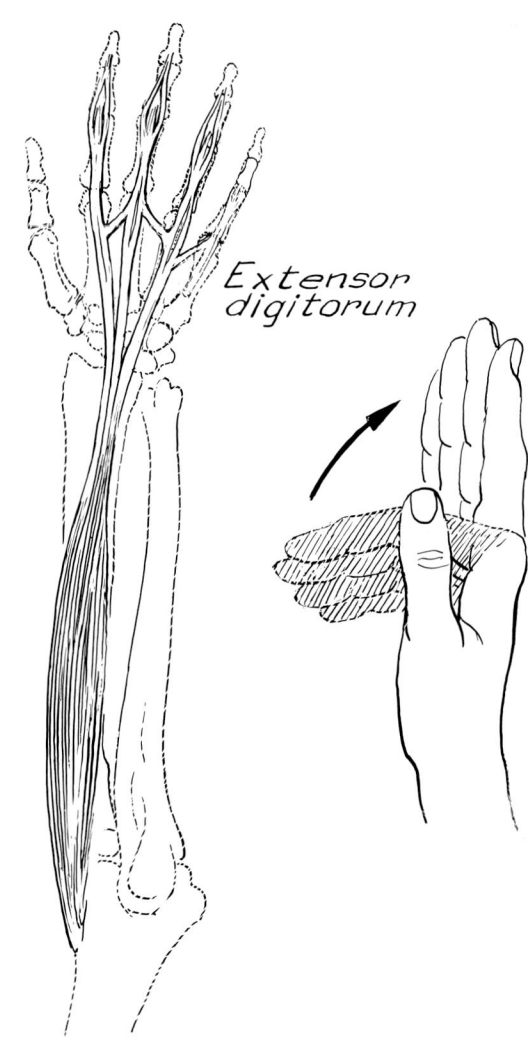

H

General Principles

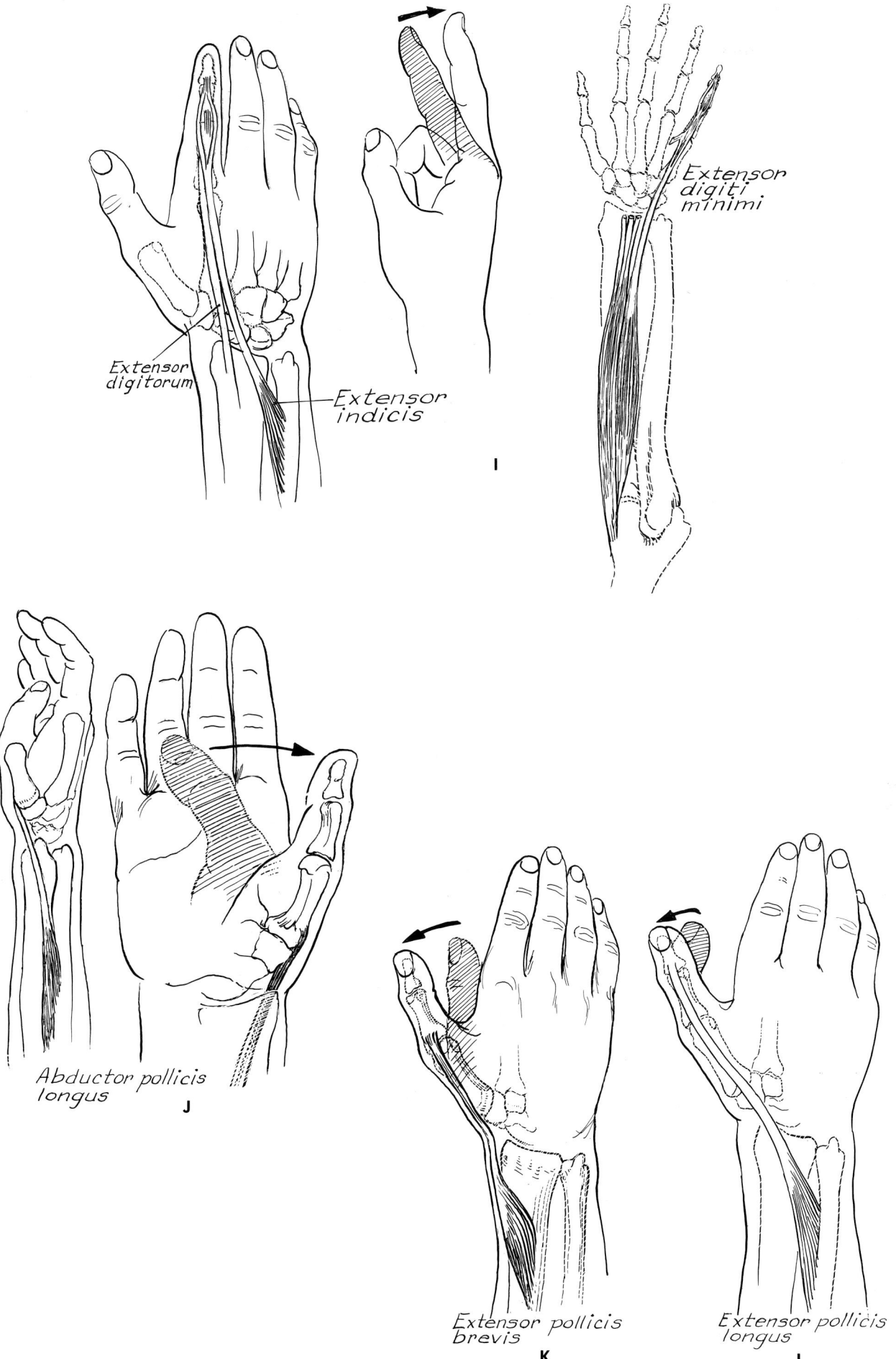

15

1 — Anatomy

Extrinsic Flexors

The flexor digitorum profundus tendon to each finger inserts on the distal phalanx. (**M**) The flexor digitorum superficialis tendon lies palmar (superficial) to the profundus tendon in the palm. It flattens then splits at the level of the proximal phalanx, and its two tails surround the profundus, decussate behind the profundus to insert on the middle phalanx.

In the finger and distal palm the flexor tendons pass through a fitted fibrous flexor sheath which has thickened areas proximal to the metacarpophalangeal joint and each of the interphalangeal joints. (**N**) The tendons at this level are surrounded by synovial sheaths.

The flexor digitorum profundus is the only muscle which flexes the distal interphalangeal joint. Testing for profundus function requires observation of active flexion of the distal interphalangeal joint. (**O**)

Since a muscle-tendon unit affects every joint between its origin and insertion, the flexor digitorum profundus also may flex the proximal interphalangeal joint. This makes the diagnosis of nonfunction of the superficialis more difficult. Each superficialis flexor has its own muscle belly and each acts independently of the others. The profundus flexors are not as independent since there is a common muscle for the profundus tendons of the long finger, ring finger, and little finger, and a variable degree of interconnection between these and the profundus of the index finger. The diagnosis of disruption of flexor digitorum superficialis function is confirmed by check-reining the profundus by holding the other fingers in extension while the patient actively attempts to flex the finger whose superficialis is being tested. Flexion of the finger at the proximal interphalangeal joint while the distal interphalangeal joint remains loosely extended confirms the functional integrity of the flexor digitorum superficialis. (**P**)

Selected flexion of one or more of the metacarpophalangeal joints or of either the proximal or distal interphalangeal joint depends on stabilizing fixation of the remainder by flexor-extensor interplay. Elimination of any single motor element reduces selective adaptability of a finger.

As noted above, a muscle may positively influence any joint between its site of origin and its insertion. The flexor digitorum profundus muscle originates in the forearm, and its tendon, therefore, bridges the wrist joint, the metacarpophalangeal joint, the proximal interphalangeal joint and the distal interphalangeal joint before it inserts on the distal phalanx. It may flex any of these joints depending upon dynamic fixation of the others. Fixation of the distal interphalangeal joint converts the profundus tendon into a functional superficialis tendon by recessing its prime site of action to the proximal interphalangeal joint. By combined fixation of any of the joints, the profundus tendon may primarily flex any selected one.

It is intriguing to realize that under certain conditions the flexor profundus may accentuate extension of the proximal interphalangeal joint. The profundus pulling primarily at the distal interphalangeal joint may flex it acutely. In flexing the distal interphalangeal joint, the insertion of the extensor mechanism is advanced distally. This advancement combined with either a contraction or fixation of the lateral bands results in extension of the proximal interphalangeal joint. This effect is easily aborted by the intact flexor superficialis, whose prime flexion function is exerted on the proximal interphalangeal joint. Absence of the superficialis, whether occasioned by injury or following tendon graft replacement of the profundus only, results not infrequently in flexion of the distal interphalangeal joint with recurvatum deformity at the proximal interphalangeal joint. This can be corrected by fusion of the distal interphalangeal joint, making the profundus a functional superficialis or by tenodesis or capsulodesis of the proximal interphalangeal joint in mild flexion. It is wise to keep in mind the innumerable functional circumstances which can be created by selective interplay of multiple motor forces exerted through a series of interdependent joints.

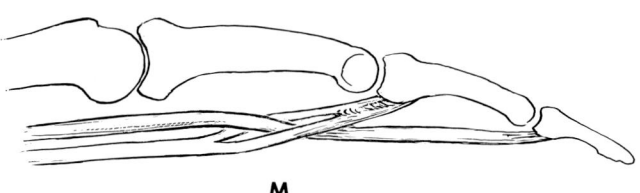

M

General Principles

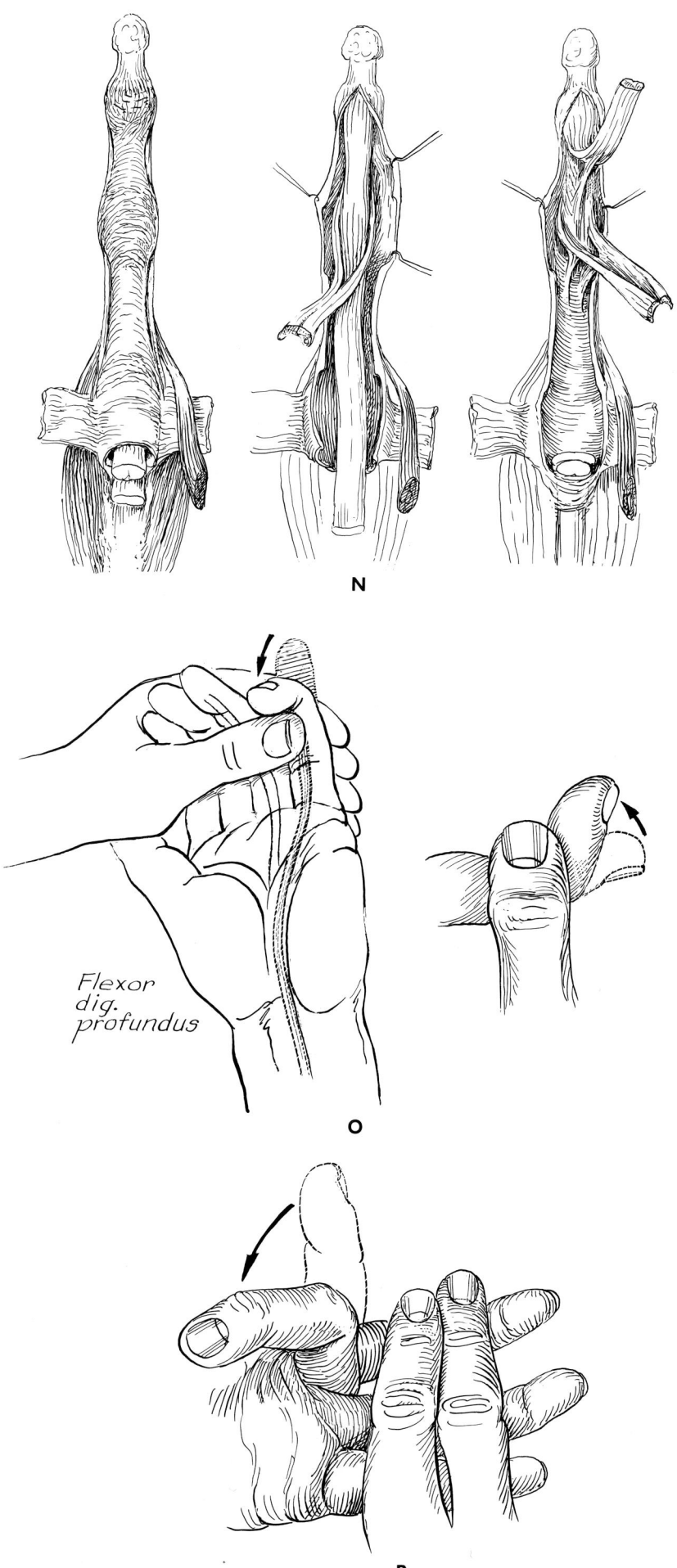

17

1 — Anatomy

The thumb, with only two phalanges, has no need for two long flexor tendons. The single flexor pollicis longus bridges all the thumb joints and the wrist joint. (**Q**)

Because the flexor pollicis longus bridges all of these joints, it may influence any one by selected fixation of the others. Like the profundus, it may extend its sphere of action beyond that of pure flexion. For example, acute flexion of the interphalangeal joint by the flexor pollicis longus may potentiate an opponens pollicis transfer inserted into the thumb extensor mechanism. It does so by moving the insertion of the opponens transfer distally, thereby increasing its total effectiveness.

The flexor profundi to the third, fourth, and fifth fingers work from a common muscle belly. Acting in unison, they fit the architectural concept of this unit as a stable vise for grasping objects. The independent function of the index profundus frees the index finger for use with the thumb to manipulate an object grasped by the viselike ulnar unit. Independence of action is well developed in the superficialis muscles and the intrinsic muscles.

The tiny lumbrical muscles harmonize function between the lateral band interphalangeal extensor mechanism and the flexor digitorum profundus. They have a moving site of origin from the profundus tendon and are generally innervated by the same nerve which innervates the corresponding profundus (the ulnar two are innervated by the ulnar nerve and the radial two are innervated by the median nerve, as are the profundi). As the flexor profundus contracts, the lumbrical origin moves proximally. (**R**) At the same time the lumbrical insertion moves distally as the extensor is advanced by interphalangeal flexion. The effective separation of its insertion and origin makes the lumbrical more effective in flexing the metacarpophalangeal joint. Conversely, with a change in balance of power, the lumbrical tends to pull the profundus distally as it shortens the lateral bands. This combination of profundus relaxation and lateral band pull results in extension at the interphalangeal joints.

The interosseous muscles function as ulnar and radial deviators of the fingers as well as flexors of the metacarpophalangeal joints and extensors of the interphalangeal joints. The dorsal interossei act as abductors from the axis of the hand, which falls in the middle of the long finger. The long finger moves both radial and ulnar under influence of dorsal interossei. The abductor digiti minimi is the dorsal interosseous equivalent of the little finger. (**S**)

The palmar interossei adduct the fingers to the hand axis. (**T**)

The pull of all the interossei palmar to the axis of the metacarpophalangeal joints and dorsal to the interphalangeal joint axis acts to flex the metacarpophalangeal joints and extend the interphalangeal joints. (**U**) The position assumed is called the "intrinsic plus" posture.

A study of the balance of motors around the digital joints is not only fascinating but most rewarding as it leads to a better understanding of the changes in adaptability caused by selective paralyses.

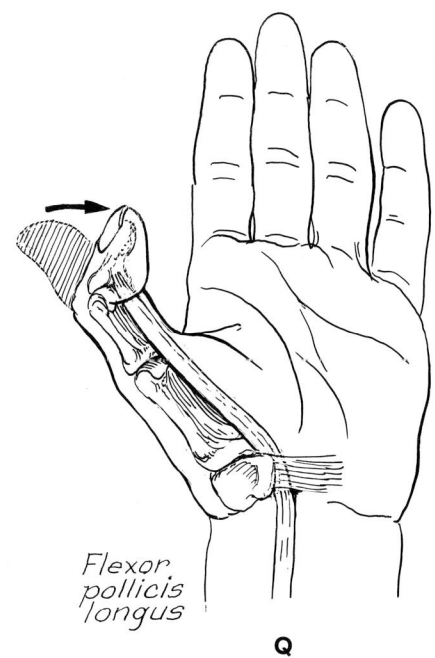

Flexor pollicis longus

Q

General Principles

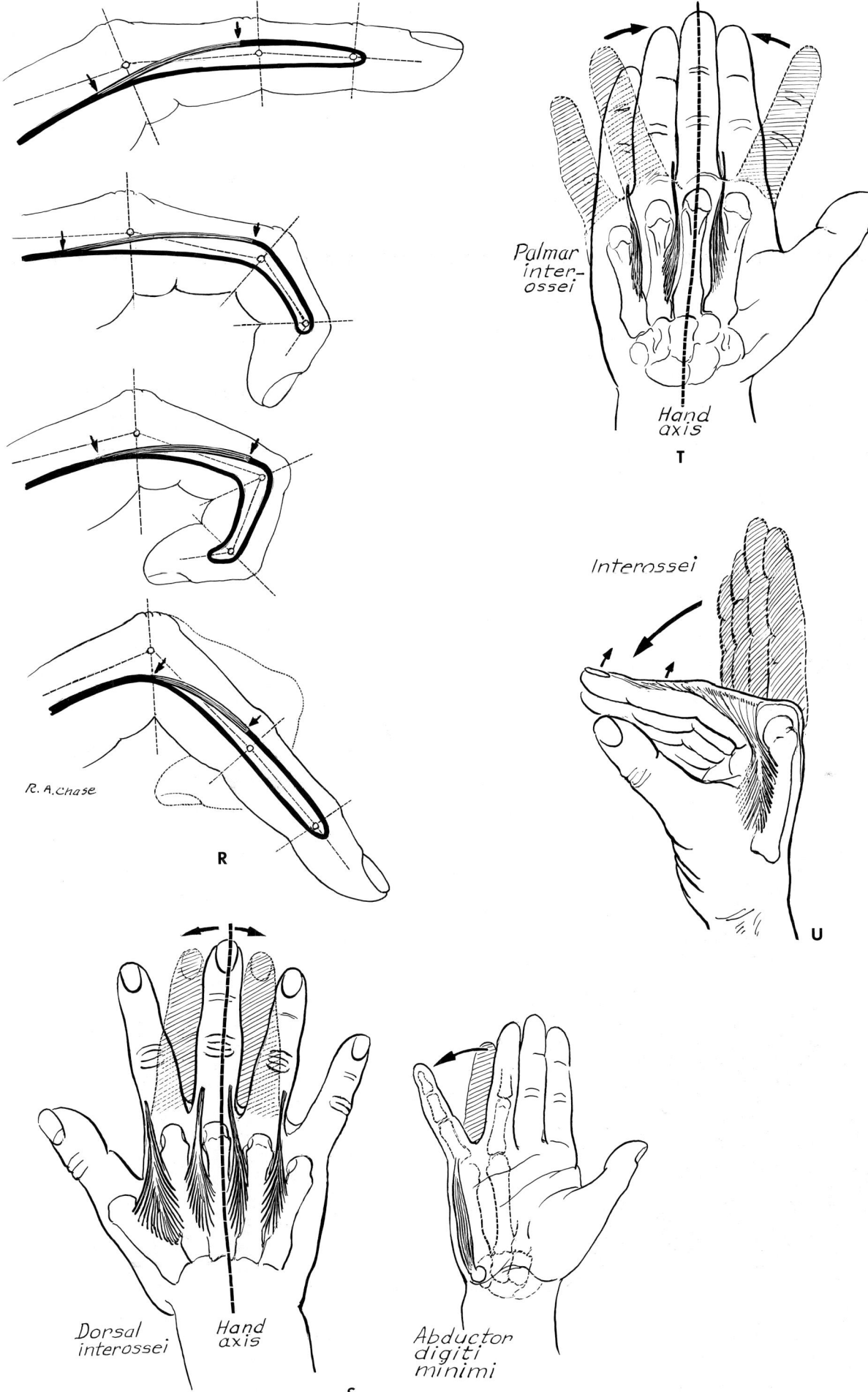

19

1 — Anatomy

SENSIBILITY IN THE UPPER EXTREMITY*

The work of Elliot Smith (1912) made us aware that a low order of mammal gains its first impressions of the world by its sense of smell; it tests the world with its nose. The olfactory sense demands a large share of cortical representation but the tactile sensations of the snout region, the lips and the tongue are soon added as sources of information concerning the outside environment. Wood Jones (1942) emphasized that when certain primitive mammals took to an arboreal life, the eyes replaced the nose as the dominant special sense organ. The hands, emancipated from the duties of bodily support, became the great testing members of the body. Primitive arboreal animals learn of the world and test objects with their eyes and hands. In the human brain the relatively large area representing the hand in the cerebral cortex signals man's dependency on his hands as a perceptive sensory organ.

Sir Charles Bell (1834) stated:

"We find every organ of sense, with the exception of that of touch, more perfect in brutes than in man. In the eagle and the hawk, in the gazelle and in the feline tribe, the perfection of the eye is admirable; ... in the dog, wolf, hyaena, as well as in birds of prey, the sense of smelling is inconceivably acute; and if we should have some hesitation in assigning a more exquisite sense of taste to brutes, we cannot doubt the superiority of that of hearing in the inferior animals. But in the sense of touch, seated in the hand, man claims the superiority; and it is of consequence to our conclusion that we should observe why it is so."

It is ontogenetically interesting that the general epidermal covering of the embryonic body develops into the mid-dorsal depression or neural groove. It becomes buried in the tissues beneath the general surface of the body and becomes the hollow primitive neural tube. The rest of the surface covering is important in giving rise to special sense organs and finally to the skin and all its adult derivatives. In essence, our brains, the whole of our nervous systems and the entire surface covering of the body arise from the same ectodermal layer.

Wood Jones (1942) stated:

"It would seem that we should not unduly strain the logical deductions that may be drawn from a study of embryology if we regard the central nervous system as no more than a buried portion of skin, or alternatively we may look upon the skin as an exposed portion of the central nervous system. Certainly we shall be upon safe physiological grounds when we regard the skin as the greatest and most ancient sense organ of the animal body."

Everything we wish to learn about a novel object which we cannot glean from our other sense organs we learn by hand testing. We learn of its surface texture, whether it be smooth or rough. We learn its shape and its dimensions; we estimate weight and draw conclusions as to its consistency, hard or soft; and we appreciate the fact that it is either hot or cold. These senses, highly developed in the blind man, make it possible for him to learn a great deal about an object by subjecting it to examination with his fingers. The thumb, index, and third fingers are the primary digits of exploration. Their contact surfaces are median nerve territory. We may, therefore, conclude that the median nerve is the channel by which a large bulk of informative sensory stimuli is carried to the brain. In the more primitive mammals the fifth cranial or trigeminal is the great informative nerve. In the arboreal animal, and especially in man, the prime function of the fifth nerve is usurped by the median. Coupled with visual sensibility, a double sense in the extremity is exercised in arriving at the truth in the evaluation of objects. The first component of this double sense is the superficial sensation felt by contact of the skin with the object. The second component is the sense of muscular effort made to reach it, grasp it, and support it with the fingers, that is, proprioceptive sensibility. These two sources of sensory perception combine centrally to create the conscious picture of the object being explored.

The extreme sensibility of the skin, even in the slightest injury, suggests that the pain should be more severe, the deeper the wound. This, of course, is not the fact. Any surgeon will attest to the fact that once the skin is incised, the most severe pain is over. One may operate under relatively light anesthesia for a period of time then turn to take a skin graft and find that the patient is quite sensitive to skin incision at the same level of anesthesia which is adequate for deep dissection. The skin with its exquisite sense of touch and pain, then, guards the deeper, less sensitive, structures. Such structures cannot be reached except through the sensitive skin. The most delicate skin is, in fact, a more effectual cover by virtue of this sensibility than is the thick and resistant hide of a rhinoceros, because it forces us to avoid injury by avoiding resultant pain. Thus, sensibility is protective. Lack of such protective sensibility in nerve palsies may result in injury and destruction of parts. Sensibility in the upper and lower extremities is, therefore, critically important to man in helping him both to evaluate his environment and to protect himself from injury.

---

*The pattern of sensibility in the upper extremity is depicted on pages 203 and 211.

2 Records

Maintenance of proper and complete records is essential in hand surgery. A metal or plastic hand stencil is useful in constructing diagrams for recording the physical findings. (**A**)

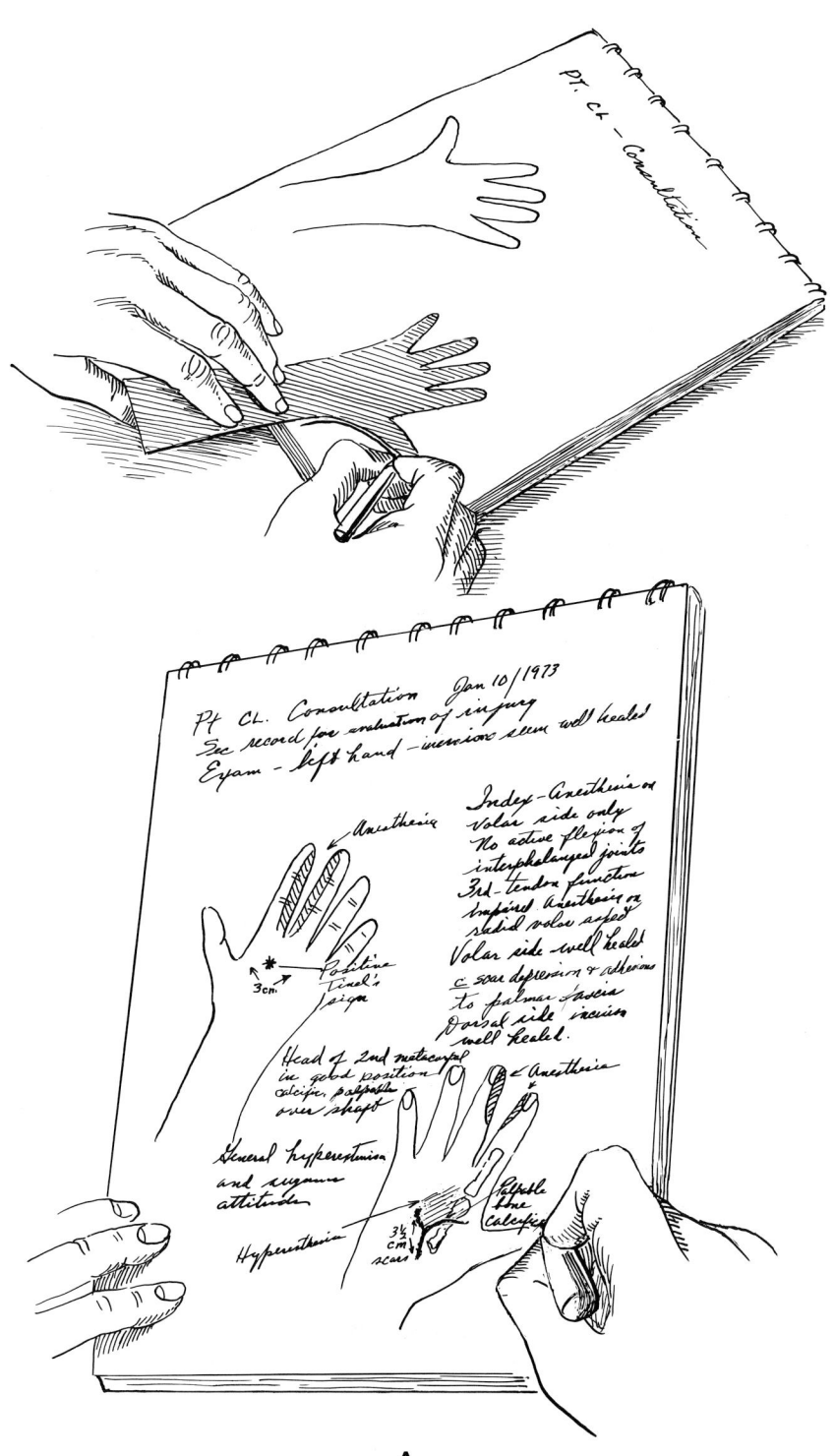

A

3 Tourniquet

The pneumatic tourniquet, properly used, is an essential adjunct in hand surgery. The precise anatomical dissection essential in most operative procedures on the hand requires a quiet, bloodless field. Meticulous attention to detail in use of the tourniquet will prevent possible complications.

Technique of Tourniquet Use

Soft sheet wadding or Webril* is applied to the upper arm over its muscular portion prior to application of the pneumatic tourniquet cuff. (**A**) Smooth application without bunching or wrinkling is essential to avoid pressure points or skin pinching by the cuff.

The proper size pneumatic tourniquet cuff is wrapped smoothly around the arm as snugly as possible. (**B**) Care is taken in application to have the air and guage outlet on the lateral aspect of the arm to avoid kinking of the tubing by arm pressure when the hand is positioned for the operation.

Prior to tourniquet inflation the hand and arm are emptied of blood by distal to proximal wrapping using a rubber bandage (Esmarch). (**C**) A wad of mechanic's waste or gauze sponge in the palm allows the hand to be wrapped with digits flexed for even pressure on the fingers and thumb. Should the tourniquet fail during the procedure, it should be fully deflated, after which the arm is re-emptied of blood before tourniquet reinflation. Reinflation with the arm vasculature filled with blood increases the danger of intravascular thrombosis.

The tourniquet should not be left inflated for more than 90 minutes without a period of restored blood flow for a 10- or 15-minute "breathing interval." After this the process of emptying the arm of blood and reinflation may safely be done. In adults the inflated pressure should be about 300 mm of Hg and in children 200 mm of Hg pressure is sufficient and safe. *The manometer should be checked at regular intervals against a mercury column to assure pressure accuracy.* A special tourniquet test gauge is made for this purpose.** A special automatic self regulating gas chamber provides air pressure to the inflatable arm cuff.***

At the end of the operation it is critically important that preparation be made to remove the tourniquet and underlying padding immediately after deflation. To leave the tourniquet cuff or its circumferential padding in place creates a venous tourniquet effect and may cause unwarranted hemorrhage in the wound.

The rules for use of the tourniquet should be displayed on the gas chamber as a check list.

Tourniquet: Rules for Use

1. Check equipment
   a. Gas supply
   b. Gauge accuracy against a mercury column or special test manometer
   c. Leaks in system
   Leave up overnight on stable device or Under water check
2. Use proper cuff size
3. Smooth application of sheet wadding
   a. Free of wrinkles
   b. Keep dry during prep
4. Apply smoothly and snugly (venous tourniquet)
   a. Proper placement of tube outlet
5. Check and set gauge at proper level
   a. 200 mm Hg for children
   b. 250–300 mm Hg for adults
6. *Do it yourself!*

---

*Kendall Corporation, Hospital Products Division, Chicago, Illinois 60606

**Zimmer, Warsaw, Indiana.
***Walter Kidde & Co., Inc., Belleview, New Jersey.

General Principles

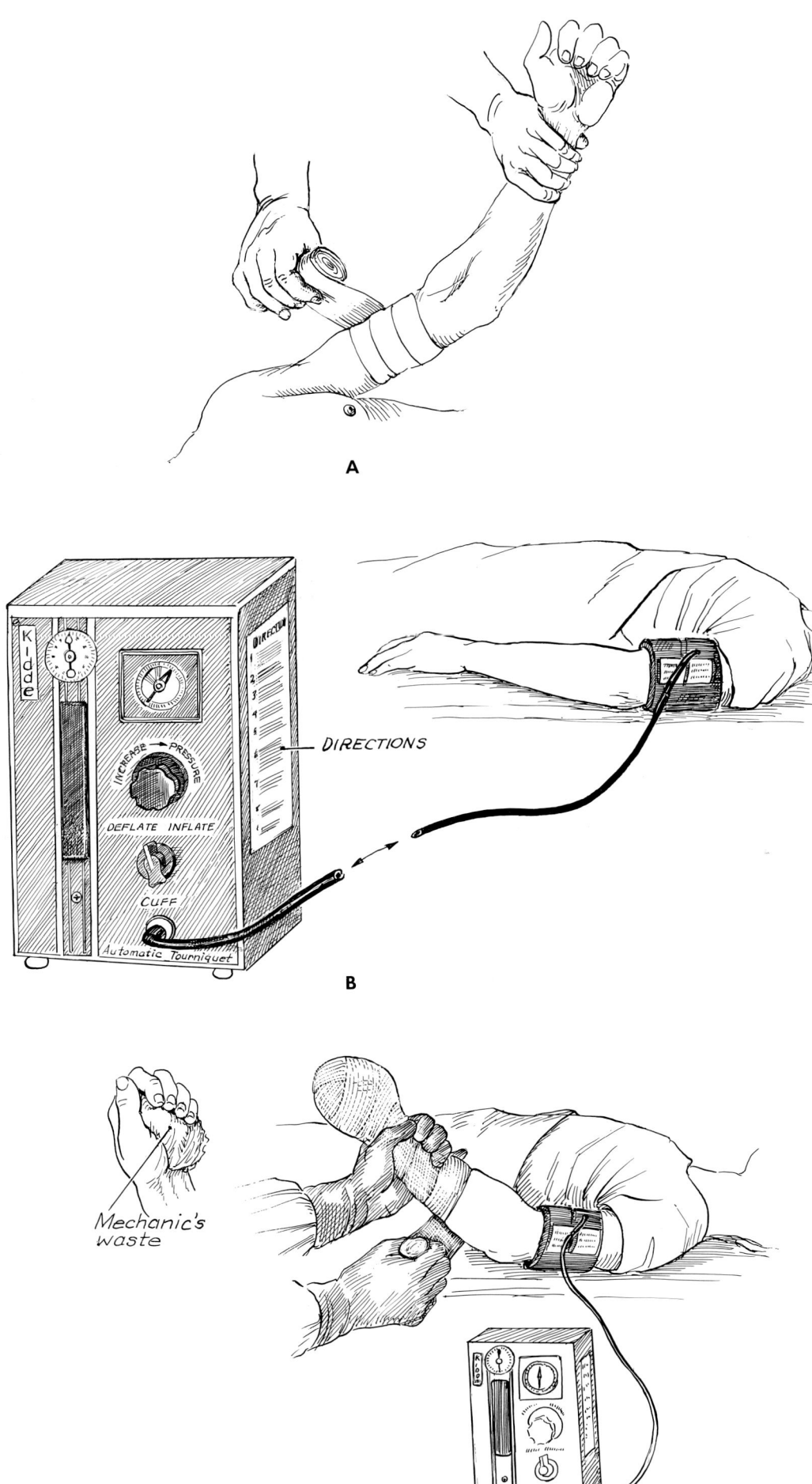

23

4

Nerve Block Anesthesia

Wrist Block: Median Nerve

Palpate the space between the palmaris longus and flexor carpi radialis. Independent flexion of the index finger will allow palpation of the index superficialis deep in this interval. The median nerve is just superficial to the index superficialis and beneath flexor investing fascia. (**A**)

In the absence of the palmaris longus the important landmark is the flexor carpi radialis. A skin wheal of local anesthetic agent is made about 2 cm proximal to the distal wrist crease between the palmaris longus and flexor carpi radialis. (**B**)

A fine short hypodermic needle is then gently inserted just through the deep fascia. With the syringe held like a pen or pencil, the needle is gently jiggled as exploration is made to produce a median nerve paresthesia. Generally such a paresthesia is obtained over the median nerve. When paresthesia is experienced the anesthetic agent is injected (about 1.5 ml of 2% xylocaine). Commonly, the hypodermic needle is inserted too deep, placing the point beneath the median nerve. If a paresthesia is not experienced the needle should be withdrawn to a more superficial level and exploration reinstituted.

General Principles

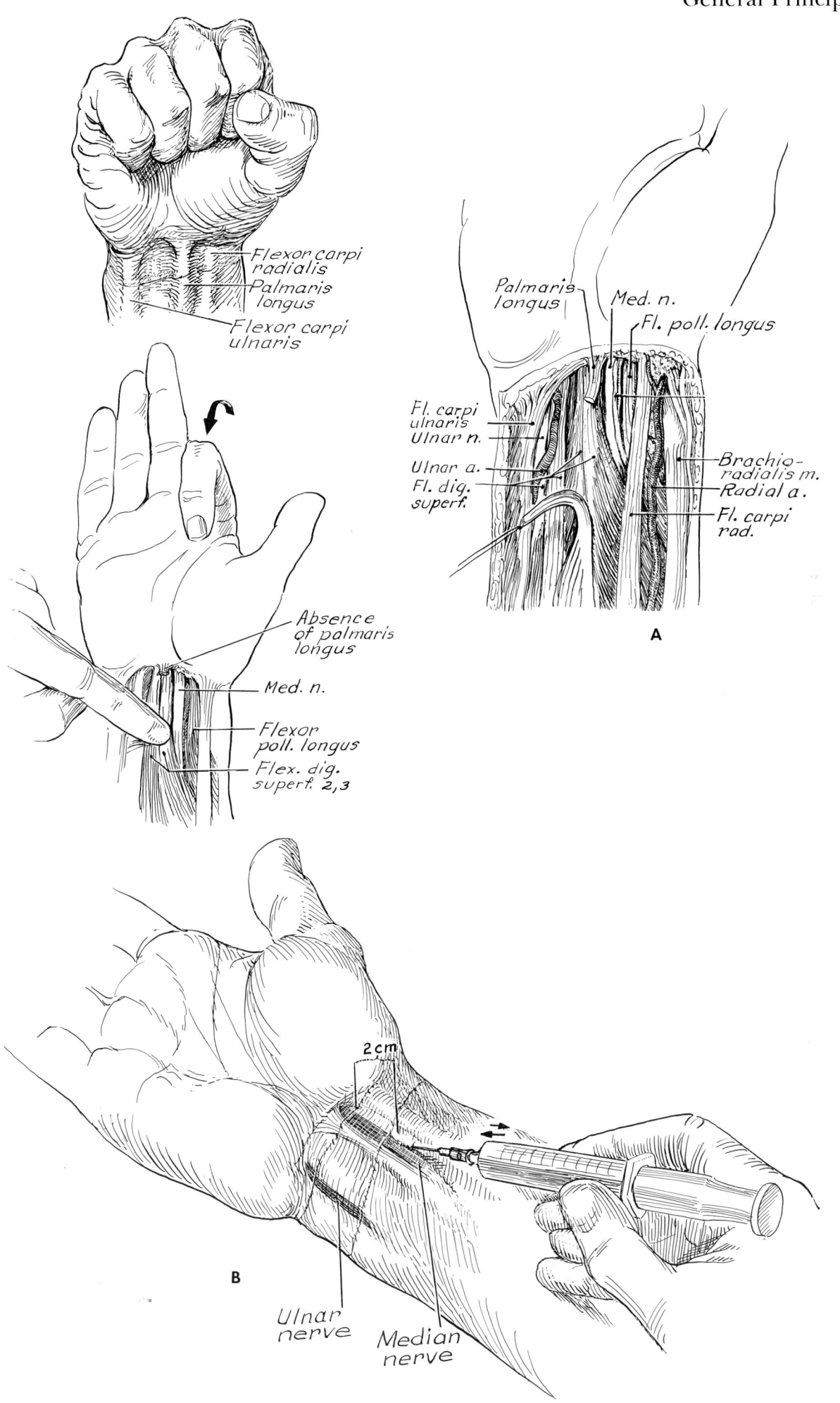

25

4 — Nerve Block Anesthesia

Wrist Block: Ulnar Nerve

The flexor carpi ulnaris is easily identified and palpated after asking the patient to spread or abduct the little finger. (**C**) The flexor carpi ulnaris automatically tenses.

The ulnar nerve is just radial to this tendon and it courses superficial at the wrist. Injection is made using the technique described for the median nerve at the proximal wrist crease just radial to the flexor carpi ulnaris or the prominent pisiform bone which the tendon surrounds as though the pisiform were a sesamoid. (**D**)

Paresthesia may be more difficult to obtain during needle exploration for the ulnar nerve at the wrist than it is when exploring for the median nerve at this level.

If surgery is to be done on the dorsal and palmar aspect of the ulnar side of the hand, it may be wise to block the ulnar nerve at the elbow to secure anesthesia over the area served by the dorsal branch as well as that served by the palmar sensory nerves. (See Elbow Block, p. 28.)

Wrist Block: Dorsal Nerves

The small dorsal branches of the radial and ulnar nerves lie in the subcutaneous tissues and may be blocked at the wrist by superficial infiltration. The dorsal branch of the radial nerve courses across the "anatomical snuffbox" between the extensor pollicis longus and the extensor pollicis brevis. A subcutaneous injection of local anesthesia across this area is adequate to block the nerve and its branches. (**E**)

The ulnar nerve courses dorsally at the distal one-third of the forearm and it may be blocked by subcutaneous infiltration over the ulnar dorsal skin at the dorsal wrist area. (**F**)

General Principles

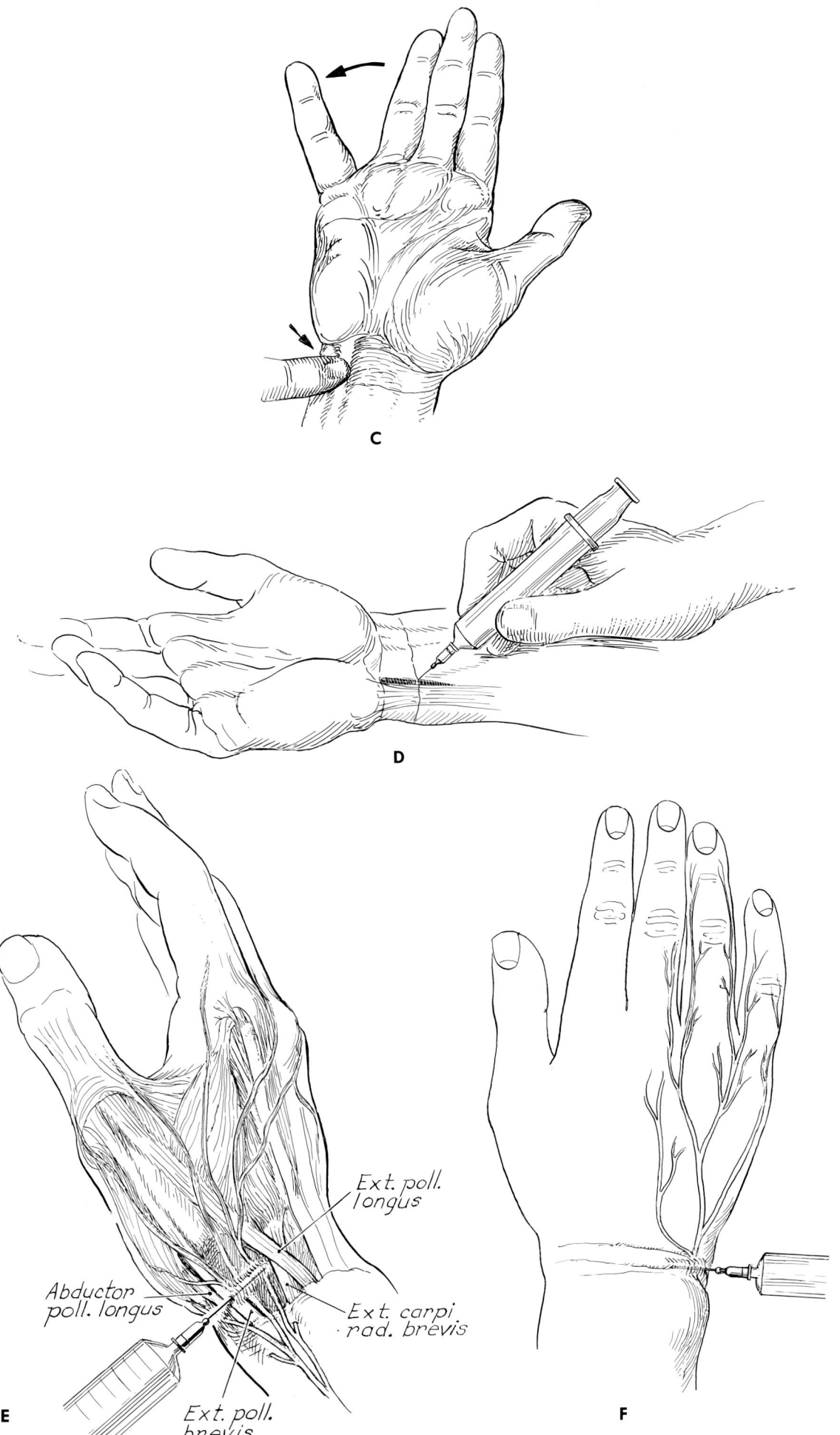

27

4 — Nerve Block Anesthesia

Elbow Block: Median Nerve

The median nerve at the elbow lies on the ulnar side of the easily visible and palpable biceps tendon. (**G**) Palpation in this area will readily reveal the pulsations of the brachial artery as it enters the anticubital fossa. The median nerve is immediately adjacent to it and on its ulnar side at this point. Gentle fine needle exploration frequently will produce a median nerve paresthesia. Injection of local anesthetic agent at this site will give good median nerve anesthesia. (**H**) It has no great advantage over a more easily performed block of the median nerve at the wrist, for surgery over the median innervated area of the hand.

Elbow Block: Ulnar Nerve

The ulnar nerve at the elbow is fixed in its compartment behind the medial epicondyle of the humerus. (**I**) Although it would seem by virtue of this to be an easy nerve to block at the elbow, frequently it is not. It is best blocked proximal to its entry into the bony arch behind the epicondyle. (**J**) It may be palpated at this point, and one may get a paresthesia on needle exploration. Ulnar nerve block at this level has the distinct advantage of anesthetizing both the dorsal and palmar aspects of the ulnar side of the hand and the ulnar one and one-half fingers.

Combined Wrist and Elbow Blocks

The combination of ulnar nerve block at the elbow and radial and median nerve block at the wrist is excellent. The nerve blocks are best done prior to preparation and draping of the hand for surgery. This allows time for nerve block to render the part completely anesthetic prior to surgery. The nerve blocks must be done prior to preparation and debridement in an acute open wound. Nerve blocks and instrumentation *must not be done* prior to careful examination, mapping of sensibility, and muscle testing in such wounds. If use of an arm tourniquet is essential, an axillary brachial plexus block is best since it spares the patient the pain of tourniquet ischemia in the arm and forearm. A carefully applied Esmarch tourniquet may be used at the wrist for short procedures. The rubber bandage is wound on from fingertips to wrist, then unwound to the wrist leaving the last few turns as compression over the vessels at the wrist level.

Patience is a specific and particular virtue if one intends to perform surgery under local or block anesthesia. After injection of the anesthetic agent the surgeon must wait for anesthesia to be complete before any manipulation or incision. In the case of local anesthesia used in the area of surgery a five-minute wait (by the clock) will pay dividends in time saved later. Repeated testing, pinching, stabbing and pricking immediately after injection will only shatter the patient's confidence and make him less cooperative during the rest of the procedure. Following nerve block, a similar waiting interval should be observed prior to testing for anesthesia. As one blocks nerves more proximal than the wrist, the waiting interval should be extended to allow for diffusion of the agent into larger nerve trunks. A minimum wait of 10 or 15 minutes is proper before testing after a brachial plexus block.

Patience and truthfulness in explaining to children who are facing procedures under local anesthesia may make the difference between success and failure. One must take time to allow a child to develop confidence. Then a careful explanation of what is going to happen, what hurts, and how, will allow the child to sustain that confidence throughout the procedure. This is more important than pharmacologic sedation in the child from 4 to 12.

General Principles

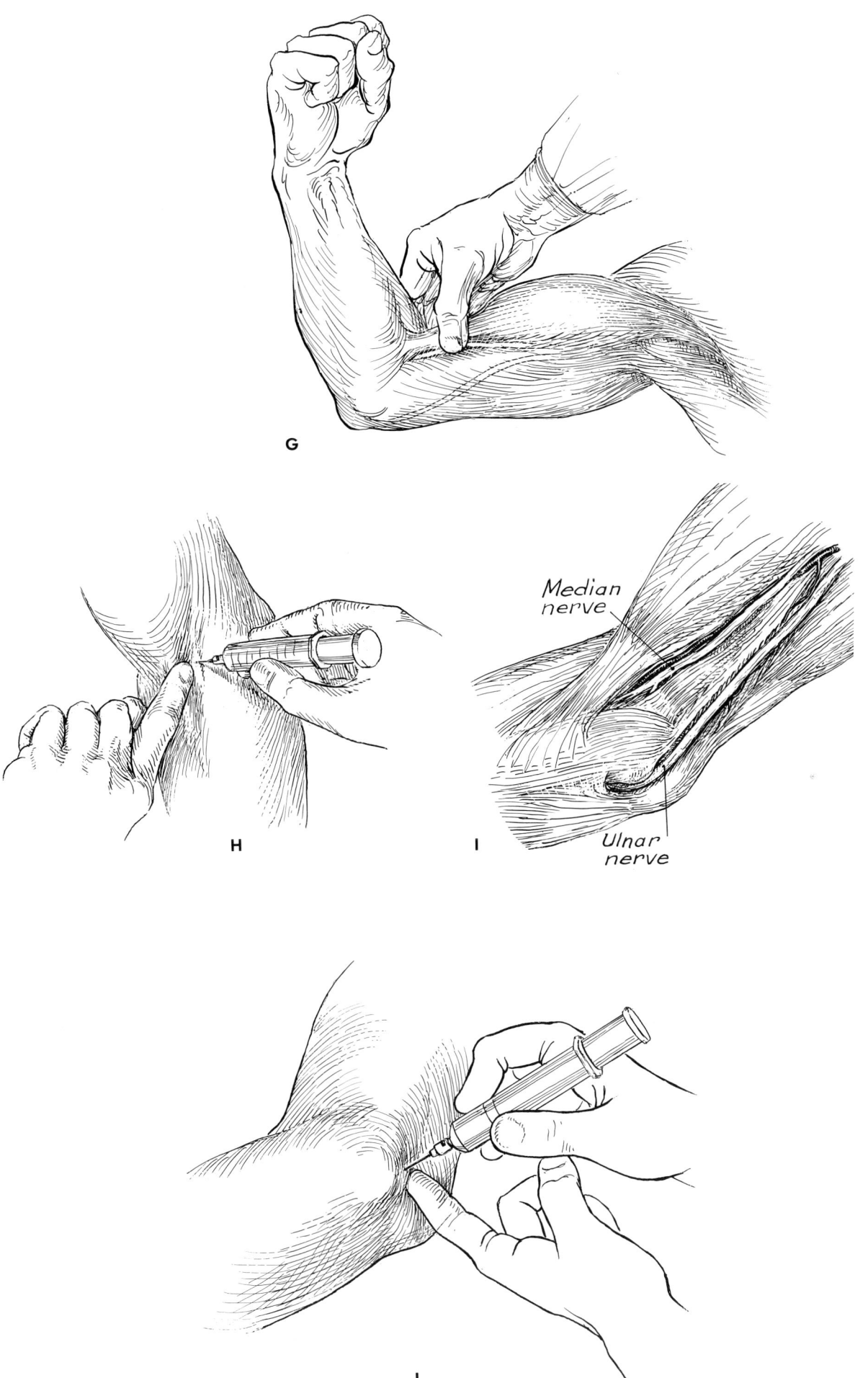

4 — Nerve Block Anesthesia

Axillary Brachial Plexus Block

Axillary brachial plexus block is very effective for use in hand surgery. The technique is simple and the dangers are minimal. With the patient supine and the arm abducted on an arm rest or table the axilla and upper arm are prepared with appropriate solutions. One may readily palpate the brachial artery as it leaves the axilla where it lie subcutaneous and against the humerus. (**K**) Using a short fine bore (25- or 23-gauge) needle, the overlying skin is penetrated. One may feel the resistant fascial sheath over the brachial artery and brachial plexus nerves with the exploring needle. Passage of the needle just through the sheath frequently results in paresthesia over the sensory distribution of a main nerve trunk. The plunger is checked to make sure that the artery has not been entered. During injection of the anesthetic agent, pressure with the thumb over the axillary sheath just distal to the injection site will direct the solution proximal in the axillary sheath and around the circumference of the artery, where it will bathe all of the major nerves. (**L**) Injection of 40 or 50 ml. of 1% carbocaine within the sheath generally results in total anesthesia of the extremity in about 20 minutes.

Once there is evidence that anesthesia is developing in the radial ulnar and median distribution, the tourniquet may be applied, but it should be left deflated while the arm and hand area is prepared for surgery.

Nerve Blocks for Individual Fingers

Effective anesthesia of a single finger is best achieved by blocking the digital nerves at the level of the metacarpophalangeal joints just distal to the intermetacarpal ligaments. A dorsal skin wheal of anesthesia is made between two adjacent metacarpal heads, and subcutaneous infiltration is carried across the dorsum of the metacarpophalangeal joint area of the finger to be anesthetized. (**M**)

A small bore needle may then be passed toward the palm through the anesthetized dorsal skin and subcutaneous tissue. (**N**) It is aimed in the web area toward the anatomical site of the neurovascular bundle of the finger. If one places a finger on the palmar skin as the needle is passed, he will feel the needle as it approaches the resistant dermis. (**O**) Occasionally the patient may experience a paresthesia down the finger. Whether he does or not, the bilateral deposits of a small quantity (0.5 to 1.0 ml.) of anesthetic agent *without adrenalin* will anesthetize the finger. A ten minute wait after injection is important.

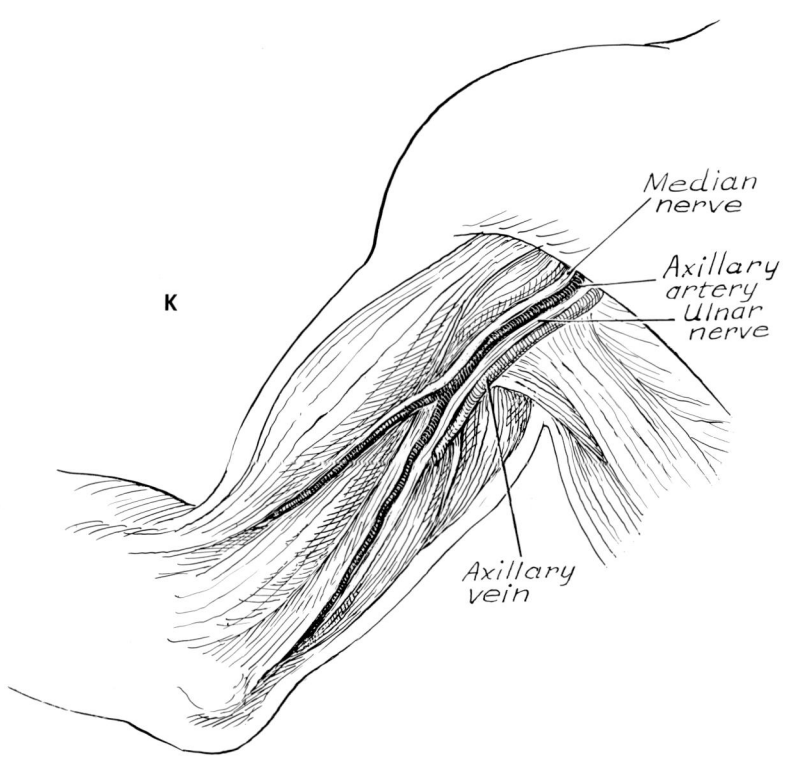

General Principles

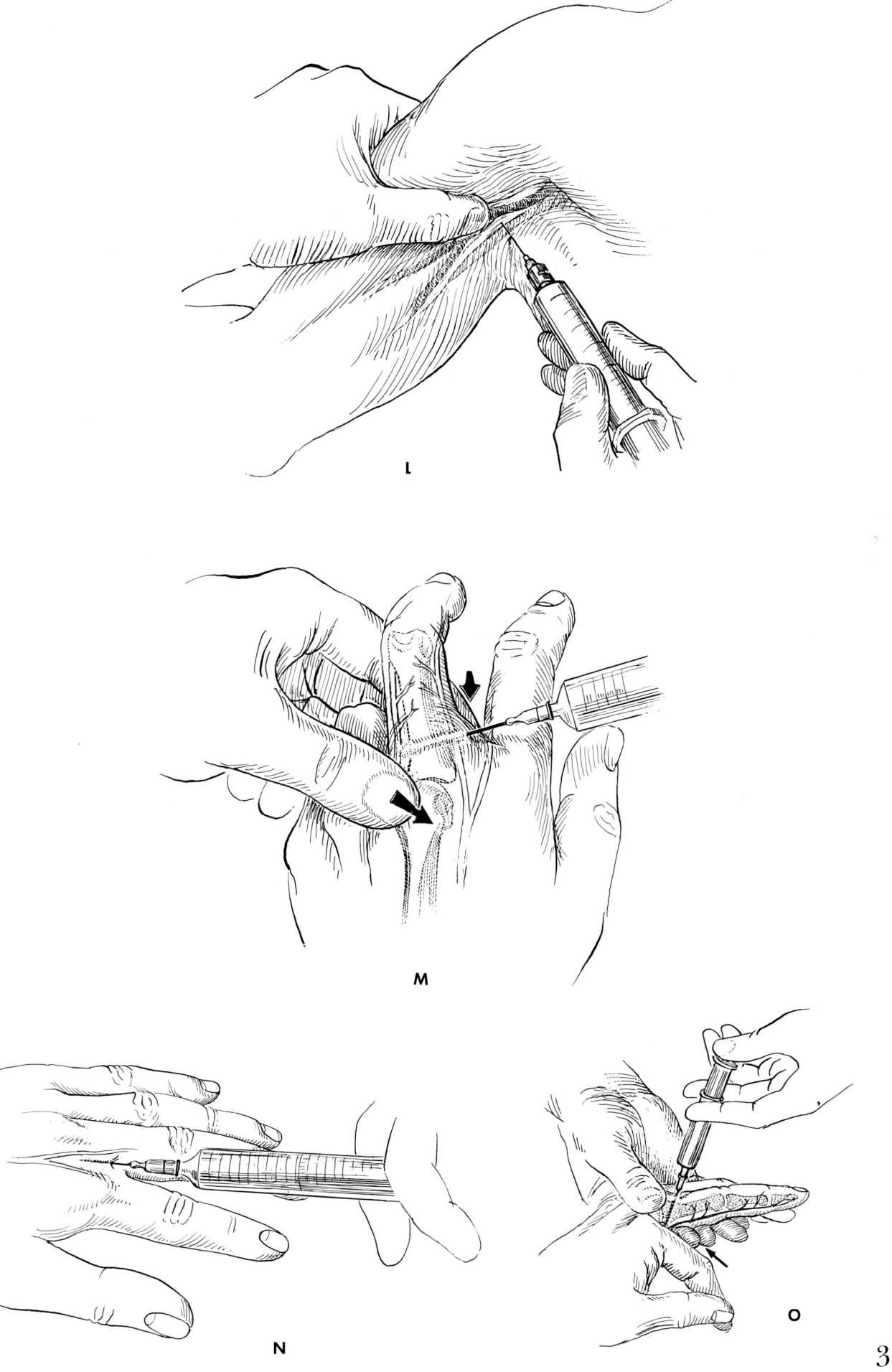

31

5

Skin and Subcutaneous Tissue

Dorsal Skin

Skin covering the dorsum of the hand is soft, pliable, thin, and elastic. (**A**) The underlying loose areolar fascia overlying the extensor tendons and their investing fascia allows the skin a wide range of mobility.

Translated into surgical principles, the combination of thin mobile skin with loose supporting fascia explains why:

1. Avulsion injuries lifting skin from the hand in the areolar plane are common.

2. When swelling occurs in the hand from injury, infection, or any other cause, it is evident first and most prominently over the dorsum.

3. Incisions and lacerations in the dorsum of the hand without loss of tissue do not cause scar contractures because of the adaptation possible by virtue of the skin's mobility.

4. Adhesion of skin to the extensor tendons with their relatively short excursions after injury or repair generally does not limit function. The adherent skin may move through the full range of tendon motion because of the mobility of the skin adjacent to the scar adhesion.

5. Surgical dissection in the subcutaneous plane is easily done and separation of the skin from underlying parts may be carried out in part by blunt dissection. (**B**)

6. The pliable elastic dorsal skin may be shifted about surgically with ease to cover an area in need of pedicle skin.

7. Dorsal skin avulsed in a severe injury may be thinned on its deep surface and be replaced as a free skin graft with the expectation that it will survive.

Palmar Skin and Palmar Fascia

Skin on the palm of the hand is thick, inelastic, and packed with sweat glands. Its external surface has a heavy cornified layer, and skin ridges are prominent. The skin's dermis is fixed to the palmar fascia by innumerable tiny fascial fibers that sharply limit movement of the palm skin over the underlying fascia. This accounts for the fixed creases in the palm skin at sites where the immobile skin must fold with flexion of the movable elements of the hand.

The *palmar fascia* is a special aponeurosis extending peripherally from the palmaris longus (when it is present) to the level of the middle phalanges of the fingers. Its longitudinal fibers are concentrated into four thickened coalescences, one passing to the palmar subcutaneous area of each of the four fingers. (**C**)

Longitudinal fibers coursing toward the thumb seem to blend into the abductor pollicis brevis suggesting that this intrinsic muscle is part of the palmar fascial mechanism. The vertical fibers of the palmar fascia are numerous and they bind the skin dermis to the fascia. The spaces between these fibers are filled with special fibro fat. The vertical fibers on the deep aspect of the flat palmar fascia coalesce into septa. These septa pass deep into the palm between the longitudinally directed structures to the fingers. These septa make up compartments for the tendons, vessels, and nerves going to the digits. One of the septa is particularly prominent and important. It passes from the palmar fascia to the deep fascia overlying the third metacarpal. There is no septum to the second

General Principles

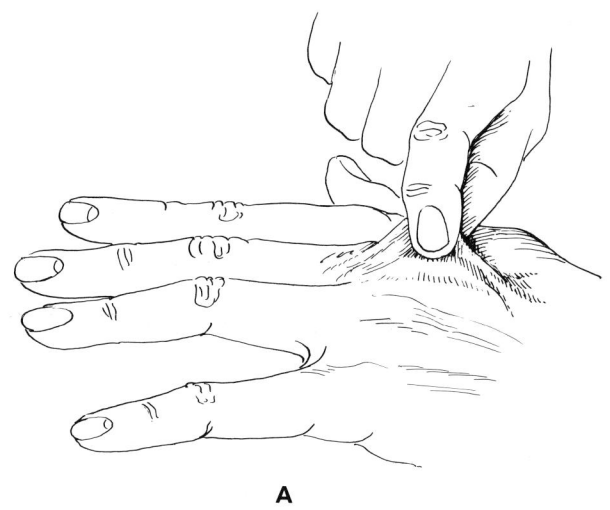

A

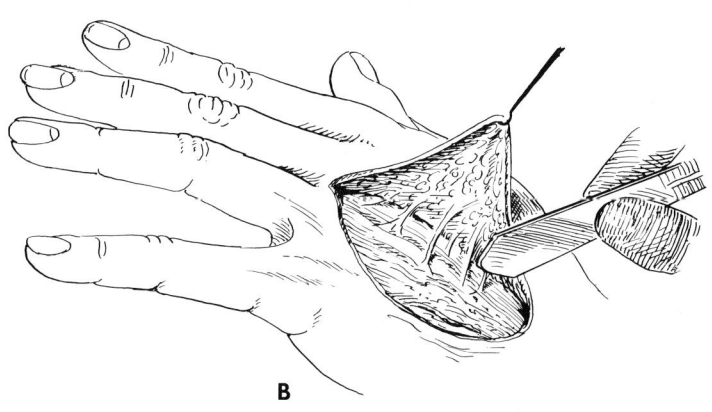

B

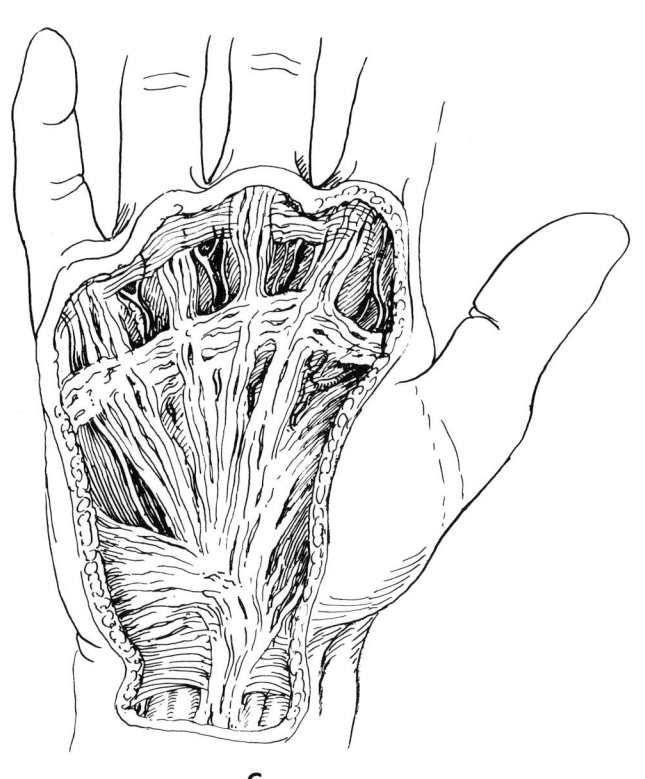

C

metacarpal since the adductor pollicis muscle crosses the area from its origin on the third metacarpal. The prominent septum to the third metacarpal may represent the coalescence of the septa to the second and third metacarpal. This thick septum divides the deep subtendinous space of the hand into the mid-palmar space and the thenar space.

A translation of characteristics of palm skin similar to that done for dorsal skin would reveal that such thick, inelastic skin fixed by rigid palmar fascia explains why:

1. Avulsion injuries require massive force, and palmar fascial elements may be torn off with the skin.

2. The skin's stability, special sensibility, and sudomotor capability make it an excellent surface for a hand which manipulates, grasps, pinches, and has a large share of responsibility for man's assessment of his environment.

3. Swelling in the subcutaneous palm is sharply limited and despite lack of visible evidence of swelling, pressure extensive enough to cause skin and subcutaneous ischemia and necrosis may occur.

4. Incisions and lacerations which cross flexion creases or are otherwise placed across areas of changing length will result in scar contracture. The inability of surrounding skin to stretch and adapt results in contracture as a wound contracts in healing. Great care must be exercised in planning incisions on the palm of the hand and fingers.

5. Adherence of a flexor tendon to palm skin and palmar fascia dooms it to immobility since the skin and fascia are immobile.

6. Surgical dissection of palm skin from its underlying palmar fascia is possible only by sharp transection of the fibers from the fascia to the dermis. (**D**) It is particularly difficult in Dupuytren's contracture since the fibers shorten, making dermis and palmar fascia difficult to separate.

7. Palm skin when avulsed has a tendency to reassume the contour it had prior to avulsion. Its very thick cornified layer and the fixed skin ridges make it comparable to the top of a derby hat or moulded plastic with a memory. The use of such skin as a free graft frequently fails because the semi-rigid skin will not adapt to the fine wound interstices. Dead space develops, plasmatic circulation of nutrients to the graft is prevented, and the grafted cells die. It is possible to peel the superficial rind from palm skin and then to thin its deep surface and expect it to take; however, this procedure is so tedious that most surgeons would choose to obtain split thickness skin from another site.

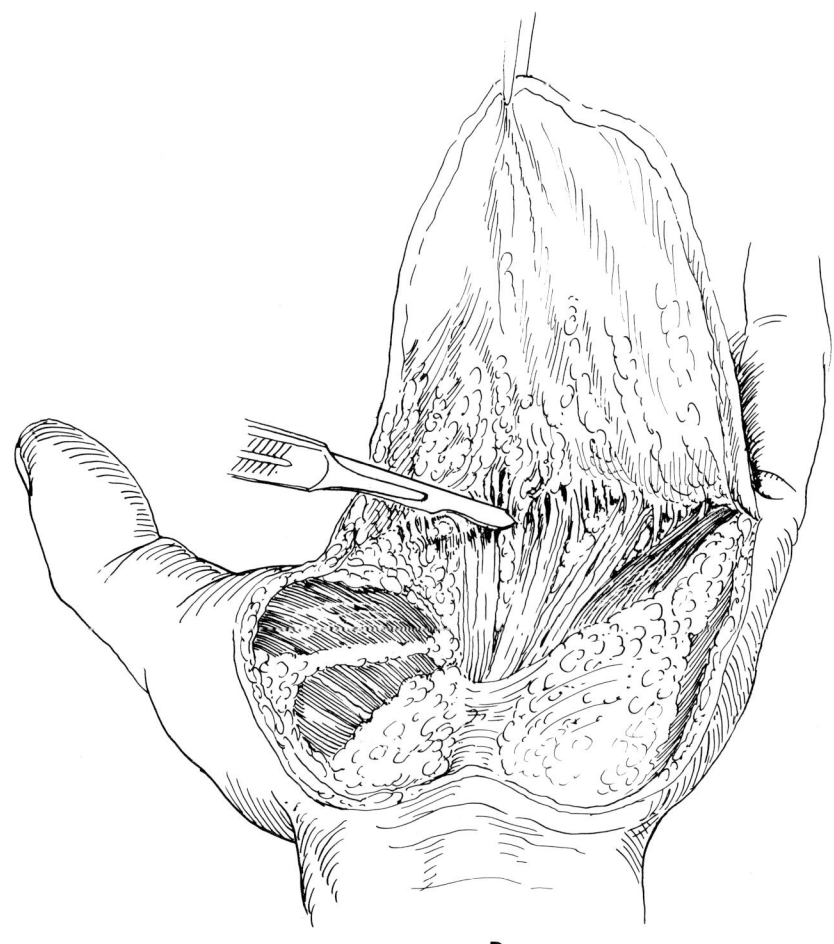

D

6

Elective Skin Incisions

Elective incisions in the hand must be planned to avoid contractures and to avoid scars in an area of maximum sensory perception. Littler has pointed out the troublesome areas on the flexor surface of the hand where motion results in folding of the skin.

In maximum flexion, skin folding results in skin-to-skin contact in diamond-shaped areas. Any incision which crosses from one-half of the diamond to its contact area in the other half may result in flexion contracture as the wound heals.

In each of the fingers the contact areas may be seen by flexing the finger, marking the dorsal extent of each skin crease (a, b, and c) and marking the point of contact in the palmar midline where skin from all three finger segments meets. (**A**)

Extension of the finger and connection of these marks by lines makes visible the contact triangles. (**B**)

Any longitudinal incision crossing from proximal to distal triangle across flexion creases may result in flexion contracture. (**C**)

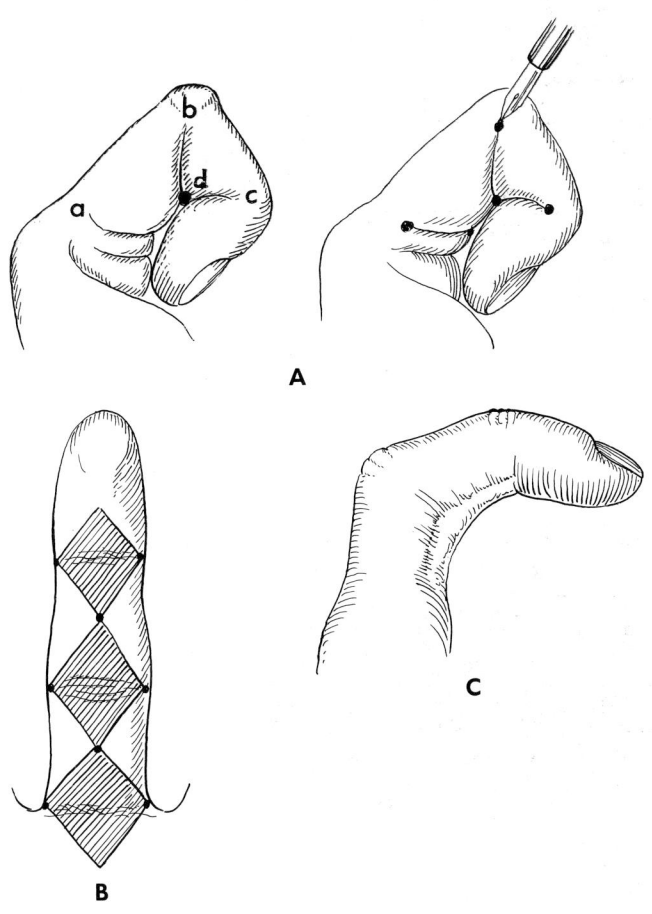

6 — Elective Skin Incisions

Similar contact areas for the thumb and the junction of the thenar eminence with the rest of the hand may be worked out in a similar manner. (**D**)

The same incision principles must be adhered to in contact areas at flexion creases in the hand and wrist if contracture and concomitant scar hypertrophy are to be avoided. (**E**)

Free choice of incision may then be made as long as none of the diamonds resulting are crossed from contact surface to contact surface. (**F**)

The prime areas of touch perception over digit tips should be avoided whenever possible in making elective incisions. This is particularly important in the prime perceptive digits, the thumb and index finger. (**G**)

In acute injuries of the finger where linear skin disruption occurs across flexion creases, a primary Z-plasty is indicated. (**H**) If the skin and soft tissue at the site of such a laceration is good, there is no better time to perform the Z-plasty than at the time of primary repair.

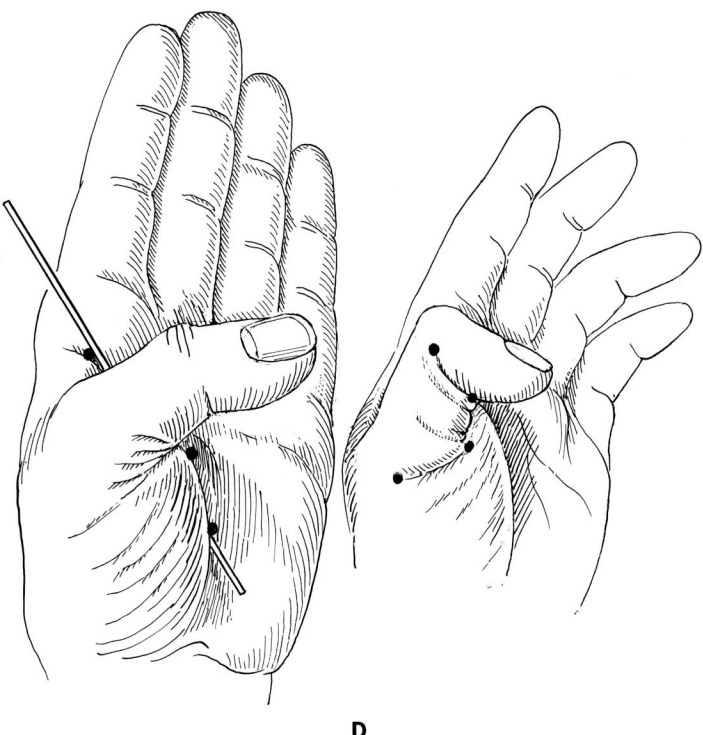

D

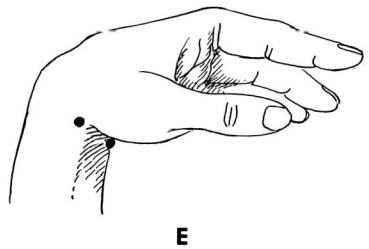

E

General Principles

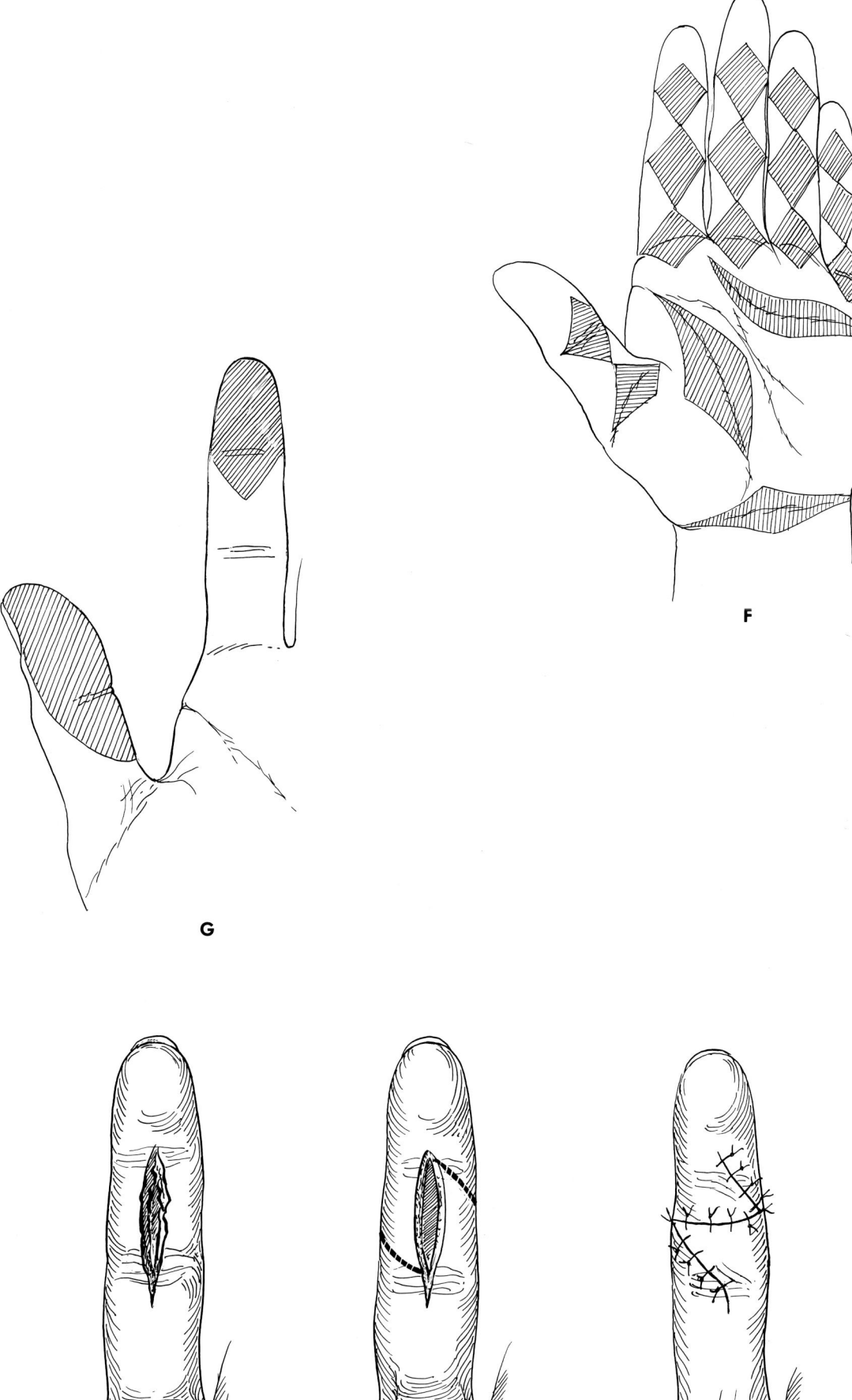

37

6 — Elective Skin Incisions

Z-plasty may be used to correct an established contracture if excision of the hypertrophic scar leaves sufficient skin and subcutaneous tissue to effect a shift without undue tension. (**I**) If skin involvement is such that Z-plasty cannot comfortably be done, a transverse release and implantation of a free skin graft is best. (**J**)

When a scar in the hand violates the principles above by crossing one of the diamonds from contact surface to contact surface, contracture and scar hypertrophy occurs. One may revise such a scar and plan the direction of the new scar by using a planned Z-plasty.

A scar crossing the thenar crease may be revised to place the new scar along the crease itself by outlining the desired line for the new scar (dotted line) then drawing parallel lines to the scar itself to create a Z-shaped wound. (**K**)

As the flaps are interchanged, the new scar line will fall along the thenar crease. (**L**)

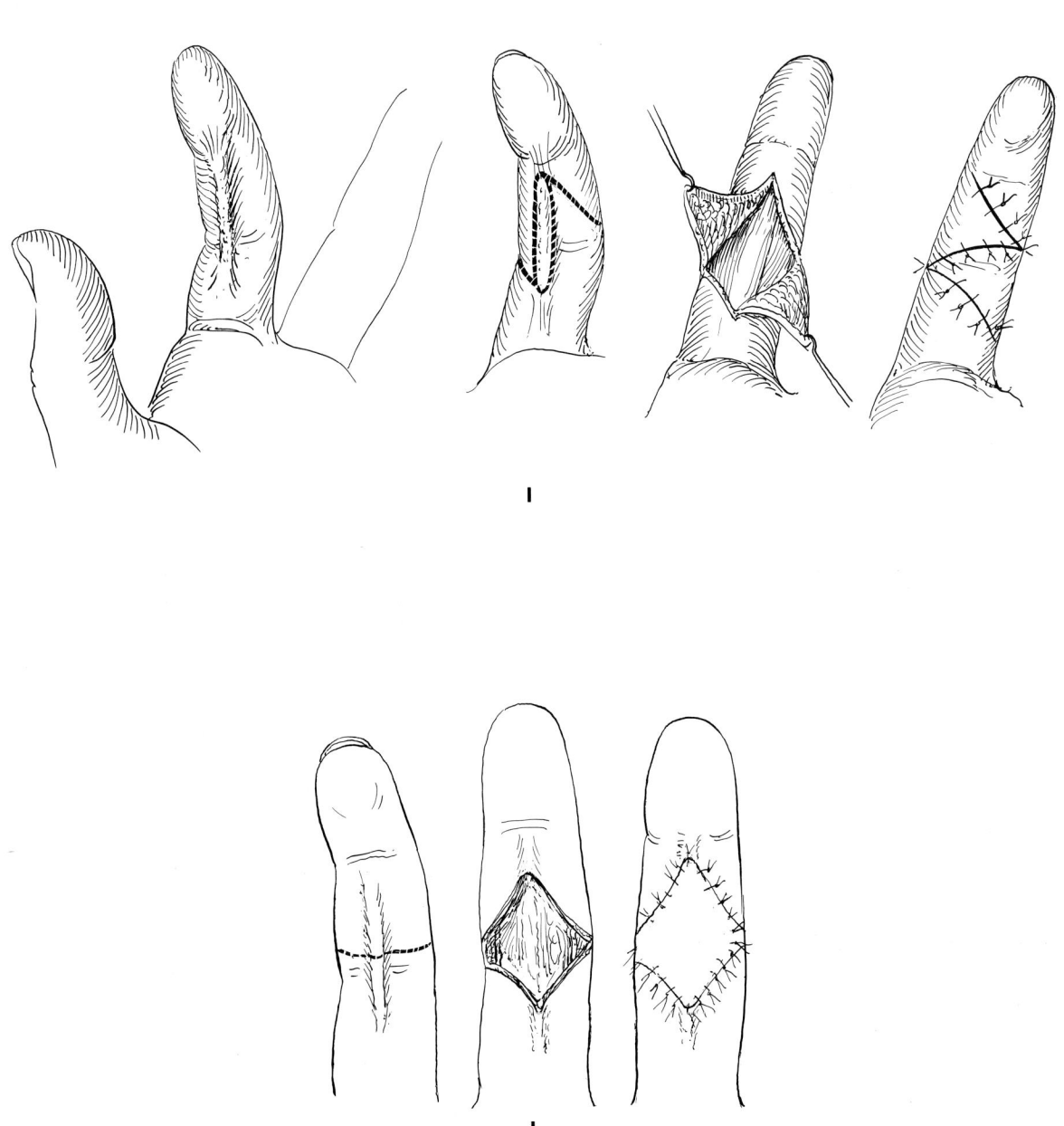

General Principles

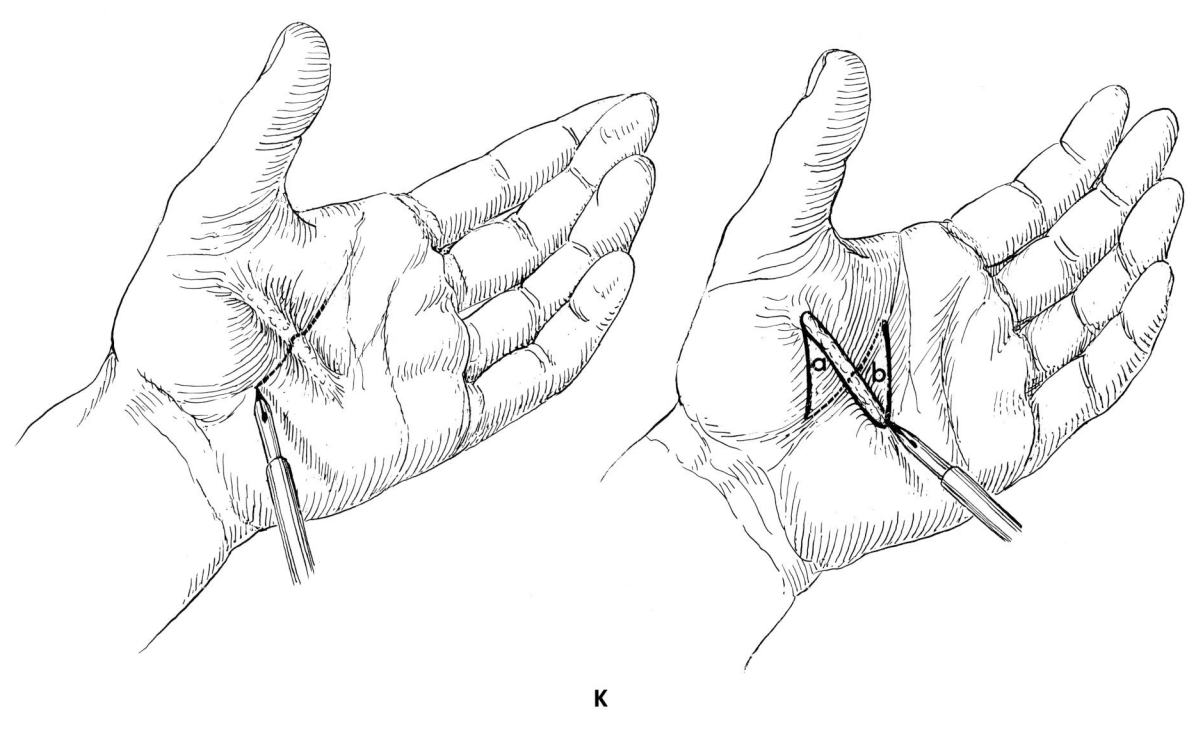

K

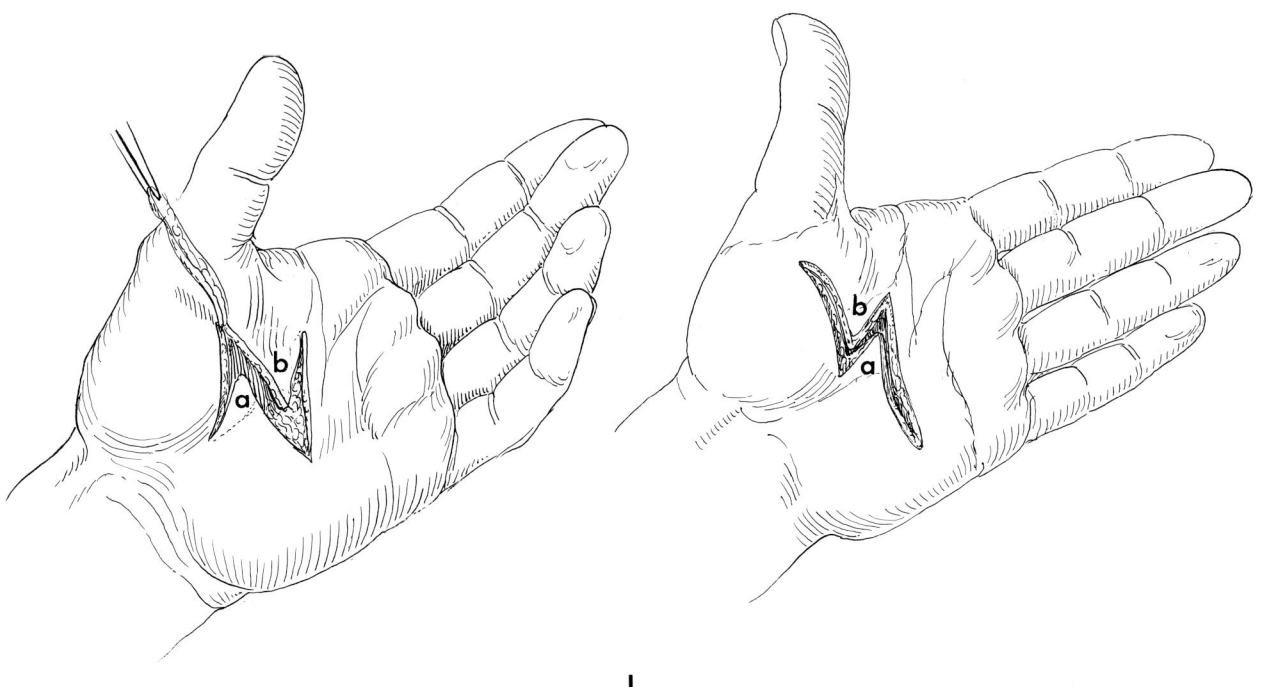

L

39

7
Skin Grafting

FREEHAND GRAFT

The quickest and most readily available means of acquiring a free split thickness skin graft is to take the graft with a freehand blade. A Weck blade 8 or 10 inches in length is the only instrument required. Such a blade may simply be hand held or one may prefer to use the special handle manufactured for the purpose. After appropriate anesthesia is induced and the skin is prepared, a small amount of lubricant (vaseline) is applied to the skin and then most of it is wiped away. The knife or blade backing is similarly lubricated as is a tongue depressor or other flat straight object used to flatten the skin as the graft is being cut. The skin-flattening instrument is dragged across the donor site several times to get the feel of the pressure and pull required. As the instrument or tongue depressor is dragged across the skin, the blade is laid on the skin and moved forward and back at the high point in the skin behind the flattener. (**A**) Once the blade has reached proper depth it may be switched forward and back quite widely resting the back of the blade against the donor site. Once the graft cut is started, the flattening implement is dragged forward and the skin cut continues at the summit of the mound that follows the flattener.

A sharp blade, previous practice, and confidence are prerequisites to successful cutting of a freehand graft.

Small area split thickness skin grafts may be taken with simple instruments in an emergency room or operating room for ambulatory patients.

The Weck blade with or without a special Ferris-Smith handle is the simplest instrument for this purpose. (**B**)

The Silver dermatome* is a small device which uses ordinary three hole razor blades. (**C**) The handle has an outrigger with a small roller which smooths the skin first in front of the blade and still allows forward and back blade motion in cutting. Depth of the graft is regulated both by the roller adjustment and the handling of the instrument by the surgeon. The Humby knife is a larger instrument which relies on the same principle.

The Davol/Simon disposable dermatome** is less difficult to use in taking a small graft for a fingertip. (**D**) A little practice with the device rapidly builds confidence, and use of complex dermatomes will not be necessary to obtain small grafts.

The Davol/Simon dermatome has a disposable sterile cutting head which attaches to the motor-containing handle. The motor handle is self-contained and cordless with rechargeable batteries. It is simply dropped into a sterile plastic bag that comes with the disposable head and the head is attached. The device is set to take a medium thickness graft (about 15 thousandths of an inch) about an inch and a quarter in width. The handle is kept in a wall charger between uses.

---

*Silver dermatome—Down Bros. and Mayer & Phelps Ltd., available from Codman & Shurtleff Inc., Randolph, Mass. 02368

**Manufactured by Davol Inc., Providence, Rhode Island 02901. Blade No. 3295; Handle, No. 3291.

General Principles

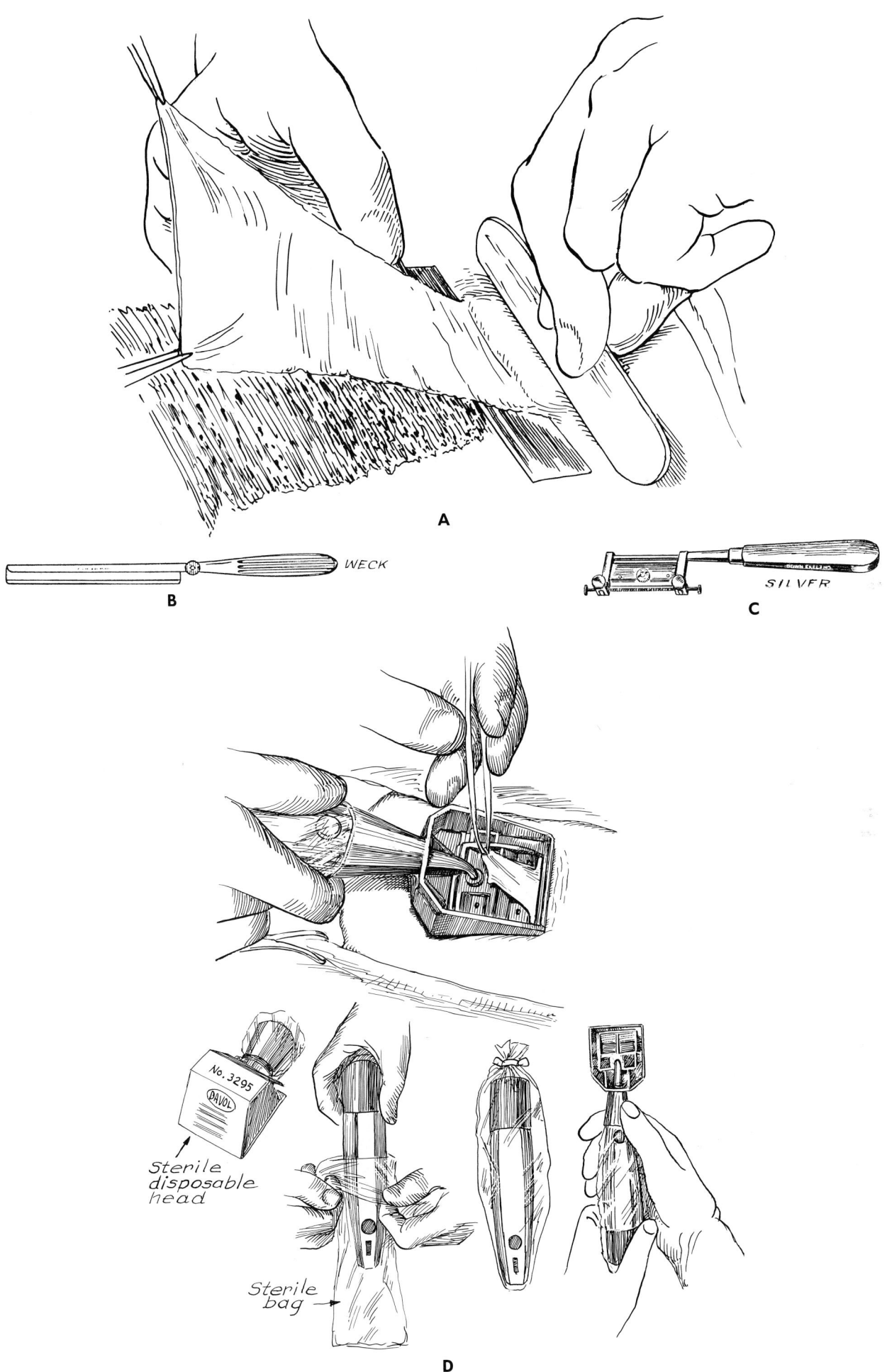

41

7 – Skin Grafting

A wide freehand graft may be obtained from the thigh. (**E**) A Weck blade or Humby knife (shown here) is best adapted for this. Support of soft tissues by an assistant's hands placed beneath the thigh will help create a broad flat surface as the graft is cut.

With the soft tissues flattened, the surface is rendered smooth and tense, using a flat block pulled ahead of the blade during the cutting procedure. Control of the skin medial and lateral to the donor area is achieved during the procedure by the extent of support given by the assistant's hands under the thigh. (**F**)

The posterior thigh may be used as a donor site with the patient supine or prone. (**G**)

The lateral thigh is also available by proper leg positioning with the patient in the usual supine position. (**H**)

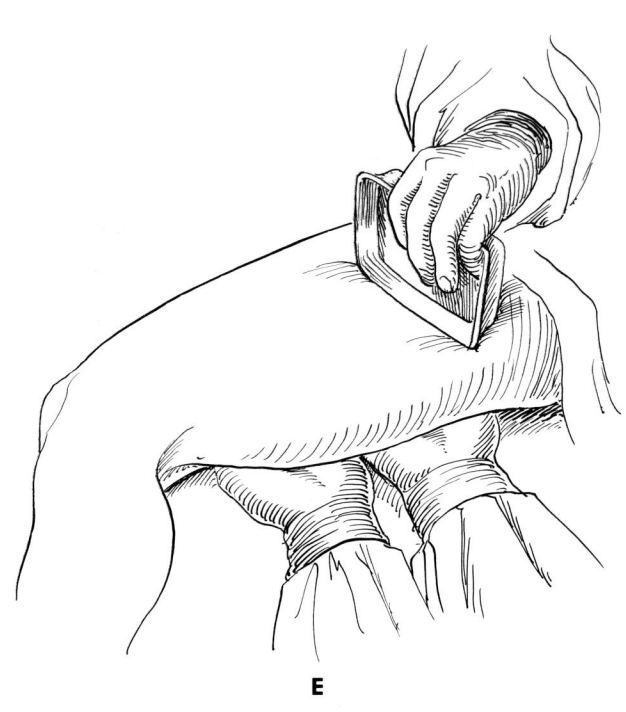

E

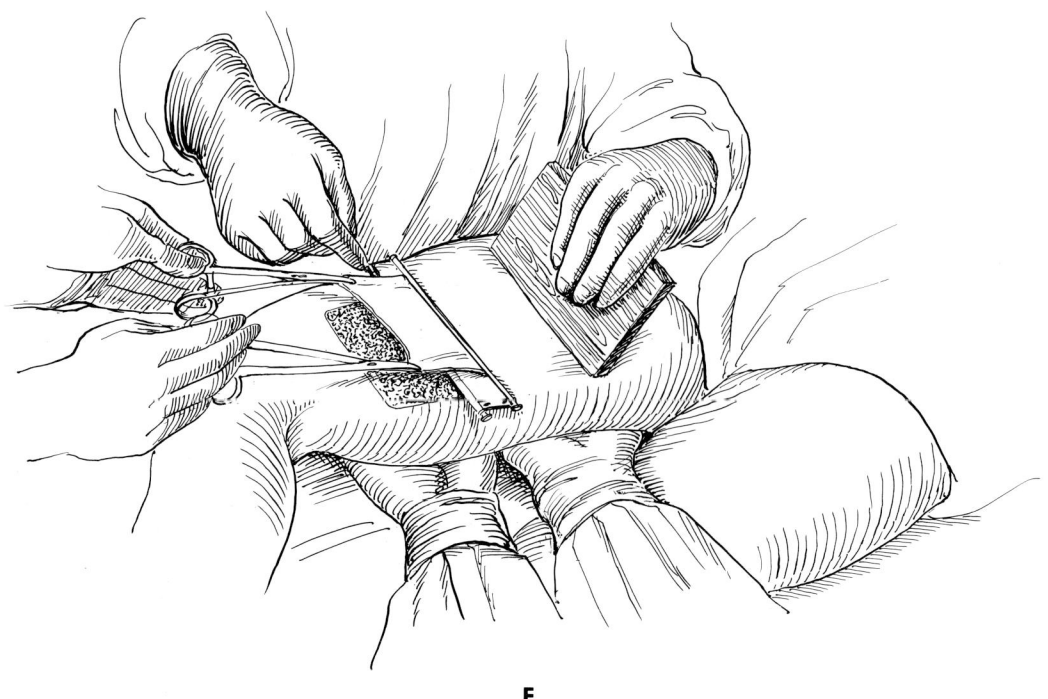

F

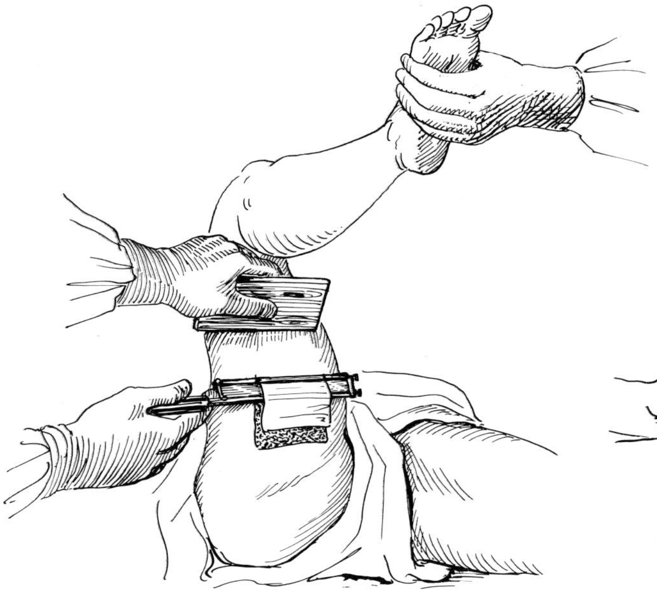

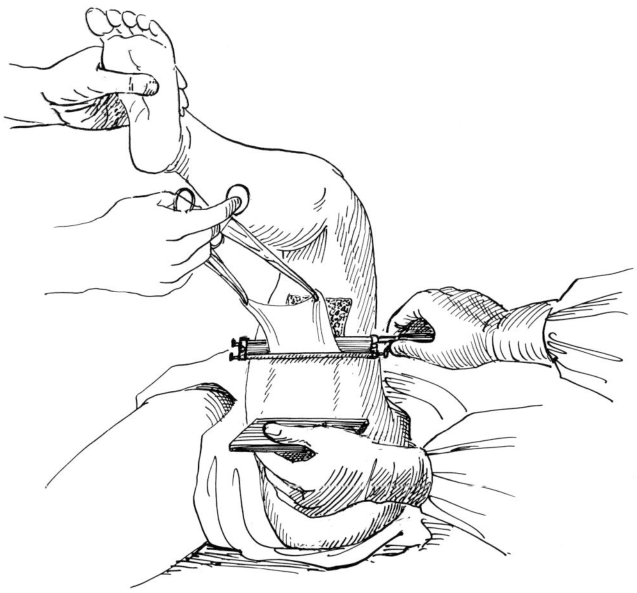

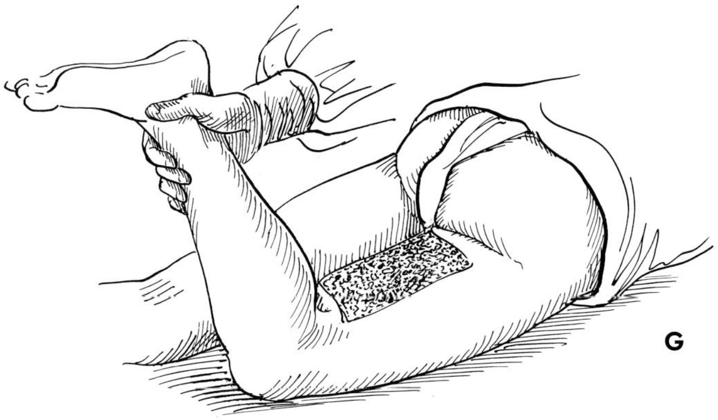

General Principles

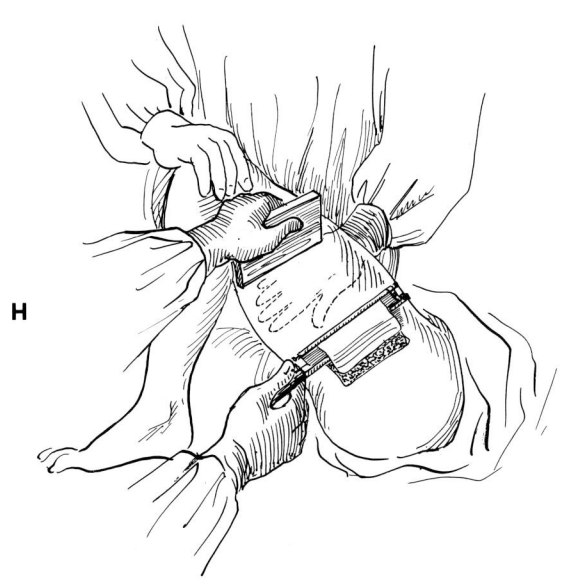

G

H

43

7 – Skin Grafting

SPECIAL DERMATOMES

There are a number of dermatomes available to aid the surgeon in taking a skin graft of reliable thickness and size.

Electric Dermatomes

Typical of electric dermatomes is the Brown-Padgett* dermatome. (**A**) Like other mechanized dermatomes, it has a removable blade which, when fixed in place, oscillates when power is transmitted to the device from an electric motor through a sterilizable cable. The thickness of the skin graft taken is regulated by turning the adjustment knob to the appropriate thickness.

The Brown dermatome is also manufactured to use compressed air as a source of power, thus eliminating the hazards implicit in use of electrically powered instruments.

The skin is prepared, using usual methods, then lightly lubricated with mineral oil. After adjustment of the instrument to take a skin graft of appropriate width, the cutting side of the instrument is pressed against the donor site. The power is turned on, using a foot pedal, and the dermatome is advanced to cut a sheet of split thickness skin. (**B**)

The electric dermatome is fast and particularly useful when one wishes to take very thin skin grafts of large area.

Similar mechanized dermatomes are available as attachments to a common source of power used for drills and bone saws. (**C**) The Hall** Air Dermatome is such a device.

---

*Brown Electro Dermatome and Brown Air-Dermatome. Zimmer, Warsaw, Indiana.

**Hall Air Dermatome — Howmet Corporation, 224 E. 39th Street, New York, New York 10016

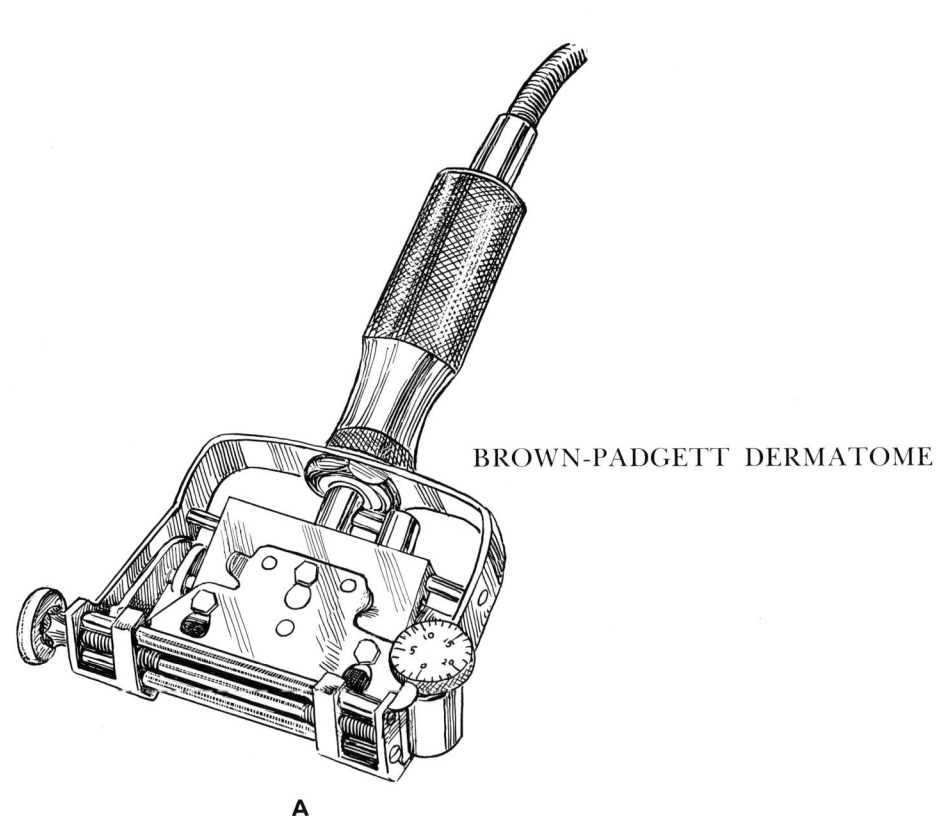

BROWN-PADGETT DERMATOME

A

General Principles

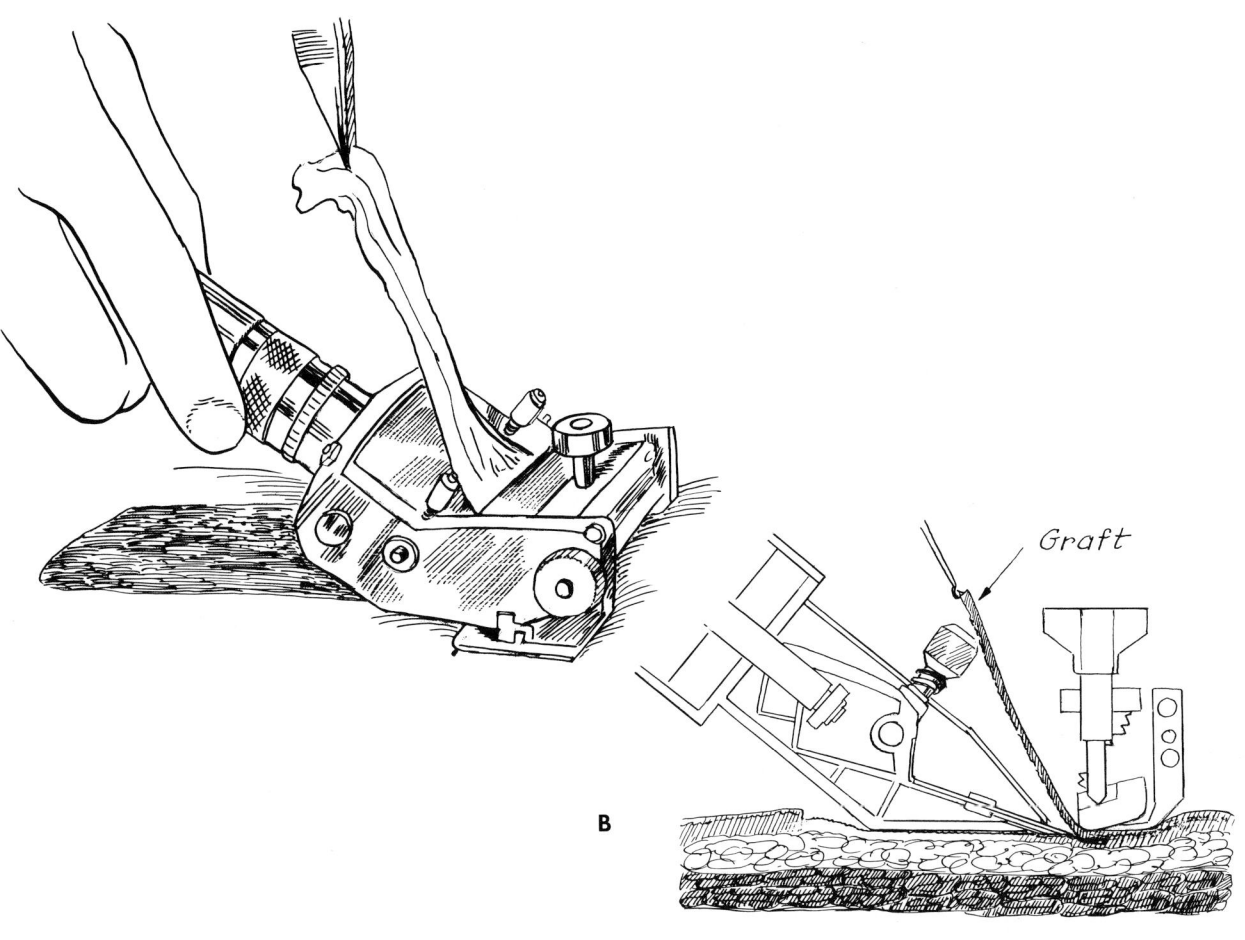

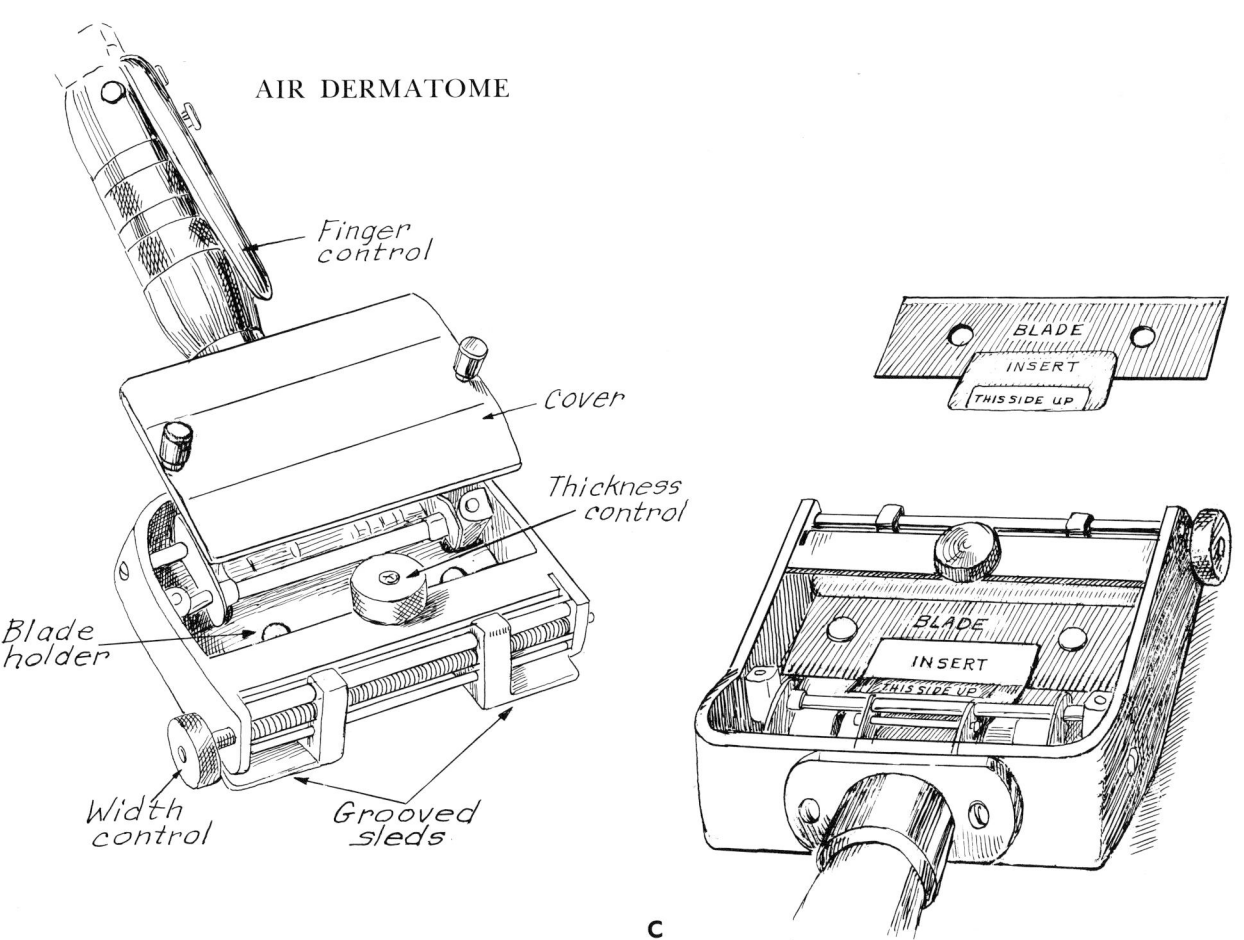

B

Graft

AIR DERMATOME

Finger control
Cover
Thickness control
Blade holder
Width control
Grooved sleds

BLADE INSERT THIS SIDE UP

C

7 — Skin Grafting

Drum Dermatomes

The Padgett* Dermatome is a drum dermatome with a swinging outrigger blade having a depth adjustment mechanism. It may be used by applying dermatome cement on the drum and the skin or it may be used with special tape with adhesive on both surfaces.

The backing of the tape is removed from one surface and the tape is placed, sticky side up, on a soft surface such as a folded towel on a firm, flat table top. The dermatome is placed on the tape starting at the trailing edge of the drum and rolling it toward the leading edge. (**D**) The drum must be aligned very carefully. As the leading edge is reached, the tape is folded over the leading edge to pick up the skin firmly at the site of pick up. The backing is removed from the surface of the tape now on the drum and the instrument is ready for use. The technique for taking a skin graft with the Padgett Dermatome is the same as that described for the Reese Dermatome.

The Reese dermatome** is a drum dermatome designed to use special tape which is held in place mechanically on the drum surface. (**E** and **F**) The skin thickness to be cut is determined by insertion of shims between the blade and the base of the blade outrigger. The laminated dermatape is fixed to the surface of the drum quite precisely by folding the tape at both ends along the marks provided. With the dermatome fixed on its special stand the tape clamp bar is released and rotated up to allow the end of the dermatape to be inserted. (**G, H,** and **I**)

*Padgett Dermatome — Kansas City Assemblage Co., 4032 Broadway, Kansas City, Mo. 64111

**Reese Dermatome — Bard Parker, Danbury, Conn.

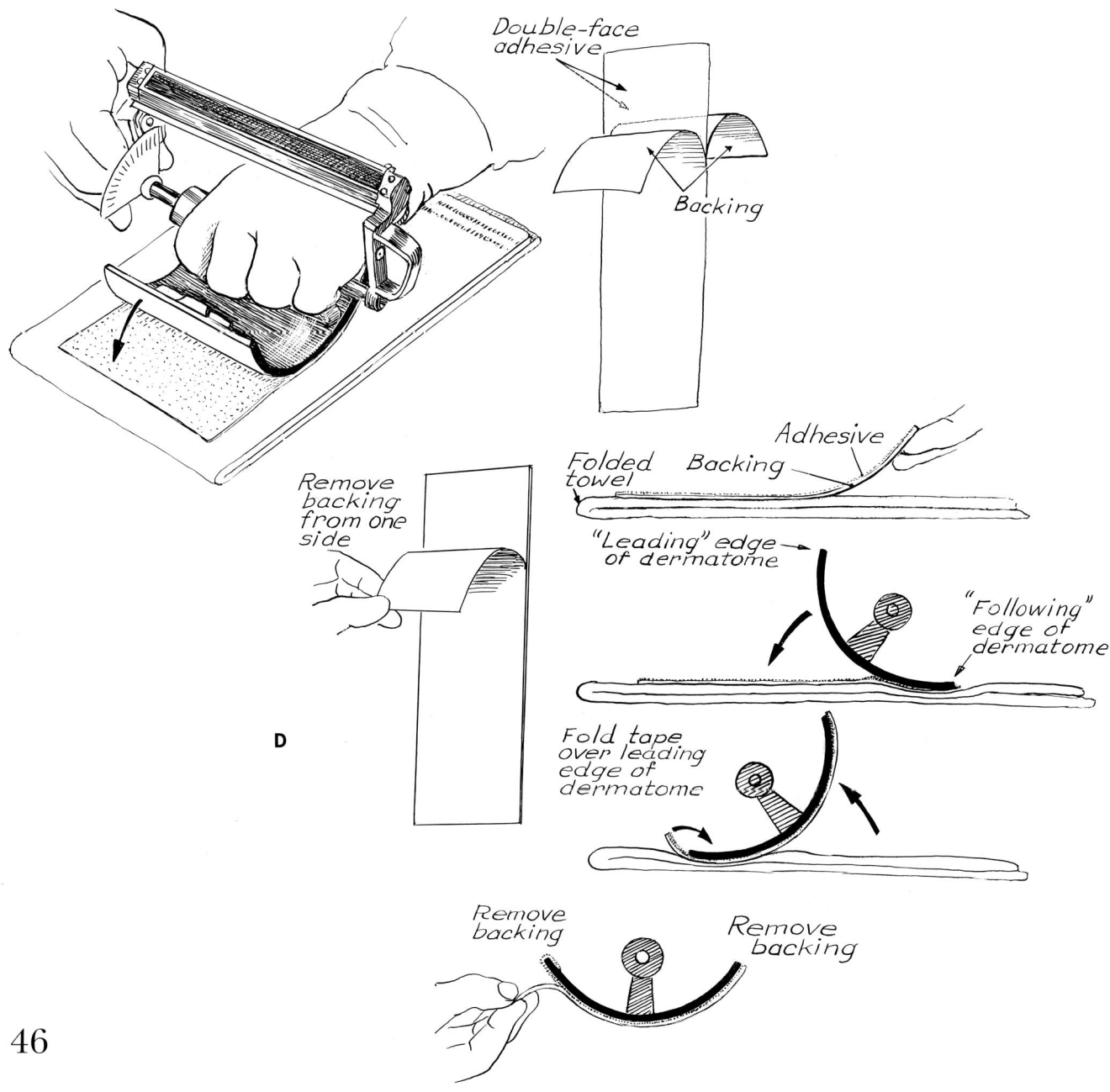

General Principles

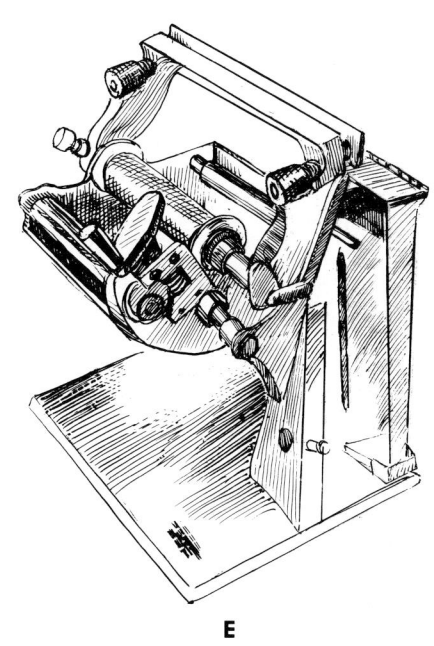

E

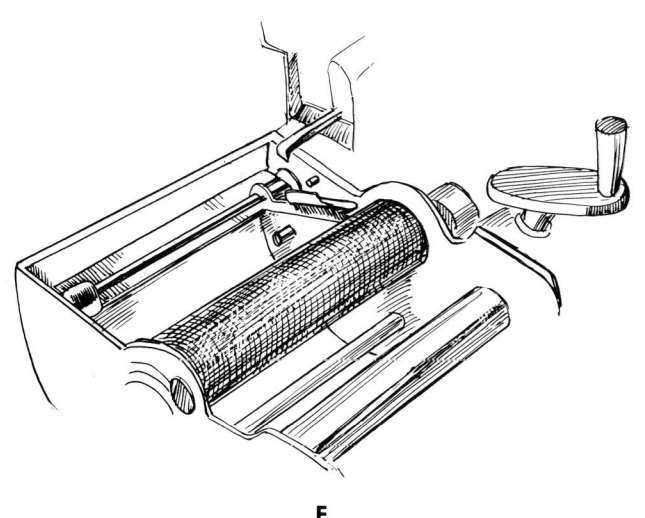

F

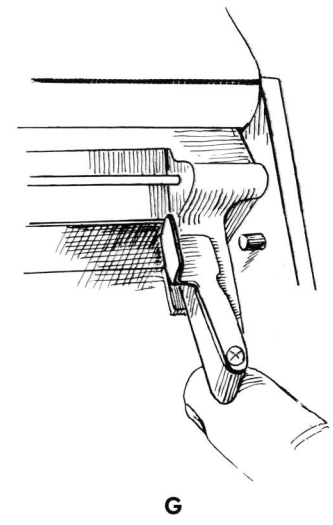

G

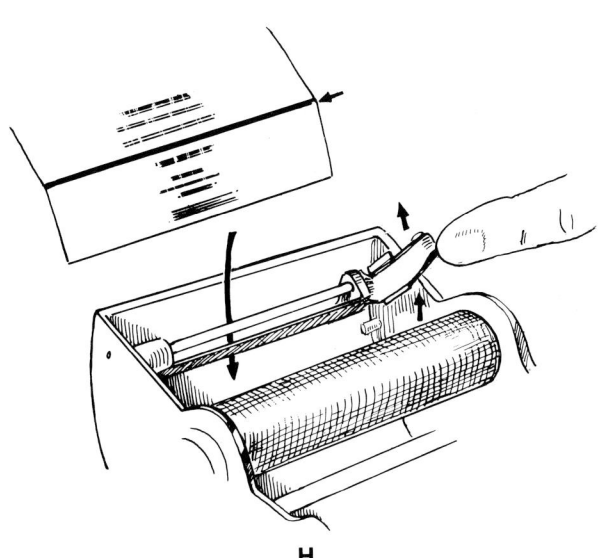

H

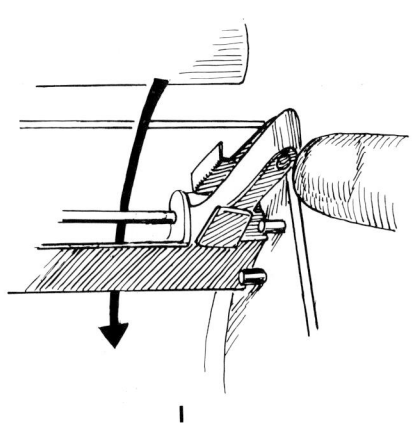

I

7 — Skin Grafting

The dermatape is inserted so that its fold is seated against the leading edge of the drum, and then the clamp bar is rotated into position to fix the tape and it is locked into position. (**J** and **K**)

The tape is pulled over the surface of the drum and the other end is inserted into the slot in the tightening spool until the fold falls flush with the spool surface. (**L** and **M**)

Using the crank provided, the spool is turned to swing the tape against the whole drum surface very tightly. (**N**)

A knife drawn lightly across the surface of the dermatape will cut through the plastic facing and it may then be peeled from the tape surface well around the leading edge of the drum where it is again sectioned for removal. (**O**)

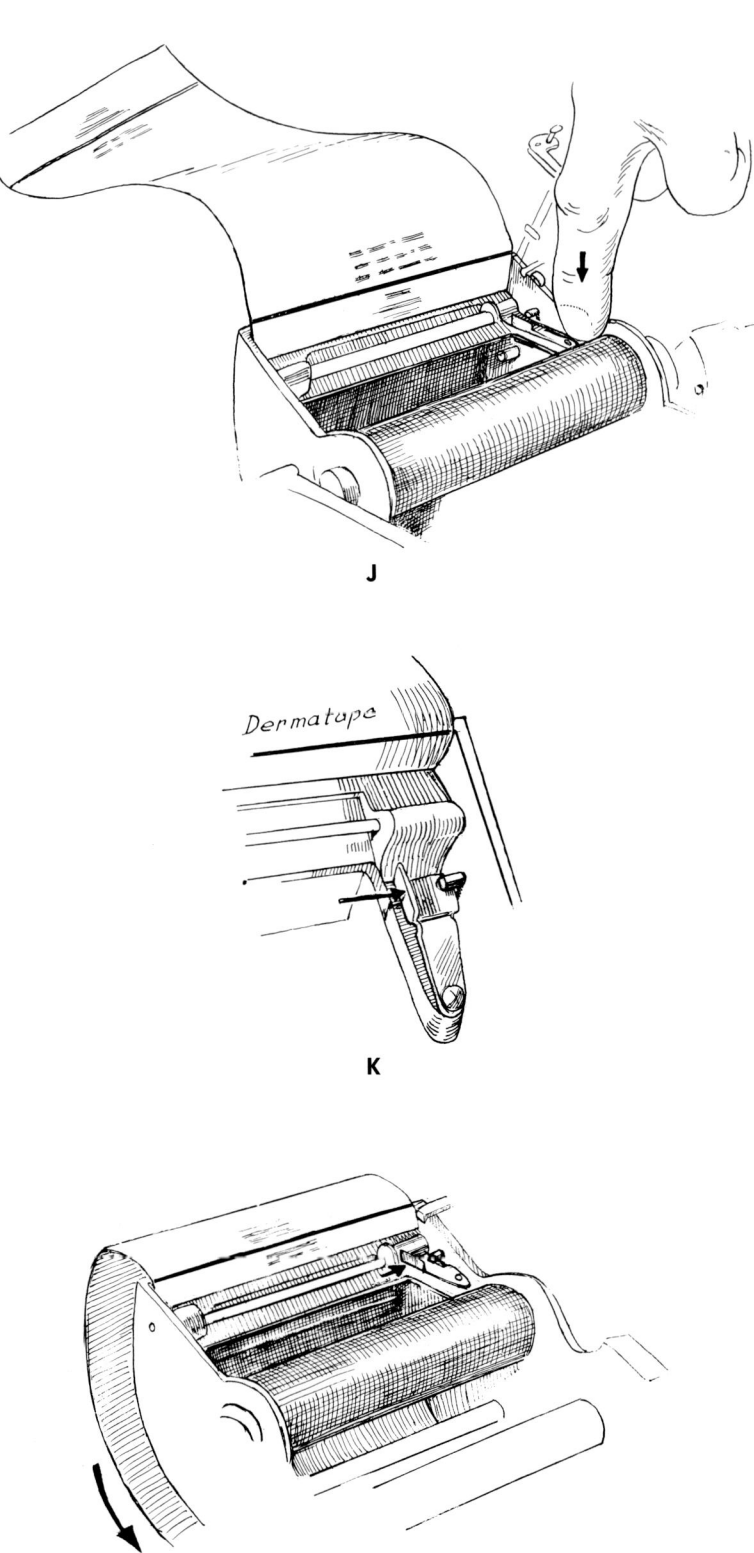

J

K

L

General Principles

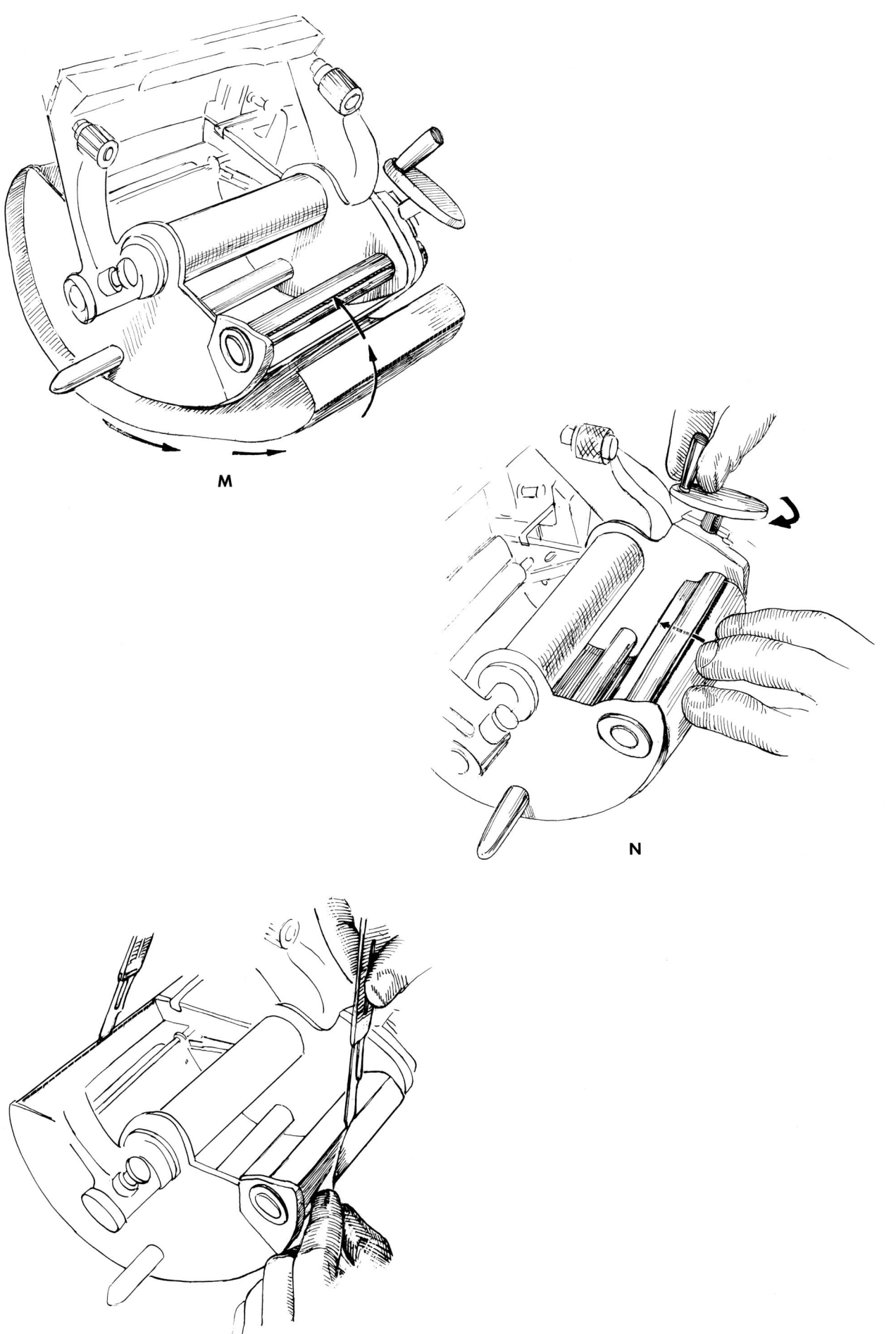

49

7 – Skin Grafting

A new blade is inserted into the blade clamp over a shim chosen for appropriate graft thickness. The knurled knobs which release and tighten the blade clamp are tightened to fix the shim and blade in place. (**P** and **Q**)

The donor area is prepared by wiping it with a defatting solvent and then it is painted with dermatome cement. (**R**) This is done with quick overlapping strokes and a brush kept wet with cement to avoid rolling and lumping of the glue which occurs when spreading is attempted during the drying period. If a small graft of specific shape is desired, an area of that shape and size only is painted. (**S**)

With the dermatome firmly held in one hand and the blade outrigger under sure control in the other, the leading edge of the drum is pressed firmly into the donor site, properly aimed to roll across the area where the rest of the cement has been applied. (**T**)

The drum is rotated slowly back until the skin adhering to the leading edge is tented up away from the plane of the donor site. (**U**) A swipe of the blade across the tented skin at the leading edge immediately increases the security of the adhesion of skin to dermatome.

The drum is rolled slowly as the skin graft is cut, and care is taken to observe the edges of the

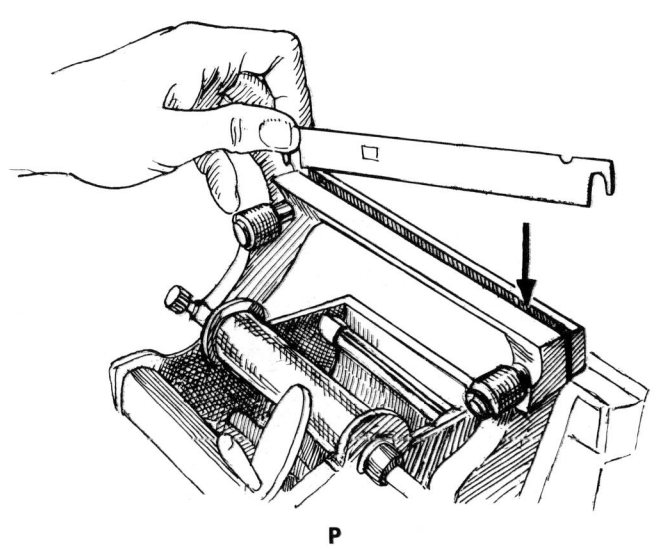

P

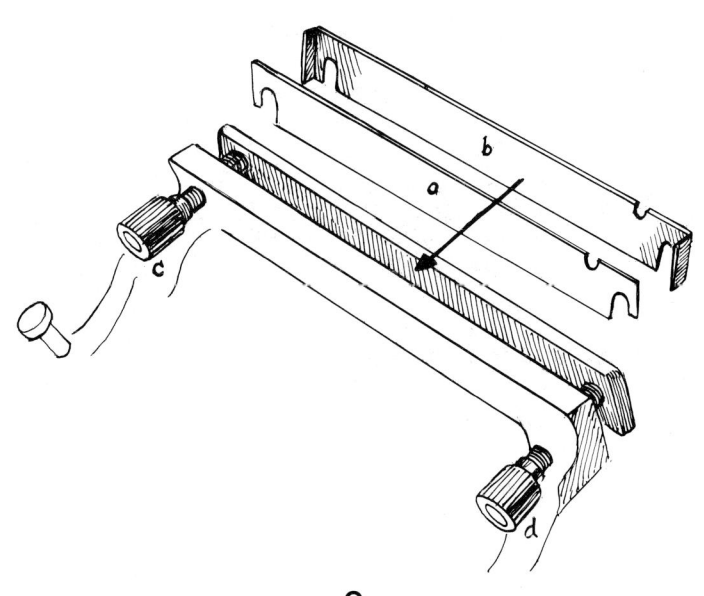

Q

General Principles

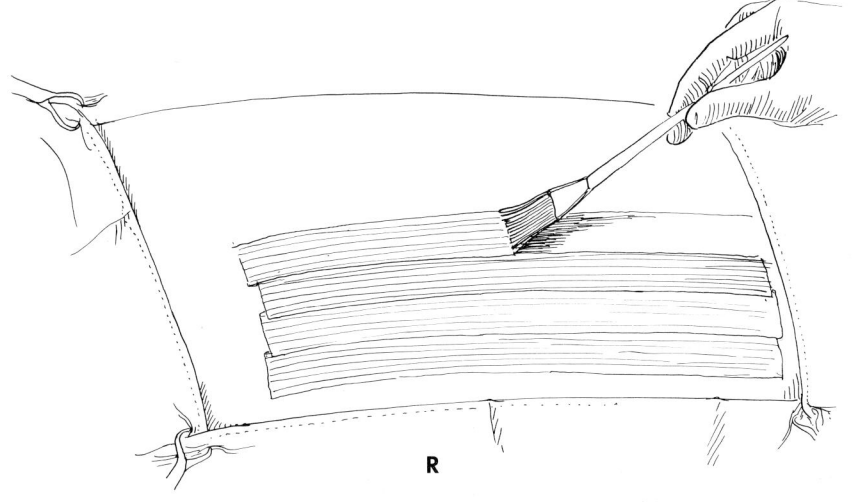

R

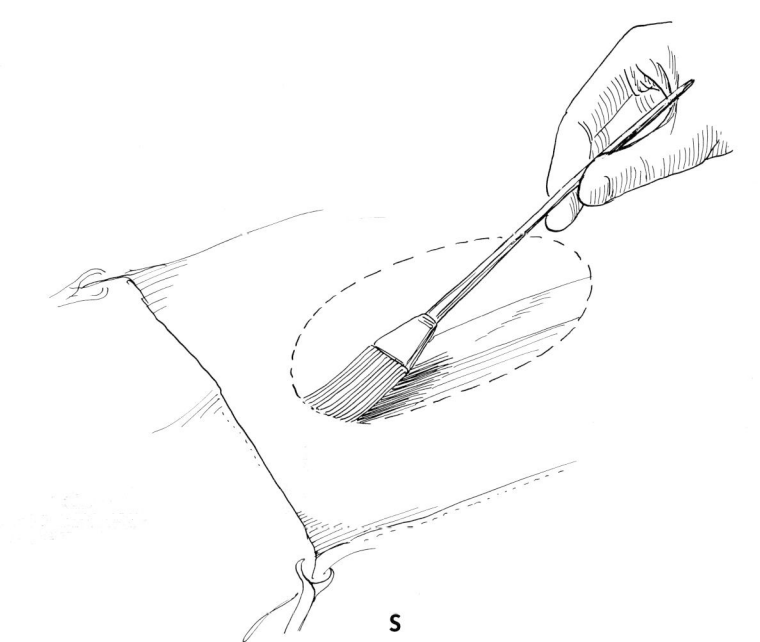

S

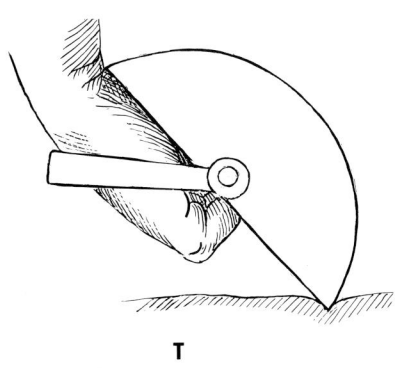

T

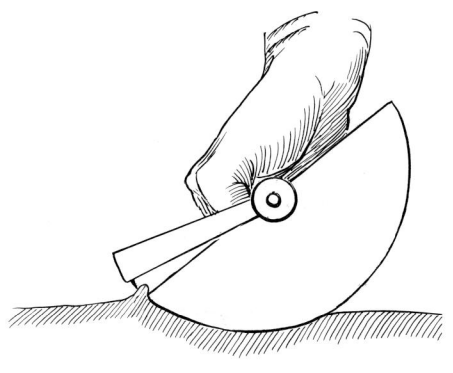

U

7 — Skin Grafting

skin graft and its junction with the donor site. (**V**) If rotation of the drum gets behind the cutting speed, the blade will cut into soft tissues beyond the drum; whereas if rotation gets too far ahead of the cut the edges of the skin may be pulled away from the drum and inadvertent narrowing of the graft will occur.

When the end of the drum is reached, the whole dermatome may be lifted to allow the surgeon to cut the graft free from the donor site at the end of the graft. (**W**)

The dermatome is placed back on the holding rack and is disarmed immediately by removing the blade. The skin graft may be removed by peeling it from the dermatome* and transferring it directly to the recipient site, or the dermatape with the skin left on it may be removed from the drum.

The laminated tape may then be split by tearing the fabric backing to leave the skin attached to the residual pliable rubber backing. (**Y**) One may wish to apply the graft to the recipient bed using the backing as a stent to hold the graft in place.

If any part or all of the graft is to be refrigerated for delayed application, it may be left on the backing for convenience. Later it may be separated and applied to the recipient site. (**Z**)

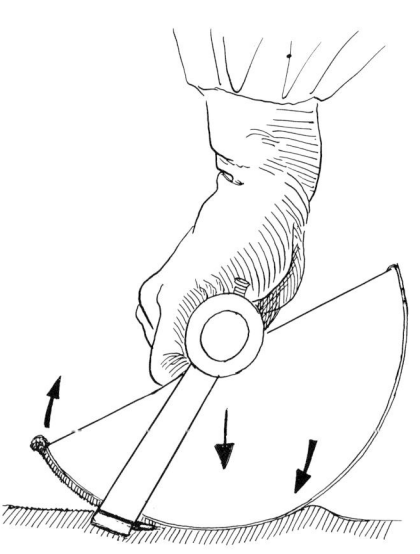

v

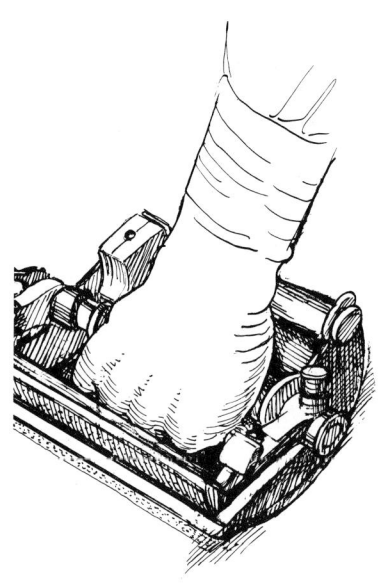

General Principles

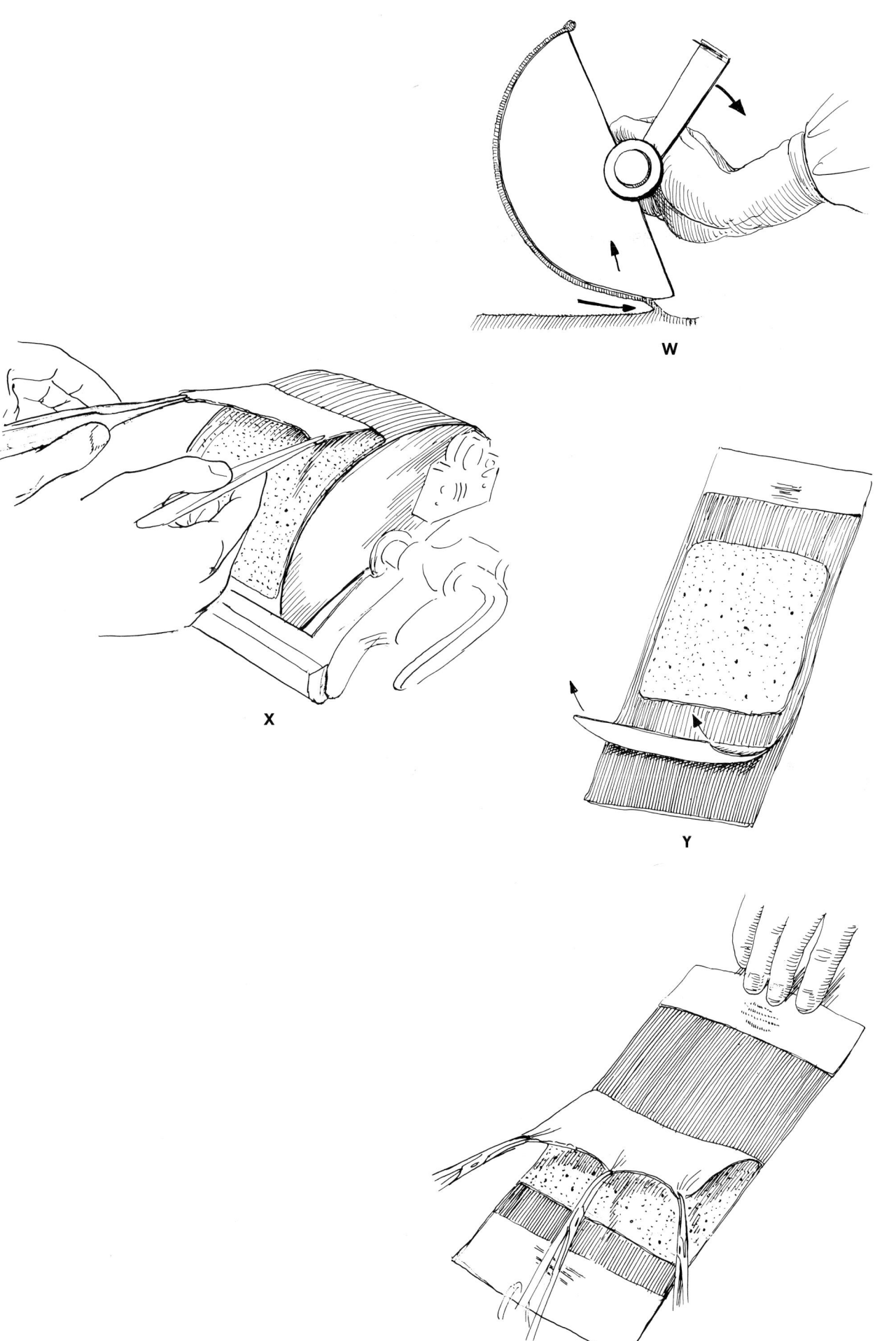

53

7—Skin Grafting

MESH GRAFTING

Various methods for efficient use of split thickness skin grafts have proved successful. Where there are limited donor sites and available skin is inadequate to cover, sheet postage stamp grafts and mesh grafts are useful.

Postage stamp size grafts may be cut from the sheet of skin and spread over the recipient site as islands of skin. As healing occurs, epithelium spreads from the postage stamp graft until re-epithelialization occurs over the residual uncovered areas. The technique is very useful when very thin grafts have been taken.

If the graft is thick enough to allow some stretching without tearing, the mesh graft technique is very useful. Expansion of the area covered is achieved by creating multiple parallel incisions in the graft which spread into diamond-shaped spaces as the graft is stretched at right angles to the incisions. (**A**) Various special devices are available to make the appropriate cuts in the graft, for example, the Tanner-Vandeput Meshgraft Dermatome.* (**B**)

A plastic skin carrier consisting of a thick and a thin layer of plastic is used to carry the skin graft through the cutter. (**C**) The skin graft is placed between the layers and the plastic skin graft sandwich is passed through the cutting device between the rollers. (**D**) Offset parallel cuts result, and, when the skin is put under lateral tension it stretches to allow nearly threefold expansion of the graft. (**E**) The resulting holes in the graft are re-epithelialized from the strips of skin making up the mesh graft.

---

*Zimmer—Warsaw, Indiana.

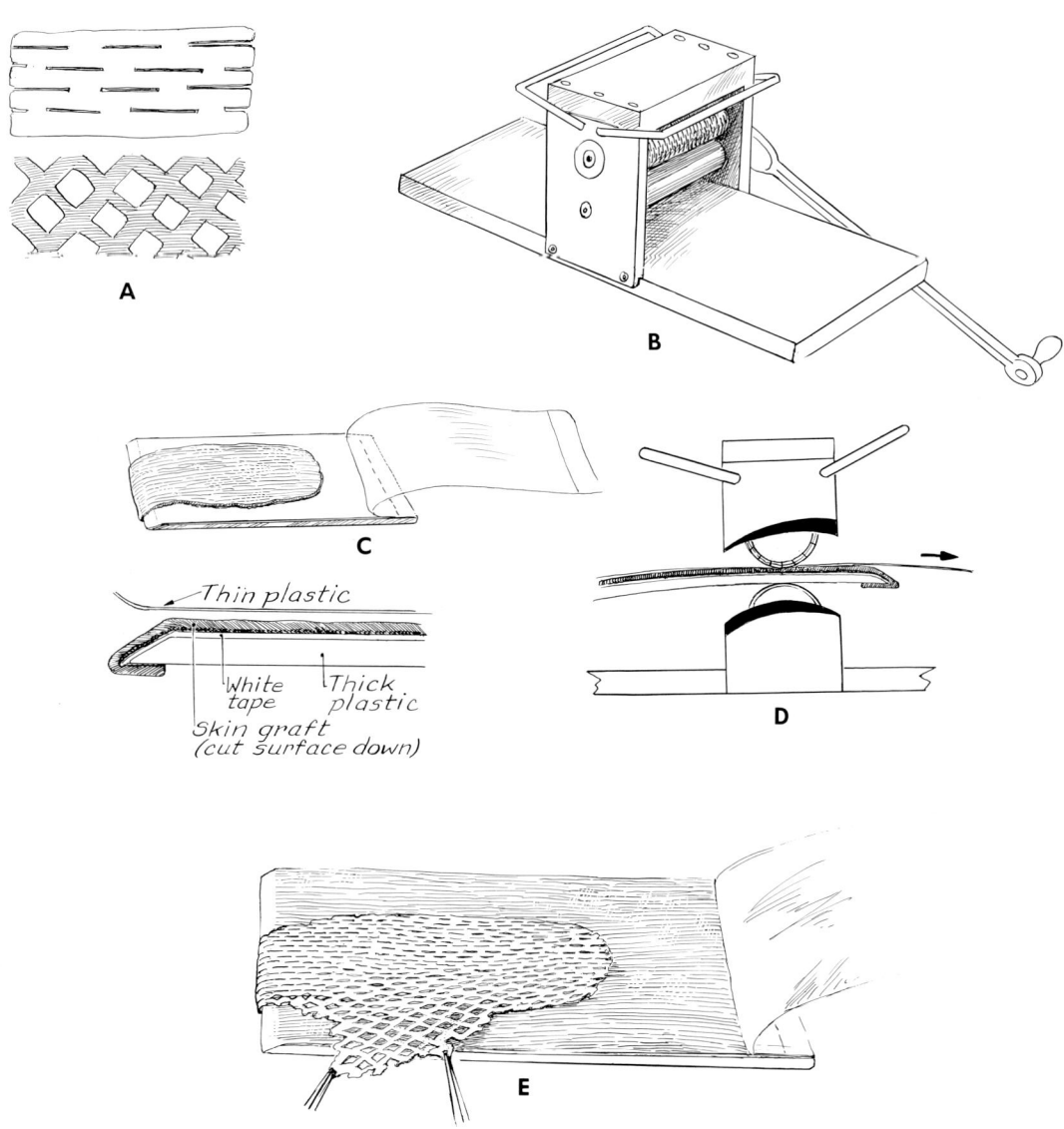

THE STENT DRESSING

Immobilization of a free skin graft over the recipient site and application of uniform gentle pressure is best achieved in some circumstances by a tie-over or stented dressing.

The sutures used to tack the skin graft to the recipient site are left long so that they may be tied over the dressing. A non-adherent gauze material such as Xeroform gauze or Adaptic gauze is cut to appropriate size and shape to overlap the recipient site by a centimeter or two on all sides. (**F**) Fluffed gauze is placed over the grafted site and the non-adherent dressing. The wound sutures are tied over the top of the gauze dressing to sutures from the opposite side. As the first knot is cinched down to create gentle pressure on the graft, it is pinched with the points of a needle holder without serrations. (Webster needle holder.) (**G**) It is held until the second knot is brought down to fix the proper tension.

The procedure is repeated until all suture ends are tied over the dressing. (**H**) The dressing is covered with additional fluffed gauze to protect it from exposure and movement. Tie-over dressings are generally left in position for five days, after which the dressing is loosened by cutting the tie-over stitches. The free edge of the non-adherent gauze is held down against the recipient site as the fluffed gauze is removed. The technique is particularly useful where dressings are difficult to apply.

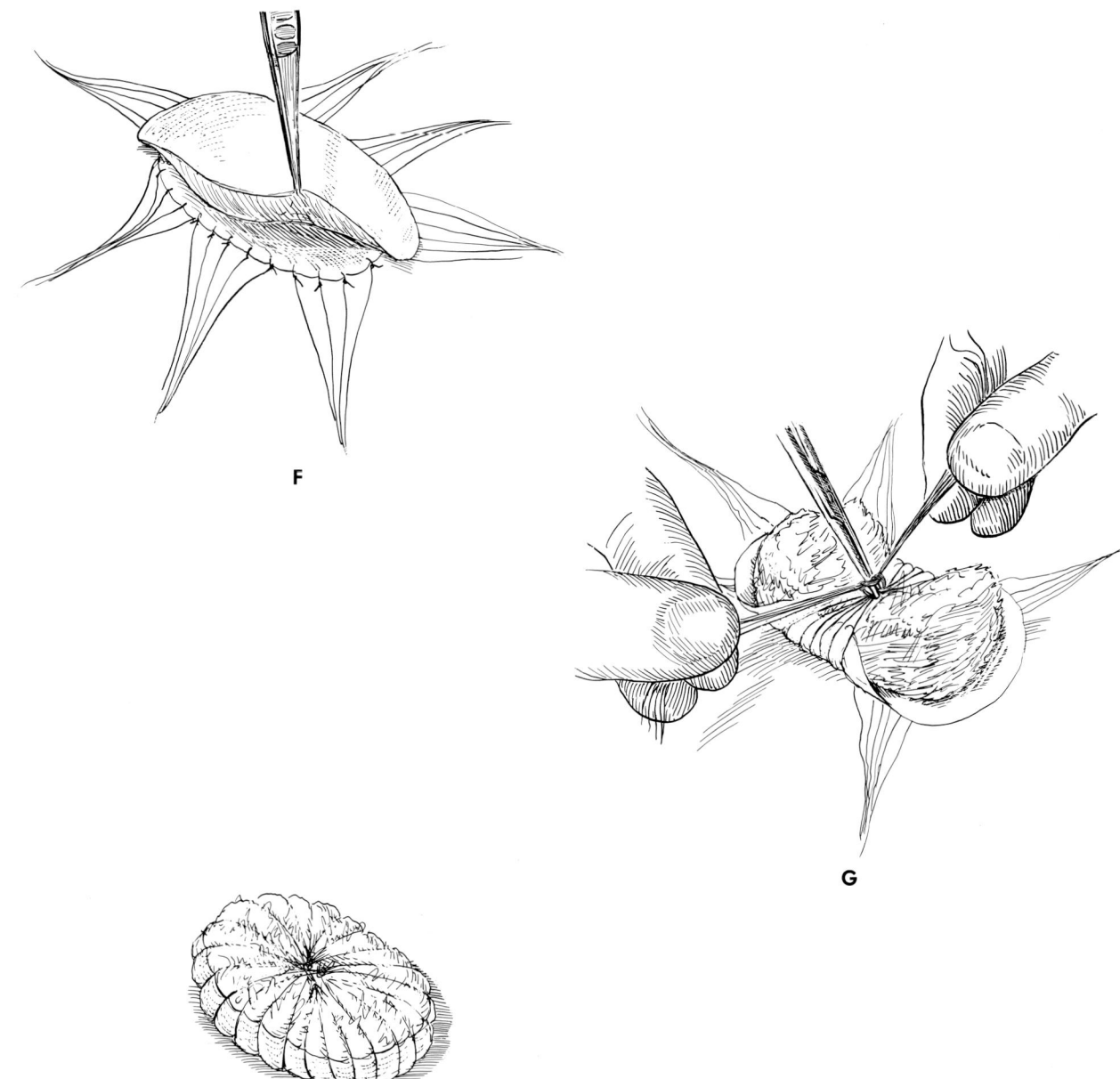

8
Infections

Paronychia

Infection around the nail bed occurs because the area is frequently subject to injury which creates a portal of entry for bacteria and also because the nail juncture with soft tissues is a weak area of defense against local invasive infection. The initiating cause may be hangnails, ingrowing nails, manicure trauma, unclean subungual areas, steel-wool slivers, or other foreign bodies. Once the paronychia is established, the cornified nail acts as an intrinsic foreign body perpetuating the infection. Staphylococcus is usually the offending organism. Combined infection with staphylococcus and streptococcus is resistant to treatment and requires not only incision and drainage but appropriate antibiotics and intensive soaking.

Surgical drainage of the paronychial abscess is best performed through an incision proximal to the corner of the involved nail. (**A**)

If the abscess extends around the nail base or lateral margin, the base or margin should be excised to assure adequate drainage and removal of nonviable nail which serves as a foreign body. (**B**) The fingernail will regenerate from the nail bed.

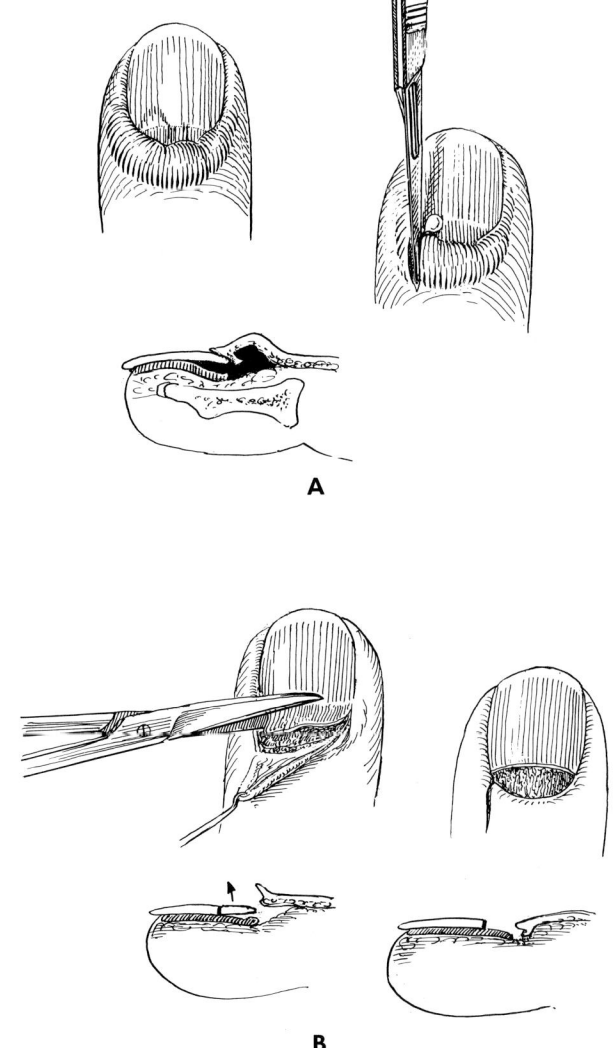

Felon

Infection which involves the pulp of a finger tip is called a felon.

The fibrous tissue septa in the finger pulp lends it stability and tethers the skin to the distal phalanx to limit skin slippage and mobility.

When infection occurs in the soft tissues where swelling is limited by the fascial septa entrapment, an increasing pressure develops with the inflammatory response. This is particularly painful in the finger tip because of the high concentration of sensory receptors there. Evidence of infection coupled with pain is a clear indication for incision and drainage of a felon. If the felon is left without decompression, deep soft tissue necrosis develops and osteomyelitis of the distal phalanx is almost inevitable. The infection follows the course of least resistance and may progress to the flexor synovial sheath to initiate serious hand space infection. All of this may occur without spontaneous drainage to the finger surface.

The surgeon's role is clear. He must provide external drainage before deep necrosis and progressive infection start. Incision and drainage should be performed through an incision which will not leave a scar on the working surface of the fingertip. (**C**) An incision on the ulnar side of the tip of the index, long, or ring finger is appropriate. Incision on the radial side of the little finger is best. Choice of side on the thumb may depend on the individual's use of his thumb in his occupation. The incision may be extended beneath the free nail edge across the tip to obtain wide-open drainage and debridement in more advanced infections.

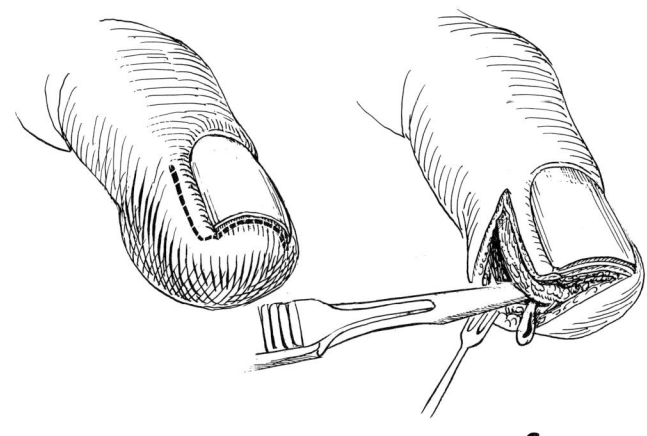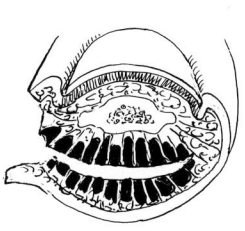

C

8 — Infections

Synovial and Space Infections

A knowledge of the classical anatomy of the synovial sheaths and potential anatomical spaces in the hand is essential for proper diagnosis and treatment of serious hand infections. (**D**)

The flexor tendons are shrouded in synovial sheaths, particularly where there is flexion mobility in the longitudinal arch of each ray and at the wrist. The synovial sheath of the flexor pollicis longus generally extends from the flexor insertion to a point proximal to the wrist flexor retinaculum. The same is true of the synovial sheath around the little finger flexors, but as the little finger sheath approaches the proximal palm just distal to the carpal tunnel, it expands to encompass the flexors of the ring, long, and index fingers. At this point it is referred to as the ulnar bursa. Each index, long, and ring finger has a flexor synovial sheath from the point of insertion of the profundus tendon to the level of the distal palmar crease in the palm. The deep space beneath the flexor tendons is divided into two compartments by the heavy vertical septum from the palmar fascia to the third metacarpal. Ulnar to the septum is the midpalmar space, and radial to it lies the thenar space. The thenar space straddles the adductor pollicis muscle like two legs extending between the adductor and deep flexors on the palmar side and between the adductor and the first dorsal interosseous on the dorsal side.

Infections starting in the digital synovial sheaths may extend to the deep palmar spaces.

Infections in the digital synovial sheath should be diagnosed when signs of infection occur, such as pain, redness, and fever. The digit is held in a flexed posture. Pain is elicited on passive gentle extension. Such an infection may be obvious if the patient has a paronychia or felon or other identifiable source of contamination.

Synovial sheath infections should be treated promptly by decompression, incision, and drainage along the mid-lateral surface of the digit. Appropriate antibiotics should be prescribed after material is obtained from the digit for smear and culture.

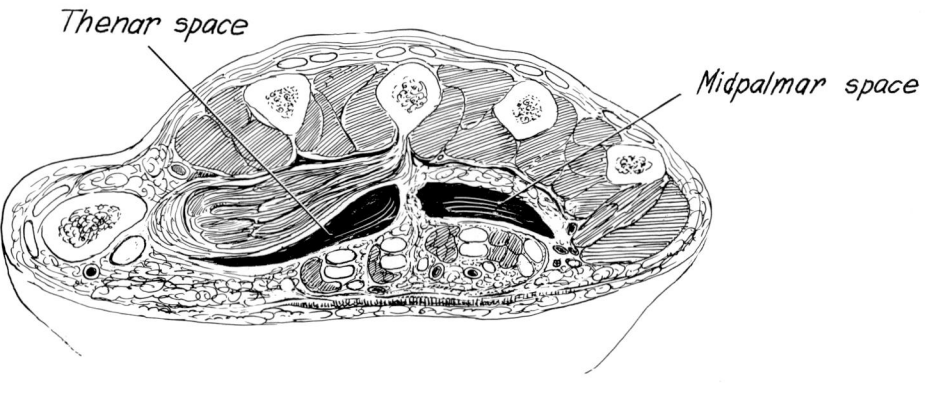

D

General Principles

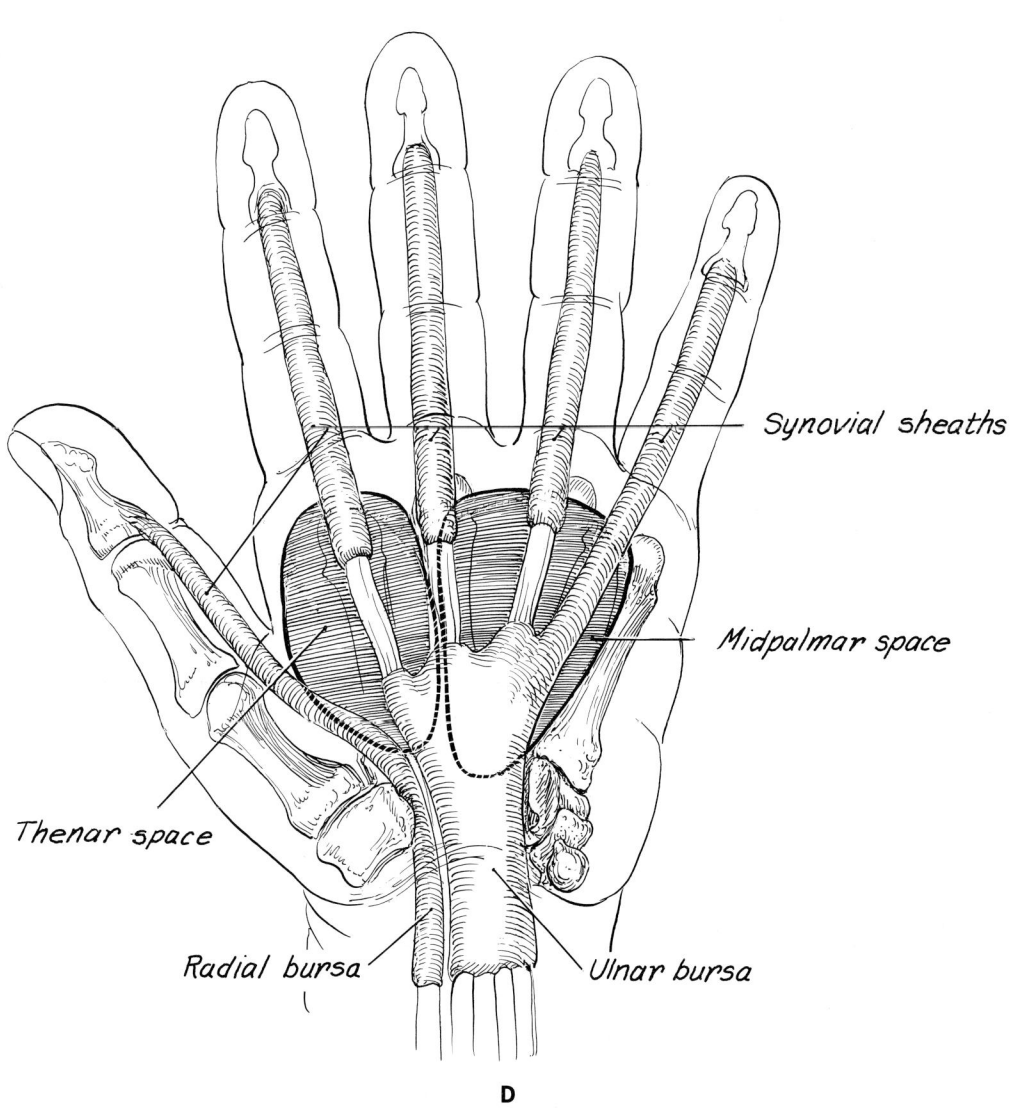

D

8 – Infections

Collar Button Abscess

A synovial sheath infection may, at its proximal end, extend to the palmar subcutaneous tissue. The infection may then course through the lumbrical canal to dorsal soft tissues. (**E**)

Superficial infections starting in the distal palm at sites of trauma, calluses, and cracking also frequently penetrate through the palmar fascial openings and point dorsally in the intermetacarpal spaces. (**F**) A double abscess develops—one palmar and one dorsal—with a narrow connnecting neck. Proper drainage of such a "collar button" abscess is only achieved by incision and drainage, both on the dorsum and in the palm. Generally, a short transverse palmar incision and a longitudinal intermetacarpal dorsal incision will adequately drain this commonly occurring infection. (**G**)

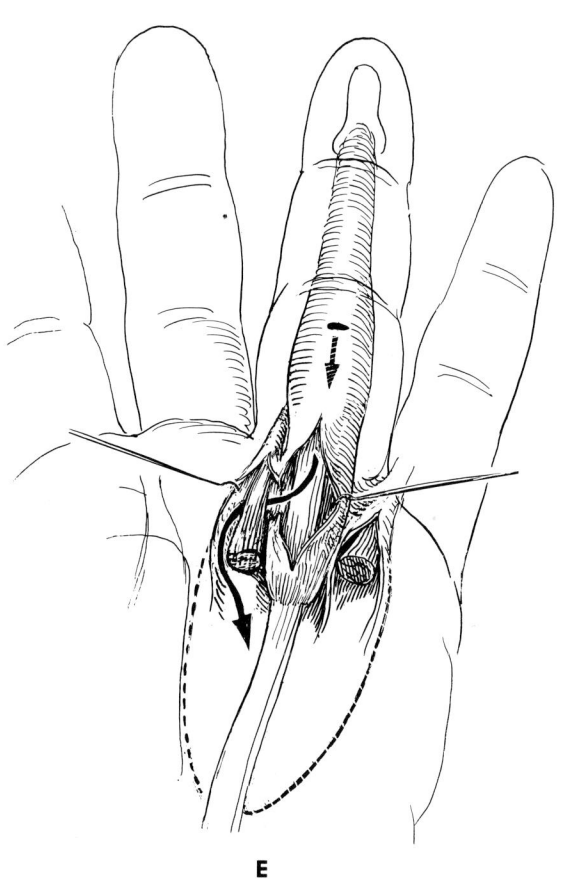

E

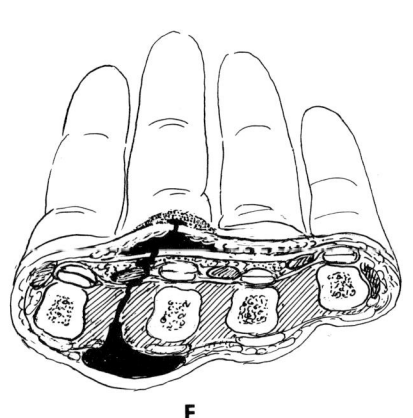

F

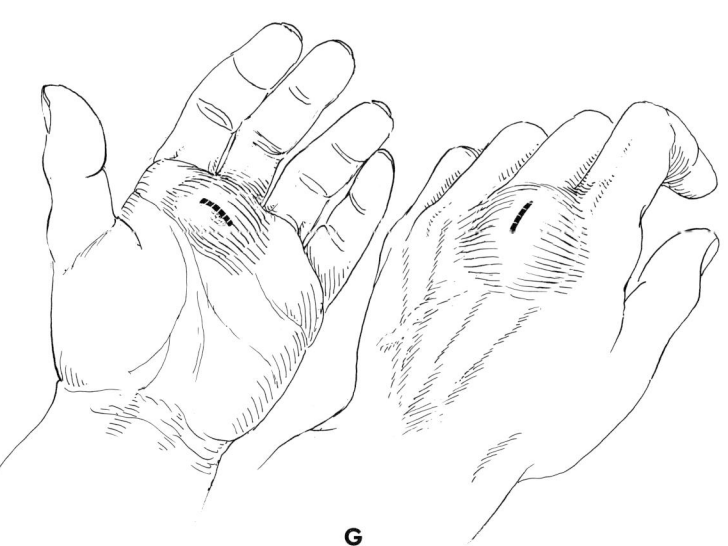

G

Fingertip Injuries

9
Minor Soft Tissue Loss

Principle

When skin and soft tissue alone are lost in fingertip injuries, one may restore the finger without loss of length using a free skin graft. If the defect is large enough so that wound contraction will not easily restore full-thickness skin coverage, then a thick split thickness (0.018 to 0.020 inch) or a full thickness free graft may be used. The split graft leaves dermis and skin appendages at the donor site and healing of the site will occur by re-epithelialization. Full thickness removal requires surgical closure of the donor site.

When a fingertip injury is sustained which leaves a relatively small defect limited to soft tissues, wound contraction will result in closure with good full thickness coverage and intact sensibility. Such wound contraction takes many weeks during which the patient suffers all of the problems incidental to having an open wound.

One may achieve wound closure and still not stall the desirable contraction of the wound if a thin (0.008 to 0.010 inch) split thickness skin graft is used to cover the wound.

Example

A young male kitchen worker sustained an amputation of his left long finger tip from a broken glass. (**A**) There was loss of soft tissue only, and it appeared that the palm soft tissue could cover the tip if it were allowed to heal by wound contraction. In this case it was desirable not to carry out any additional dissection to mobilize the palm flap but it was important to achieve wound closure.

A free skin graft was taken as thin as possible with a free-hand blade. (**B**)

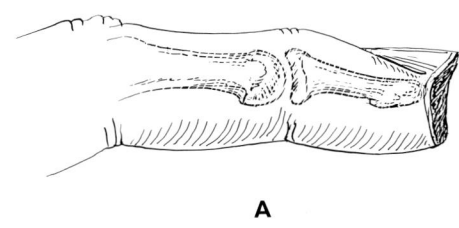

A

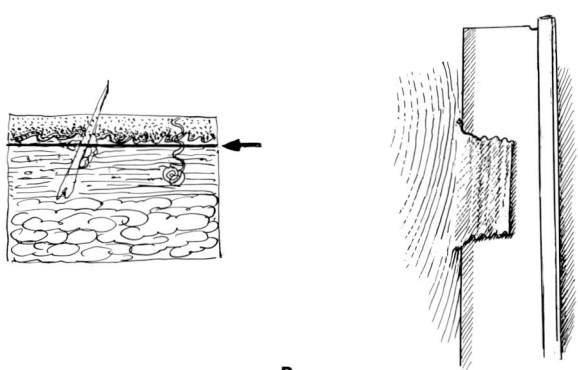

B

9 — Minor Soft Tissue Loss

The thin bit of skin was draped over the raw fingertip. (**C**)

A non-adherent gauze cut to the size of the defect was applied. (**D**)

The uninjured part of the finger was painted with Ace adherent. (**E**)

A bulky gauze dressing was applied and fixed securely in place. (**F**)

There was no need to change the dressing for 10 days at which time the wound was healed. In the weeks that followed, the inadequate coverage furnished by the thin graft was replaced by advancing full thickness skin and soft tissue from wound contraction.

Six months after injury, the graft occupied a very small area beneath the protective nail. (**G**)

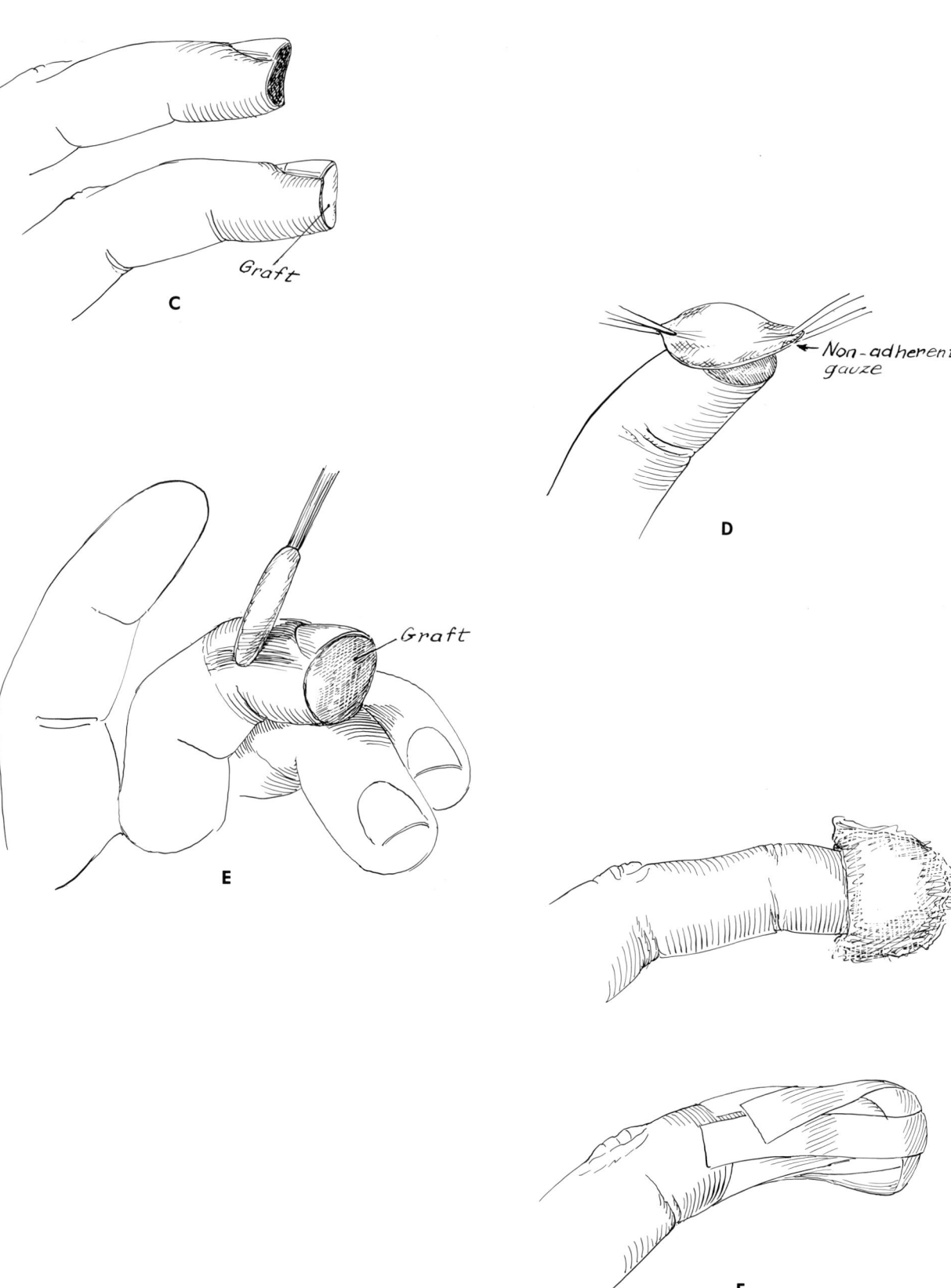

Fingertip Injuries

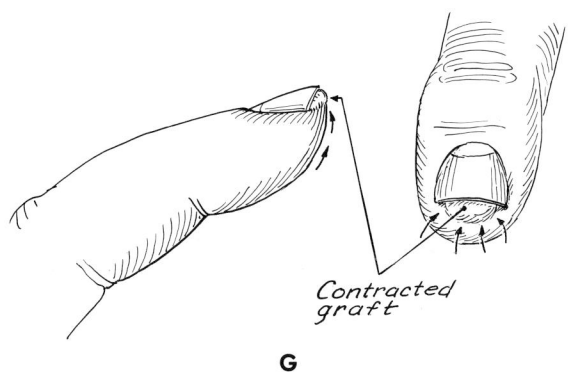

G

INJURY THIN SKIN GRAFT

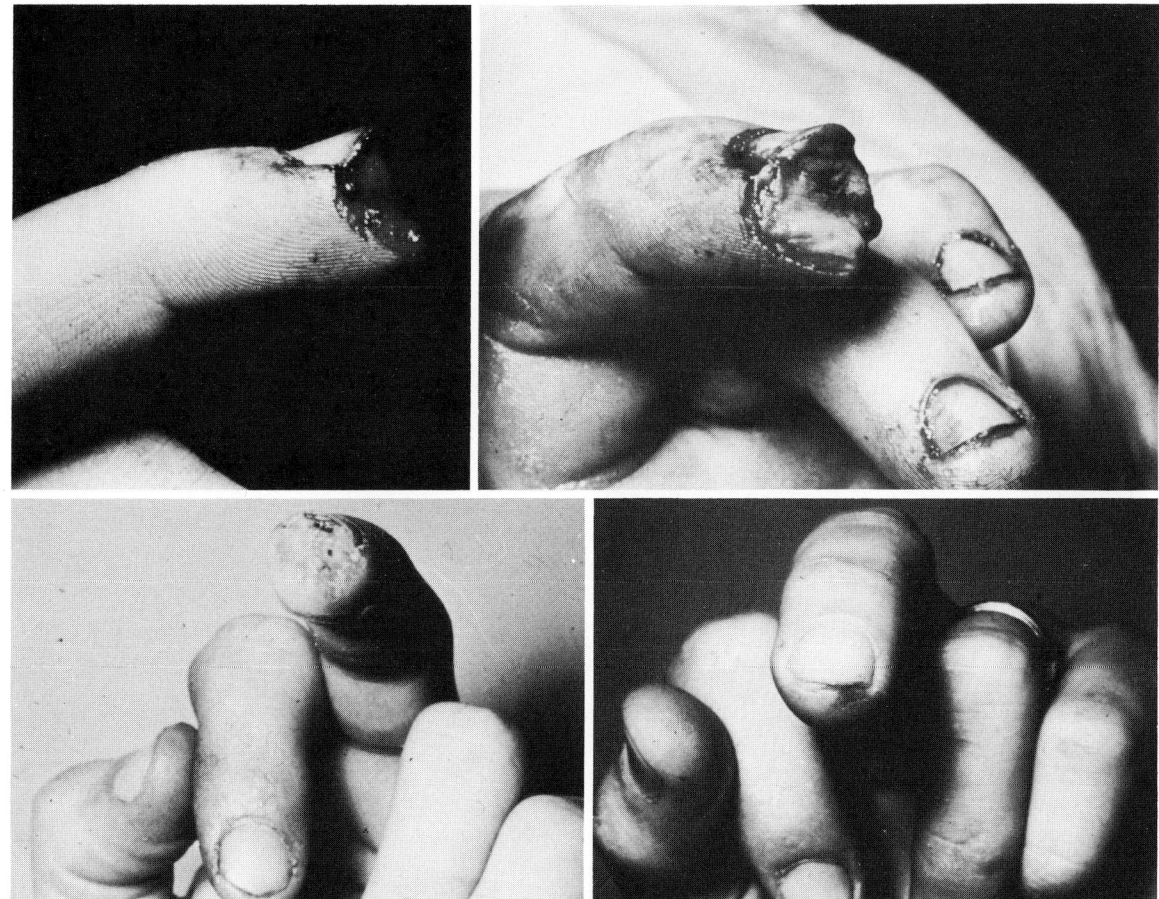

10 DAYS 6 MONTHS

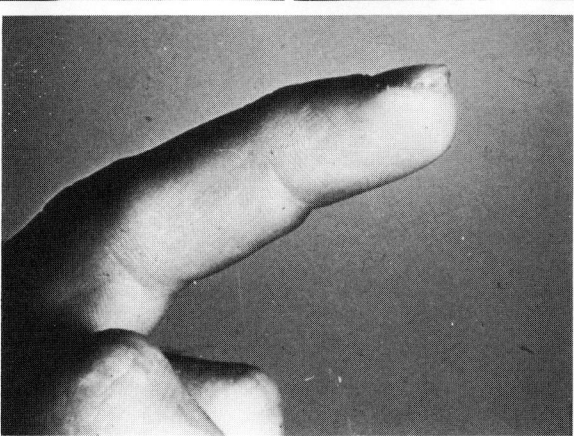

RESULT

10

Extensive Soft Tissue Loss

Principle

When the fingertip skin loss is extensive enough that wound contraction would not result in restoration of full thickness coverage, a free graft of full thickness or thick split thickness (0.020 inch) skin is most appropriate.

Example

A fruit merchant caught his left long finger tip on the tailgate of a pickup truck as it drove away. He sustained an avulsion amputation of the skin of the entire pulp of the finger. The loss was too extensive to expect that contraction of the wound would result in full adequate skin and soft tissue restoration. There was no exposed bone. (**A**)

Since fingertip loss was extensive enough that wound contraction would not result in restoration of full-thickness coverage, a free graft of thick split-thickness (0.020 inch) skin was considered most appropriate. (A full-thickness free graft is an excellent alternative.) (**B**)

Such restoration may be adequate as permanent coverage for a digit of secondary importance but where subcutaneous pulp to restore contour and padding is essential a vascularized flap must be used.

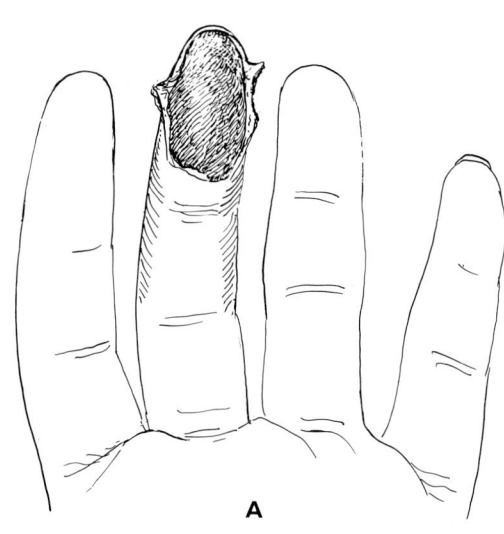

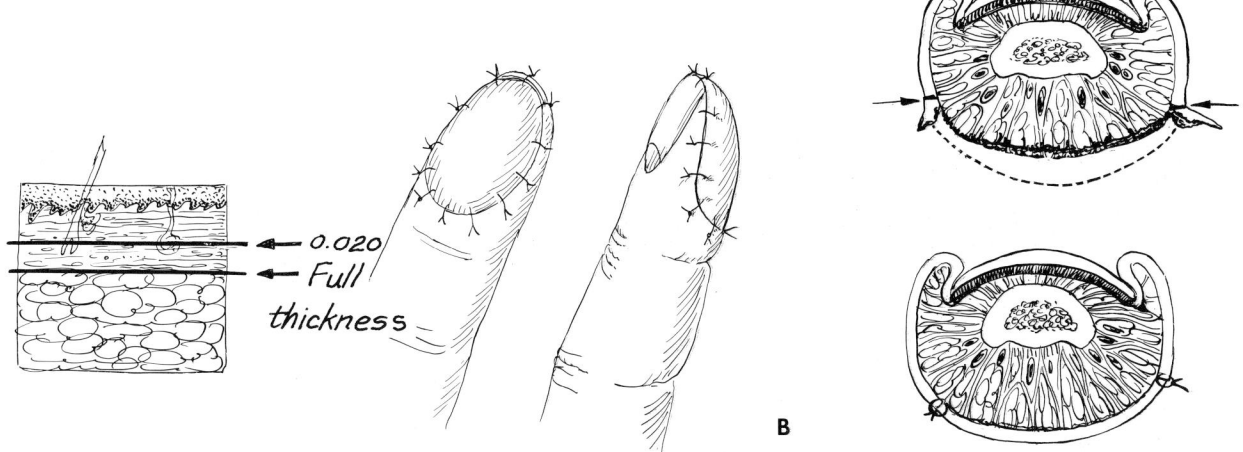

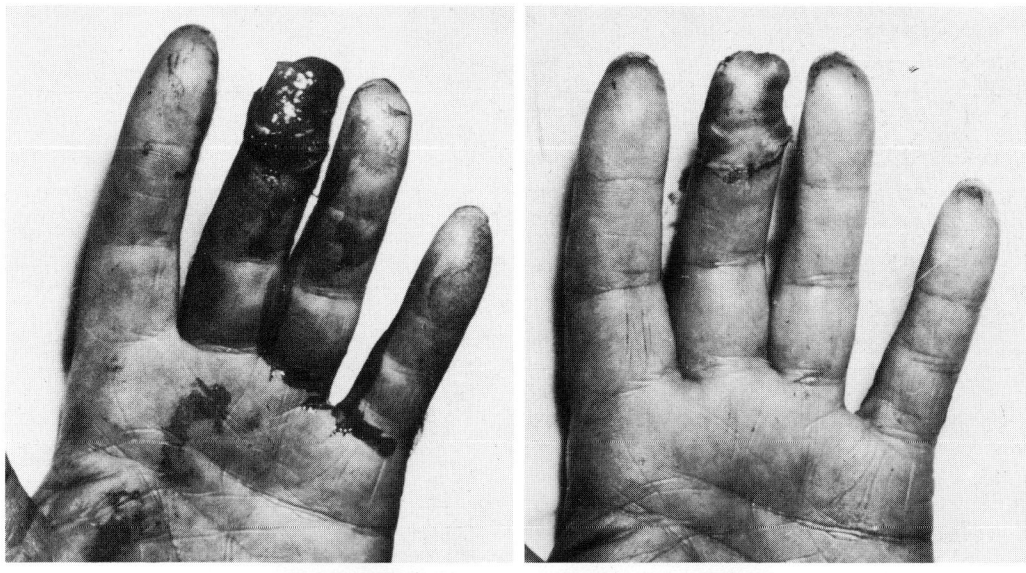

INJURY | THICK SPLIT GRAFT

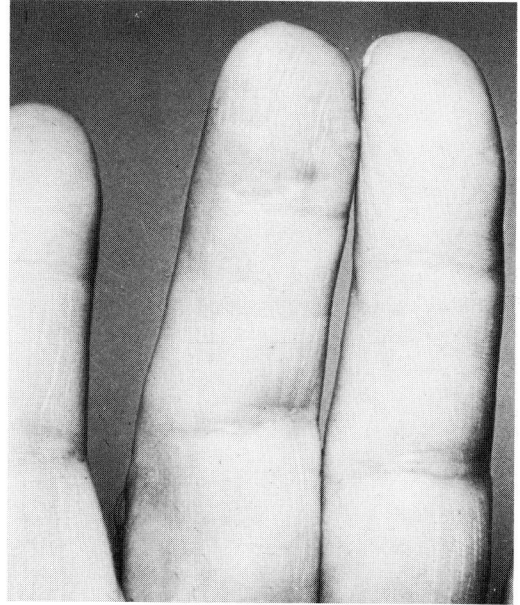

RESULT

11 Replantation of Fingertip After Amputation

Principle

There is a strong temptation to replace a totally avulsed fingertip. After such replacement, however, the incidence of failure is very high in adults and the harm that may come from the attempt makes it better judgment not to try. An exception should be made for children since the incidence of successful survival of a replanted composite fingertip graft is high enough to warrant the minimum risk.

The basis for failure after replantation of a free composite fingertip is that circulation cannot be restored soon enough to assure survival of the composite parts. Less obvious is the basis for failure of replantation of the tip skin alone after the bone, nail bed, and fat have been removed from the graft. The character of fingertip skin accounts for failure of such a graft to survive.

Observe fingertip skin once all fat and other tissue are removed from its deep surface. It spontaneously reassumes the shape of the fingertip as the dome of a derby hat assumes its contour again and again. (**A**) The thick cornified layer of the surface epithelium and the anatomical riblike ridging give it this characteristic.

If one peels the ridged cornified rind from the external surface of the fingertip graft, it becomes limp and pliable and it may survive. (**C**)

If the fingertip skin is replanted without peeling the external layer, the dermal surface will not adjust and settle into the small wound irregularities to acquire plasmatic nutrition and new blood supply. The resulting dead space regularly results in nonsurvival of the graft.

When non-survival is the result the graft becomes an adherent slough and sets the stage for infection, delayed healing and protracted disability.

All too often the patient may have unnecessary periods of absence from his occupation only to end up with a result far worse than if replantation had not been attempted. Worse still, the complications which may arise can result in loss of a part or all of the finger.

Example

A salesman demonstrating farm machinery lost the tip of his long finger by catching it in a moving belt. Replacement of the tip was attempted but the replanted tip did not survive. (**B**)

In this case example the finger healed by secondary intention. The soft tissue coverage of the tip was inadequate, unstable and the tip was tender. (For secondary correction see Section 16.)

Fingertip Injuries

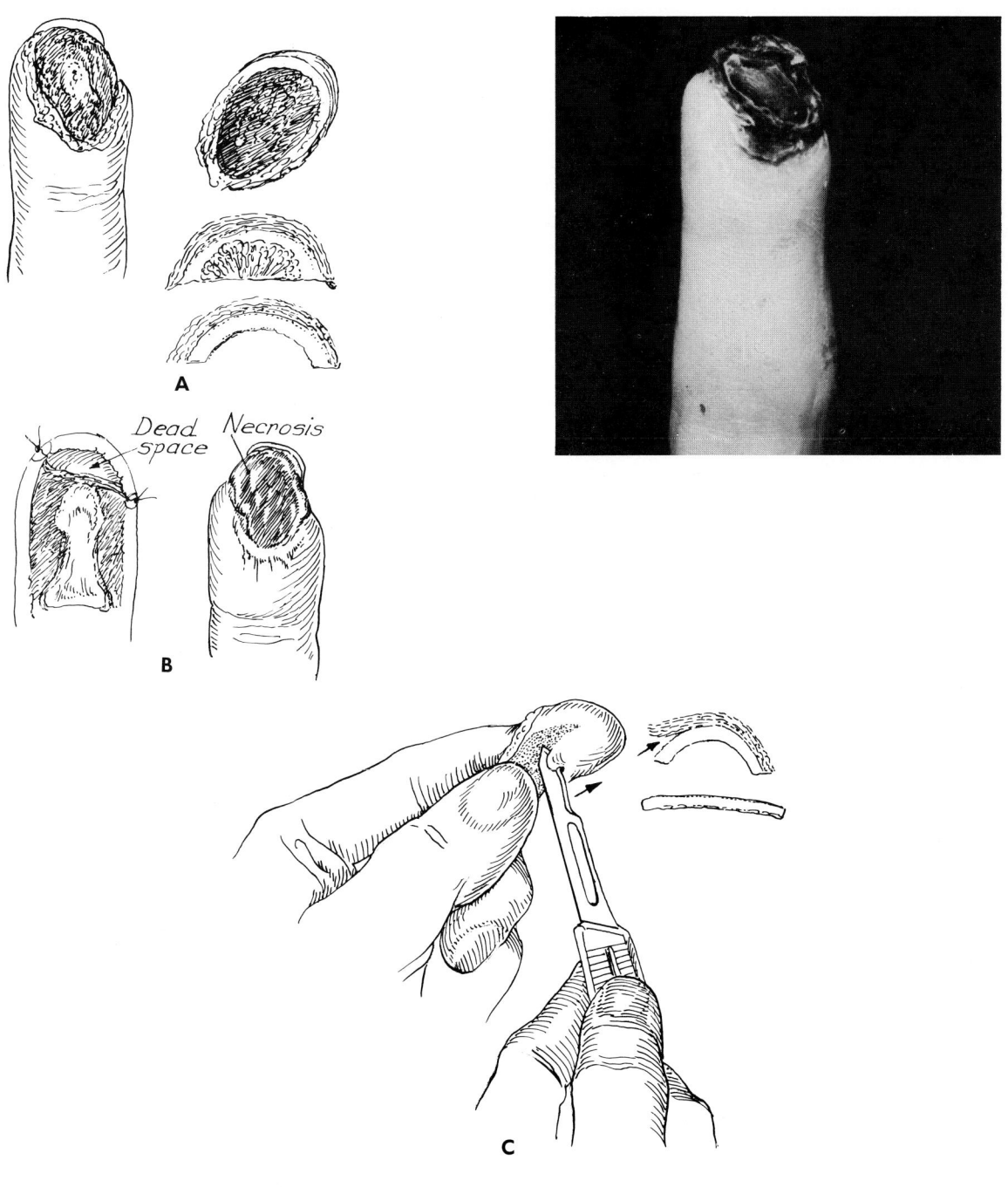

12

Fingernail Injuries

Principle

Treatment of avulsion and crush injuries of the fingernail requires careful reduction and immobilization of disrupted and displaced nail elements. The offset separation in a nail bed may be treated like a skin laceration after the nail is completely removed. (**A**)

Coaptation of nail bed wound edges with fine absorbable sutures or monofilament nylon will help to avoid late deformity of the nail when it regrows. (**B**)

Coincidental loss of dorsal skin proximal to the nail may be overcome by undermining and advancement of the dorsal skin. (**C**)

If the deficit is too large, a free skin graft may be required.

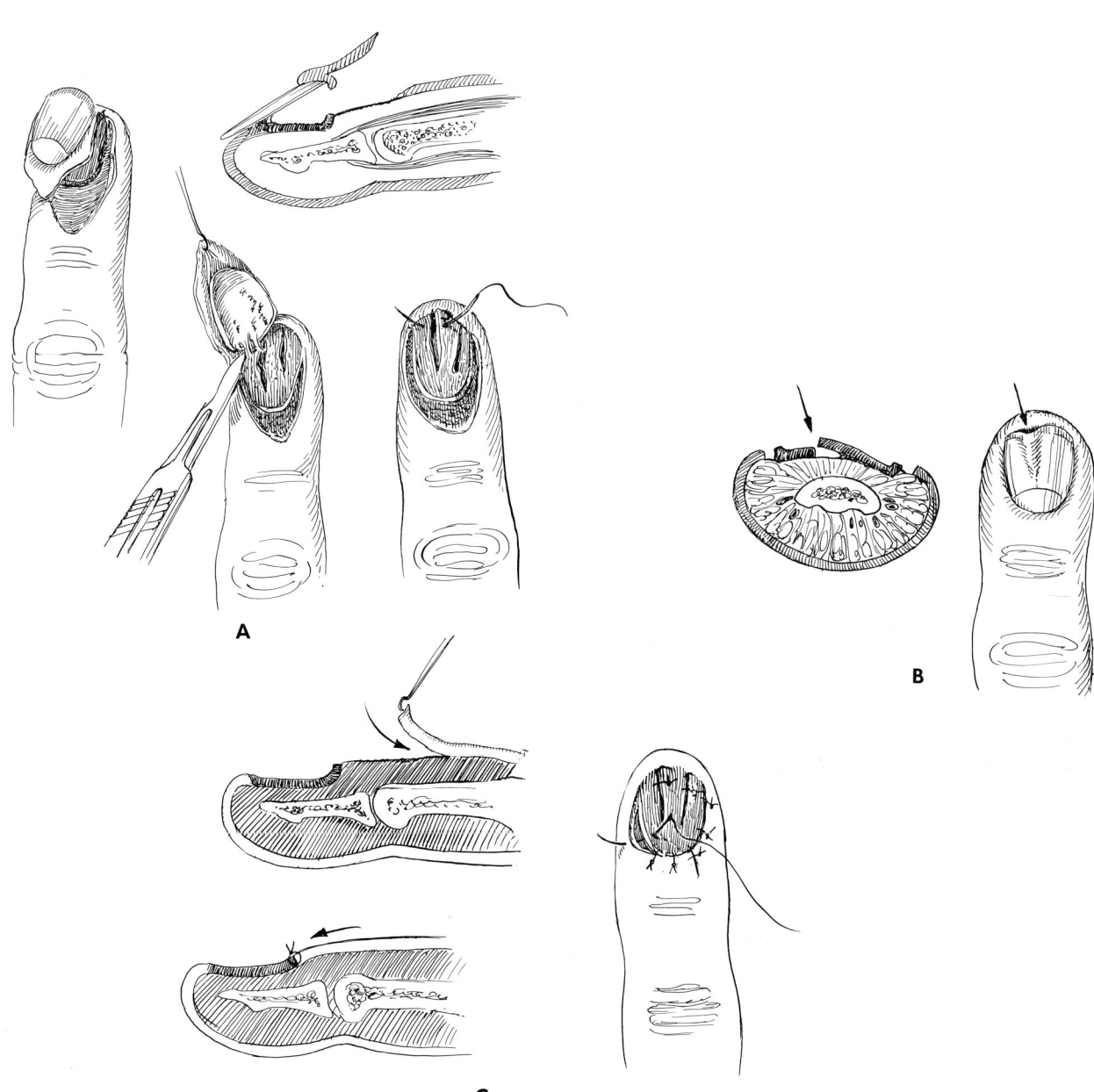

13

Cross-Finger Flap

Principle

Loss of digital pulp from a digit of prime importance to the patient requires replacement of the skin, the underlying subcutaneous tissue, and the potential for precise sensibility. A free graft is inadequate for good restoration of contour with a cushion of soft tissue.

Skin and subcutaneous tissue losses which result in loss of proper padding and contour, particularly on the thumb or prime fingers, should be replaced by vascularized pedicle flaps. When possible, such soft tissue replacements should either bring nerve supply (sensibility) with them or they should consist of skin and subcutaneous tissue most likely to regain good sensibility after regeneration of recipient bed nerves. Shifted skin and subcutaneous tissue never regains two-point discrimination superior to that in the donor area. Since the hand has highly developed sensibility, skin and soft tissue obtained from the hand is superior to skin from the trunk or elsewhere. Specialized sensory end organs carried from the donor finger are later spontaneously reinnervated to restore digital sensibility to a level of discrimination nearly equal to that which existed in the donor site.

Additional advantages of local pedicle flaps from the injured hand itself are not only that the soft tissues have proper characteristics but also that there is no need for attachment and immobilization of the hand to another area of the body. Adjacent pedicle flaps, interpolated pedicle flaps, cross-finger pedicle flaps, and island pedicle flaps all have a place in supplying necessary padding, sensibility and sudomotor function.

The necessity of immobilizing the arm by attachment of the finger to the trunk or contralateral extremity is avoided by use of a local pedicle flap. One local pedicle which is uncomplicated, useful and reliable is the cross-finger pedicle flap.

Example

An 18-year-old college girl sustained amputation loss of the pulp and a bit of the distal phalanx of her left index finger when a heavy door closed on the finger. A skin graft was applied and uncomplicated healing occurred. Loss of pulp contour and an inadequate functional pad on this important finger prompted the use of a cross-finger pedicle flap from the long finger. The procedure might properly have been done at the time of the original injury except that the long finger also was crushed and use of it as a donor finger was contraindicated. The defect in the index finger was re-created by excising the skin graft and releasing all scar contracture.

A precise pattern to fit the defect was cut from a piece of gauze material. The side which fitted against the donor finger was left long to represent the pedicle base. (**A**)

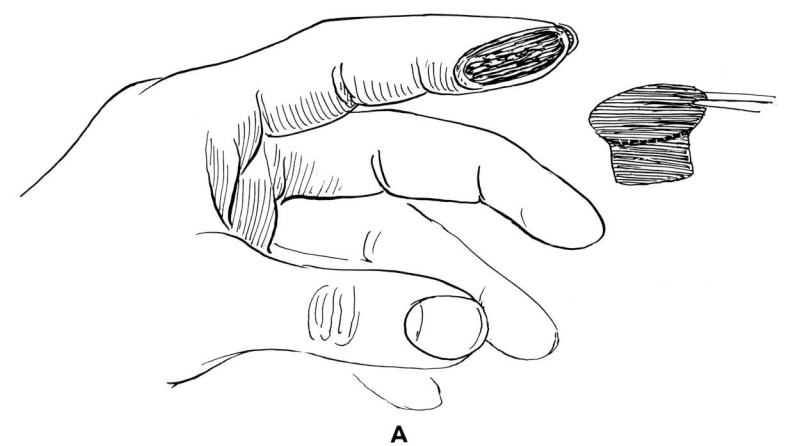

A

13 — Cross-Finger Flap

With the recipient finger positioned comfortably against the donor finger, the pattern was adjusted and it was then held by the pedicle portion against the donor finger. (**B**)

As the recipient finger was withdrawn, the pattern fell against the donor finger, showing the surgeon exactly the site from which the flap should be surgically elevated. (**C**) The skin was marked with methylene blue in preparation for raising the skin and subcutaneous tissue flap.

The flap was elevated by incising the sides of the flap, leaving the base pedicle intact. (**D**) The dissection of the flap from the donor finger was made in the areolar plane just superficial to the extensor tendons. Mobility was not complete until the ligamentous fibers from the skin at mid-lateral plane of the finger to the phalanx were cut (ligaments of Clelland).

The pedicle was based palmar since it is preferable, though not essential, that the base of the pedicle be toward the digital neurovascular bundle (proper digital nerve and artery). (**E**)

The donor site for the flap was immediately covered with a free full thickness skin graft (a split thickness graft would do). The fingers were fixed to one another with adhesive tape to avoid tension on the pedicle.

Within three weeks after application of the flap to the recipient finger healing was adequate so that the carrying pedicle was transected. (**F**) The pedicle was transected in such a way that it would supply just enough tissue on the recipient finger to fill the original defect. The neurovascular bundle was carefully preserved on the donor finger.

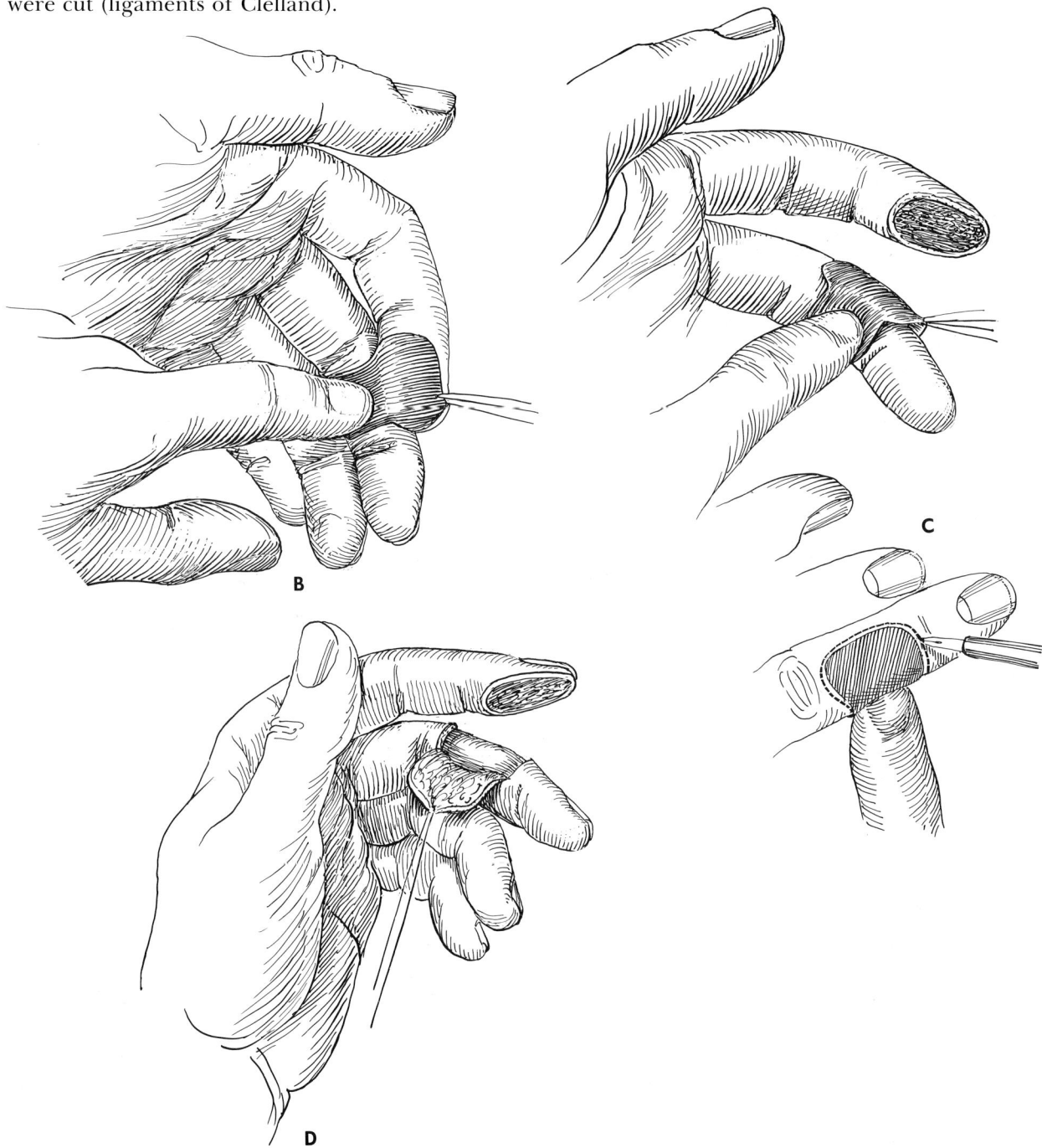

Fingertip Injuries

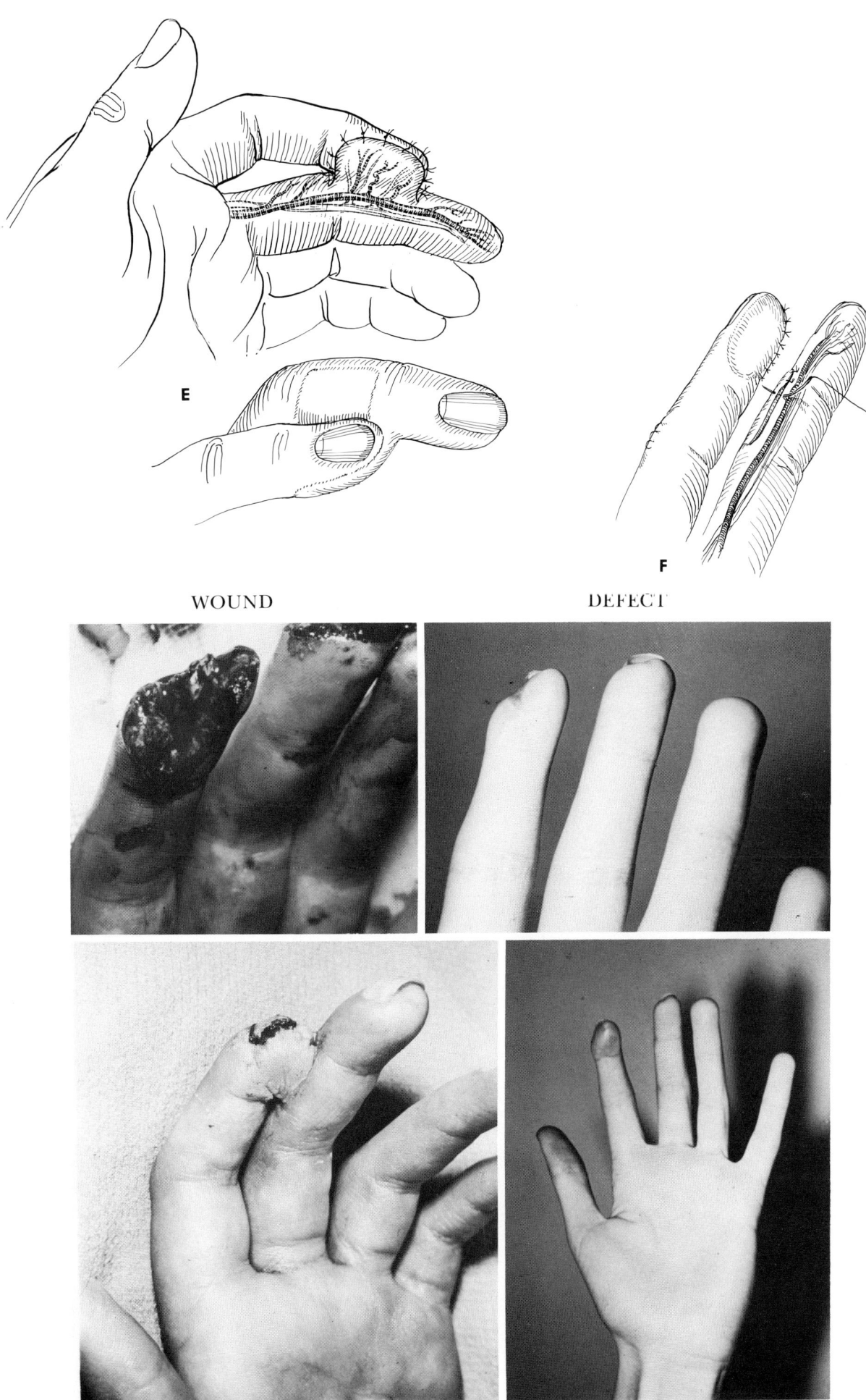

WOUND DEFECT

CROSS-FINGER FLAP RESULT

73

14

Finger to Thumb Pedicle Flap

Principle

Thumb tip injuries with loss of pulp should be treated by immediate reconstruction to restore proper protective cushioning and contour and the potential for perceptive sensibility. Such a defect requires reconstruction with vascularized composite tissues. Local skin and subcutaneous tissues from the hand carried on a nutrient pedicle best serve the purpose. A finger-to-thumb pedicle is one efficient method of repair. It avoids the need to immobilize the hand and arm as is the case with a distant pedicle flap.

Example

A 40-year-old butcher sustained a meat slicer amputation of his right thumb pulp. (**A**) The distal phalanx tuft was exposed but was intact. No other injuries occurred. Decision to restore proper skin and soft tissue contour by primary treatment with a cross finger flap was made.

A pattern of the defect was fashioned from fabric (any pliable material available in the operating set-up may be used). (**B**) The predicted carrying pedicle was left long.

The pattern was placed over the thumb defect with the thumb against the long finger. (**C**)

The index finger was *not* used so as to avoid a scar on its radial side. (The whole hand is protected by skin sensibility on the radial side of the index finger. The working side of this capital finger should not electively be violated when other, more desirable alternatives exist.)

With the base of the pattern held against the donor finger, the thumb was moved aside, allowing the pattern to fall in place on the side of the donor finger. (**D**)

The pattern was traced with a skin marker to outline precisely the flap necessary to fill the thumb defect. (**E**)

The flap was surgically elevated in the areolar plane over the extensor tendons by blunt and sharp dissection avoiding injury to the extensor tendons and neurovascular bundle. (**F**)

A free full thickness skin graft was used to cover the flap donor site. (**G**)

The flap was carefully sutured to the thumb pulp defect. Sutures of monofilament nylon were placed through the thumb nail and bed to

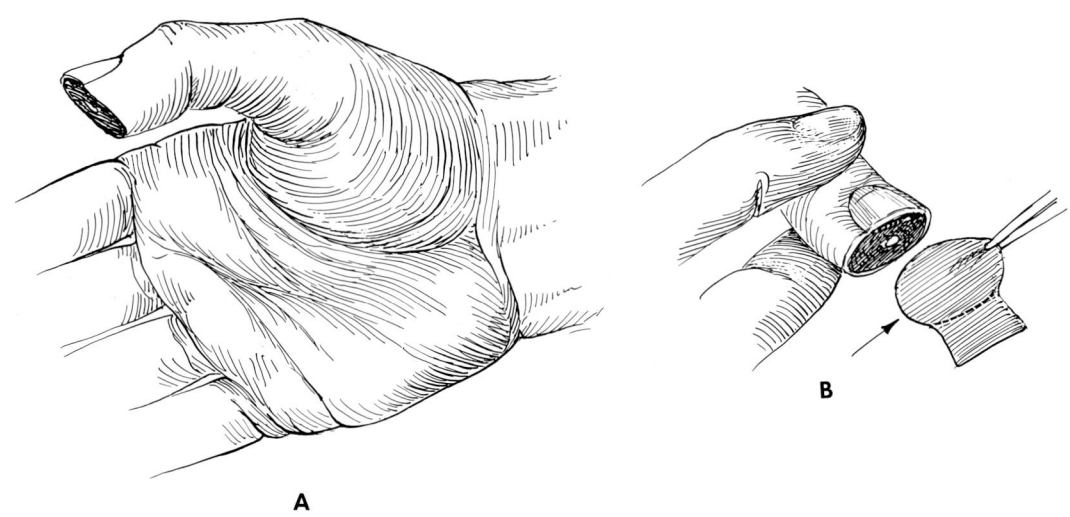

Fingertip Injuries

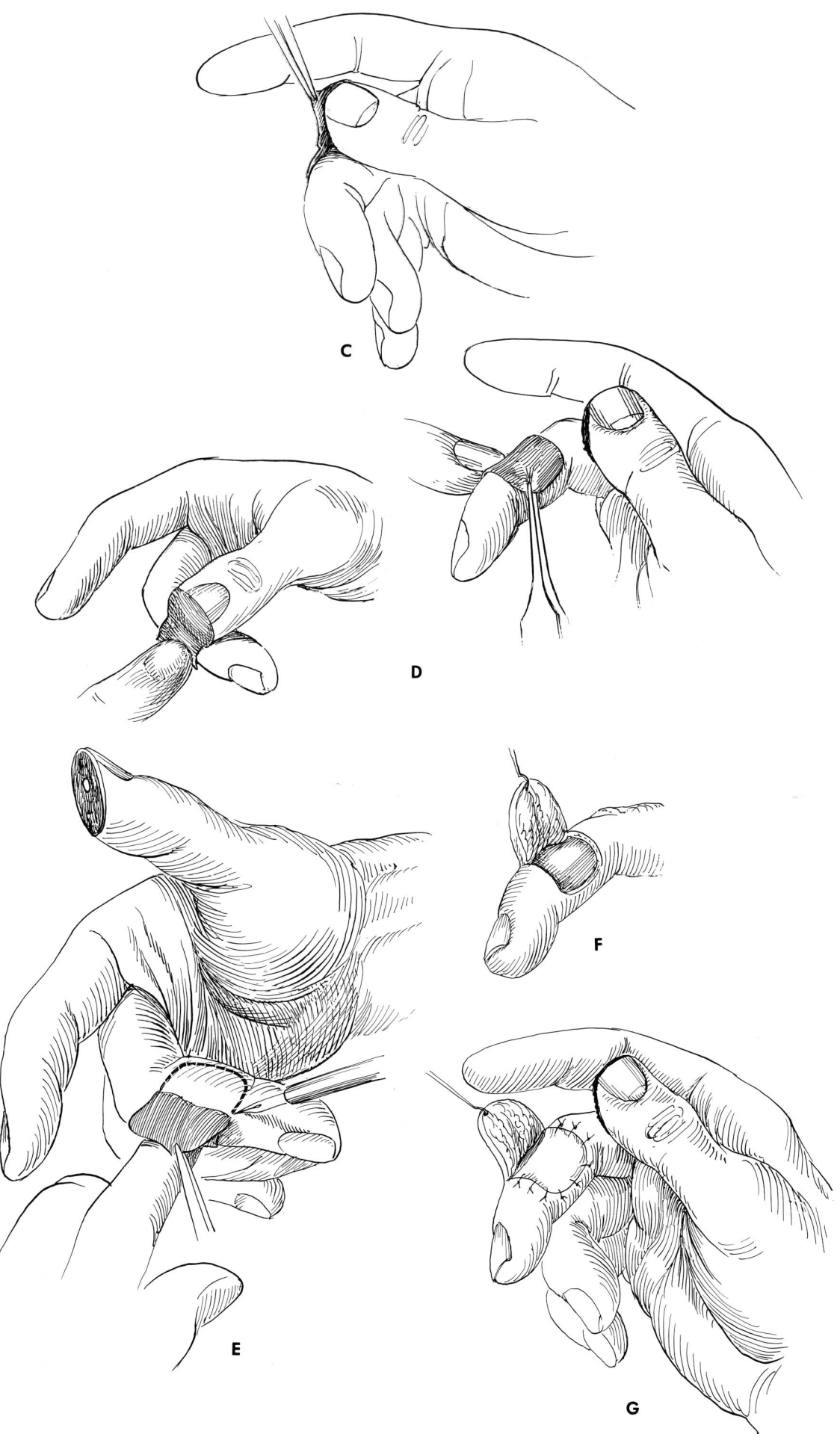

75

14 — Finger to Thumb Pedicle Flap

achieve secure closure at the junction of the nail defect and flap. (**H**)

A small, fitted, fluffed gauze pad over non-adherent gauze was placed between the thumb and the grafted donor site. (**I**)

Immobilization and fixation of the thumb to the donor finger was achieved with adhesive tape applied to the skin which was painted with tincture of benzoin. (**J**)

Ten days after surgical application of the flap, the skin sutures were removed. Twenty days after surgery the carrying pedicle was sectioned, separating the digits. (**K**)

This technique restored good thumb tip padding and brought to the thumb tissues the potential for return of good sensibility.

Good sensibility did return over the six month period of follow up.

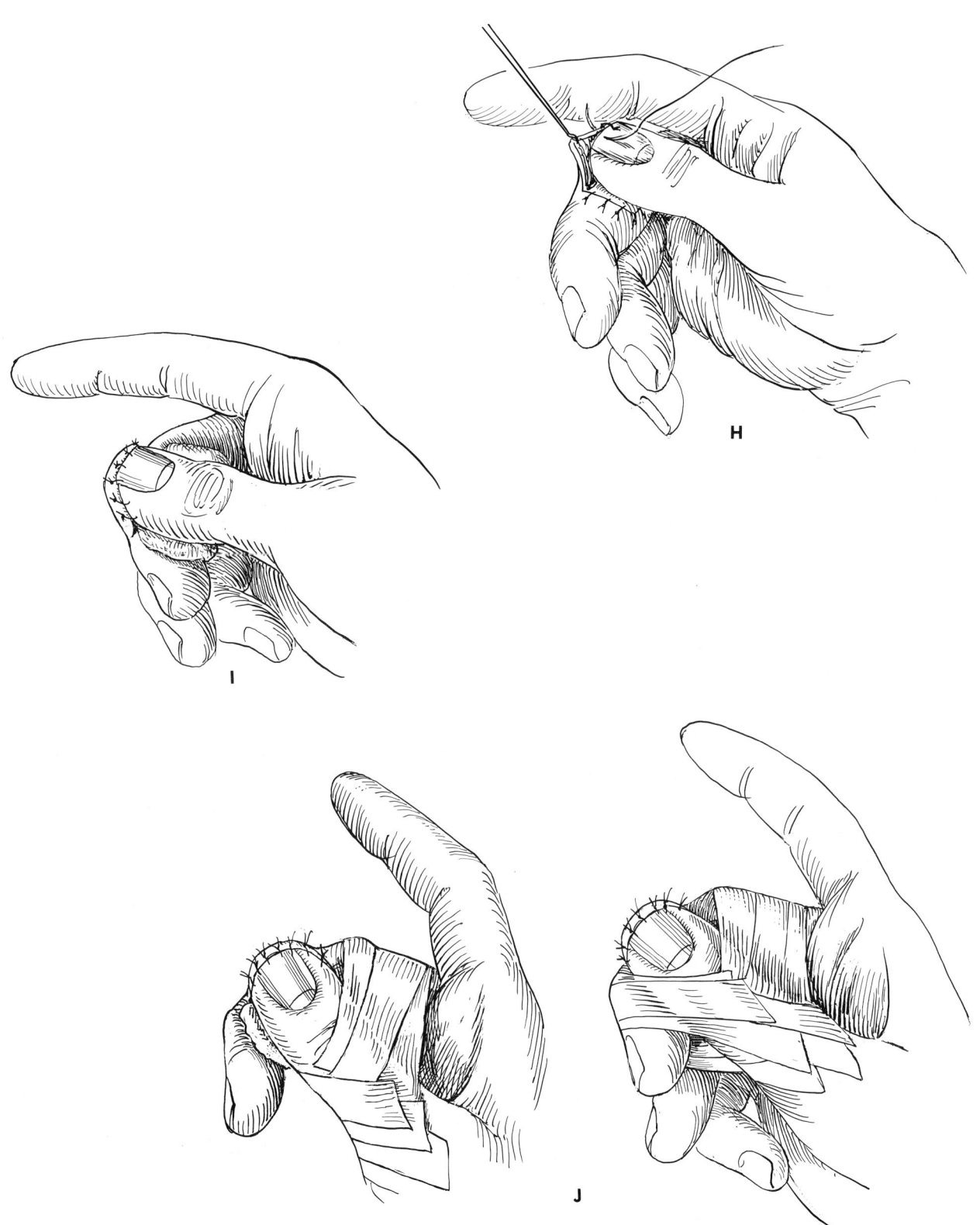

Fingertip Injuries

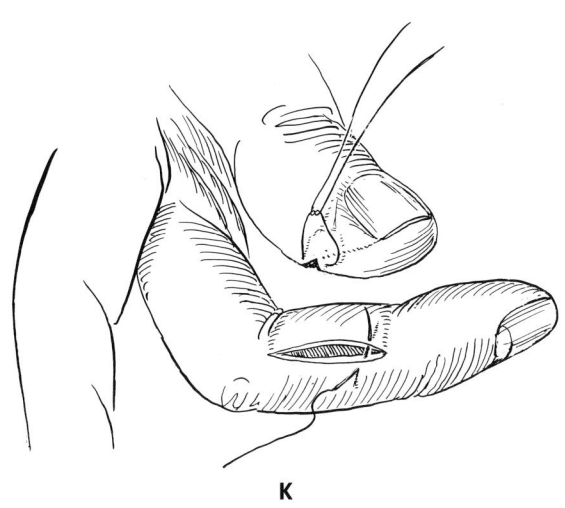

K

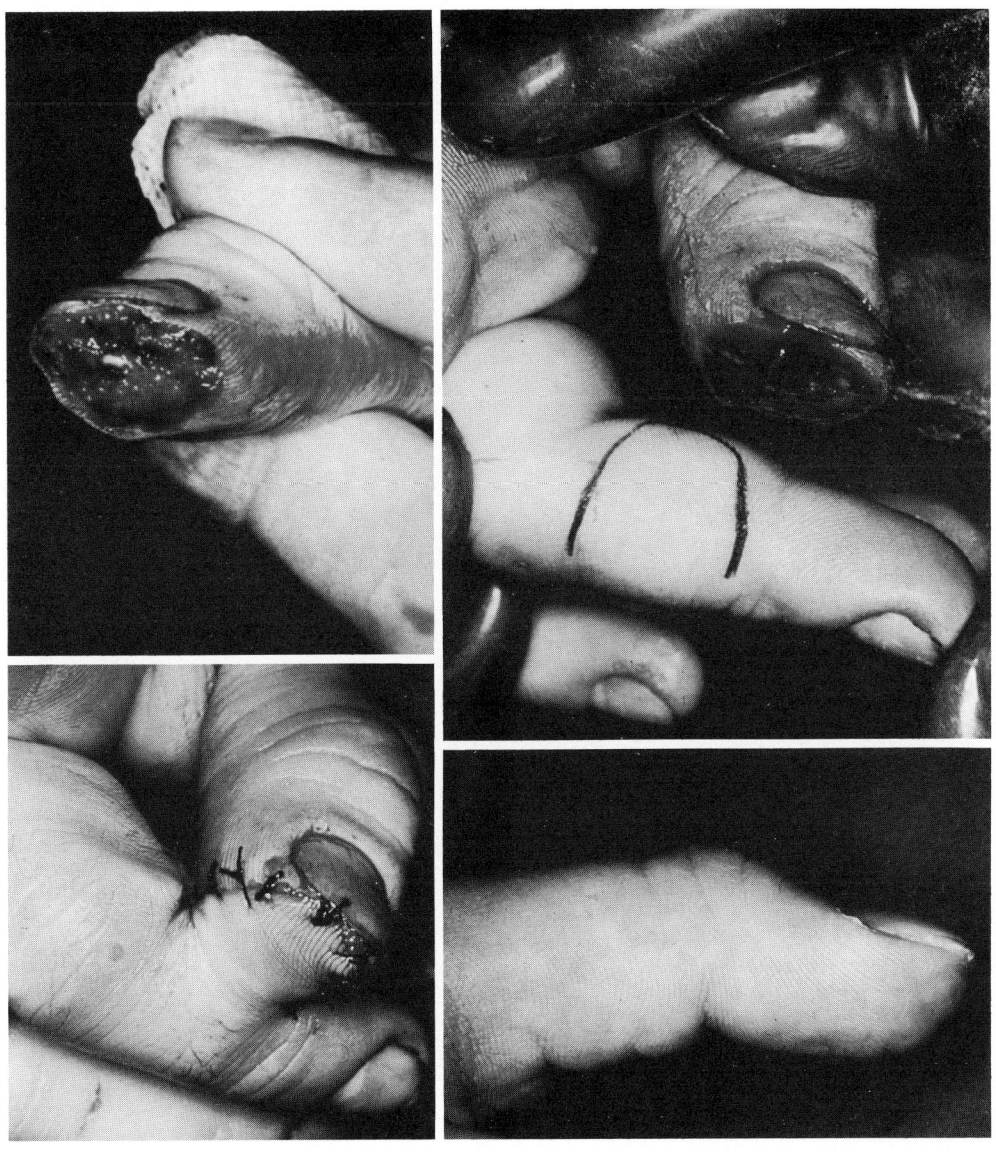

15
Island Pedicle Flap for Fingertip Loss

Principle

Reconstruction of the thumb tip and pulp with local composite tissues may be done in a single stage using a primary biological flap carried solely on its neurovascular bundle. This rather sophisticated procedure should be performed by surgeons accustomed to precision hand surgery.

The neurovascular anatomy with orientation of vessels radiating from the palmar arch lends itself well to island pedicle transfer. A flap of tissue well distal on one side of the donor finger and of appropriate size to fit the thumb defect may be transferred with permanently intact blood and nerve supply.

Example

A 38-year-old telephone lineman sustained a severe crush avulsion injury of his thumb tip. Initial treatment left the patient with an intact thumb tip having poor skin coverage and loss of sensibility. The pulp contour was lost and unstable epithelialized scar covered the palmar aspect of the distal phalanx.

The tip injury defect was re-created by excising the epithelium and scar over the thumb tip. (Had conditions been appropriate, a primary island pedicle flap could have been elected as appropriate management.)

An island pedicle flap donor site was outlined on the ulnar side of the long finger, and a curved incision was planned in the palm proximal to and continuous with a mid-lateral incision in the finger. The common digital vessels and nerves to the adjacent sides of the long finger and ring finger were exposed to make certain the anatomical arrangement was appropriate for neurovascular bundle transfer of the outlined island of skin and soft tissue. (**A**) The island flap was then dissected from the finger in the areolar plane over the tendon sheaths and phalanges. The neurovascular structures entering its proximal end were carefully preserved.

As the vascular bundle was dissected into the palm, the vascular branches to the adjacent finger were ligated and cut. The common digital nerve was split by slitting its sheath, thus preserving innervation to both the flap and the normal adjacent finger. (**B**)

Fingertip Injuries

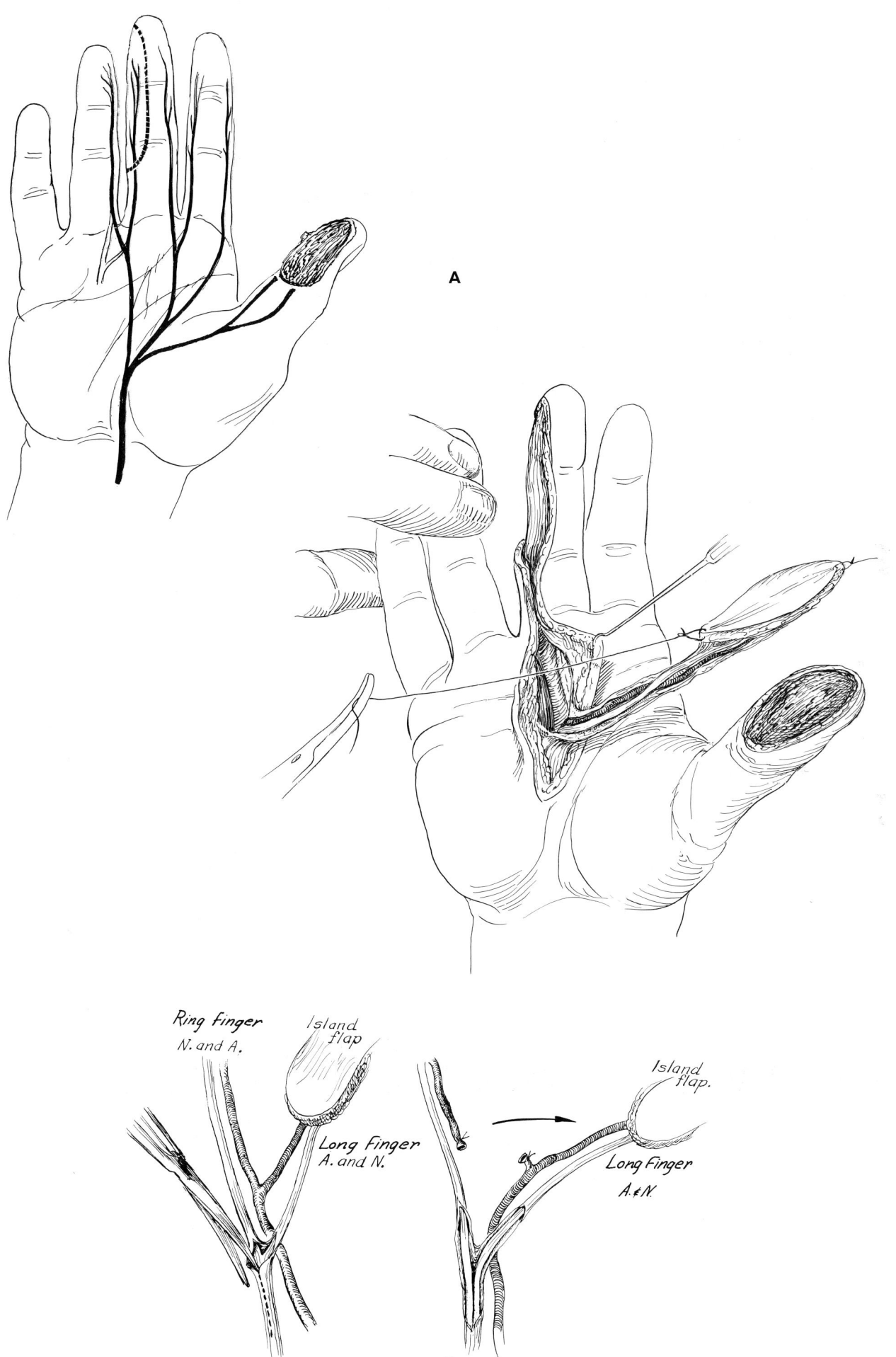

15 – Island Pedicle Flap for Fingertip Loss

The composite island, now tethered only by the proper digital vessels and nerve, was prepared for passage to the recipient area through a tunnel bluntly dissected just deep to the palmar fascia. (**C**) A suture through the distal end of the island and another through the proximal end made passage or retrieval of the island possible without risk of injury to the nutrient pedicle. After checking to see that the pedicle length was adequate by laying the island down on the recipient site with the vascular tether outside the skin, the island was eased through the subfascial tunnel.

It was sutured in place and a free full thickness skin graft was placed over the donor site. (**D**)

Darts of the graft inserted into transverse palmar incisions to break up the mid-palmar straight line incision may be necessary if the island pedicle is longer than a single phalanx length.

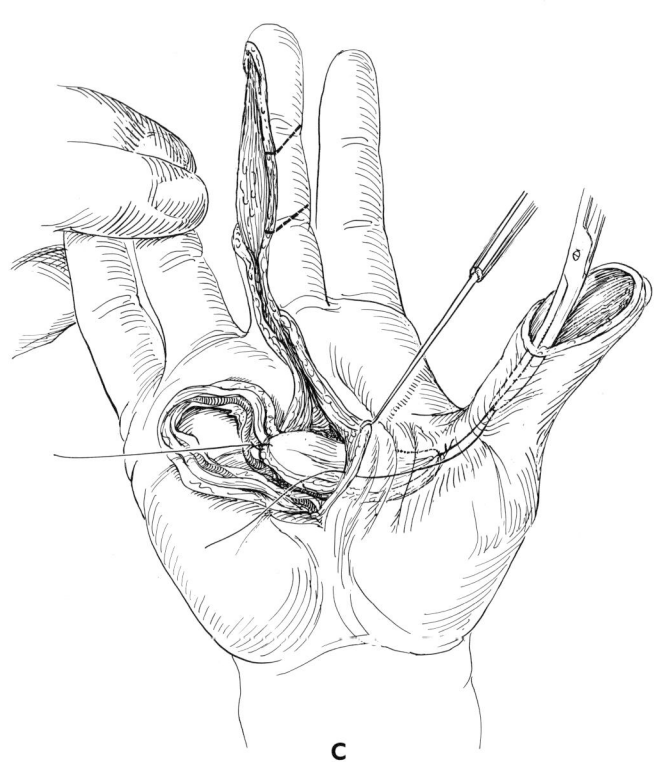

C

D

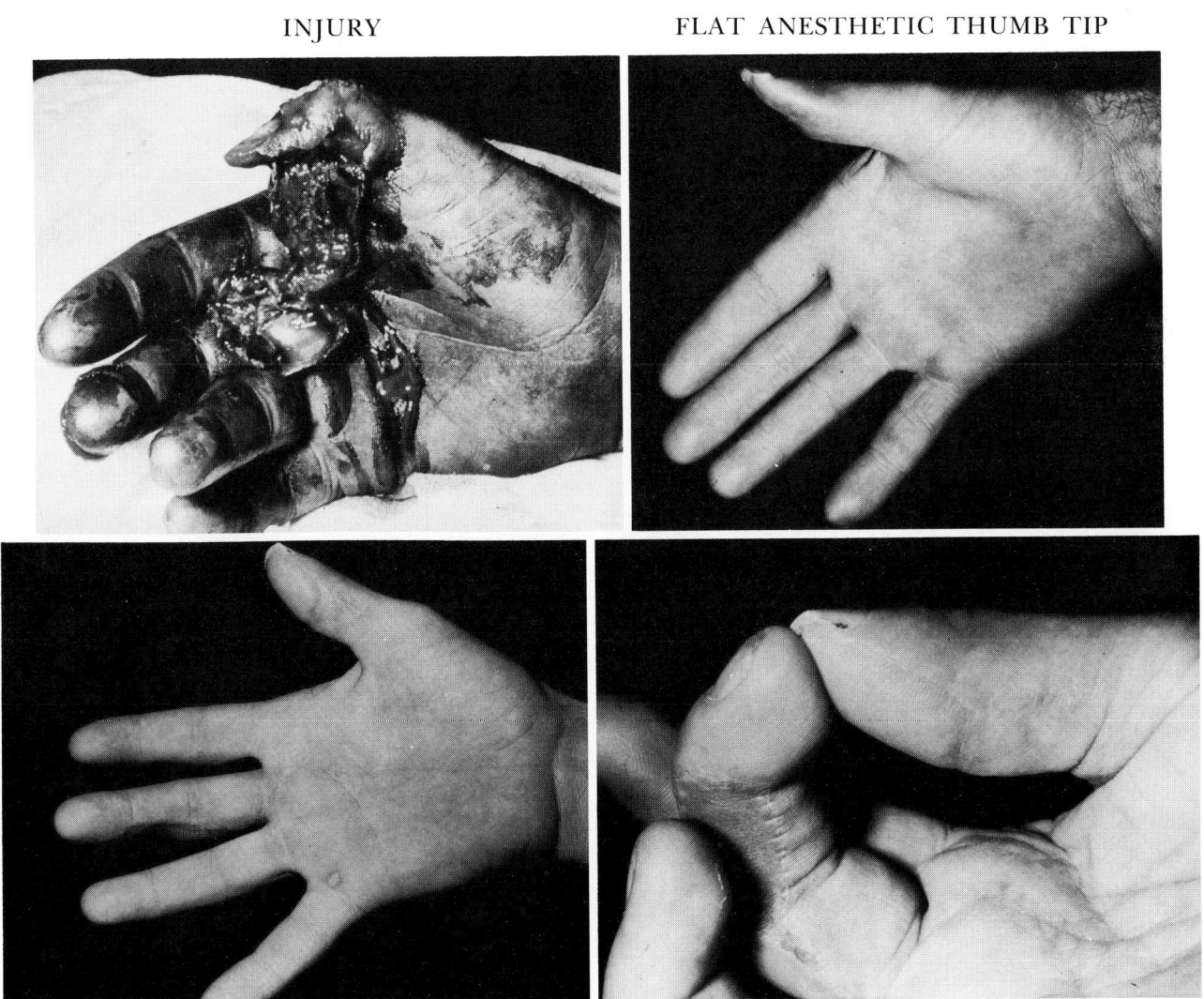

INJURY — FLAT ANESTHETIC THUMB TIP

RESULT AFTER ISLAND PEDICLE TRANSFER

16
Advancement Flap for Fingertip Loss

Principle

Faced with a tip pulp amputation of a finger where padding and sensibility are very important one should consider advancement of full thickness skin and subcutaneous tissue as a vascularized flap. The palm skin may be advanced 1.5 to 2.0 cm. by releasing it from the finger preserving its nerve and blood supply.

Example

A salesman demonstrating farm machinery lost the tip of his long finger by catching it in a moving belt. Replacement of the tip was attempted but the replanted tip did not survive and the finger healed by secondary intention. The soft tissue coverage of the tip was inadequate and unstable, and the tip was tender. (**A**)

The defect was re-created by excision of the scar. (The initial defect could logically have been treated by advancement of palm skin in the manner elected for correction of the re-created defect.)

Incisions were outlined in the mid axial plane on both sides of the finger. A transverse incision for possible use was planned and outlined on the skin over the proximal phalanx to connect the two mid axial incisions. (**B**)

These incisions were made and the palm soft tissues were elevated with the neurovascular bundles. The transverse skin incision across the flap at the proximal finger level was necessary to allow mobility of the skin flap. (**C**)

The local island flap was then advanced over the tip of the finger. (**D**)

A free full thickness skin graft was planted on the open donor area on the proximal finger. (**E**)

The technique produced a finger tip with full sensibility and permanent intact blood supply. Sudomotor function was also preserved.

CAUTION: This procedure carries some risk to the dorsal skin of the finger. Other local flaps should be used where possible.

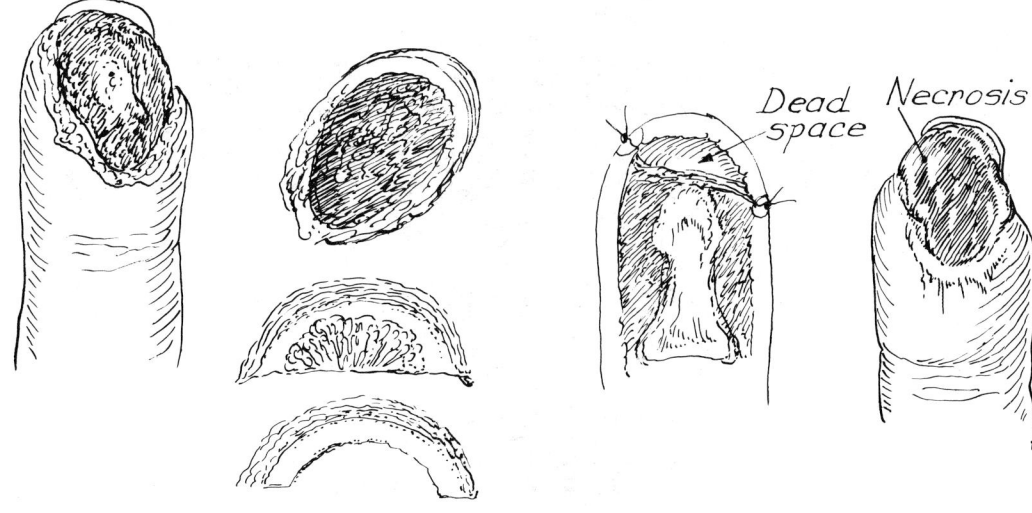

A

Fingertip Injuries

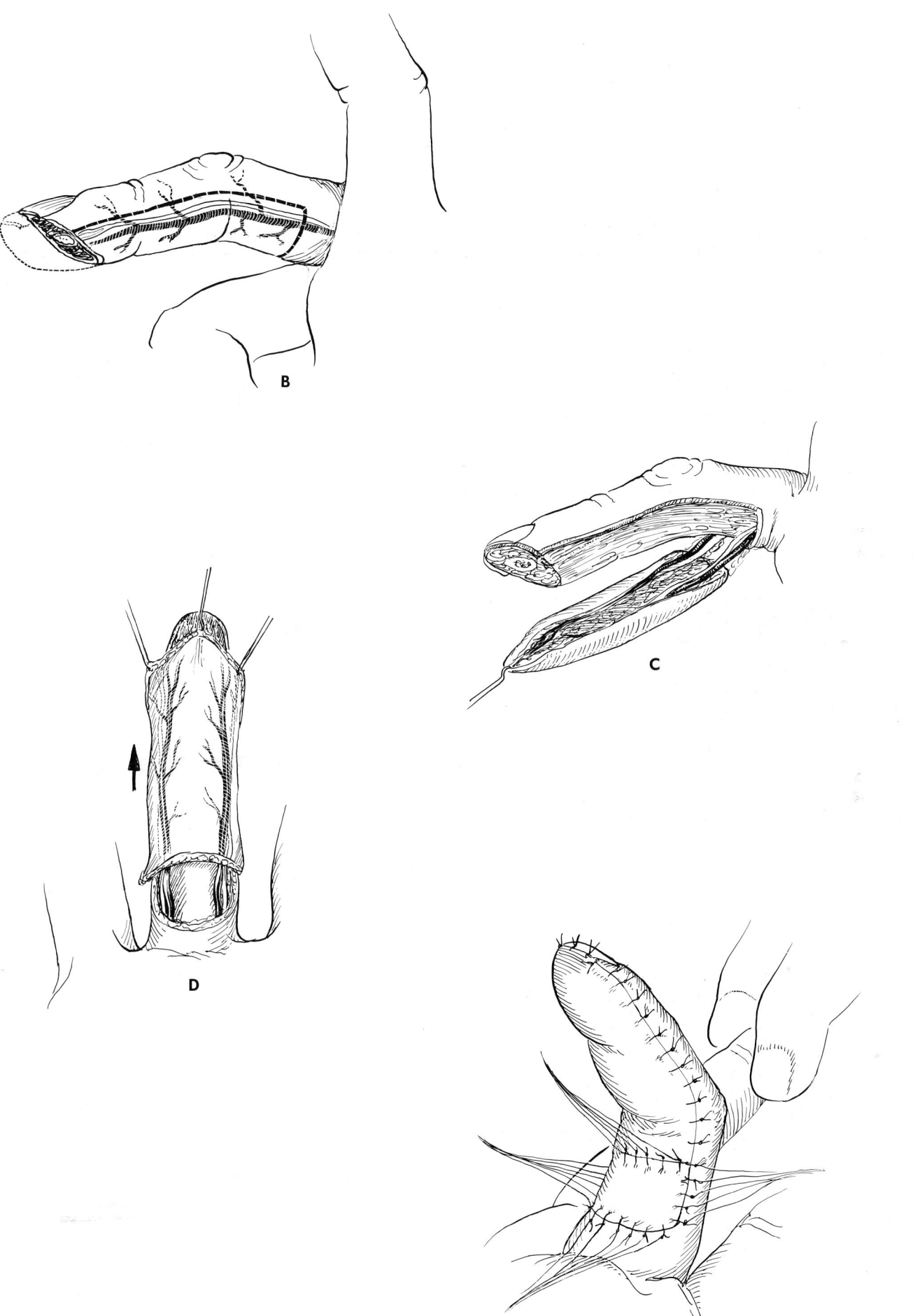

83

16 — Advancement Flap for Fingertip Loss

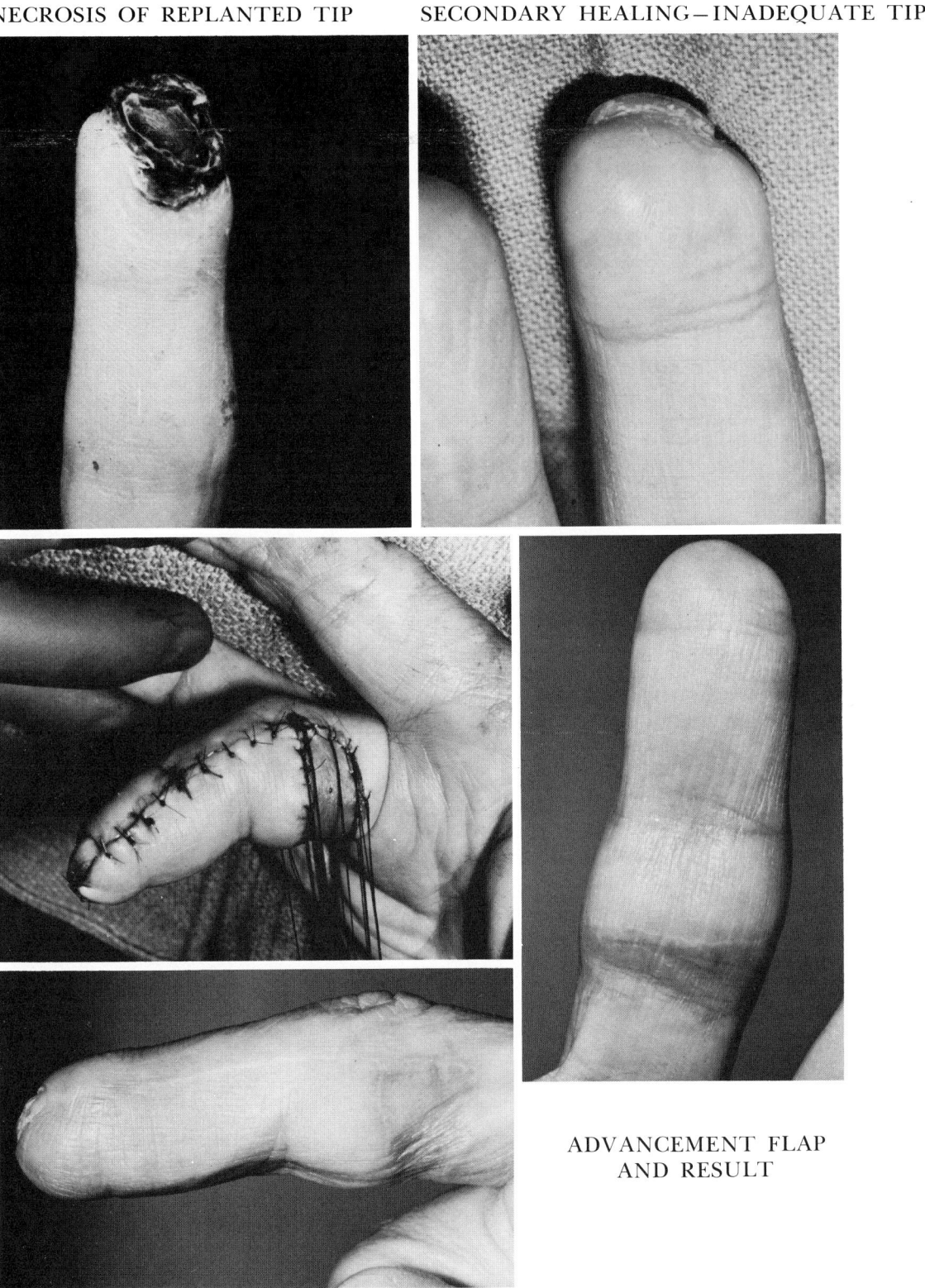

NECROSIS OF REPLANTED TIP

SECONDARY HEALING — INADEQUATE TIP

ADVANCEMENT FLAP AND RESULT

Skin and Soft Tissue Losses

FREE SKIN GRAFTS

17

Skin Grafting on the Palm of the Hand

Principle

Commonly, skin grafts are required on the palm of the hand after excisional surgery or traumatic skin losses. Thick split thickness or full thickness free grafts are most adequate for replacement after such losses. Excisional release of a scar contracture results in a defect several times the size of the resected scar. A scar crossing the thenar crease will result in scar contracture which pulls the first and fifth metacarpals into palmar abduction. If the scar crosses a metacarpophalangeal joint crease, it also produces flexion contracture of the joint. In such cases excision of the scar and replacement of the skin deficit with a skin graft is appropriate treatment.

Example

A 10-year-old girl sustained a burn of the left palm which after skin grafting and healing left her with a thickened scar from the mid-palmar aspect of the little finger across the palm to the base of the thumb. (**A**) Contracture developed which prevented full spread of the palm across the thenar crease and the little finger was held in mild flexion.

An incision was planned to excise the scar and to create side cuts for release of the contracture. (**B**)

Skin and Soft Tissue Losses

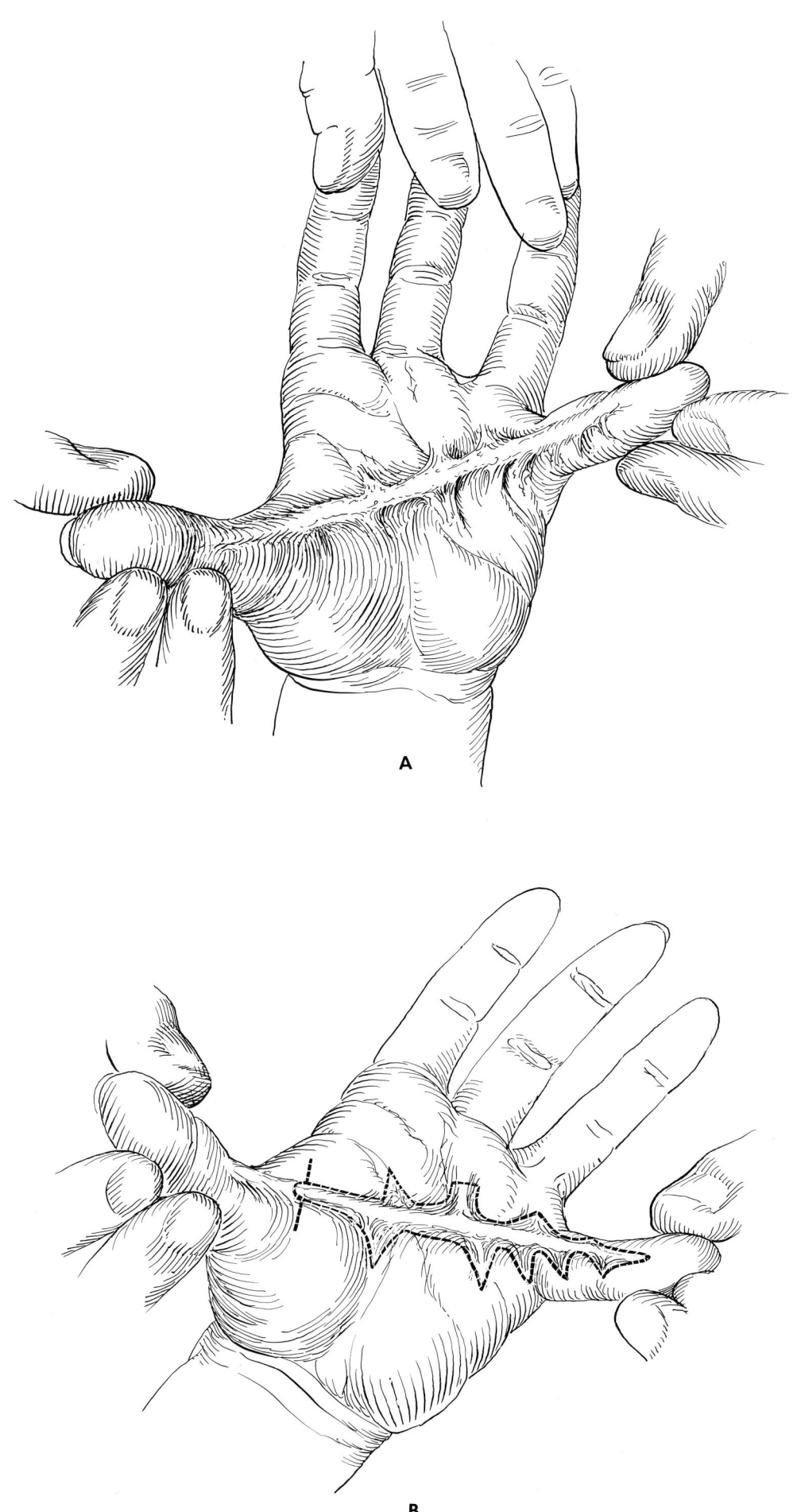

87

17 — Skin Grafting on the Palm of the Hand

As the contracture was released the true skin deficit became evident and the surgeon could judge how much skin would be required to replace the loss. (**C** and **D**)

A free thick (0.018 inch) split thickness graft of skin was draped over the defect and fixed in place with single sutures at the extremes of the defect. (**E**)

Once key sutures were in place the skin graft was cut to fit the deficit precisely, placing additional sutures to fix each angle in place. (**F**)

A bulky pressure dressing and plaster shell was applied to the hand.

The first dressing was done after five days and the graft appeared to be taking well without hematomas. The hand was re-dressed and immobilized for 10 days after which sutures were removed and progressive activity was initiated. The patient gained a great deal of range of motion.

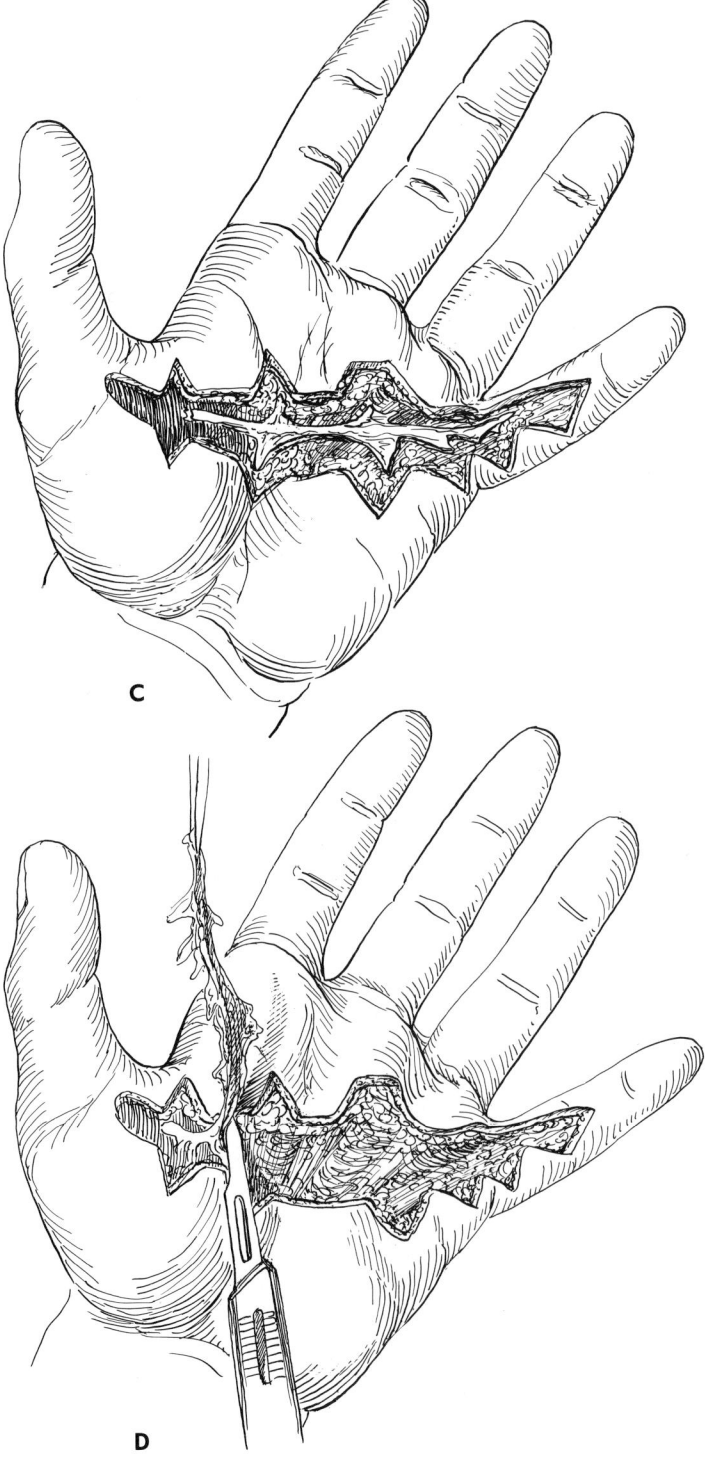

C

D

Skin and Soft Tissue Losses

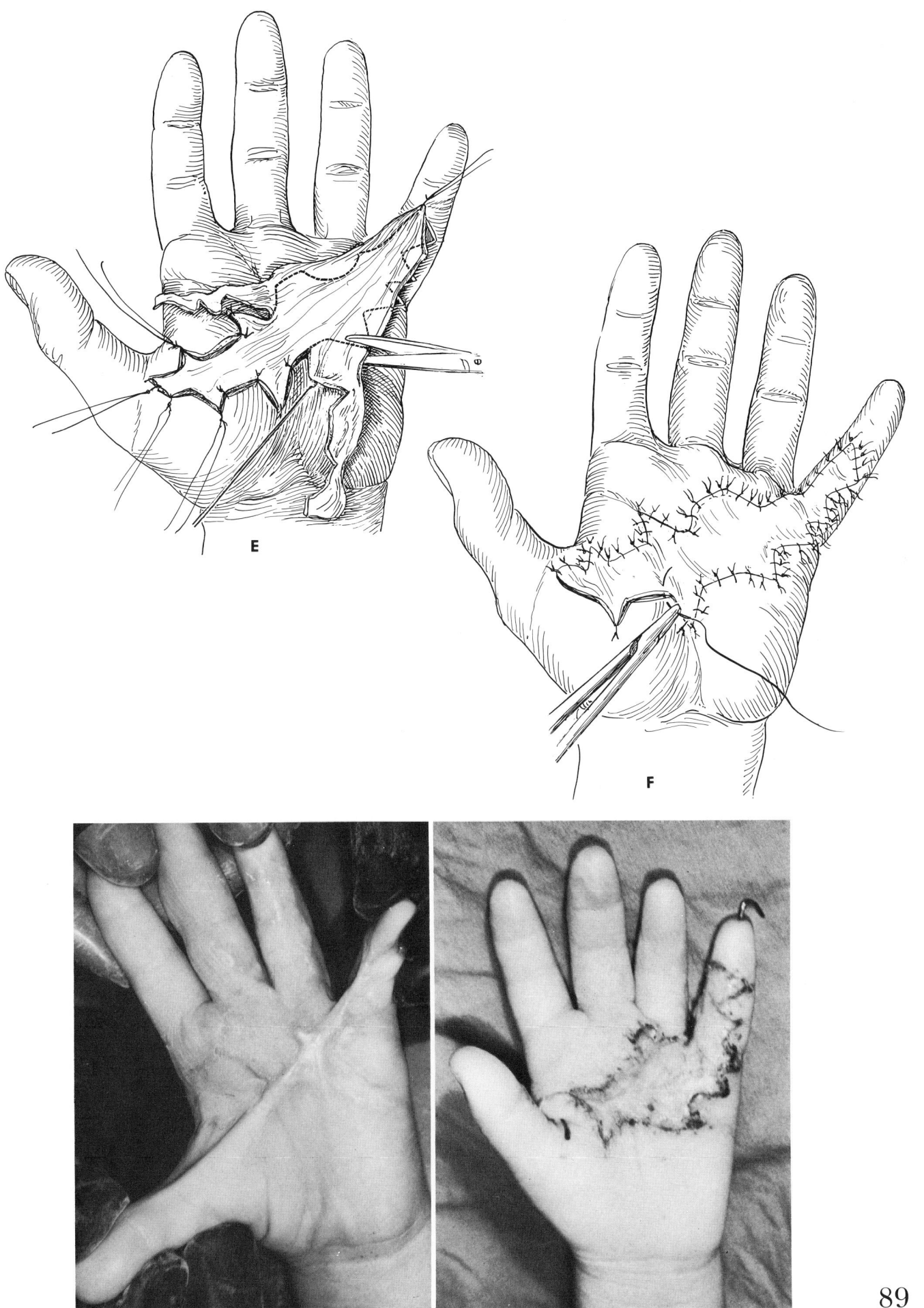

89

18 Free Plantar Skin Graft to Palm

Principle

To replace large area losses of palmar skin with a free graft, one may choose any standard donor site and expect to get a good functional result. To replace a small area of skin loss on the palm with skin of similar characteristics, the surgeon may choose a donor area with those characteristics. The plantar surface of the foot is such an area. (**A**) A thick split thickness skin graft can be taken from the non-weight bearing, longitudinal arch area of the foot for use on the palm. (**B**) This is particularly useful in black patients since skin grafts from any other source end up as noticeable jet black patches on an otherwise lightly colored palm.

Small full thickness skin grafts may be taken from the ulnar aspect of the hypothenar area to achieve the same objectives of matching color and palm skin characteristics.

Example

A verrucous lesion required excision of a 5 by 4 centimeter area of skin proximal to the little finger in a black female patient.

The lesion and skin were excised leaving a palm defect which required skin graft replacement. A plantar donor site was elected. A split thickness (0.020 inch) graft was obtained using an electric dermatome.

The graft took well and achieved the objective of coverage with skin appropriate for the recipient palm.

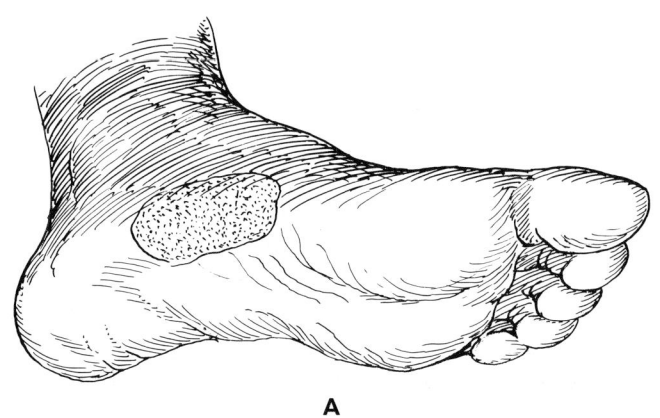

A

Skin and Soft Tissue Losses

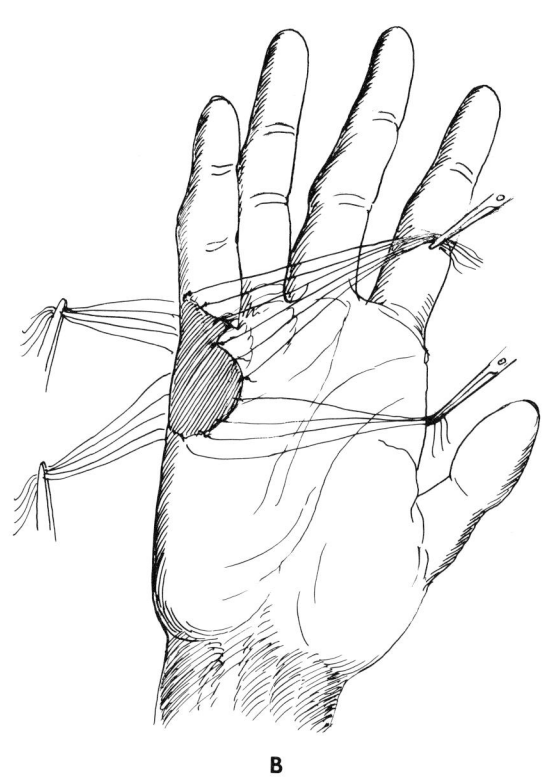

B

PREOPERATIVE   POSTOPERATIVE

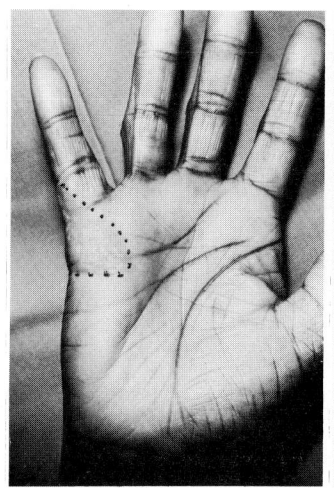 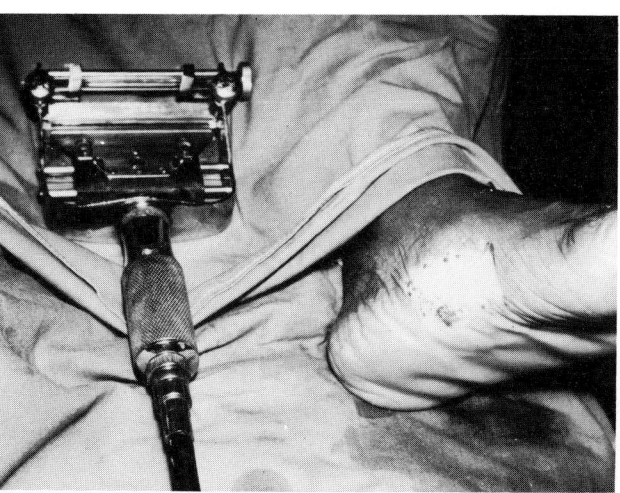 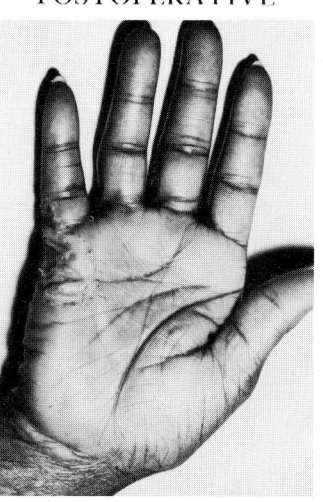

91

19

Skin Grafting on the Dorsum of the Hand

Principle

When man assumes a protective position for an impending injury or accident, he generally exposes the dorsal aspect of his hand to injury. The dorsum of the hand is subject to soft tissue losses from burns and avulsion injuries. The skin is resistant enough that even most third degree burns spare the underlying areolar fascia. Avulsions classically occur in subdermal plane, leaving open areolar tissue after injury. This areolar layer is an excellent recipient bed for split thickness skin grafts. Plasmatic support of the graft is immediate as the areolar tissue adapts to the newly applied skin. Blood supply is good and is readily picked up from the undemanding areolar tissue. Once the graft takes, it quickly assumes the normal mobile characteristics and the appearance of normal dorsal hand skin.

If large areas of skin are destroyed by a burn or avulsion, healing by secondary intention generates a thick plaque of scar and creates hyperextension contracture of the metacarpophalangeal joints in the hand. Fixed hyperextension of these joints then results in formation of fixed flexion contractures of the interphalangeal joints now subject to unbalanced pull by the flexor tendons.

Faced with thick plaquelike scars on the dorsum of the hand, one should urge full replacement with thick split thickness skin grafts. The whole scar plate may be movable over the underlying tendons and bone. When its removal is possible by dissection in the loose areolar plane, one may preserve the major veins and dorsal nerves at the time of scar removal. This assures a good functional and cosmetic result after skin grafting.

Attention to details in the implantation of a dorsal skin graft is very important. Particular attention must be directed to web spaces and the areas where motion is greatest. In these areas linear scars across lines of stretch must be broken up by Z-plasty and inserts of skin graft corners or tongue flaps. After surgical excision of the entire scar, one may put the hand passively through a full range of motion to detect incision lines at the edge of the excision that should be broken up or interrupted by Z-plasty or skin graft inserts. Meticulous hemostasis is essential for successful take of the graft.

Example

A 58-year-old night watchman sustained deep second and third degree burns of the dorsum of both hands from open flames in a house fire. The wounds healed over several months in part by secondary intention. In the two years that followed the scars became quite hypertrophic and post-burn dorsal syndactylism of the fingers to the level of the proximal interphalangeal joints developed. (**A**) The patient was unable to fully flex his fingers nor was he able to abduct his thumb well because of hypertrophic scar and contracture in the first web space.

After consultation the patient elected to undergo resection of the whole dorsal plaque of scar and replacement with split thickness skin grafts.

The mobile scar plaque was resected in the areolar plane, preserving a number of large veins and the dorsal branches of the ulnar and radial nerves. (**B**) Once the scar was resected, the fingers and thumb could be put passively through a full range of motion.

Skin grafts 0.018 inch in thickness were taken from the lower abdominal wall using a Reese dermatome (see Section 7). The grafts were sutured in place and, at intervals, lateral incisions were made; darts of skin were inserted to break up the straight line scars in areas of changing length. (**C**) Similar angular darts of skin were placed through the interdigital web

Skin and Soft Tissue Losses

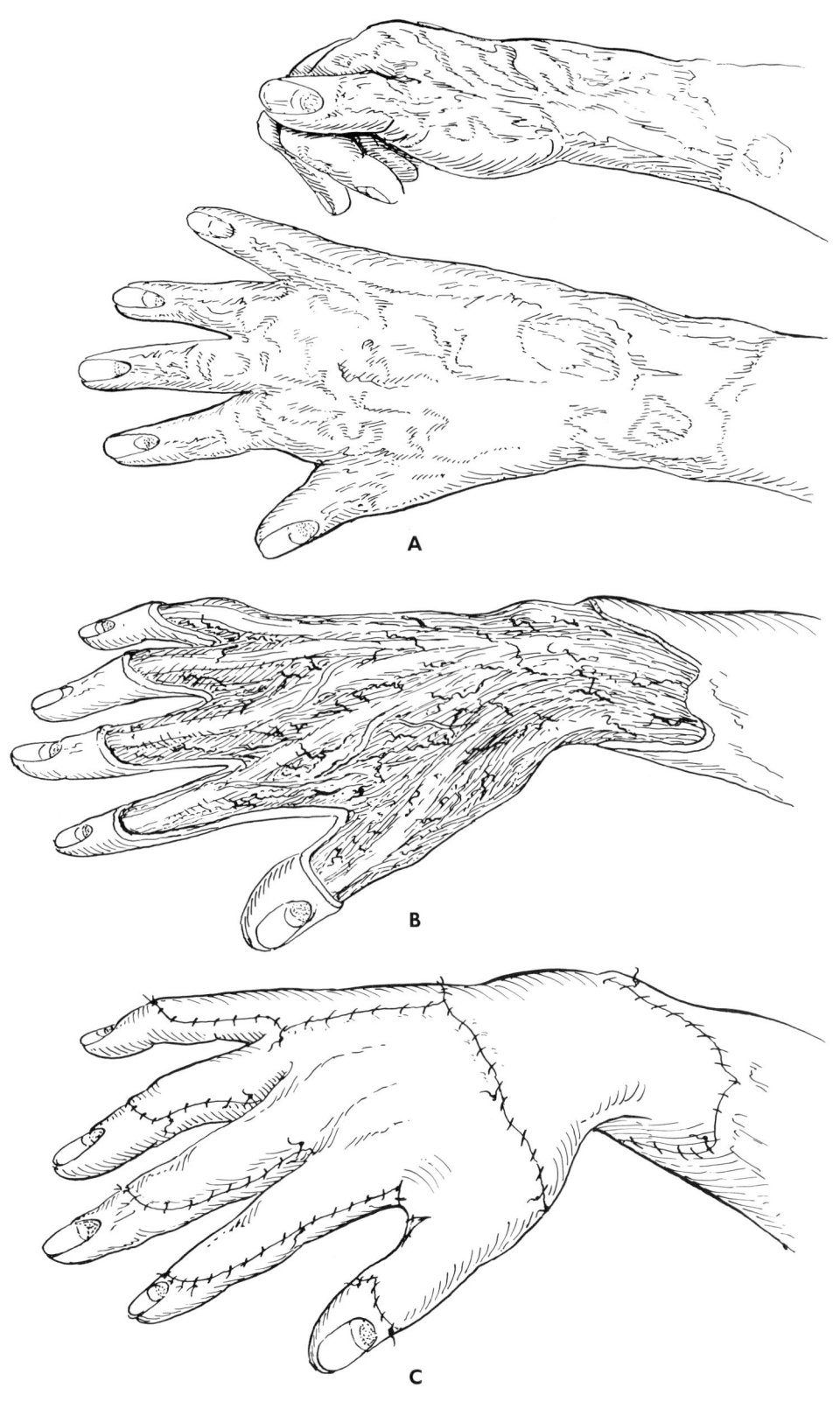

93

19—Skin Grafting on the Dorsum of the Hand

spaces to allow spreading to the fingers and thumb. (**D**)

The grafts took well and after a year all of the normal folds and markings on the fingers had redeveloped. The functional result was excellent. (**E**)

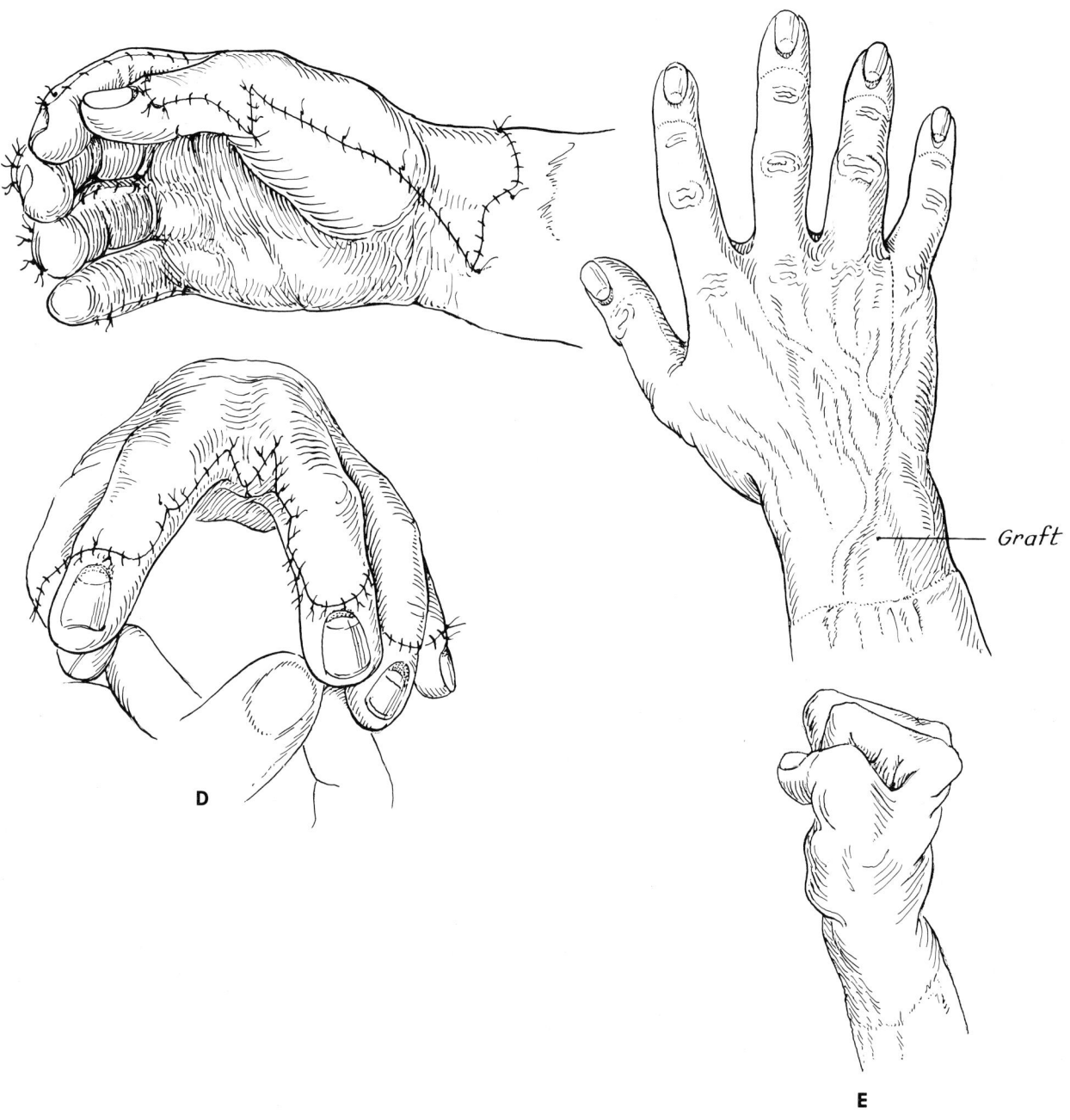

Skin and Soft Tissue Losses

PREOPERATIVE

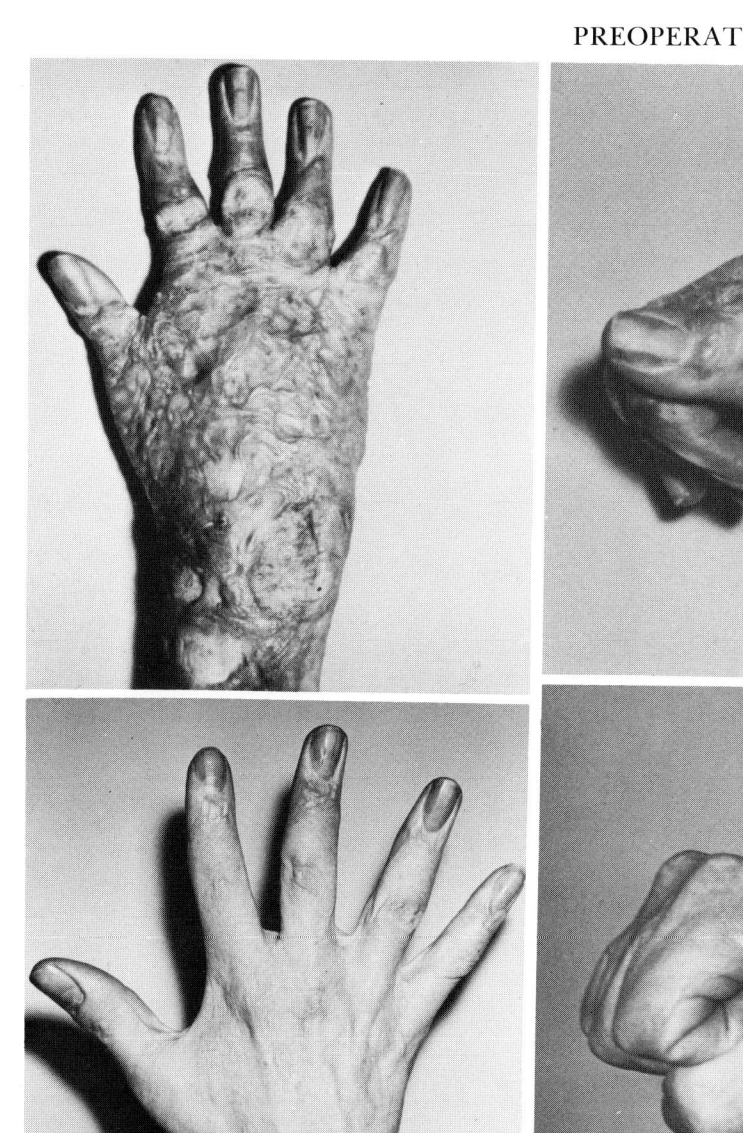
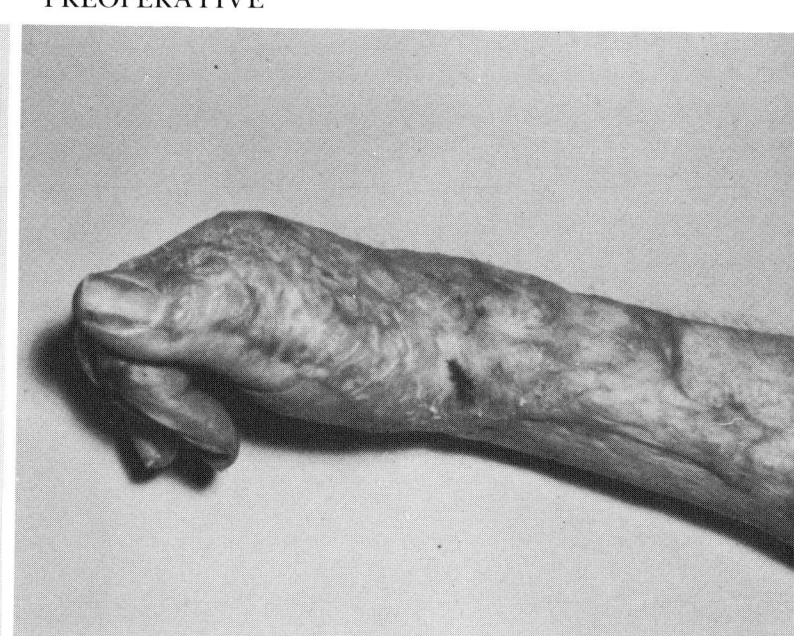
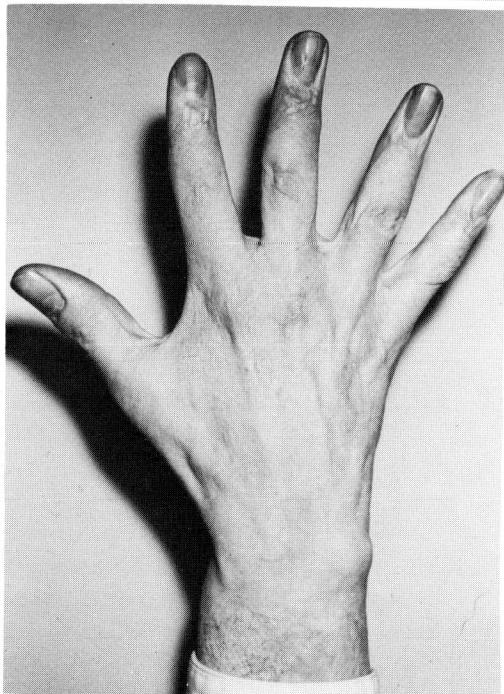
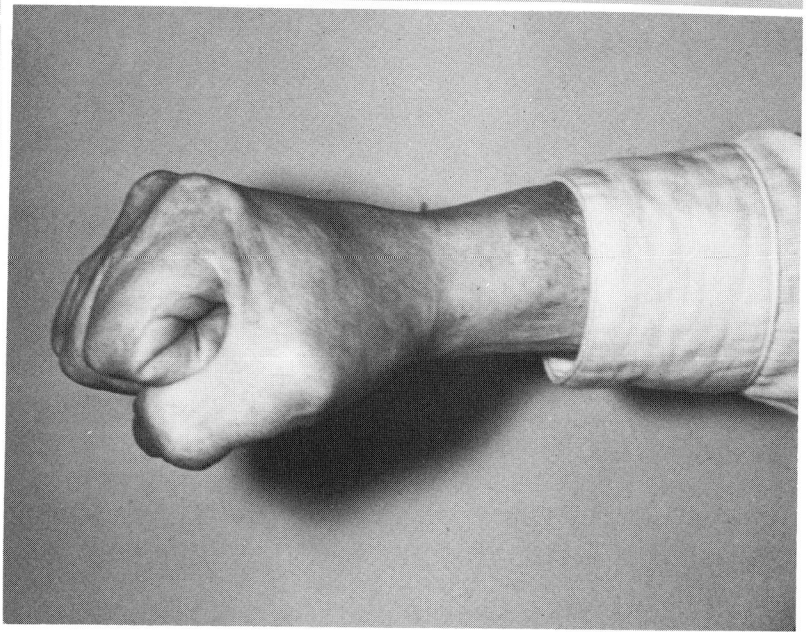

POSTOPERATIVE

PEDICLE FLAPS

20

Soft Tissue Replacement Using Vascularized Pedicles

Principles

When reconstruction of functional structures within the hand is anticipated, an area of deficit of overlying tissue must be replaced with vascularized skin with subcutaneous tissue. Split thickness skin grafts which depend for their blood supply on the whole recipient bed are generally inadequate when subsequent deep reconstruction is necessary. Structures such as tendons will become adherent to a graft without subcutaneous tissue. Only if subcutaneous tissue is already present on the recipient site will a split thickness graft be appropriate.

A free graft which has taken well on a recipient site devoid of a blanket of subcutaneous tissues cannot be shifted about by Z-plasty or flap without a serious risk of loss of the flaps. The blood supply is parasitized from the whole recipient bed rather than from the edges via the subdermal plexus and thus any shift will succeed only if the shifted flap takes as a new skin graft, not by survival through the base pedicle.

Any structure used in reconstruction which itself does not have intrinsic blood supply may be responsible for necrosis of an overlying skin graft if it is placed beneath it.

When reconstructive procedures are anticipated in an area of skin deficit, it is good judgment to utilize a vascularized pedicle flap for skin coverage. Such soft tissue may be permanently vascularized from the donor site in the case of local soft tissue shifts or island pedicle flaps. Even if this is not the case in instances where the carrying pedicle must be sectioned, the skin with its underlying subcutaneous tissue picks up most of its blood supply from the margins of the recipient site. One may then work beneath the replaced soft tissue without fear of loss of the overlying skin. The skin may also be shifted about with impunity with the expectation that it will survive on the blood supply from the margins via the subdermal plexus.

Pedicle-carried soft tissues may be obtained locally from the hand or from distant sites such as the chest or abdominal walls.

Local pedicle flaps have the advantages of bringing hand skin to the defect, and elimination of the need to immobilize the hand to another part of the body. Some local flaps bring with them a permanently intact blood supply.

Whenever a digit is to be amputated, it should be inventoried for components which might be useful in reconstruction or repair of other parts of the hand. Frequently a digit which itself is too severely damaged for reconstruction is an excellent source of skin and subcutaneous tissue, bone, nerve, or tendon to repair other injured parts. These elements may be used as pedicle transfers or free grafted parts. Particularly useful is skin and soft tissue with good intrinsic blood supply.

LOCAL PEDICLE FLAPS

21

Cross-Finger Flaps

Principle

An area where bone or joint surgery is to be done must be covered by good skin with subcutaneous tissue. A cross-finger pedicle flap may serve the purpose well. (See *Fusion of Distal Interphalangeal Joint* in Section 66.)

A tendon graft or tendon transfer in a finger will not function well beneath a free skin graft without a good pad of subcutaneous soft tissue.

Example

A patient with a moderate flexion contracture of the long finger and a loss of flexor tendons required replacement of the skin deficit with vascularized pedicle skin and subcutaneous tissue. In the initial wound treatment, part of the finger had been surfaced by a split thickness skin graft. In preparation for a flexor tendon graft better soft tissue cover to include skin and subcutaneous tissue was needed. Since the area of soft tissue deficit was small, a local cross-finger flap seemed a reasonable source to supply adequate skin and subcutaneous tissue. The lateral base of the triangle of skin represented by the skin graft on the finger was toward the index finger making it the logical donor finger for a local cross-finger flap. The previously grafted site was marked out for incision with the base toward the donor index finger. (**A**)

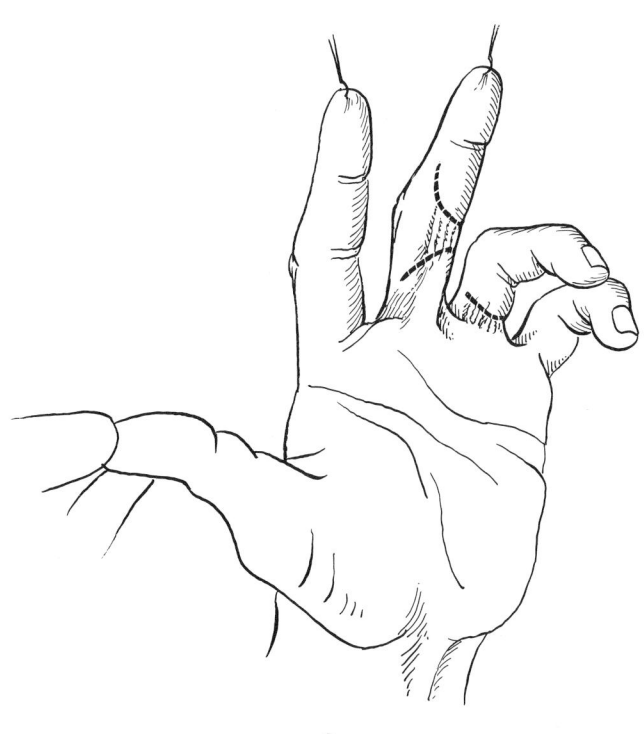

A

21 — Cross-Finger Flaps

The old healed skin graft from the recipient long finger was elevated by dissection from the lateral apex to the base, leaving the base attached to the finger. (**B**) This flap was swung up onto the dorsum of the adjacent index finger to help outline a triangular flap to interchange with the skin graft. (**C**)

The flap from the donor finger was dissected up from the apex to the base in the areolar plane just over the extensor mechanism. (**D**) The resulting flap of skin with subcutaneous tissue retained its blood supply since the base of the flap was left intact.

The long finger was extended and the skin flaps were interchanged and fixed in place with sutures, creating a surgical syndactylism between the donor and recipient fingers. (**E**)

The skin contracture in the adjacent ring finger was surgically released. (**F**) Since there was no tendon injury in the ring finger, further tendon surgery was not contemplated. The skin deficit resulting from release of the skin scar contracture was therefore corrected by implantation of a free full thickness skin graft.

After healing of all wounds (about three weeks) the surgical syndactylism between the index and long fingers was released, leaving the laterally based scars from section of both flaps on the mid-lateral aspect of the two fingers. (**G**) After healing, softening and remodelling of the scars, with full range of passive motion restored to the long finger, a flexor tendon graft was performed.

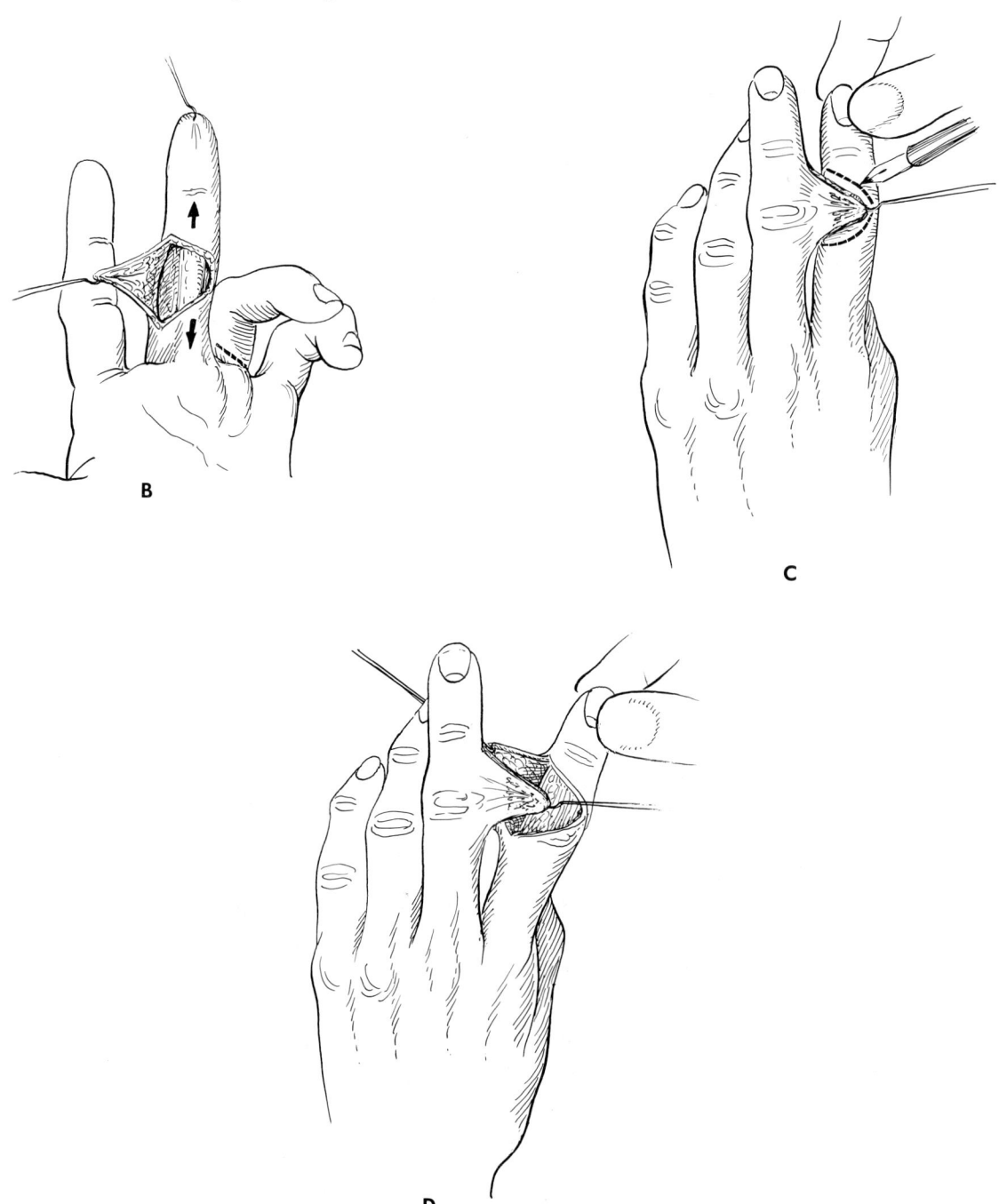

Skin and Soft Tissue Losses

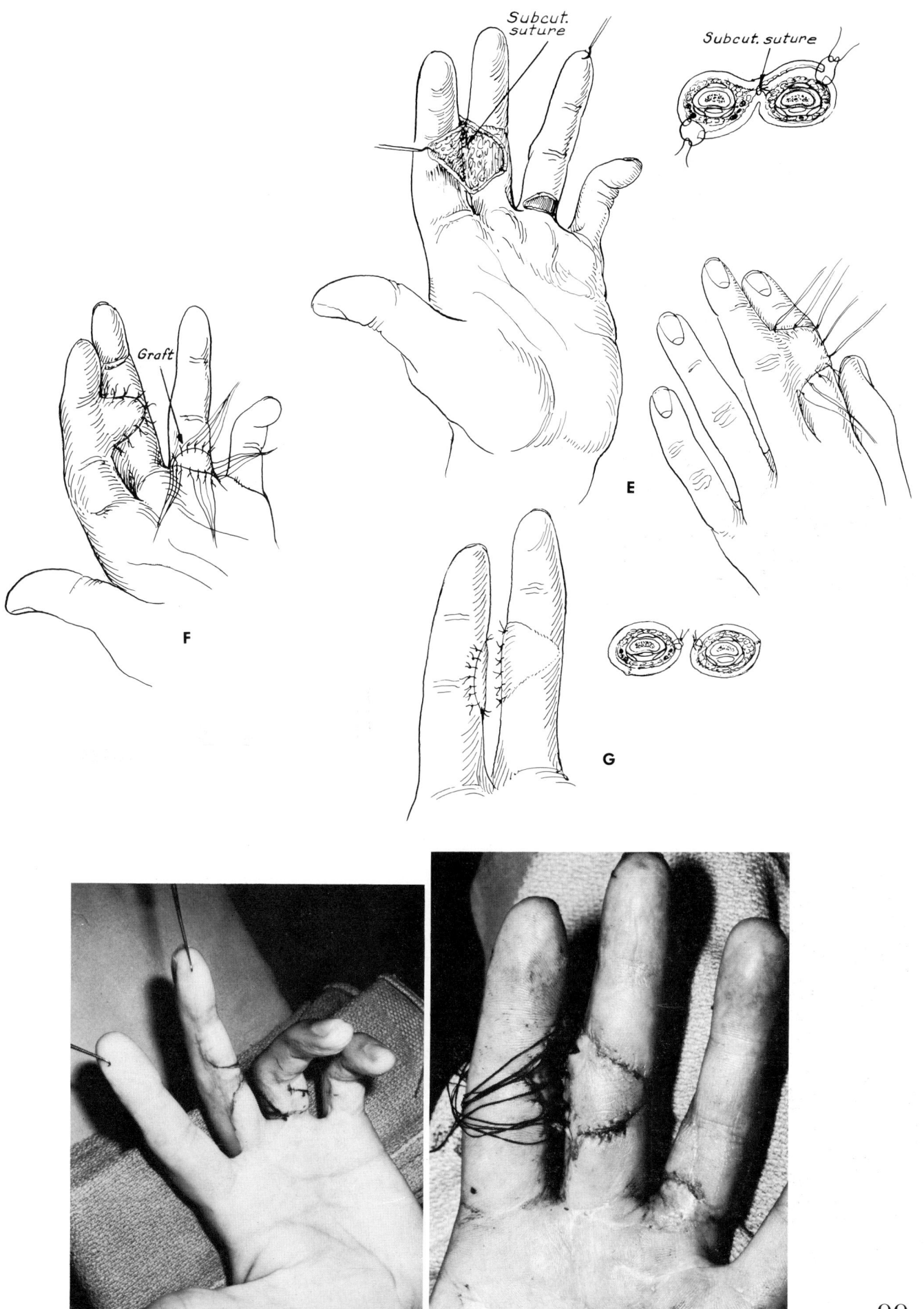

22
Local Pedicle Shift

Principle

Exposure of important structures in the hand which are devoid of intrinsic blood supply may be corrected only by covering them with skin and soft tissue which itself is adequately vascularized. Bare tendons or devascularized bone may be salvaged by acquiring pedicle flap coverage either locally or from a distant site. Permanent circulatory competence is best when the pedicle is left permanently in a locally shifted flap or island pedicle flap. Where a distant pedicle flap is essential, it must be left attached for sufficient time to assure good permanent vascular supply from the healed edges of the recipient site. An additional considerable bonus in certain local pedicle shifts and island pedicle flaps is shift of sensibility and sudomotor function.

When amputation of the thumb occurs, the surgeon is obligated to save as much of its length as possible. It is sometimes appropriate to cover the exposed bone using a local, first web space, vascularized flap. Such a flap should be planned with the carrying pedicle proximal in order to preserve flap sensibility. Using a pattern of fabric (see Section 13: Cross-Finger Flap), a flap may be designed which will cover the defect and shift without undue tension.

Example

A young laboring man sustained an injury which nearly completely amputated his right thumb through the proximal portion of the proximal phalanx. Initial treatment had consisted of an attempt to replace the thumb but gangrene and autoamputation occurred, leaving uncovered bone because of loss of soft tissue in excess of bone. (**A**) A local web space flap was used to cover the bare bone. The flap was outlined with a palmar base in the first web space. (**B**)

The skin and subcutaneous tissue just superficial to the fascia over the first dorsal interosseous muscle and adductor pollicis was raised far enough proximal to allow a shift to the recipient area without tension. Care was exercised to avoid injuring the proper digital nerve to the radial side of the index finger and the tiny filaments from it into the base of the web space flap. (**C**)

Skin and Soft Tissue Losses

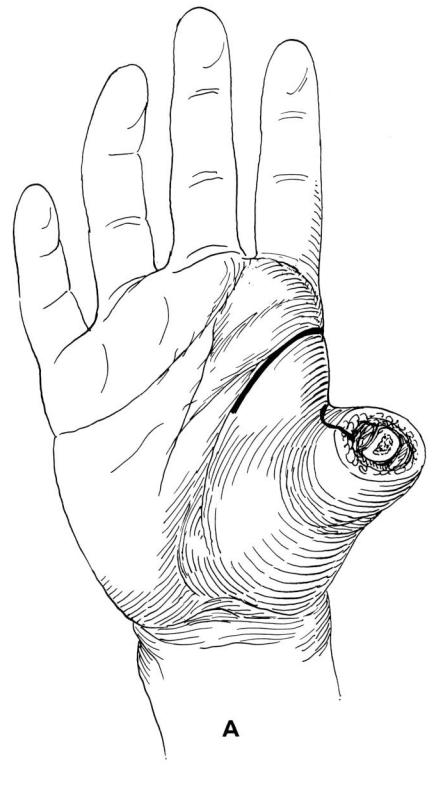

A

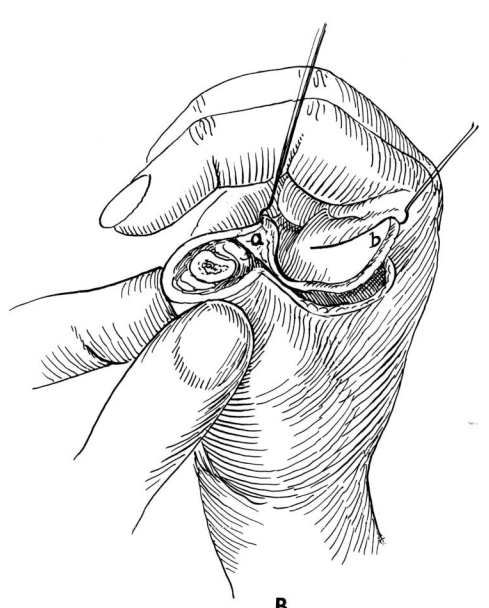

B

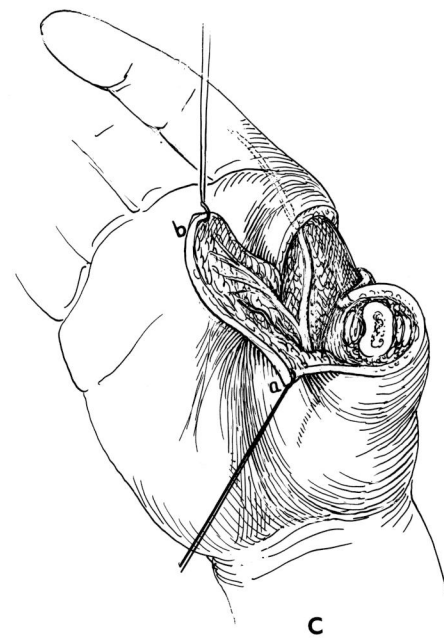

C

101

22 — Local Pedicle Shift

The bone end was trimmed back to viable bone. The padded flap was turned over the recipient area and fixed with interrupted sutures. (**D**)

A split thickness free skin graft was used to cover the donor area in the first web space. (**E**)

This local flap achieved primary wound closure without sacrifice of thumb length. The cushioned skin flap with sensibility furnished permanent coverage. The skin graft replacement of thick web space tissue deepened the web space between the salvaged foreshortened thumb and the index ray. Further reconstruction was not necessary.

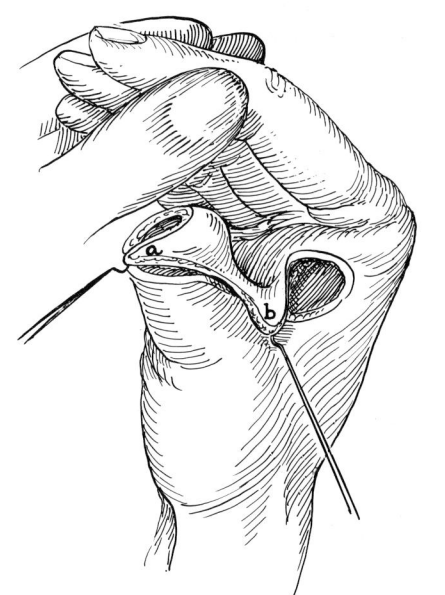
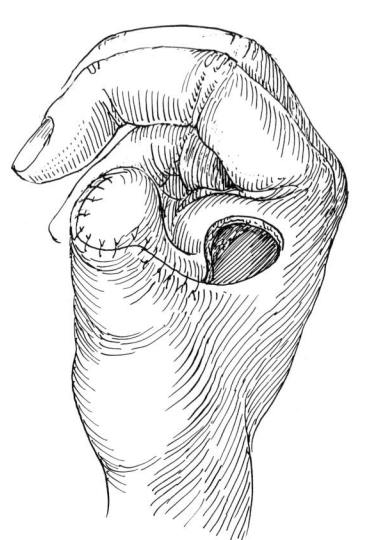

D

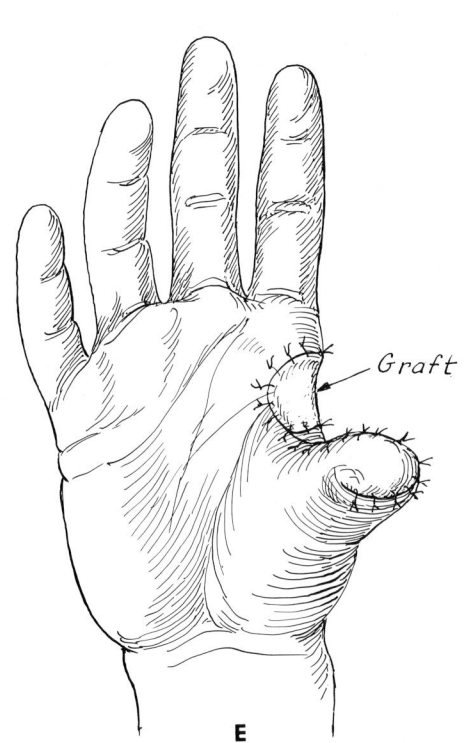

E

Skin and Soft Tissue Losses

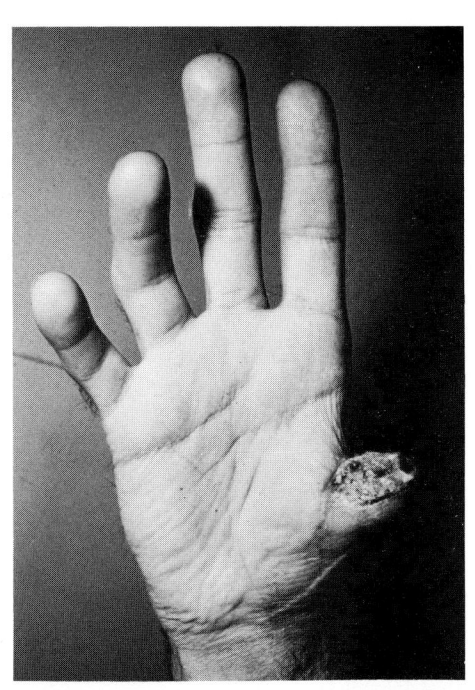
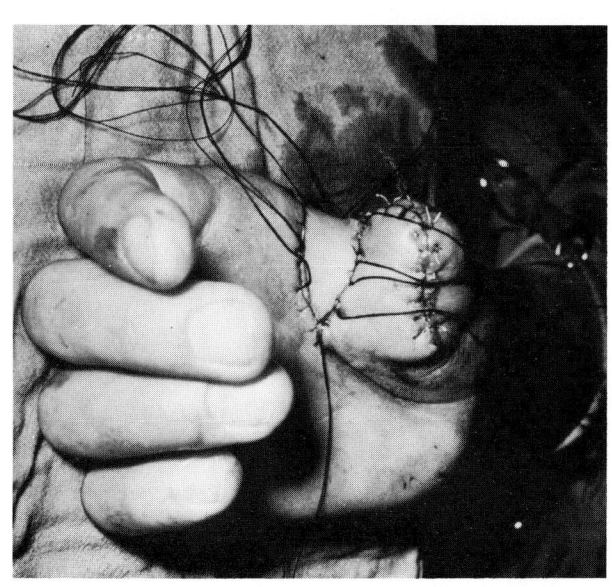
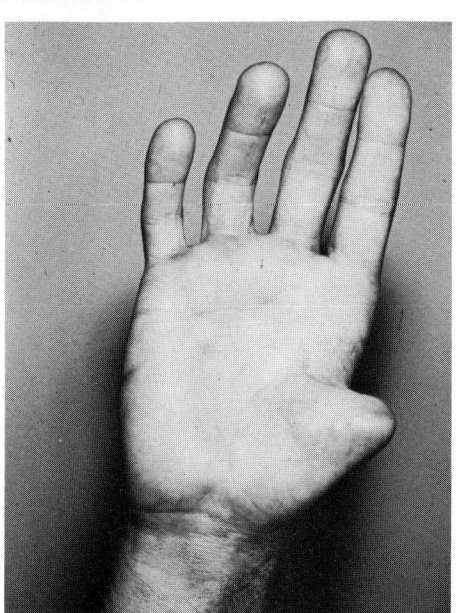

23

Secondary Digital Fillet

Principle

Frequently the vascularized soft tissues with normal sensibility in a digit about to be amputated may be very useful when transferred to an area of need. The technique picturesquely referred to as the "digital fillet" is often useful in secondary reconstructive hand surgery. For example, it may be used to resurface defects in the dorsum of the hand.

Example

A through-and-through gunshot wound of the hand destroyed the metacarpal of the right long finger, leaving the finger beyond reasonable potential for repair. (Such a finger may be left *in situ* simply as a source of elements for general secondary reconstruction or to determine its own salvageability.) This finger was detrimental to hand function by its functionless presence, fixation of tendons, and, thereby, the checkreining of tendons to adjacent fingers. The gunshot wound created a loss of soft tissue at the site of missile exit on the dorsum of the hand, leaving an unstable and sensitive scar. At the time of amputation of the long finger, the skin and subcutaneous tissues and the neurovascular bundles were preserved to allow excision of the scar and replacement by vascularized soft tissues with intact sensibility.

The dorsal scar was outlined for excision and a mid-dorsal finger incision was planned. (**A**)

The skin and subcutaneous tissues were dissected from the underlying tendinous and skeletal elements, preserving the neurovascular bundles in the flap. (**B**)

The scar was excised and the finger skeletal and tendinous elements were amputated. All tendons were pulled distally and cut short, allowing the ends to retract toward the wrist since there was no use for them as transfers to areas of motor loss in the hand. (**C**)

Skin and Soft Tissue Losses

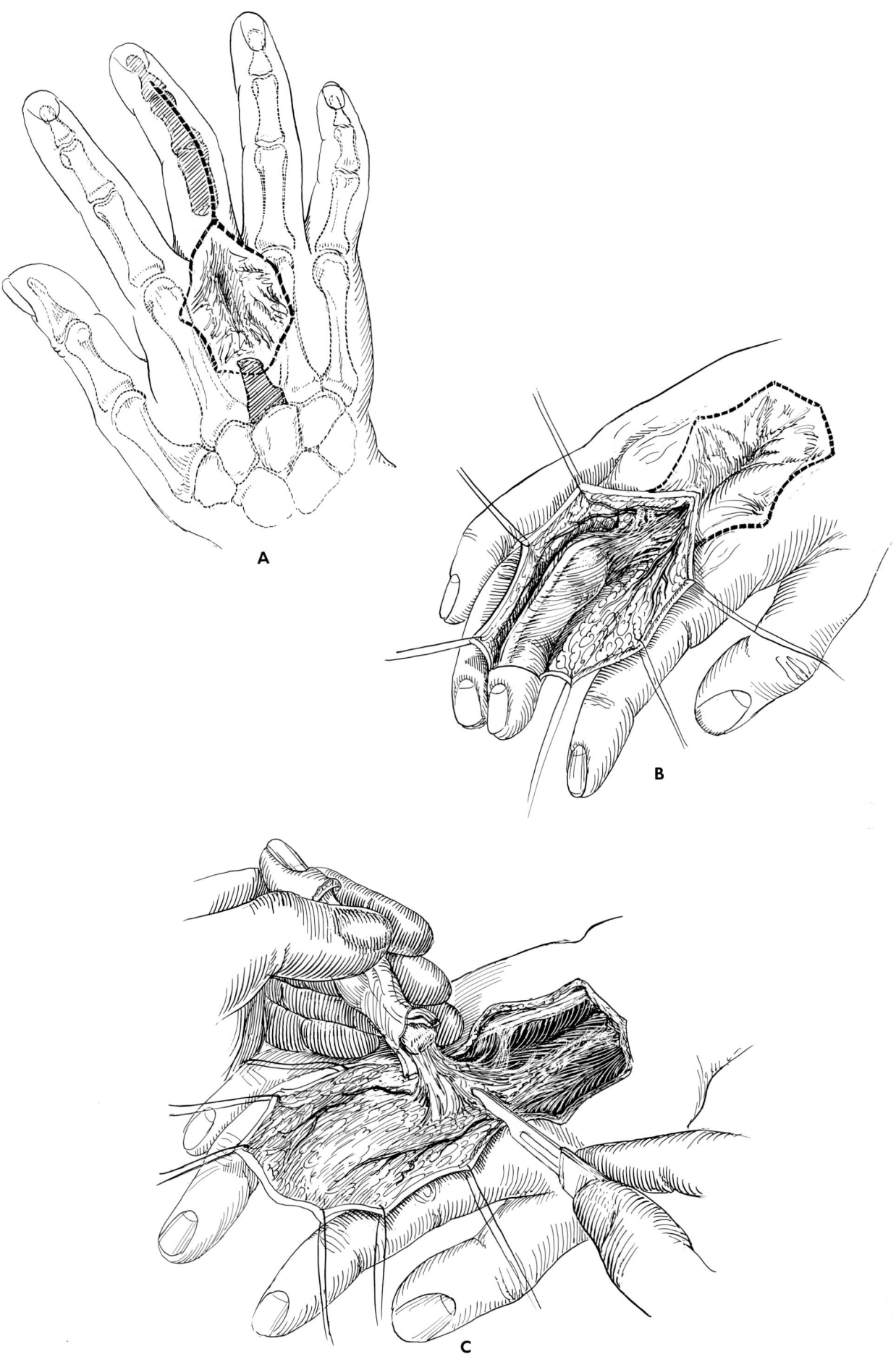

105

23 — Secondary Digital Fillet

The finger flap was fitted to the defect left after the scar was excised and the normal surrounding skin receded to its pre-injury position. (**D**)

The pedicle base in the web space was narrowed to avoid bunching of soft tissue in the web space. (**E**)

The fillet flap supplied full and thick coverage with excellent sensibility and permanently transferred blood supply. The patient at first interpreted a touch in the recipient area as a touch on the amputated finger. Function of the remaining fingers improved and the cosmetic result, though not perfect, was satisfactory.

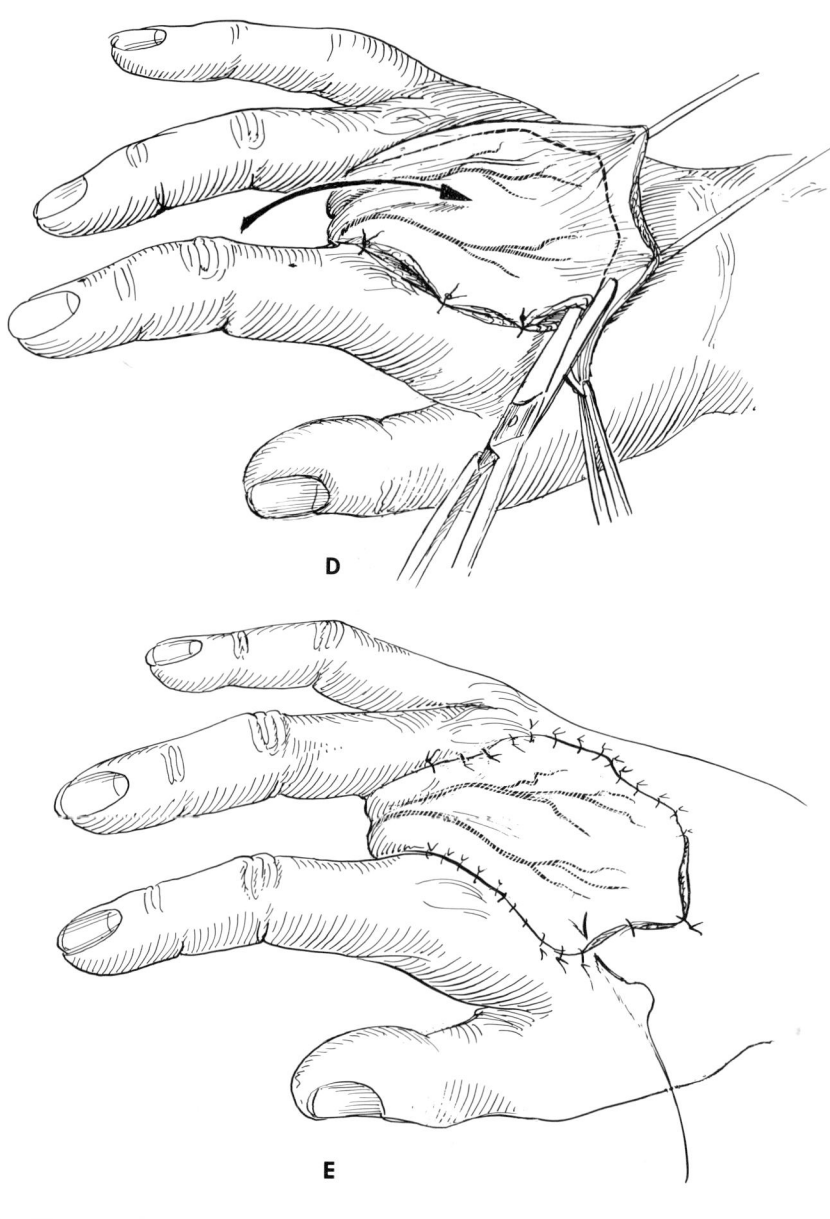

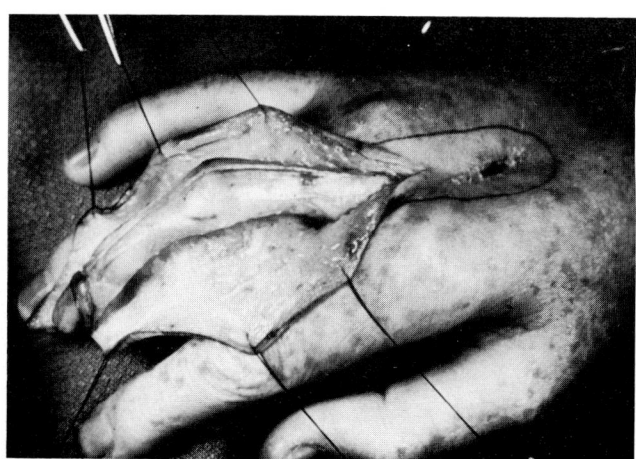

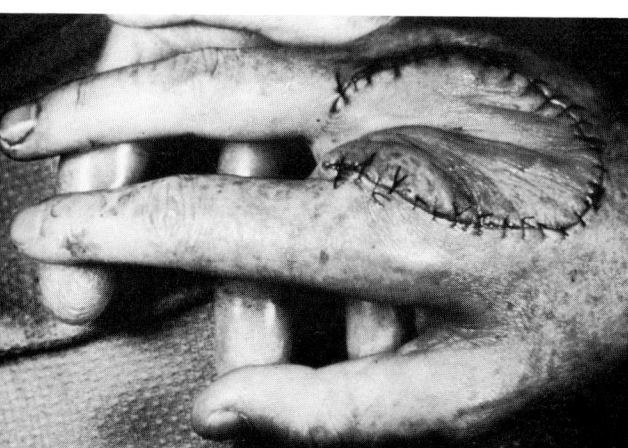

Skin and Soft Tissue Losses

Principle

The skin from a digit destined for amputation may be used to resurface the palm as well as the dorsum of the hand. Not uncommonly the injury which causes irreparable damage to the digit also creates flexion contracture of other digits by skin loss in the palm.

Example

In this instance, the filleted skin from a useless index finger folded beautifully into the palmar defect left when the soft tissue scar contracture involving the other finger's was released. (**A**)

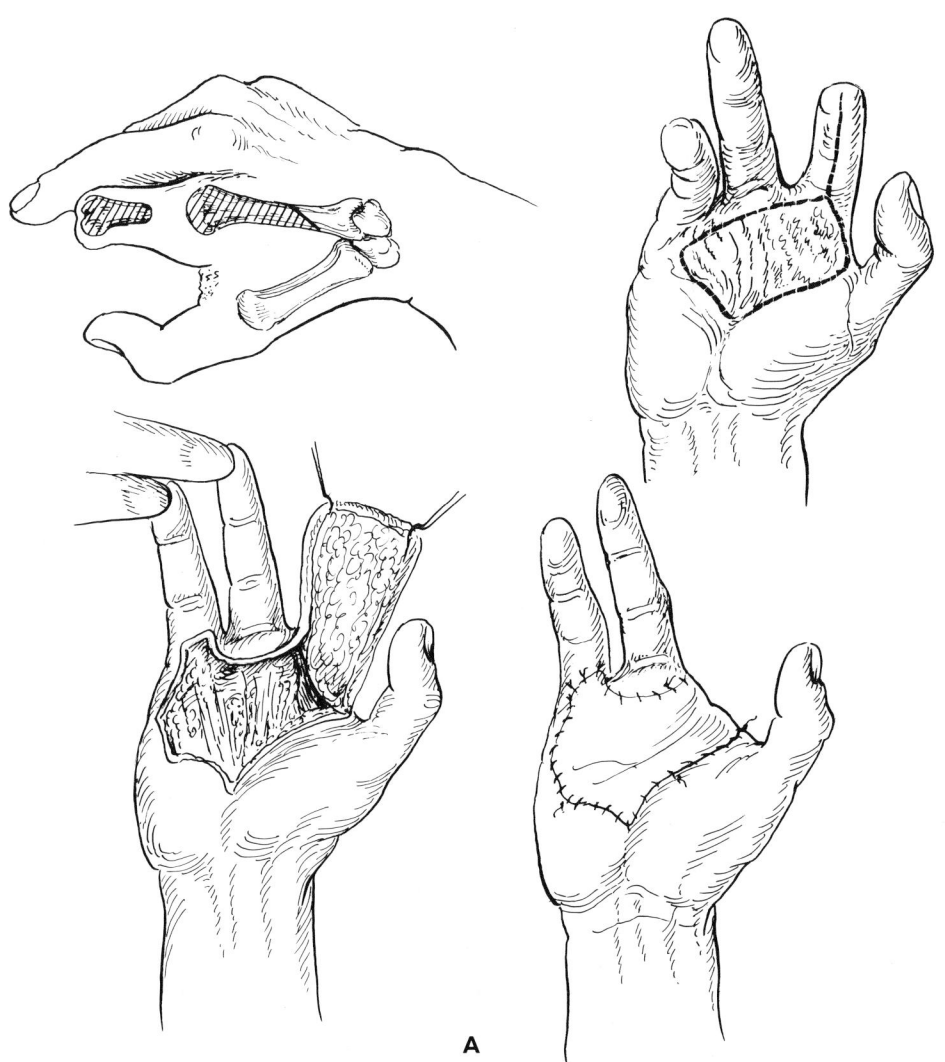

A

23 — Secondary Digital Fillet

Principle — Toe Fillet

The digital fillet technique may usefully be applied to achieve full thickness composite coverage for troublesome areas of the metatarsal head area of the plantar surface of the foot. Amputation of the metatarsal head with the rest of the toe skeleton and the use of the vascularized toe soft tissues may assure that the area of ulceration will not recur.

Example

A chronic ulcer developed in the plantar skin of the patient depicted below. Amputation after fillet was decided upon.

The incision for excision of the ulcer was combined with a mid-plantar digital incision. (**A**)

The level of amputation was planned to remove the prominent and, in this case, offending metatarsal head together with the phalanges and tendons.

After fillet of the soft tissues, the osseous and tendinous elements were amputated. (**B**)

The resulting flap was turned into the sole of the foot and fashioned to fit the defect resulting from excision of the ulcerated area. (**C**)

The toe flap sutured in place brought permanent and excellent blood supply and sensibility to the area. (**D**)

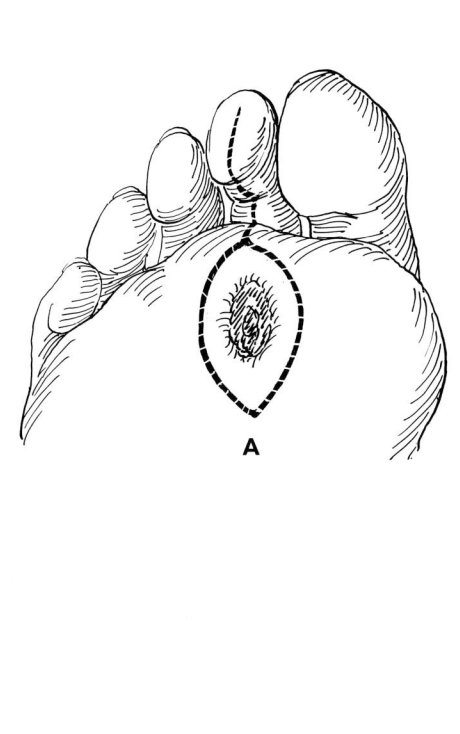
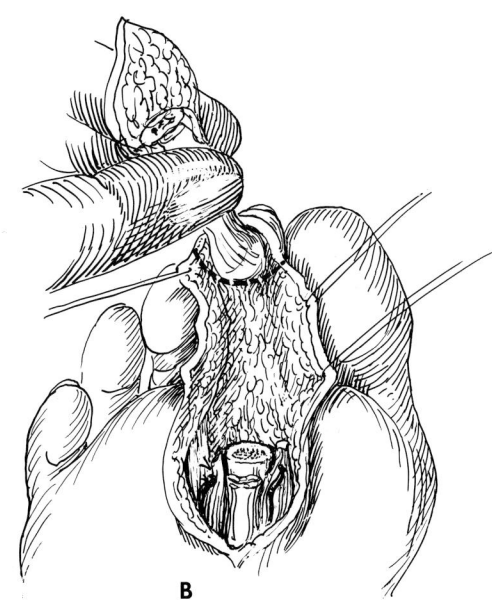
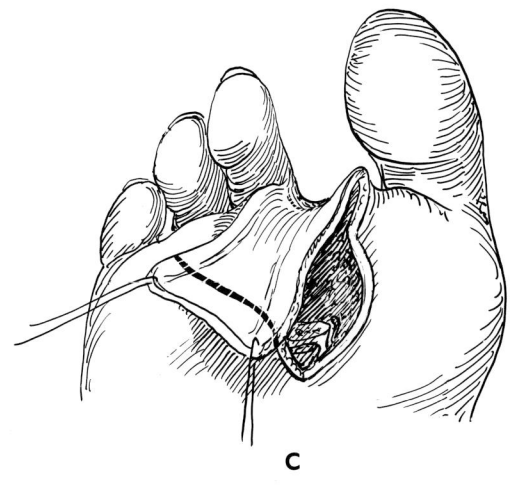
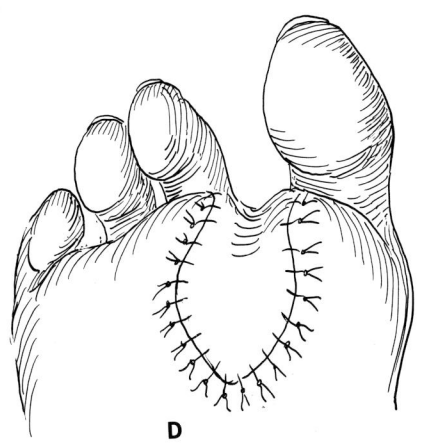

24
Finger Fillet to Resurface the Thumb

Principle

Injury of adjacent digits is common. This sets the stage for shift of useful skin and parts from one such digit destined for amputation to another which will be preserved and reconstructed.

Example

An electrical burn injury to the working palmar surfaces of the thumb and index fingers resulted in total loss of the palmar skin surface of both. The index finger additonally had suffered from tendon injury and irreversible joint destruction with stiffness.

A ray amputation (See Section 33) was done, preserving the vascularized, innervated dorsal skin. (**A** and **B**) The Z-plasty flap shift principle was applied to shift a tongue of skin across the first web space and onto the skinless working surface of the thumb. (**C, D,** and **E**) The web space flap and the dorsal index finger flap were shifted, to surface the new web between the thumb and long finger. (**F, G** and **H**)

Sacrifice of a useless index finger contributed to restoration of the thumb and to overall improved function of the hand.

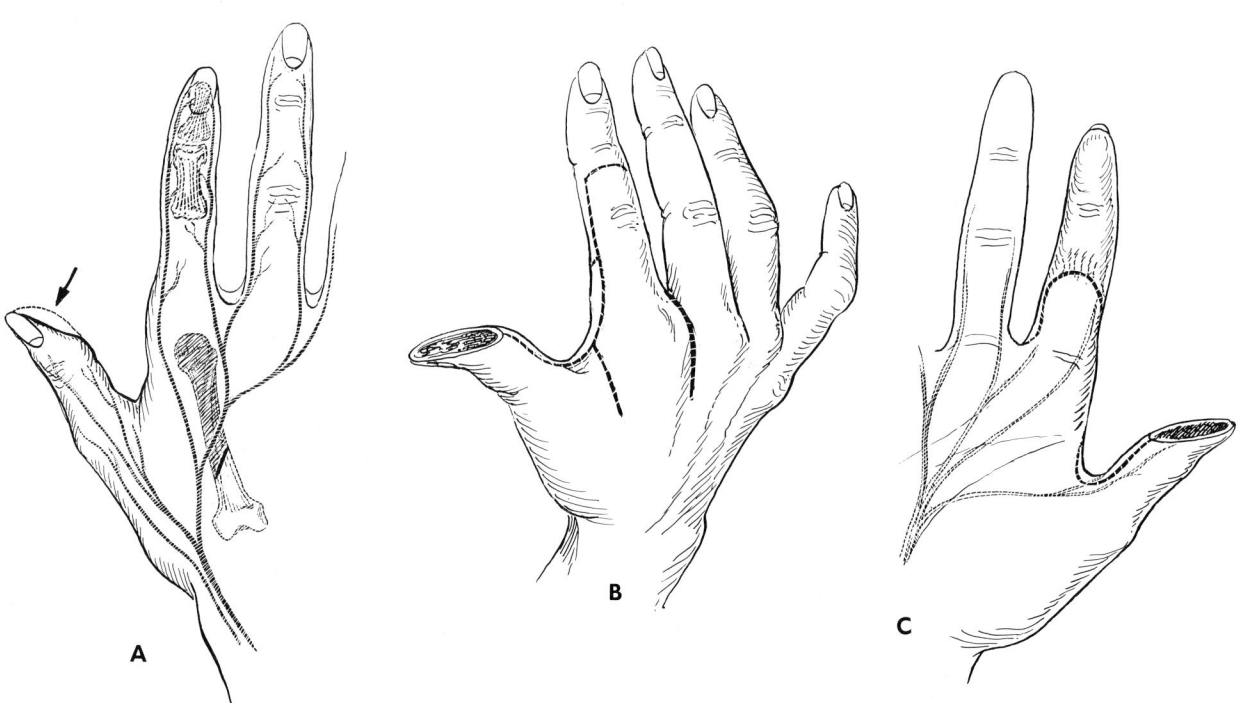

Skin and Soft Tissue Losses

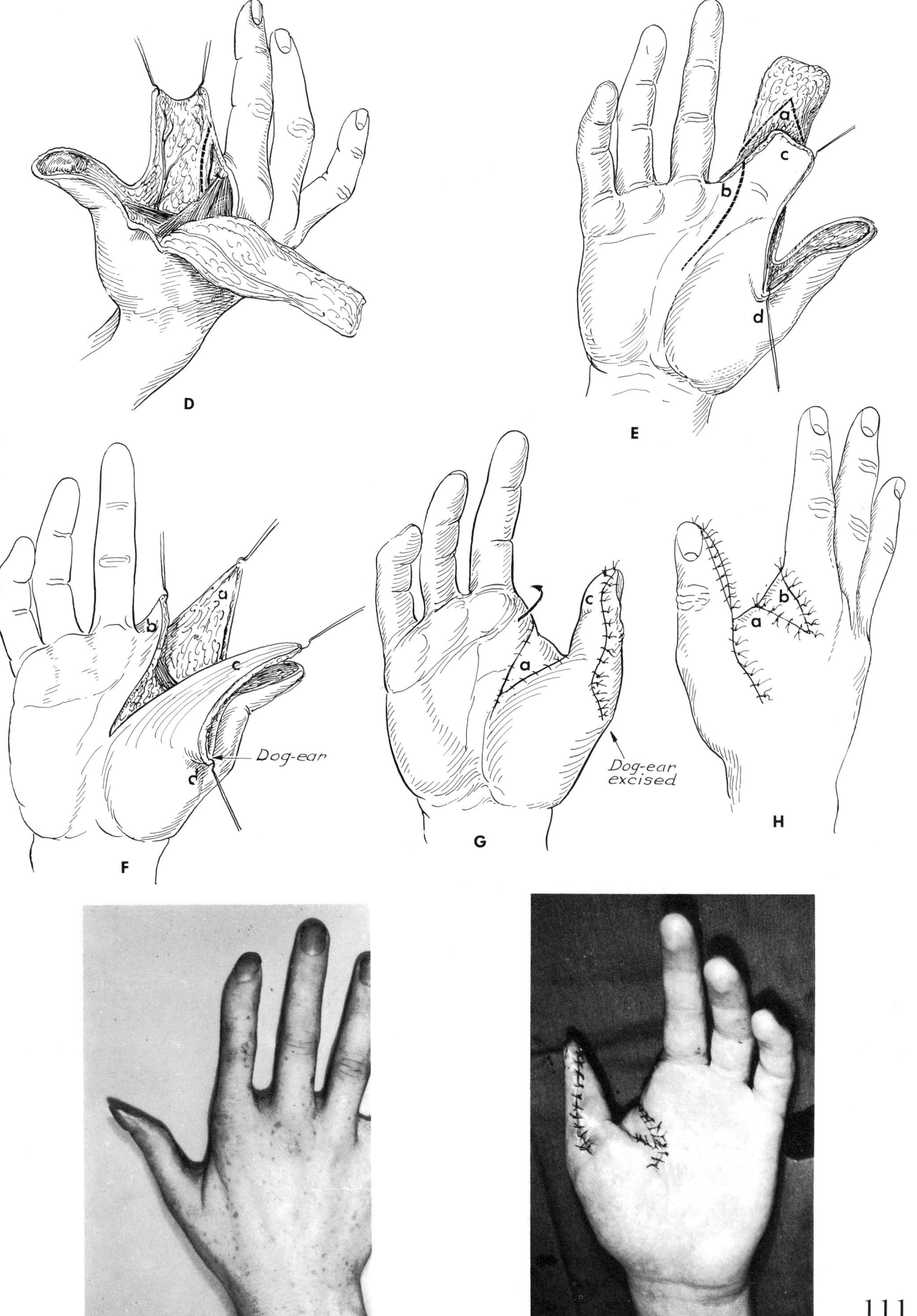

111

25

The Fillet Principle in Acute Injury

Principle

Severe mutilating injuries of the hand on initial examination frequently present an apparent degree of destruction which appears to make reconstruction possibilities hopeless. By rigorous, detailed examination of such a hand and thoughtful consideration of all the alternatives, a pattern of salvage frequently emerges which makes use of many of the surviving parts which initially seemed useless.

Example

A blast injury sustained by a construction worker literally destroyed all palmar structures between the thenar eminence and the fourth metacarpal. The index and long fingers were blasted wide open, with their structures crushed beyond recognition, and the palmar surfaces and bones were pulverized. (**A**) The thumb was blown away from the palm, and its adductor was crushed and avulsed. The thumb fell back along the forearm laying open the carpometacarpal joint. (**B**) The thumb hung by a dorsal pedicle which contained the major deep branch of the radial artery and dorsal branches of the radial nerve. The ring finger was injured but it was anatomically intact as were the structures to it and to the little finger in the palm.

An inventory of surviving parts of the index and long fingers revealed two which might be useful in the overall reconstruction of this badly damaged hand.

One useful surviving part was the dorsal skin, with its intact innervation from the dorsal branch of the radial nerve. The other was the superficialis flexor tendon to the long finger. All other hand elements proximal to the index and long fingers were removed by debridement. (**C**)

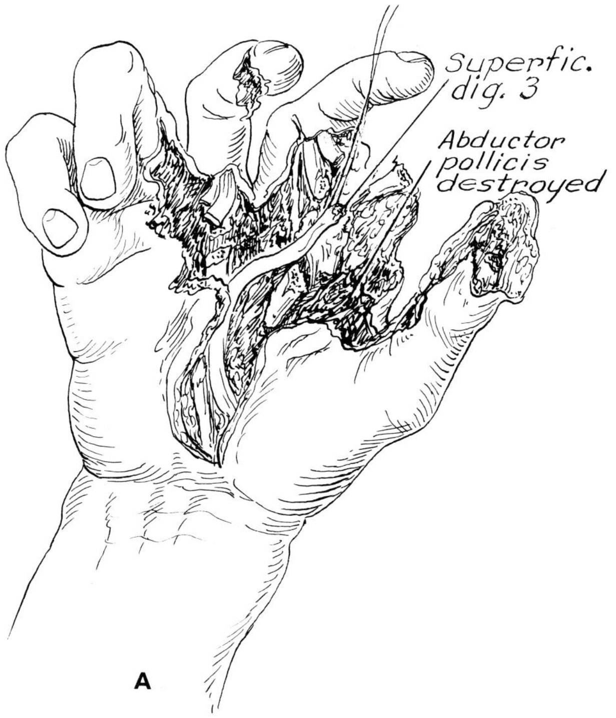

Skin and Soft Tissue Losses

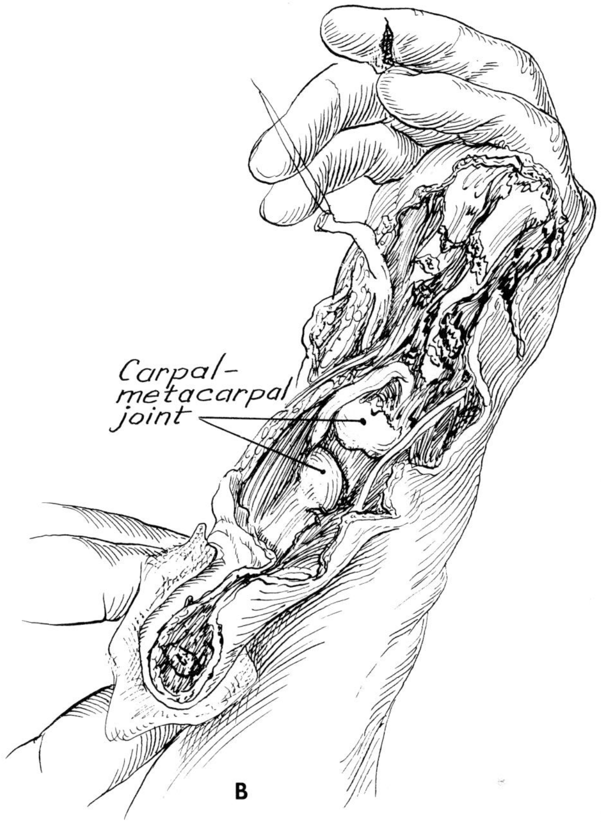

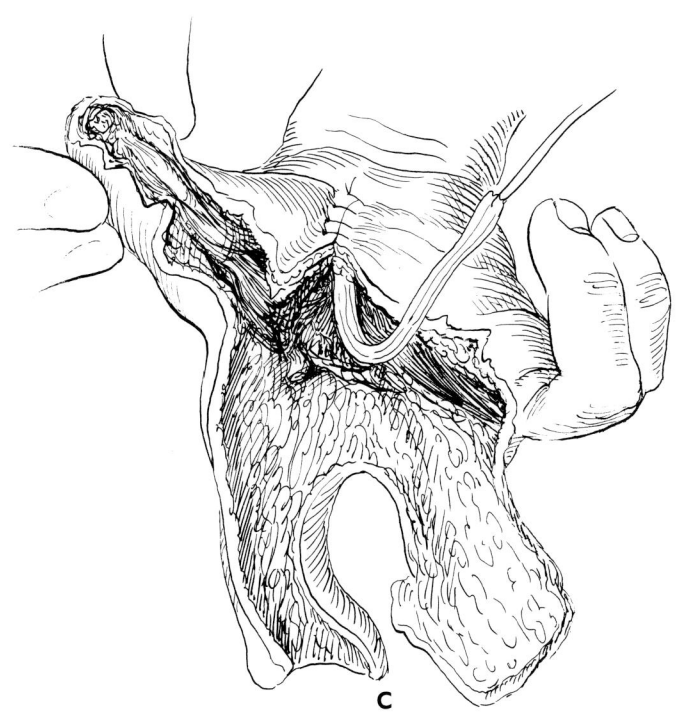

25 – The Fillet Principle in Acute Injury

The long finger superficialis tendon was transferred to the insertion of the destroyed adductor pollicis. (**D**)

The vascularized and innervated dorsal skin flaps from the index and long fingers were adequate to resurface the whole area of skin blown out by the blast. (**E** and **F**)

The functional result was satisfactory without revisional surgery. (**G**)

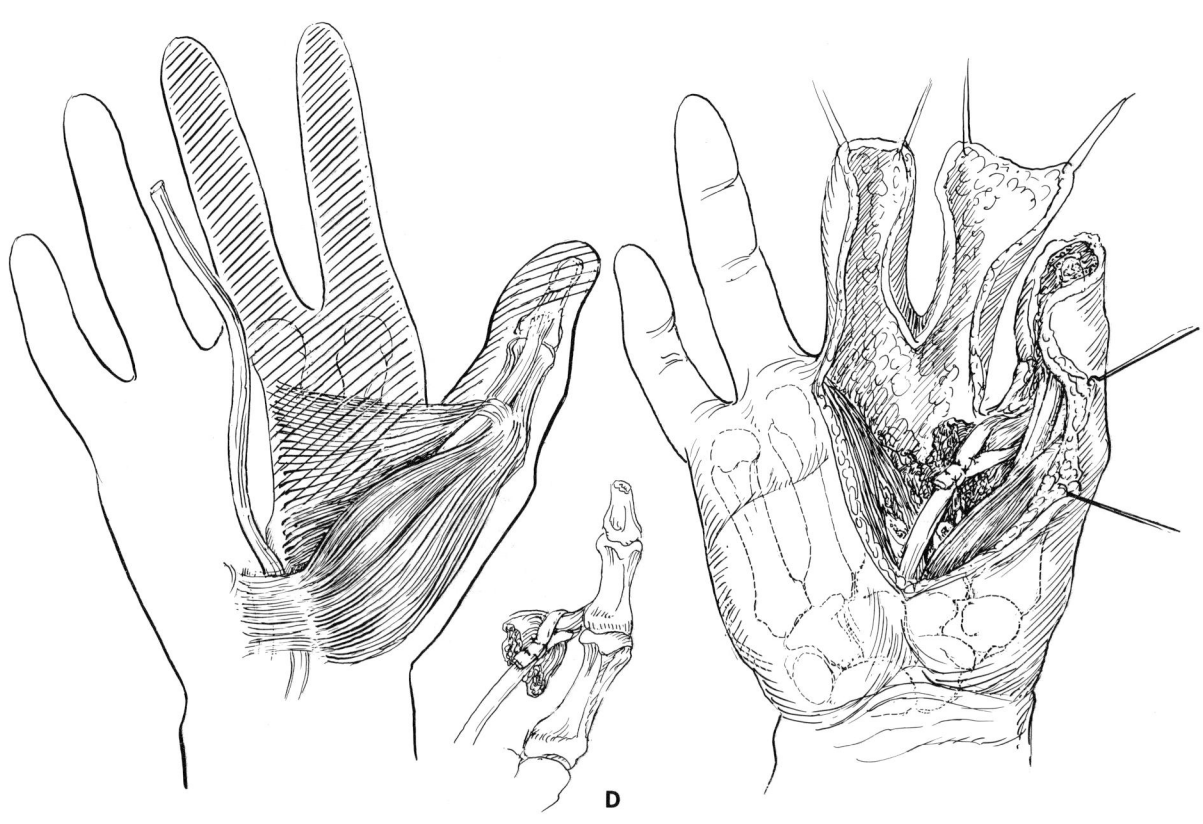

D

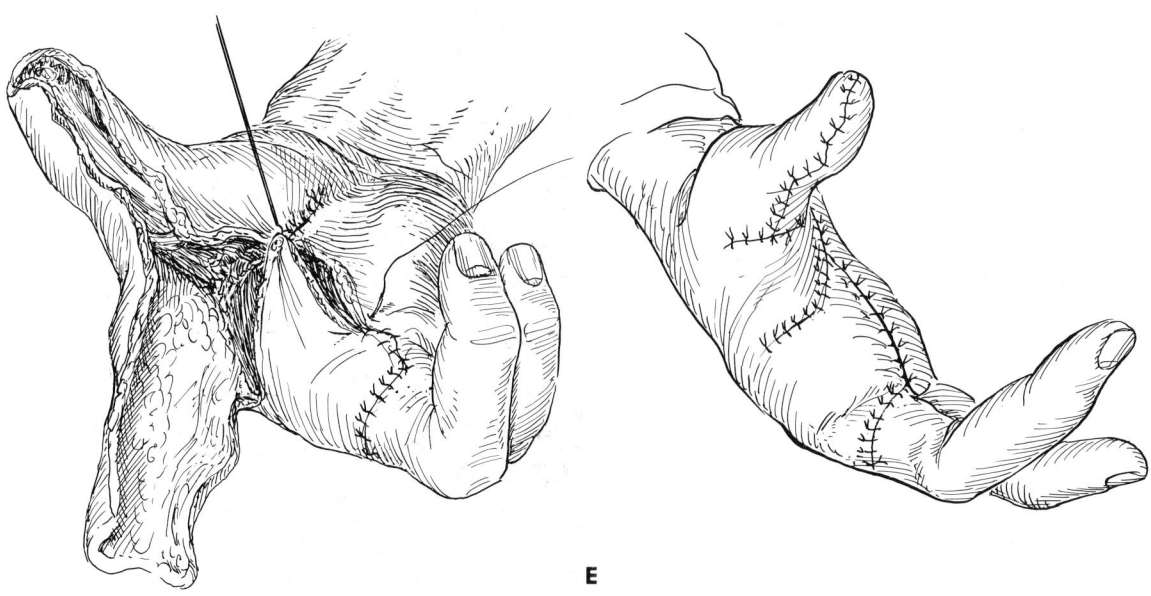

E

Skin and Soft Tissue Losses

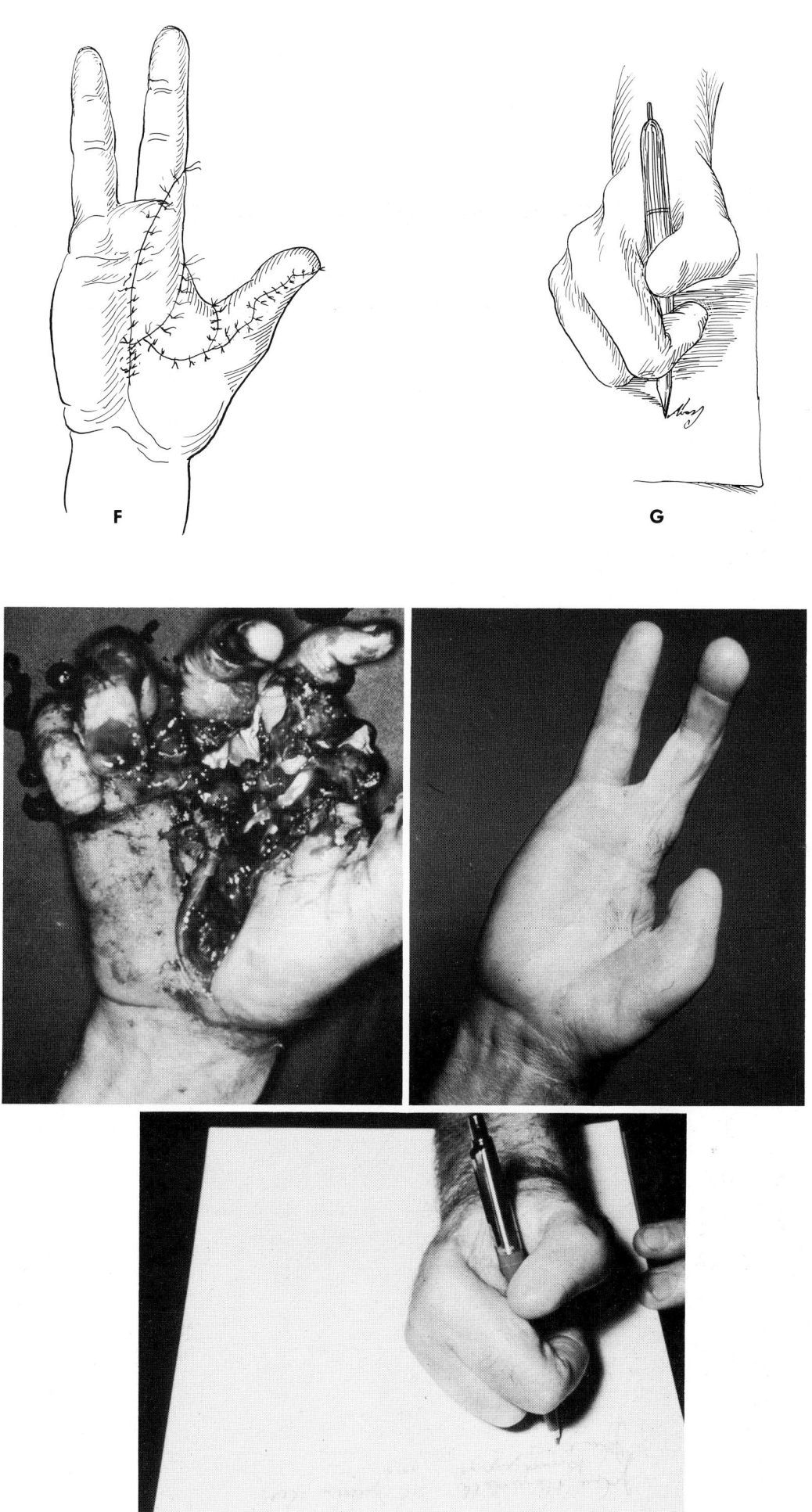

115

26

Two-Stage Amputation with Cross-Finger Flap

Principle

If additional permanent blood supply and innervation from the donor digit is not essential to the reconstruction of another digit, the use of the skin and soft tissues as a two-stage cross-finger flap as part of the amputation is very useful.

Example

This patient had an objectionable index digit nub which he wanted removed for both cosmetic and functional reasons. (See Index Ray Amputation, Section 33.) In addition, however, he had suffered a loss of soft tissue over the radial side of his thumb at the level of the interphalangeal joint. (**A**) This had resulted in a radial fixed deviation of the interphalangeal joint by scar contracture. (**B**)

To correct the deviation by fusion of the interphalangeal joint would leave a soft tissue deficit on the radial side of the thumb. The resulting exposed bone would require as a minimum a vascularized flap of skin.

A ray amputation of the index nub and metacarpal was planned in a manner that would leave the skin temporarily attached to its own bed as a flap to cover the defect in the radial side of the thumb. The flap, planned prior to ray amputation, was marked out on this nub. (**C**)

The soft tissues were filleted and the tendinous and skeletal amputations were carried out as one would perform an index ray amputation. (See Section 33, Index Ray Amputation.) The thumb scar was excised and the radial deviation was corrected by fusion of the interphalangeal joint. (**D**) The pedicle flap was trimmed to fit the defect and was sutured in place. The carrying pedicle was tubed and sutured closed. (**E**)

Skin and Soft Tissue Losses

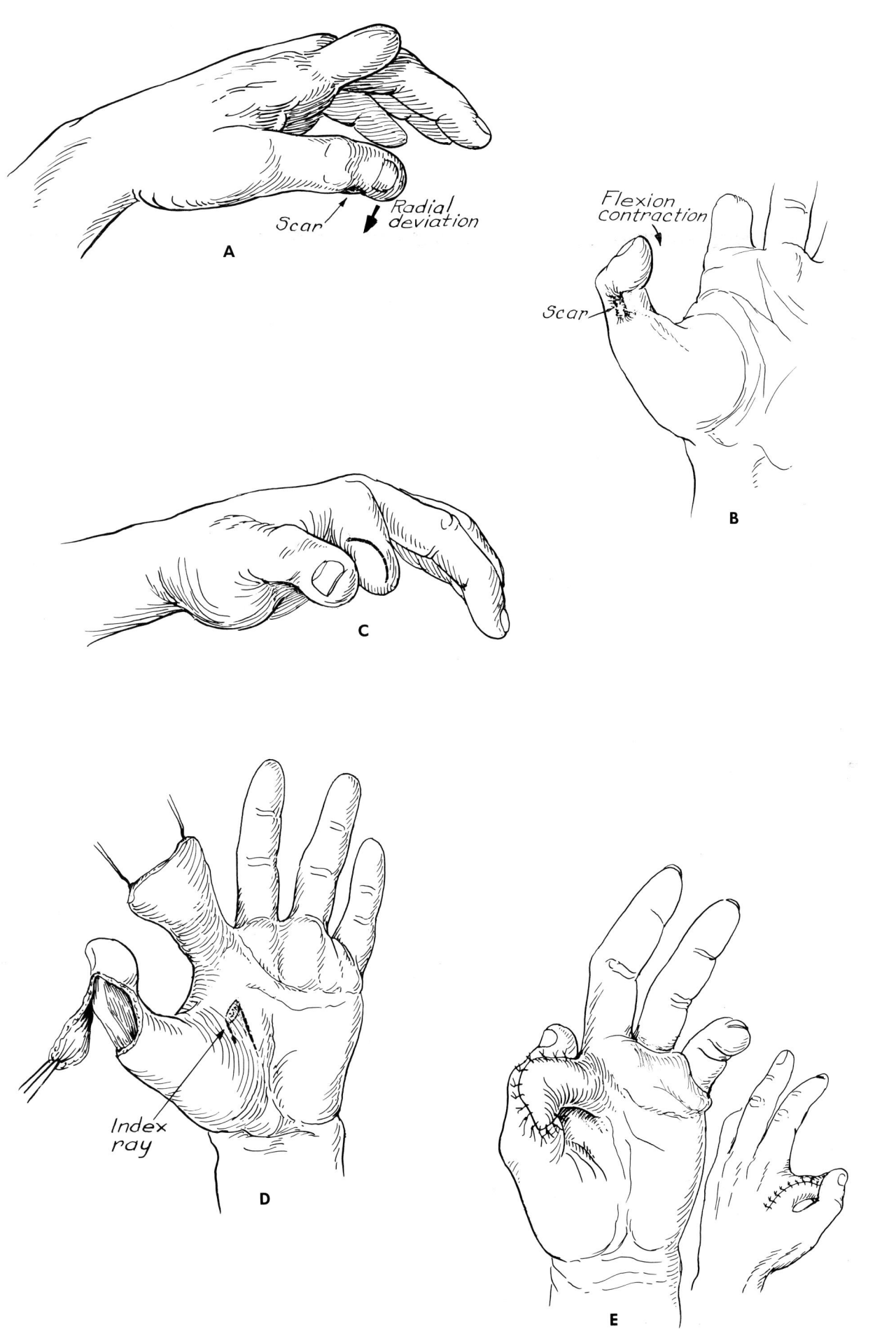

117

26 — Two-Stage Amputation with Cross-Finger Flap

After a three-week period the ray amputation was completed by tailoring the skin both at the thumb implantation site and in the web space. (**F**)

The result left the straightened thumb well covered with full spectrum soft tissue. The desirable effect of ray amputation was achieved, but not until the best use of the superfluous skin was achieved. (**G**)

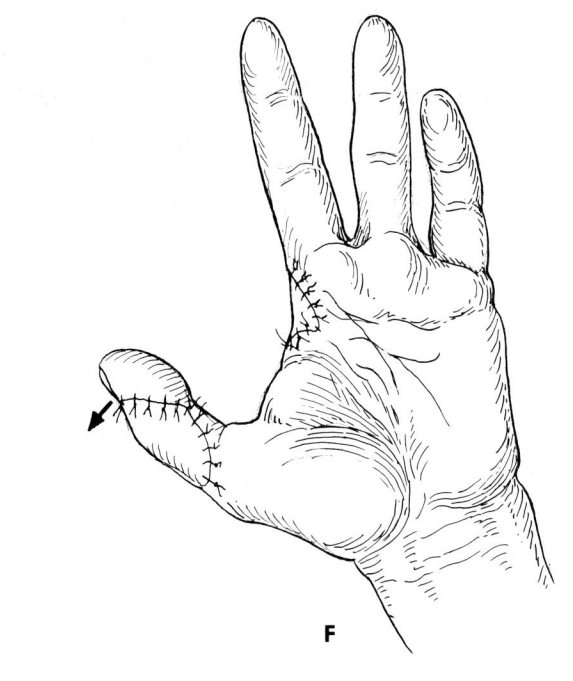

F

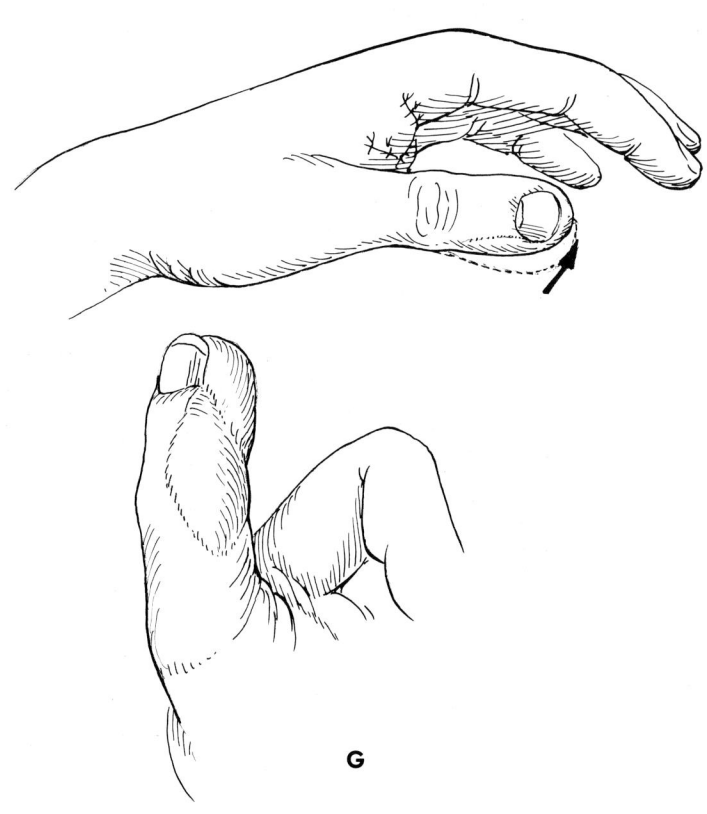

G

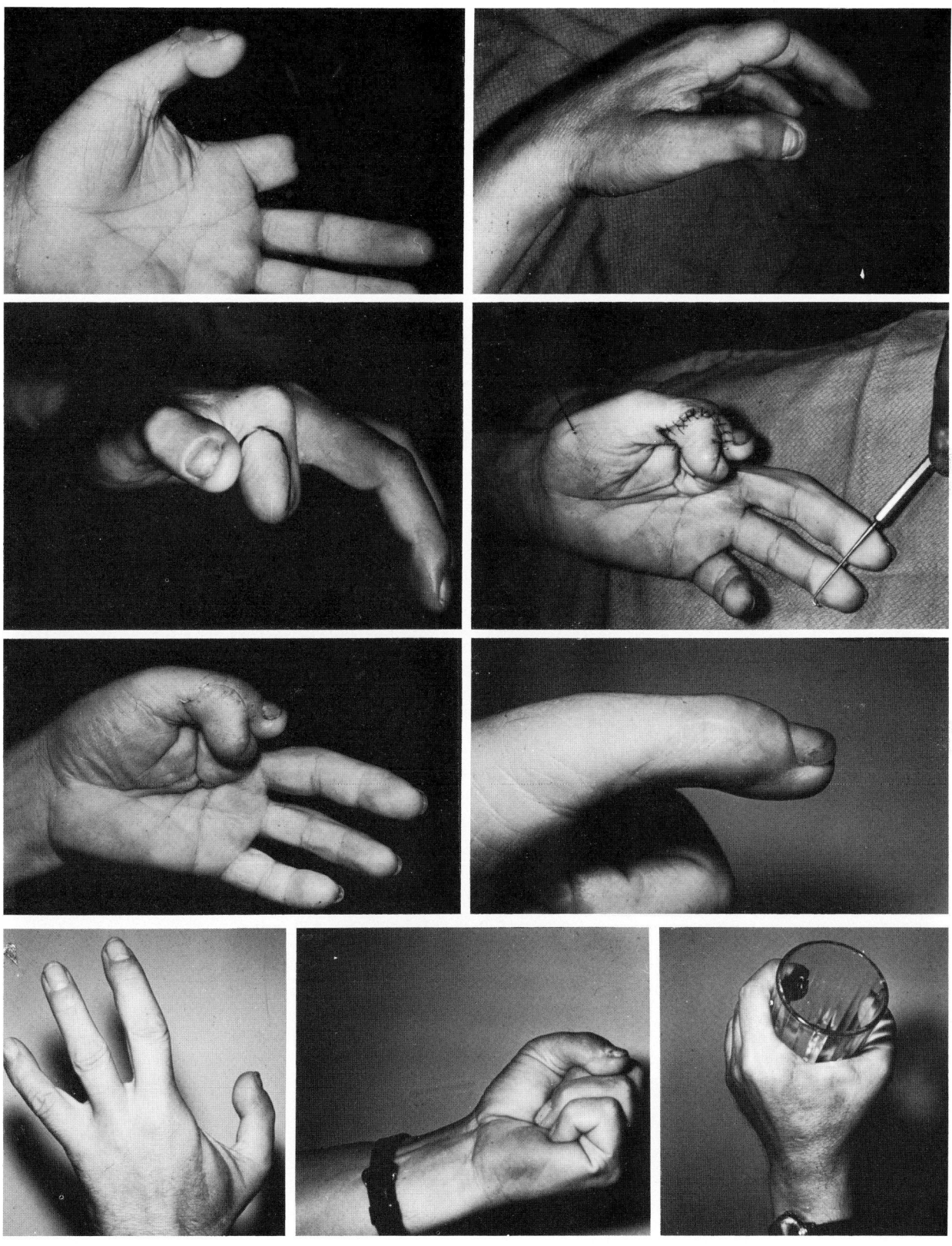

DISTANT PEDICLE FLAPS

27

Pedicle Soft Tissue from Distant Sites

Principle

Whenever possible, vascularized soft tissues for repair and reconstruction of deficits in the hand should be acquired from the hand itself.

When defects are large and pedicle flap tissue is mandatory, the surgeon is forced to use a distant donor site.

Immediate pedicle flap coverage is mandatory where the deficiency of soft tissue leaves structures exposed which will not survive on their own intrinsic blood supply. Obviously, this is true when the structures so salvaged are important in ultimate reconstruction of the hand. To put a patient through the trial of a staged distant pedicle flap procedure to salvage a part which ultimately is to be amputated is poor judgment. Even worse, however, is to lose an essential part of the hand that could have been salvaged by immediate coverage with a well vascularized distant pedicle flap.

Distant pedicle flap transfer may be delayed and done as a secondary procedure if the recipient bed will accept a free skin graft as a temporary form of closure. The distant pedicle flap is then done under better conditions of sterility and at a time of election. The justification for the secondary pedicle flap then is the need for reconstruction of structures beneath the area of soft tissue deficiency.

Large pedicle flaps are obtained from the lower chest or abdominal wall at a site which is appropriate for comfortable positioning of the arm and hand. Smaller pedicle flaps may be obtained from the infraclavicular position of the chest wall.

Using a pattern technique described in Section 13, Cross Finger Flap, a properly oriented flap may be fashioned.

Although the flap is elevated easiest in the areolar plane just superficial to the deep fascia, it should be partially defatted, leaving some fat over the subdermal plexus of vessels.

The donor site is covered, using a split thickness skin graft. The skin graft is carried onto the raw surface of the carrying pedicle to achieve a completely closed wound.

AVULSION ABRASION OF THE DORSUM OF THE HAND WITH LOSS OF SKIN AND TENDONS

Principle

If the nature of an injury with soft tissue loss on the dorsum of the hand is such that later reconstructive procedures will be necessary, coverage with a pedicle flap of skin *and* subcutaneous tissue is essential. One may choose to use the pedicle flap primarily if the circumstances of the wound, such as time since injury, contamination, and associated injuries are appropriate. Alternatively, immediate closure with a thin split thickness skin graft followed by healing, autosterilization and patient recovery will allow a deliberate well planned, secondary pedicle flap to be applied.

Example

A grinding avulsion injury over the dorsum of the hand and forearm was sustained in this case. (**A**) The extensor tendons to the fingers were destroyed *over the level of the metacarpals*.

The severity of the total injury to the patient and the nature of the wound itself contraindicated a primary pedicle flap procedure. The wounds were debrided and a split thickness skin graft was applied. (**B**)

After the wounds healed, the patient regained good function except that the metacarpophalangeal joints could not be flexed—particularly when the interphalangeal joints were in flexion. It was evident that the distal ends of the extensor tendons were adherent over the distal dorsal aspect of the metacarpals.

In order to release the extensor tendons and to reconstruct them with tendon grafts, full spectrum of skin with subcutaneous fat was needed over the area of planned tendon reconstruction. An abdominal pedicle flap was planned. The split thickness skin graft was dissected from the radial toward the ulnar side of

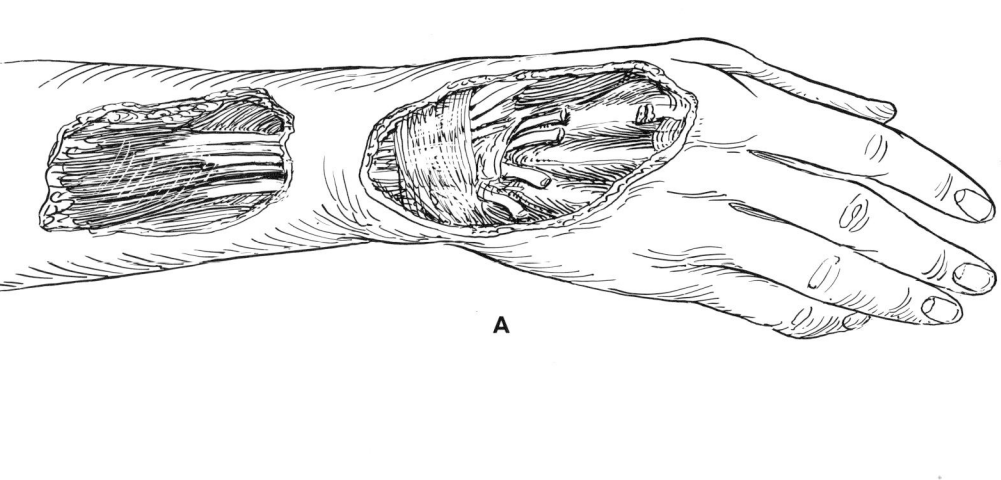

A

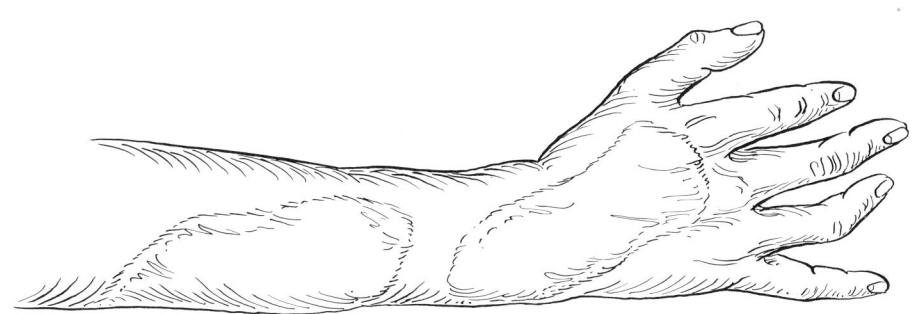

B

27 — Pedicle Soft Tissue from Distant Sites

the hand and was left attached along the ulnar border. (**C**) The extensor tendons were released from the metacarpals and the metacarpophalangeal joints were put passively through a full range of motion with the interphalangeal joints flexed.

A large, inferiorly based pedicle flap on the opposite side of the abdominal wall was planned using a pattern technique. (See Section 13, Cross Finger Flaps). The blood supply to the abdominal skin comes from each side of the abdomen toward the midline. The flap and pedicle should not cross the midline in a manner which would compromise circulation to the tip of the flap.

The pedicle flap was elevated in the avascular areolar plane over the deep fascia. The portion of the flap to be applied to the hand was partially defatted leaving a thin layer of fat over the subdermal plexus of blood vessels.

The pedicle flap donor site was covered with a split thickness skin graft held in place with silk sutures left long to use to tie over a dressing. The skin graft was carried on to the base of the pedicle flap to surface all except the part used to cover the denuded surface of the hand. Silk sutures inserted through the graft and into deep fascia of the abdominal wall were placed along the line where the pedicle flap was based. (**D**) The tie-over dressing then placed no tension on the pedicle itself.

The peeled, previously applied skin graft from the recipient hand was appropriately trimmed and sutured to the skin graft applied to the raw side of the pedicle to get a closed under surface for the pedicle. (**E**) Two incisions were made across the linear longitudinal incision on the radial side of the wound to break up the straight line crossing the wrist.

The pedicle flap was fitted to the defect with the hand and arm held loosely against the trunk. The straight line along the radial side of the wrist was broken by cutting transversely in two places and then fitting the flap to the resulting curved line. The flap was sutured in place as precisely as possible. (**F**)

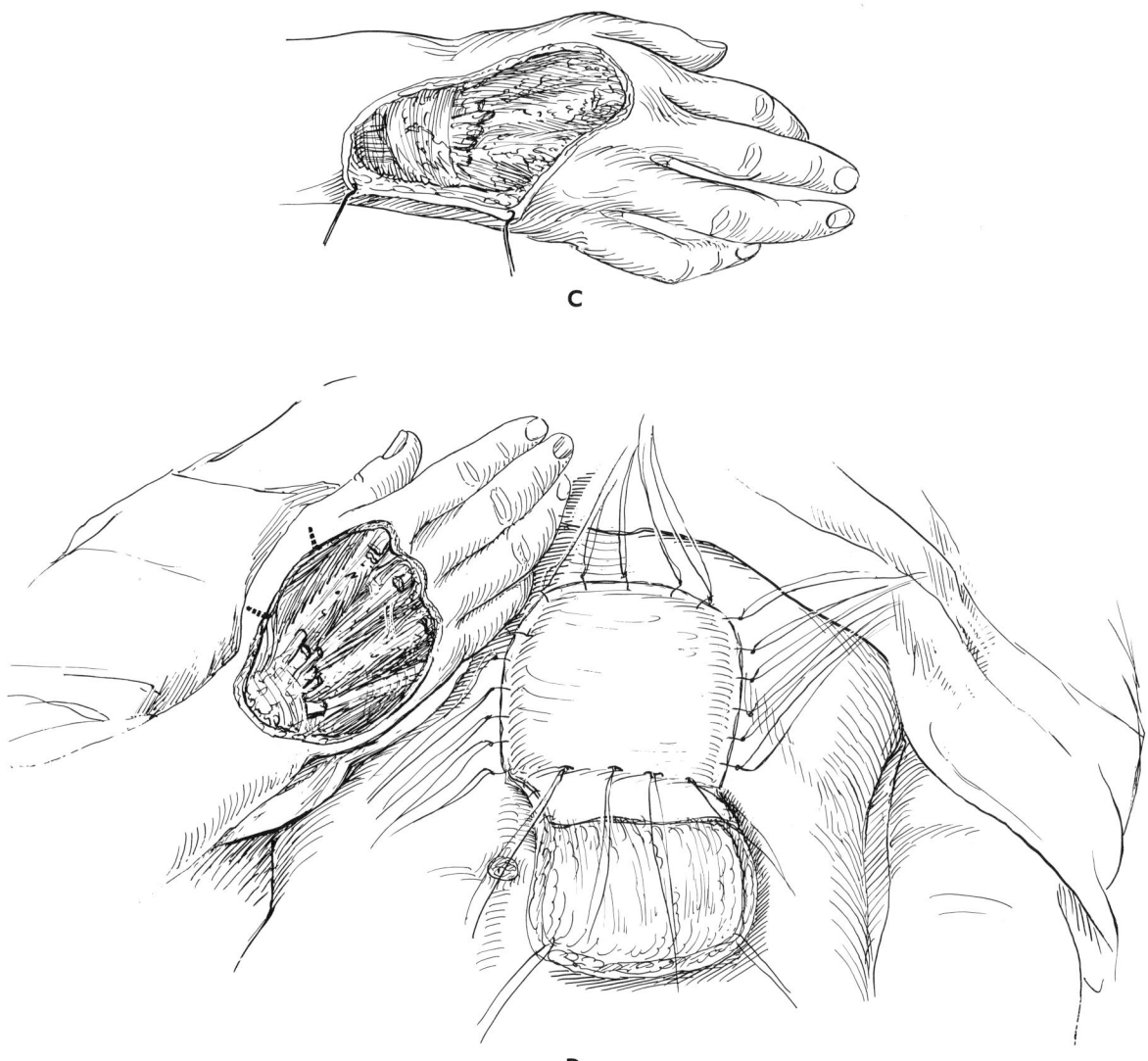

C

D

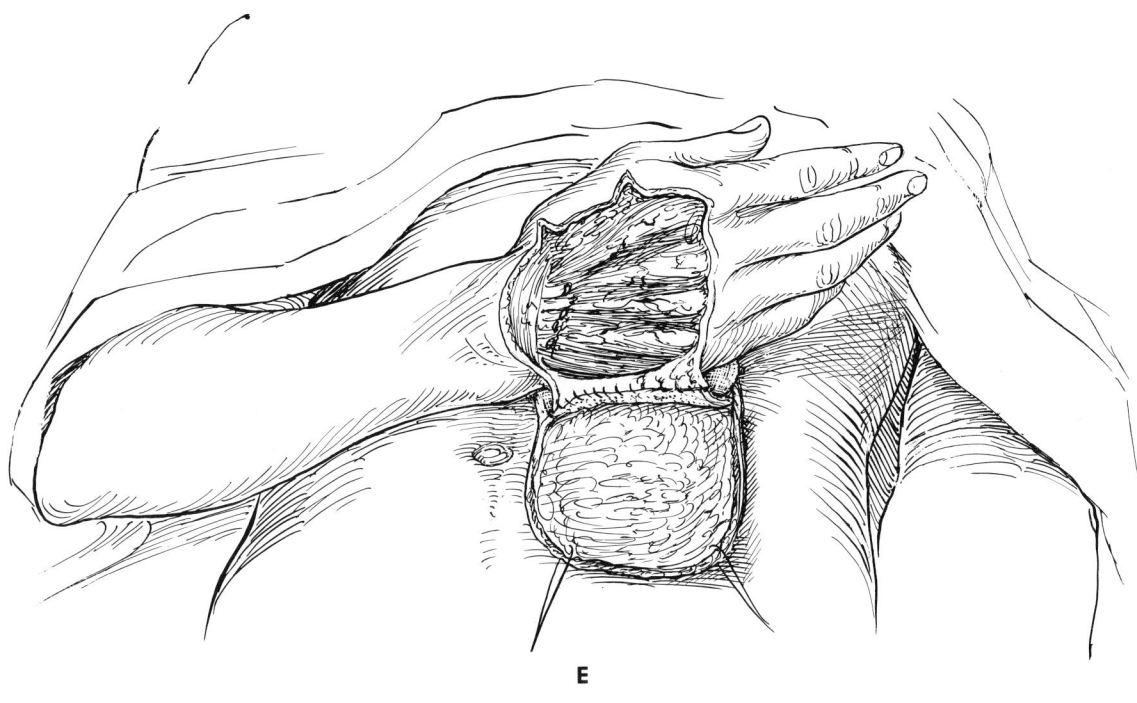

E

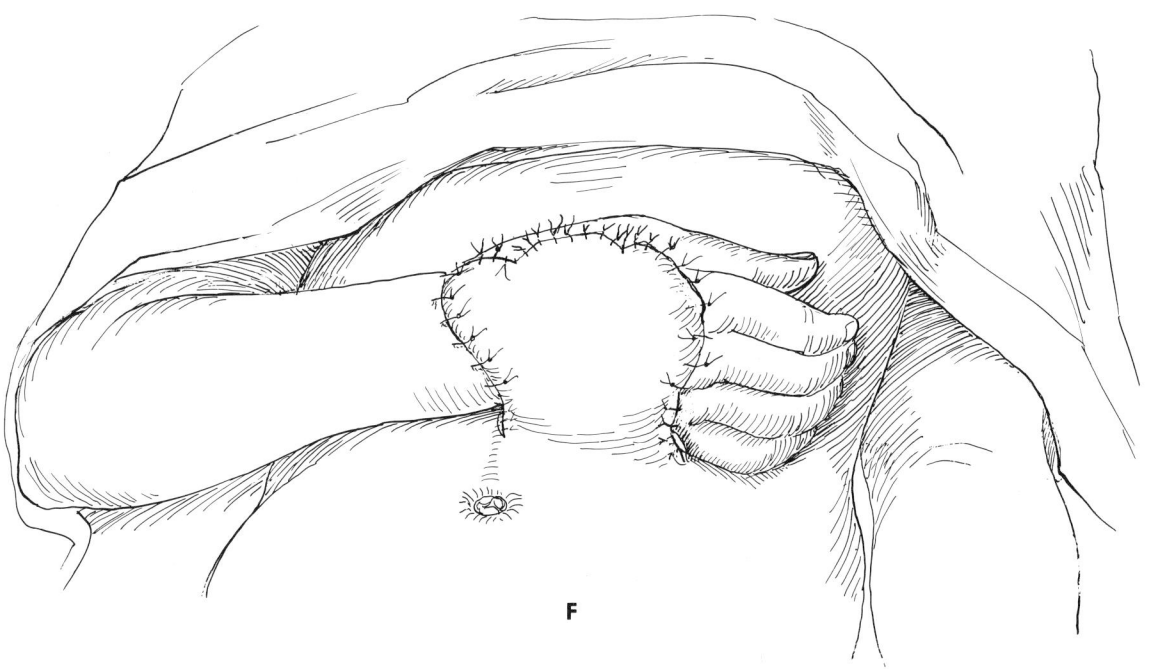

F

After three weeks of healing the pedicle was transected in curvilinear fashion along the ulnar side of the hand. The abdominal wound and hand wounds were closed leaving skin with subcutaneous tissues over the area of previous deficit.

After several months of passive and active range of motion exercises, tendon grafts to the digital extensors were implanted. The plantaris tendon and palmaris longus served as tendon grafts. An incision over the extensor mechanism at the metacarpophalangeal joint level of each finger was executed. The recipient extensor mechanism was prepared to receive a graft by exposing it at the metacarpophalangeal joint, checking its range of motion and releasing it from metacarpal adhesions where they existed.

A tendon tunneler (a neurosurgery alligator forceps may be used) was passed blindly through the pedicle flap's subcutaneous fat in a direction appropriate to achieve proper directional pull to restore long extensor tendon function. (**G**)

Separate tendon grafts to each finger were pulled through subcutaneous tunnels and the proximal ends were sutured to the extensor digitorum tendons in the case of the ulnar three fingers and to the extensor indicis for the index tendon graft.

After closure of the proximal wounds, the distal ends of the tendon grafts were woven into the central extensor tendon over the metacarpophalangeal joint and sutured after adjustment of tension. Tension adjustment was made by placing the wrist in a relaxed neutral position then fixing the graft with the metacarpophalangeal joint midway between flexion and extension. (**H**) The index finger metacarpophalangeal joint was extended about five degrees more than that of the long finger. The ring finger metacarpophalangeal was flexed about five degrees more than that of the long finger and the little finger metacarpophalangeal was flexed about five degrees more than that of the ring finger. This placed the fingers in proper functional relationship with one another. After the tendons were securely sutured, one could passively fully flex the fingers with the wrist in full extension, and wrist flexion pulled the metacarpophalangeal joints into extension.

The wrist and metacarpophalangeal joints were splinted in extension for 5 weeks after grafting and then gentle *active* motion was initiated. Passive pull on the extensor grafts was put off till 6 or 8 weeks had passed after the operation.

Skin and Soft Tissue Losses

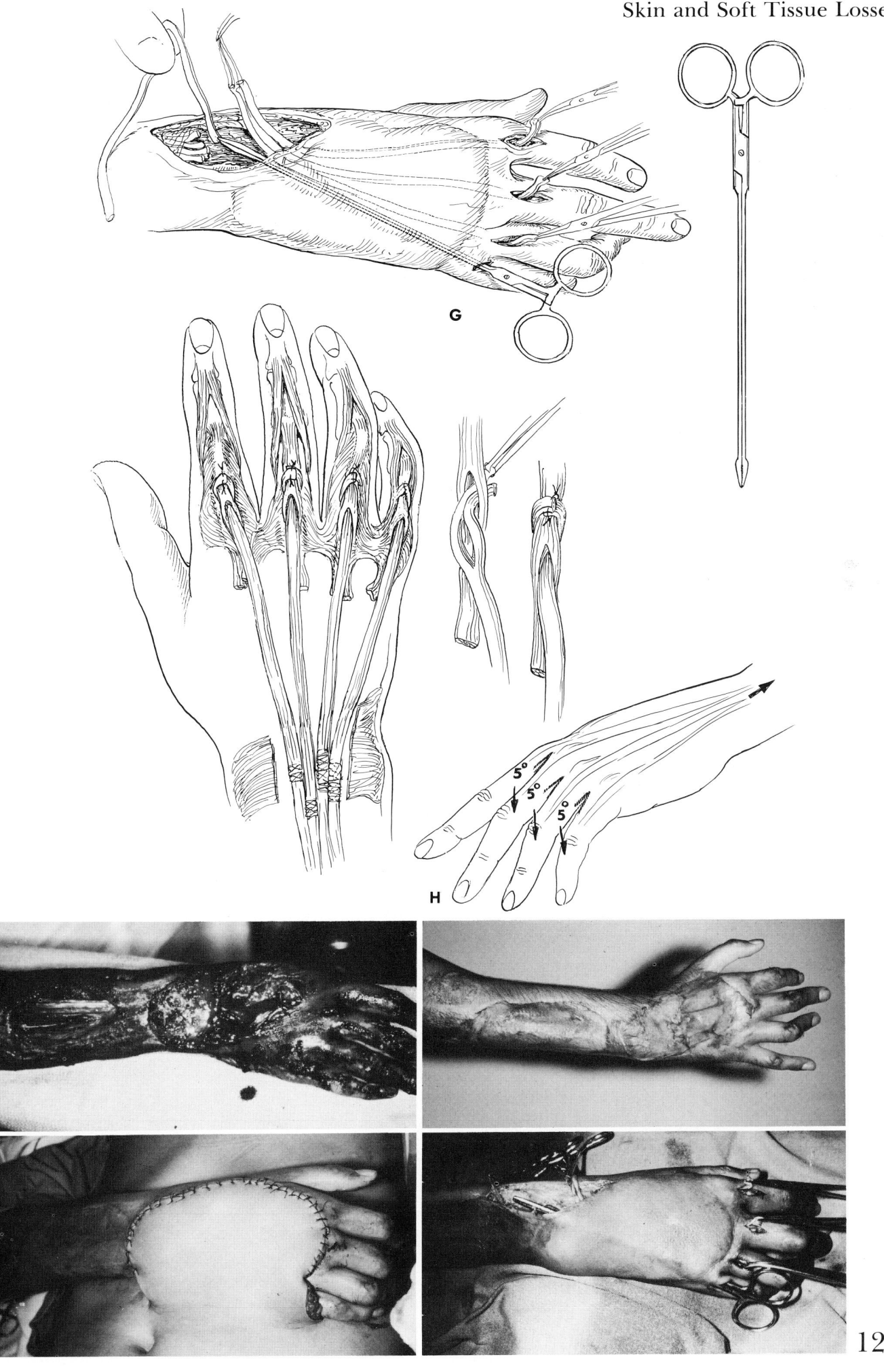

125

28

The Infraclavicular Flap

Advantages

The infraclavicular area of the contralateral chest wall is a useful pedicle flap donor site for the following reasons:

1. The skin is thin and more like hand skin than that elsewhere on the trunk.
2. The skin blood supply is excellent in this area.
3. The hand immobilized in the infraclavicular area is automatically elevated for good venous return in both the supine and upright posture.
4. The hand assumes a functional position with fingers flexed around the anterior axillary fold when the flap is used on the thumb. (**A** and **B**)
5. The position is natural and comfortable.
6. The flap may easily be tubed to cover circumferential defects or to lengthen a shortened digit.

Disadvantages

The disadvantages of the infraclavicular donor site are:

1. The size of flap obtainable from this area is limited.
2. Only the distal part of the extremity (hand) will reach the infraclavicular area comfortably.
3. The scar is left in a suboptimum position and thus the procedure is not used in female patients.
4. The area is sometimes very hairy and therefore not usable.

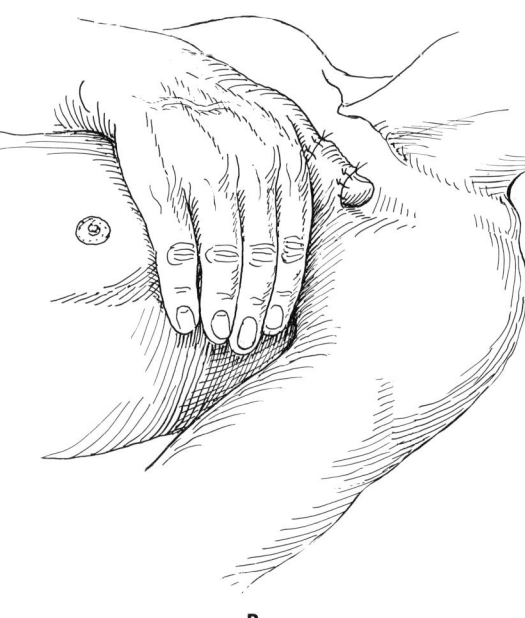

B

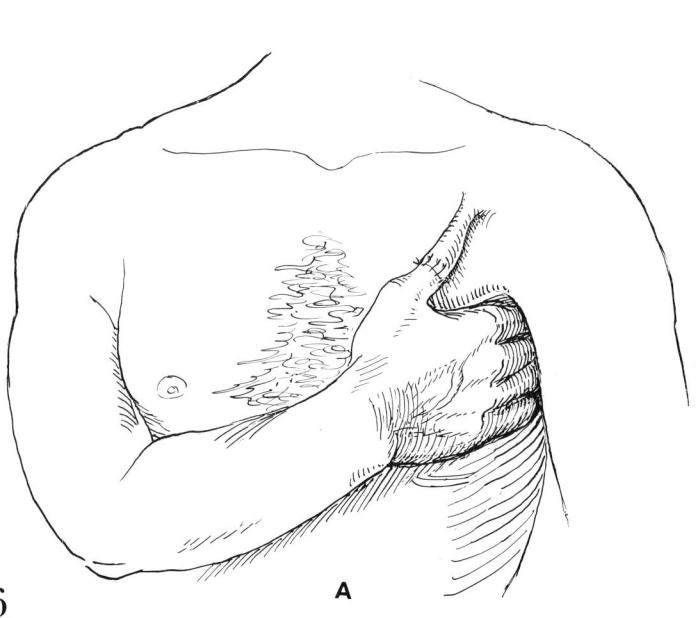

A

AVULSION AMPUTATION OF THE THUMB WITH LOSS OF SKIN IN EXCESS OF BONE

Principle

Amputation of the thumb with loss of soft tissues in excess of bone should *not* be treated by additional shortening to achieve skin closure. Vascularized skin and subcutaneous tissue must be utilized to salvage the denuded skeletal elements. If the defect is small, local vascularized flaps as transfers from the hand may be used. If the defect is large, a distant vascularized pedicle flap is required.

Example

Amputation of the thumb with loss of soft tissues in excess of bone too extensive for local pedicle flap closure required a distant pedicle flap. (**A**)

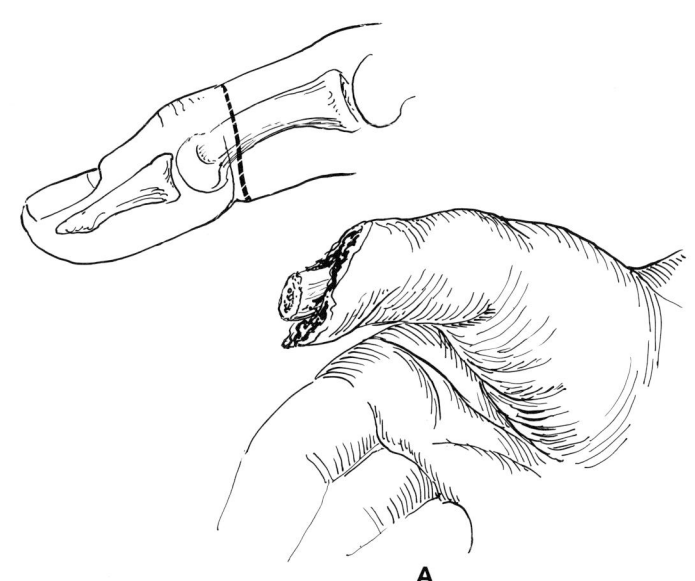

28 — The Infraclavicular Flap

A pedicle flap based in the deltoid area using infraclavicular skin and subcutaneous tissue was appropriate. The flap was outlined using a fabric pattern (See Section 13, Cross-Finger Flap), with the hand comfortably against the pectoral area and the fingers flexed around the anterior axillary fold. (**B**)

The flap was elevated in the areolar plane over the pectoralis muscle but prior to transfer it was sharply defatted. (**C**) All but a thin layer of fat deep to the subdermal vascular plexus was removed. This avoided the commonly seen bulky, flabby reconstructed thumb.

The pedicle flap was sutured to the thumb, and the carrying pedicle was tubed thus achieving a closed wound. (**D**) The skin left on the thumb was shifted to the palmar working surface. This preserved the most precise sensibility for the working surface of the thumb.

Immobilization of the hand and arm was achieved by applying tape to the arm and trunk after painting (or spraying) the skin with tincture of benzoin. Fluffed gauze and abdominal pad dressings were placed between the arm and trunk and in the axilla to avoid skin-to-skin contact. (Failure to separate skin surfaces will result in maceration and untidy dressings with increased potential for contamination and infection.)

Two or three weeks after the flap was ap-

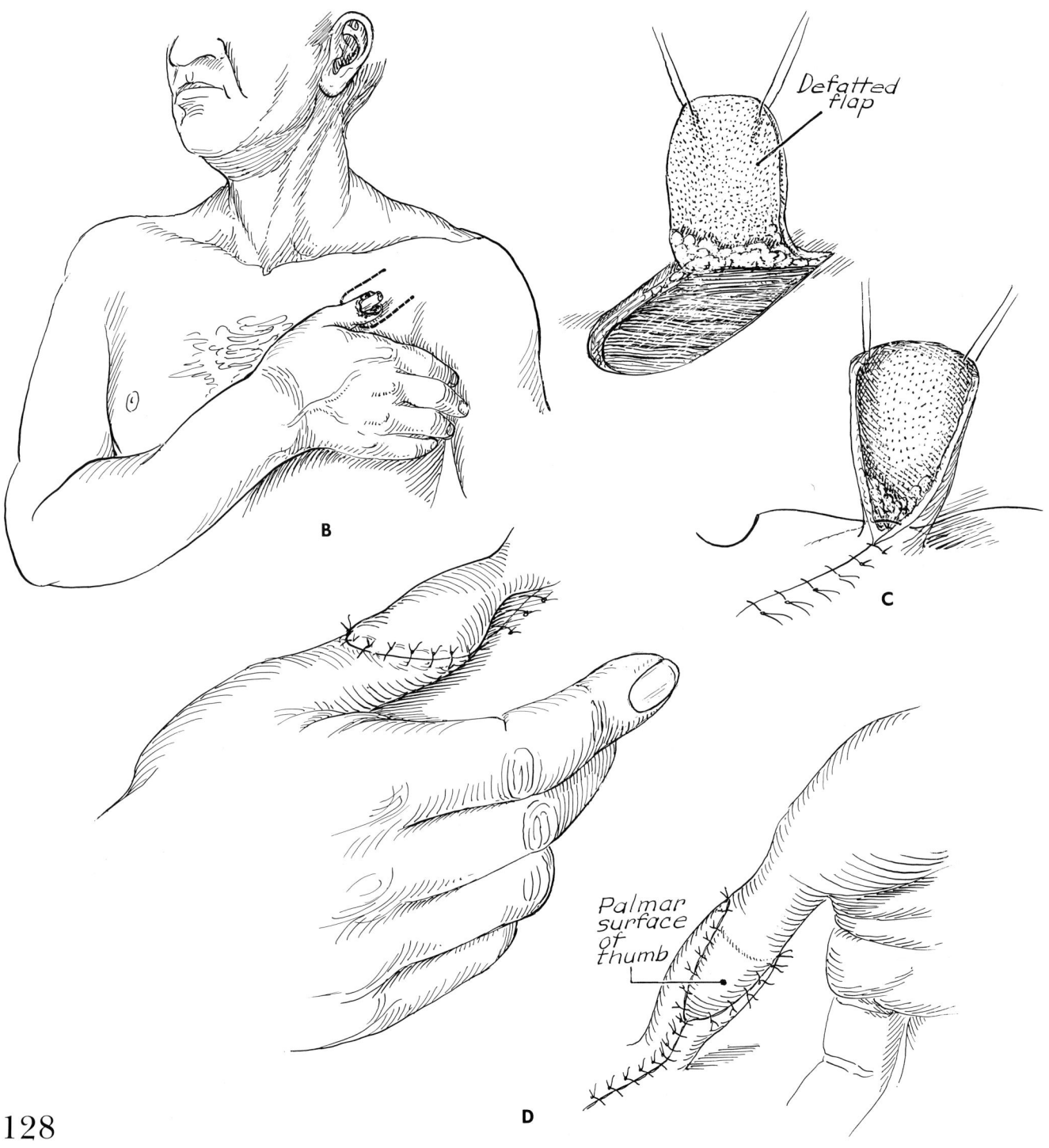

Skin and Soft Tissue Losses

plied, healing was adequate to allow separation of the hand from the chest wall, and the end of the transferred flap was fashioned to restore proper thumb contour. (**E** and **F**)

Length was preserved by the distant pedicle flap and sensibility was preserved over the working surface of the thumb.

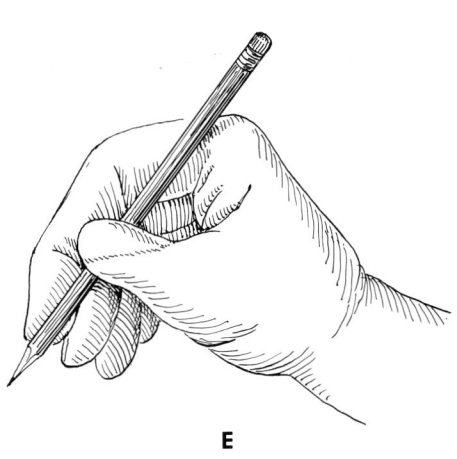

E

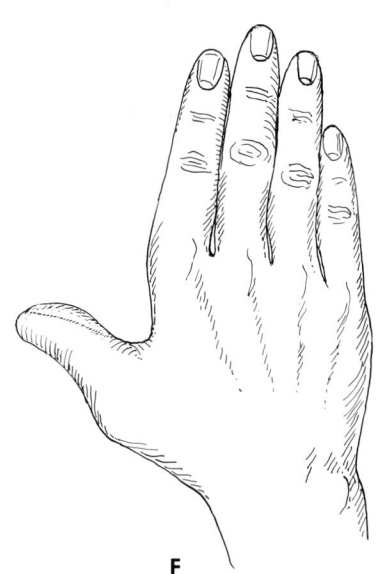

F

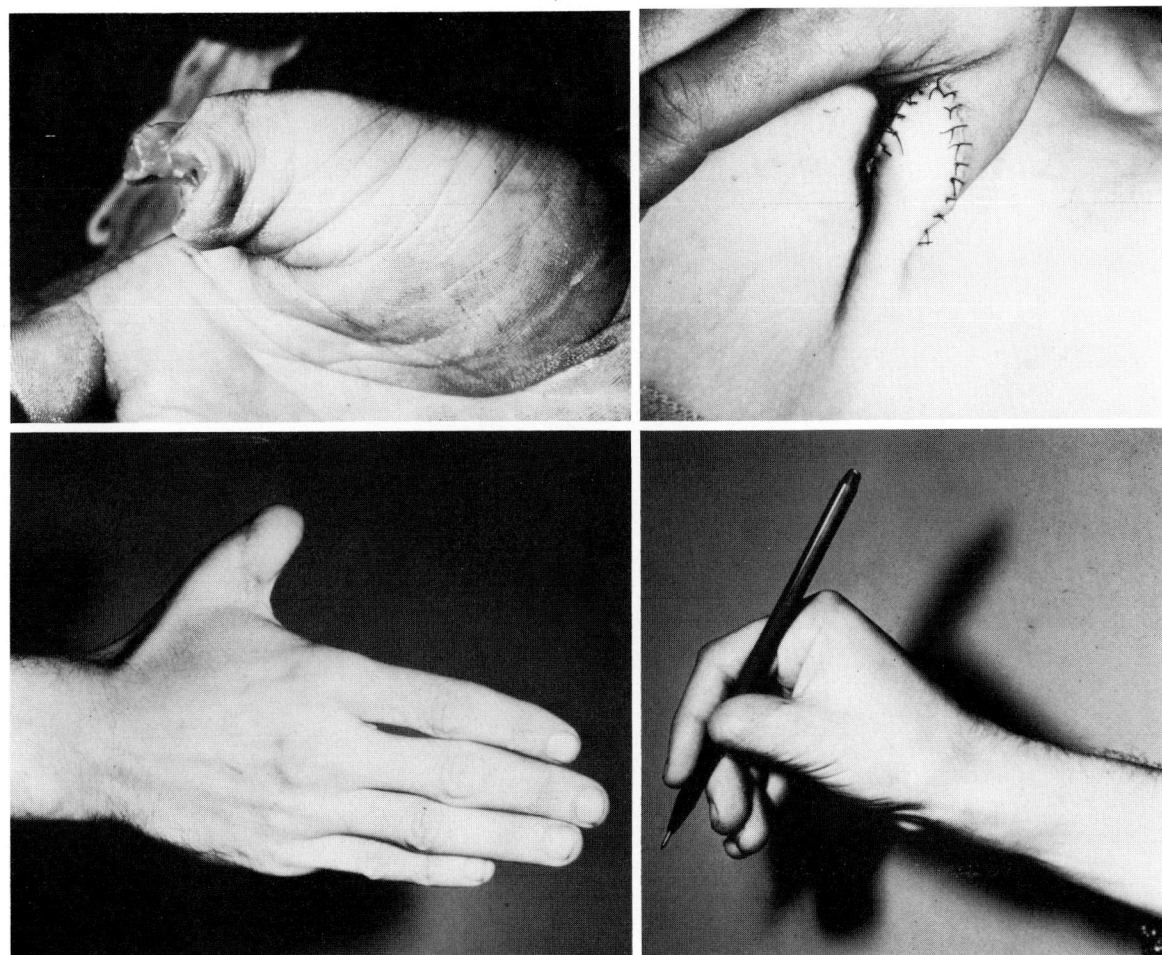

RING AVULSION OF SKIN FROM A FINGER

Principle

A ring which catches during a fall or is itself caught on a moving object may create devastating injury to the finger. Injury varies from complete avulsion amputation to severe contusion. Commonly, all dorsal soft tissues are avulsed by the ring, and the distal phalanx with all its soft tissues is also traumatically avulsed.

In general, if the dorsal avulsion is in the areolar plane over the extensor tendons, a free skin graft may be used to salvage the remaining finger. If the injury is such that a free skin graft will not take, *primary amputation is logical treatment and must seriously be considered.*

Occasionally, when there is adequate palmar skin with sensibility left on the finger, the surgeon might choose to preserve the finger using a vascularized pedicle flap.

A convenient place to obtain a trunk flap of such vascularized, thin skin and subcutaneous tissue is the infraclavicular area. A deltoid based flap planned by the pattern technique (see Section 13, Cross Finger Flap) is appropriate for skin and subcutaneous coverage for a digit.

The scar left at the donor area may not be appropriate in some patients. An alternate donor site such as the inframammary area, abdominal wall, or the opposite arm may be selected by the patient's or surgeon's preference. The donor site may be closed and the pedicle base may be tubed to achieve a closed wound at the time of application of the flap to the hand.

Example

A 32-year-old male patient caught his ring on the tailgate of a moving pickup truck and sustained a ring avulsion injury of the left ring finger. All of the dorsal soft tissue superficial to the extensors was avulsed and the distal phalanx was traumatically amputated. (**A**) Amputation of the finger was suggested but the patient refused, asking that an attempt be made to save the finger at any cost. An immediate infraclavicular pedicle flap was chosen as treatment.

A flap of skin and subcutaneous tissue tailored to appropriate proportions was raised from the right infraclavicular area. It was defatted to avoid a bulky finger. (**B** and **C**)

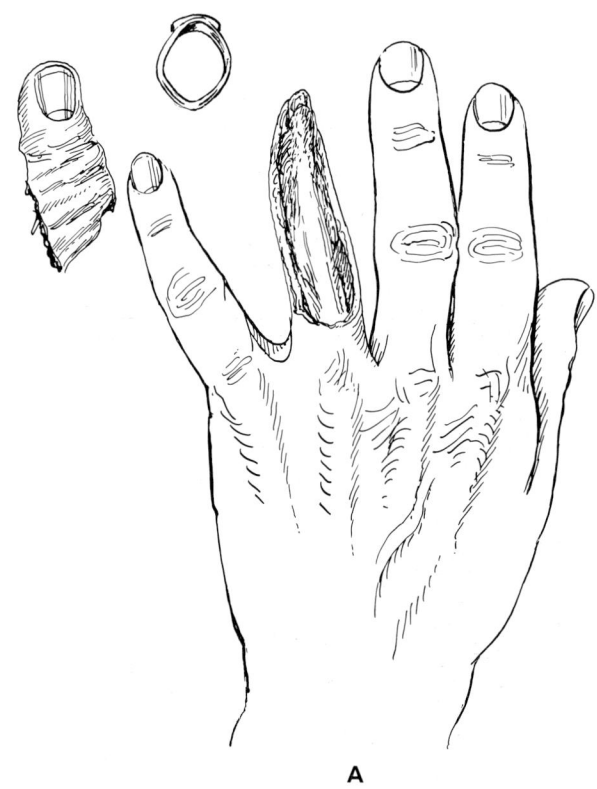

A

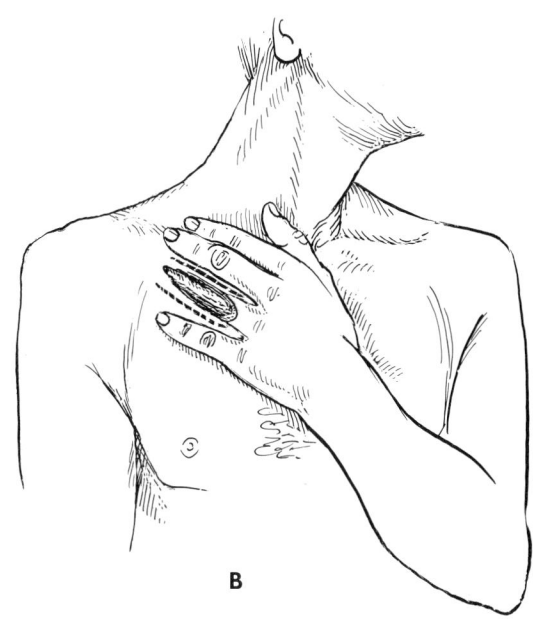

B

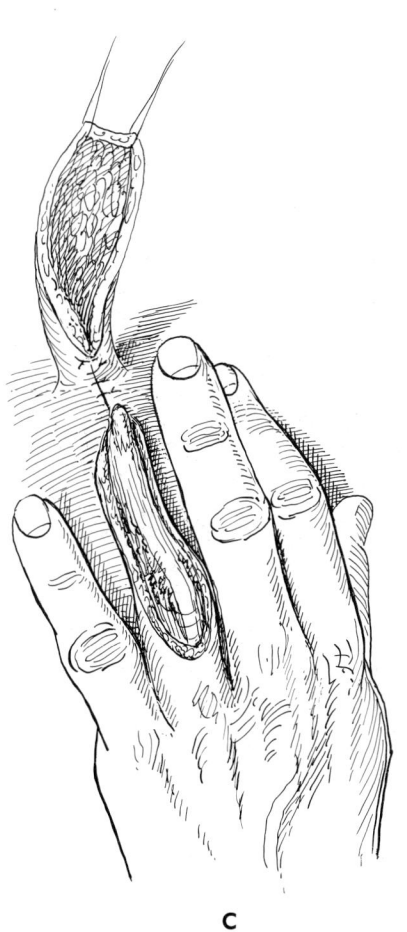

C

131

28 – The Infraclavicular Flap

The defatted pedicle flap was applied to the recipient area, carefully fitted, and sutured in place. (**D**) Light fluffy dressings were placed between the arm and trunk and in the axilla on the recipient side. The arm was immobilized by tape applied to the arm and trunk after painting the skin with tincture of benzoin.

As an experiment the nail matrix from the amputated distal phalanx was placed as a free graft over the proper place on the pedicle flap. This is not recommended and it has been eliminated from the drawings.

Two or three weeks later healing was sufficient to allow transection of the pedicle. The base pedicle was then tailored to give the fingertip proper contour. (**E**)

Although amputation of the finger is usually the first choice of therapy for ring avulsion injuries, sometimes special circumstances mitigate in favor of salvage of the finger. Distant pedicle flaps as described or various combinations of free grafts, island pedicle flaps, and cross finger flaps may be required to achieve the best possible functional result. (See page 174 for Island Technique.)

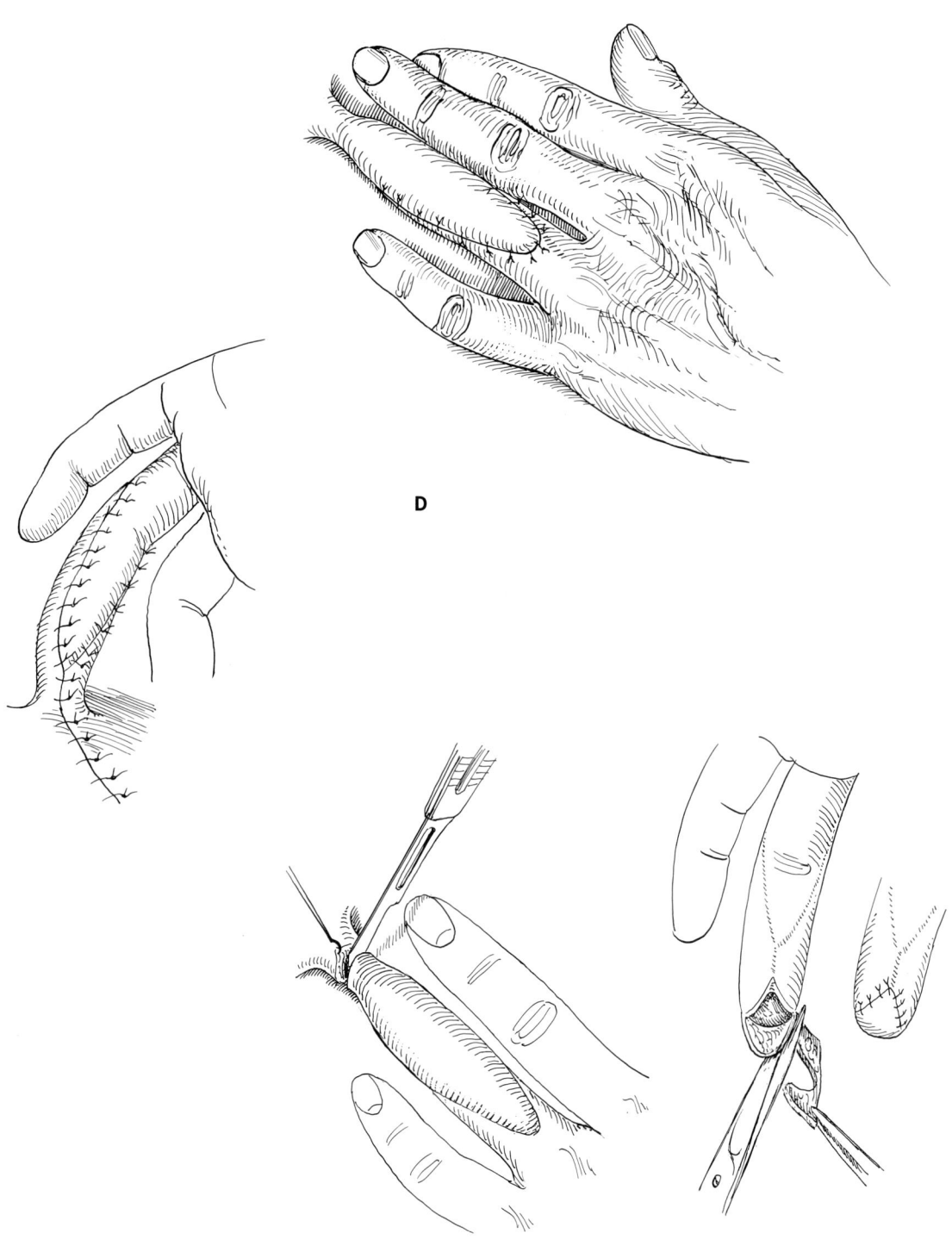

D

E

Skin and Soft Tissue Losses

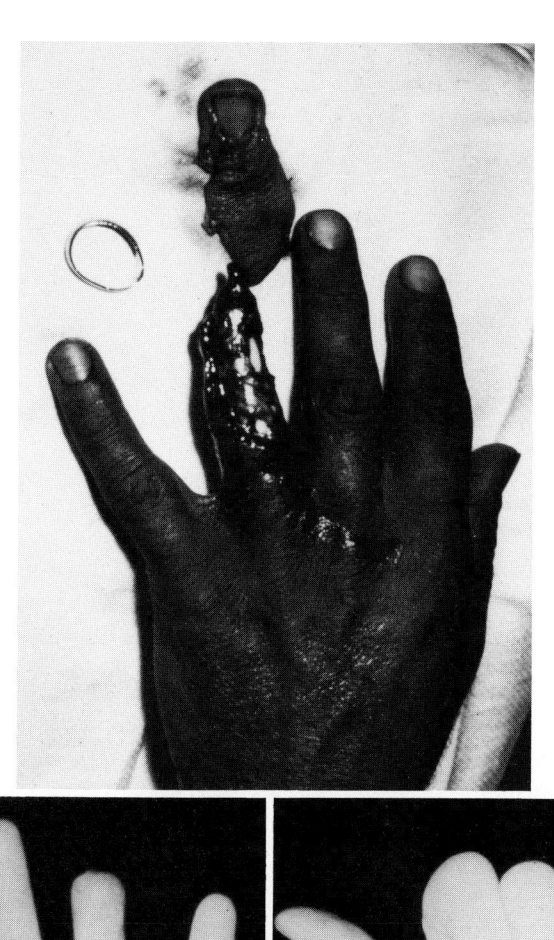
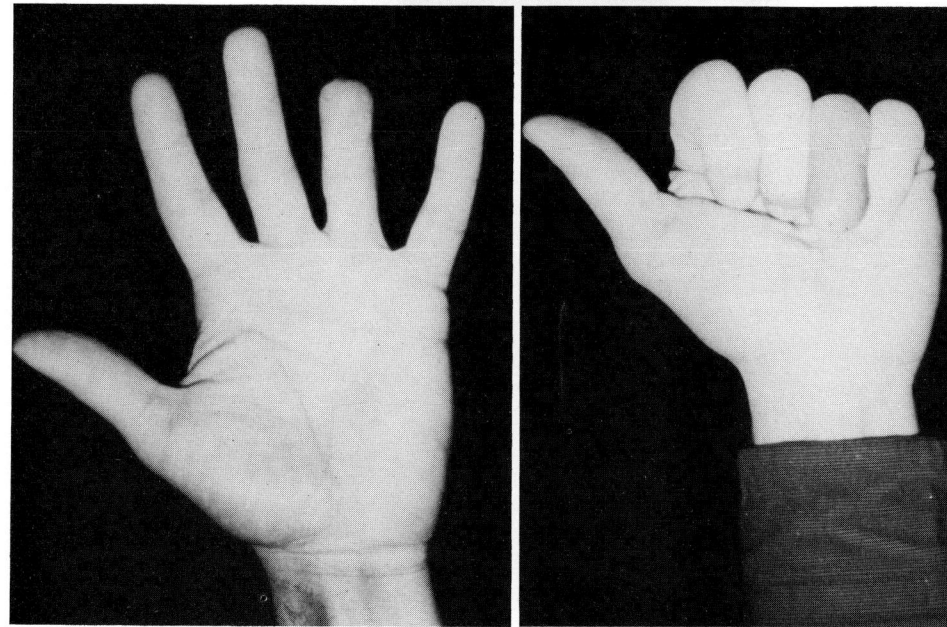

133

29

Total Hand Degloving Injury

Very severe avulsion injuries, although not common, present a challenge to the reconstructive surgeon. The detailed examination of the hand for possible salvage of functional parts is essential to answer the major overriding question: should the hand be amputated or should an attempt be made to salvage it?

Avulsion injuries confined to the hand dorsum are generally readily dealt with by resurfacing the dorsum immediately with split thickness skin. The natural plane of avulsion in the subcutaneous areolar tissue usually leaves a recipient bed that is ideal for split thickness skin grafting.

Total avulsion or degloving injuries of the whole hand present a problem which commonly tempts the surgeon to try to save too much. The hand's function is going to be sharply reduced and to try to save any elements superfluous to that functional role is poor judgment.

Degloving injuries which start proximally and avulse distally generally remove all skin, sometimes part or all of the palmar fascia, the distal phalanx of the thumb, and sometimes the distal phalanges of the fingers. (**A**)

If the thumb is shortened by the length of the distal phalanx, and tendons are exposed within the digits, one can expect, at most, to develop a functional endpiece with prehensile pinch. The distal phalanges of the fingers, if they remain, are superfluous to this function in the absence of flexor profundus function. Under these circumstances they should be amputated. Amputation of the index ray would contribute by assuring a wide and deep web space between the shortened thumb and remaining fingers. Index amputation also reduces the total skin deficit requiring coverage.

Unless some of the remaining bed consists of bare bone or open joint, one may attempt to achieve coverage with split thickness skin. Attempts to replace the intact avulsed skin glove rarely results in take. Some of the avulsed skin may be thinned and applied as a free graft but generally a thick split dermatome graft will harvest skin which is more reliable for free grafting. If it seems unlikely that the blood supply is adequate to support free skin grafts, the hand may be placed in a pedicle flap in preparation for staged reconstruction. (**B**)

If the hand ends up as a mitten hand with a thumb functioning against a composite of the ulnar three fingers, there is rarely an indication for surgical separation of the fingers. (**C**)

Skin and Soft Tissue Losses

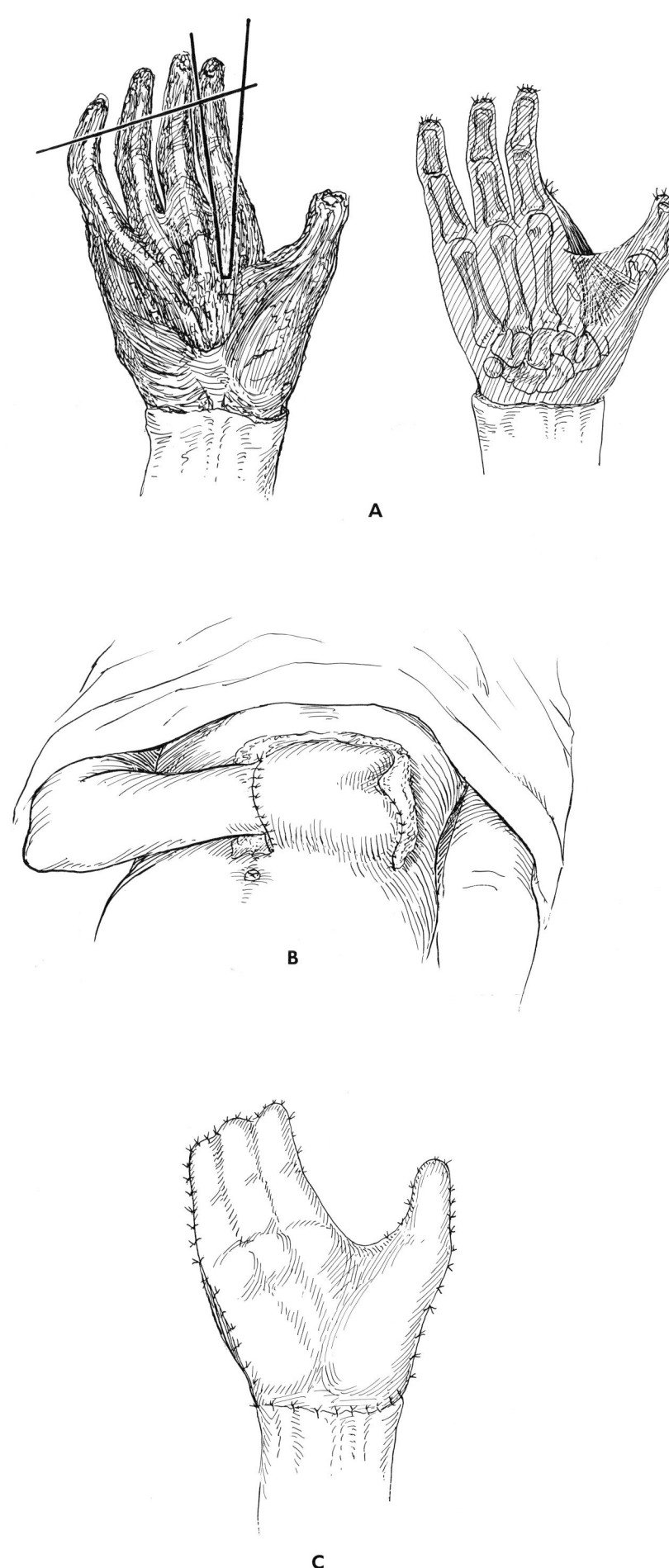

A

B

C

135

30
The First Web Space

Principles

Many surgeons routinely use a pedicle flap to resurface for loss of skin from the first web space. Frequently a thick split thickness graft is perfectly adequate to meet the need to overcome or avoid contracture in this area of capital importance in hand function.

If a skin graft is used in the first web space, it must be planned and implanted so that incision lines do not create scars that violate the scar line principles outlined. (See Section 6, Elective Skin Incisions.) The graft must lie flat against the recipient bed and not be allowed to fold upon itself as the new skin in the web space may do once its blood supply is established.

Example

A five-year-old girl sustained an electrical burn of the soft tissues in the left first web space from a bare electric wire.

The necrotic skin and soft tissue were debrided on the tenth postoperative day and a thick (0.018 inch) graft was applied.

The graft was carried down toward the root of the hand to avoid an incision transversely crossing the major thenar crease. The incision down the thumb was broken up to avoid a tethering pull on the web space skin. (**D**)

The parents were informed that the graft later would be replaced with pedicle flap skin. However the child had gone 12 years without the need for pedicle flap reconstruction when she was last seen.

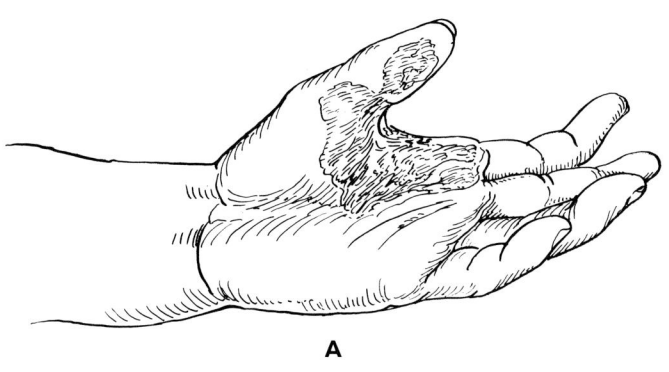

A

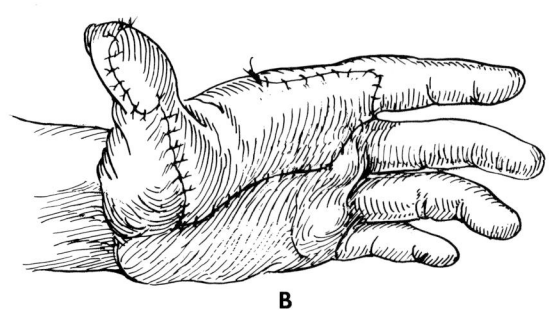

B

Skin and Soft Tissue Losses

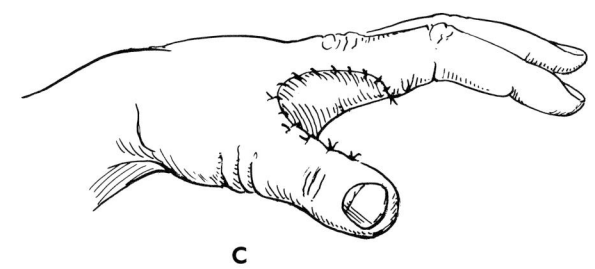
C

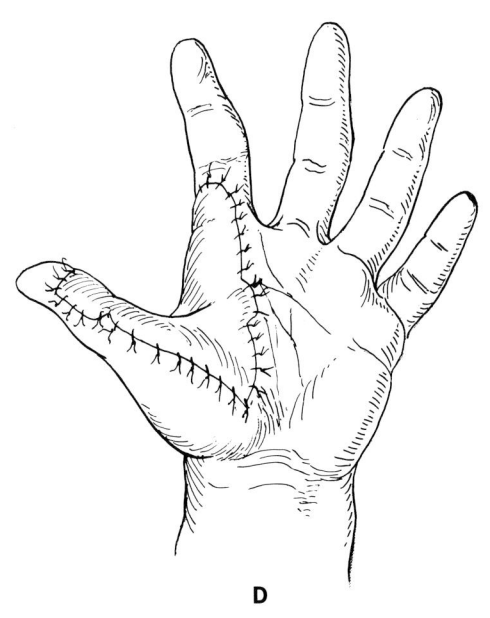
D

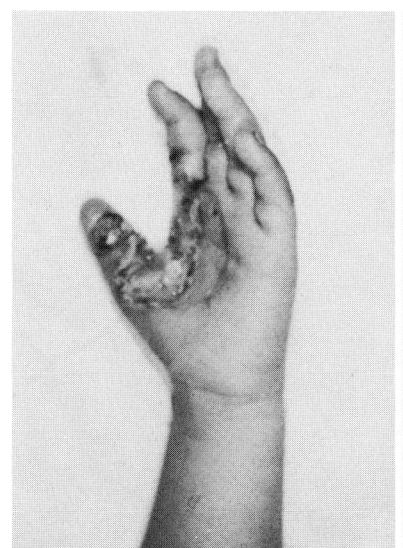 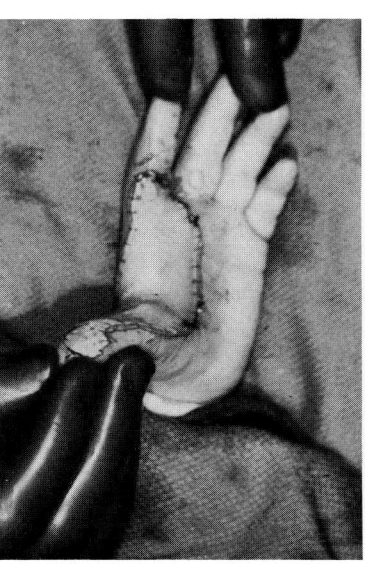 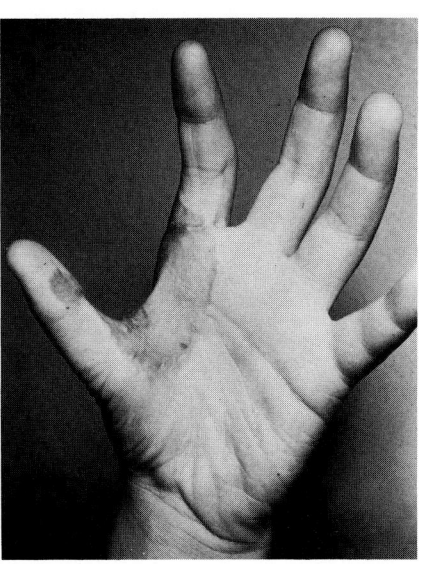

30 — The First Web Space

FIRST WEB SPACE CONTRACTURE

Using the Z-plasty principle combined with a free skin graft, a skin contracture which limits abduction of the thumb may be released.

The dorsal skin over the index metacarpal and metacarpophalangeal area must be uninvolved in scar. An incision is planned along the index metacarpal dorsally as a relaxing incision. (**A**) It is angled palmar at the level of the root of the index finger and carried on the palmar surface along the line of the index metacarpal. (**B**) The incision is made and release of the interosseous fascia is performed to gain abduction of the thumb. (**C**) The point of dorsal skin at the distal angle will fall palmar and help to delineate the location and direction of the incision to create the palmar limb of the Z-plasty. It will fall generally across the line of the second metacarpal, angling distally. After complete release the skin angles are interchanged while the thumb is abducted. (**D**)

A skin graft of full thickness or split thickness skin may be used to cover the remaining deficit which represents the necessary relaxation to regain full range of motion. (**E**)

When first web space surgery leaves a skin deficit with a residual bed which would not support a free graft, a pedicle flap is indicated. Such a flap must be patterned so that the incision lines do not cross areas of changing length. A diamond-shaped flap is planned and implanted in two stages. (See First Web Space Distant Pedicle Flap, page 140.)

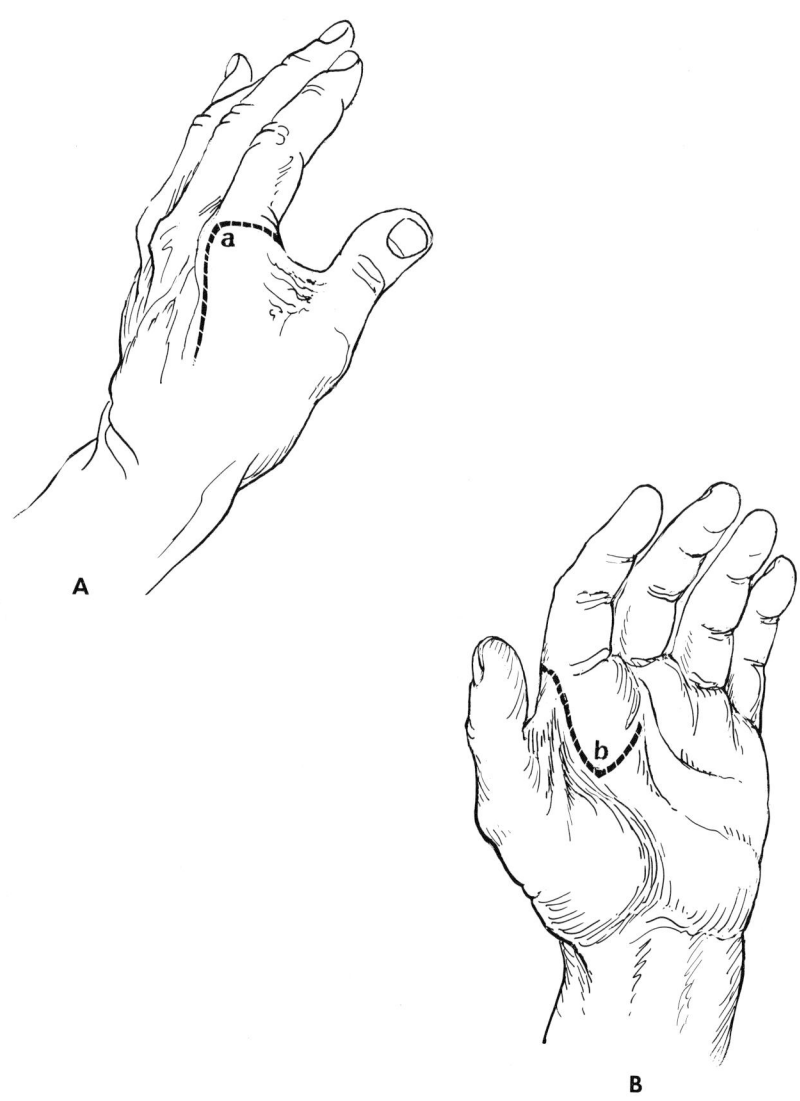

Skin and Soft Tissue Losses

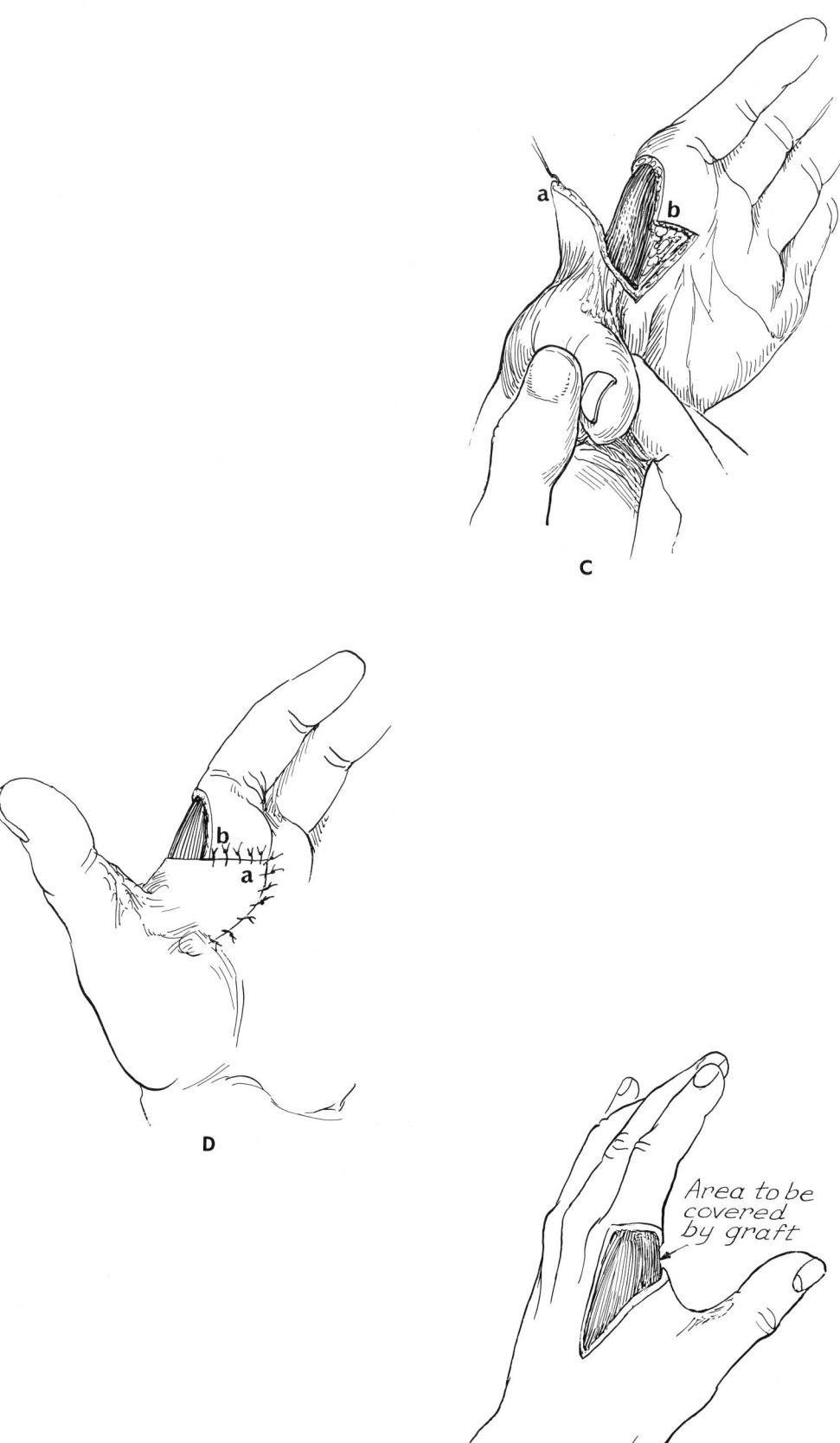

FIRST WEB SPACE DISTANT PEDICLE FLAP

To avoid an excessively deep-looking unsightly cleft between the thumb and index ray after surgical release of a first web space contracture, one may choose to cover the defect with a pedicle flap. The procedure assures one of good durable soft tissue coverage and subcutaneous filler. When a pedicle flap is decided upon, the surgeon may choose either an abdominal or chest donor site.

To avoid scars which will cross the web space and the lines of tension with thumb ray movement, the flap should be a generous one with tips that extend proximal to the apex of the angle between the first and second metacarpals on both the palm and dorsum. Such a flap will be diamond-shaped when it is complete.

Once web space release is completed by removal of skin and soft tissue scars and release of contracture in the adductor pollicis and first dorsal interosseous muscle, the skin release is checked to make sure it extends proximal enough to allow full abduction of the first metacarpal. During the period of pedicle flap application, the thumb should be kept in full abduction. This may require an external K-wire bow with ends inserted into the first and second metacarpals or simply external packing between the thumb and index finger. (**A**)

The hand is carried to the donor site and, using a pattern technique, the pedicle flap is outlined. (**B**) The full diamond for coverage is marked out to make sure that the release stage may be done within a proper donor area.

The half of the flap designed for the first inlay is elevated and appropriately thinned by removal of superfluous fat and subcutaneous tissue.

After dissecting beyond the mid length of the full pedicle flap to allow adaptation to the recipient bed, the flap donor site is loosely approximated. The flap is sutured to the hand, and the hand and arm are immobilized to the trunk by adhesive tape and dressings. (**C**)

About three weeks later the half of the diamond designed for the palm is dissected and implanted releasing the hand from the trunk. (**D** and **E**)

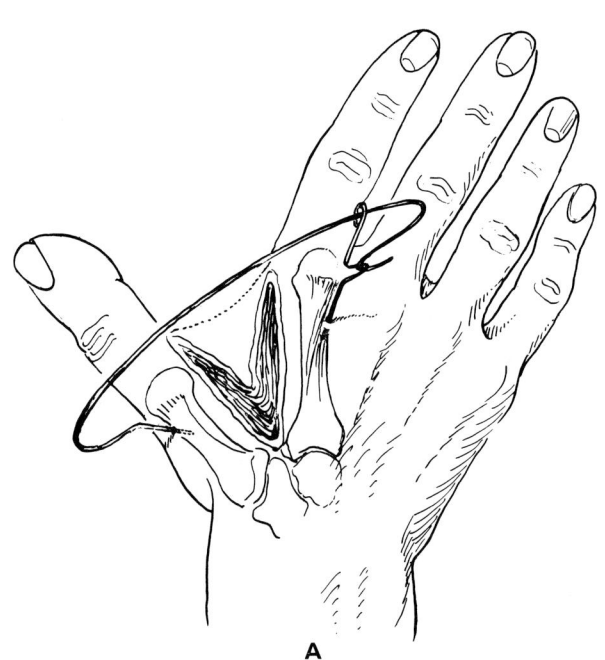

A

Skin and Soft Tissue Losses

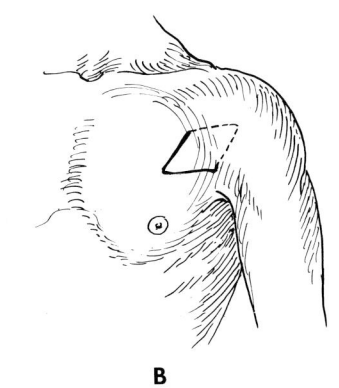

B

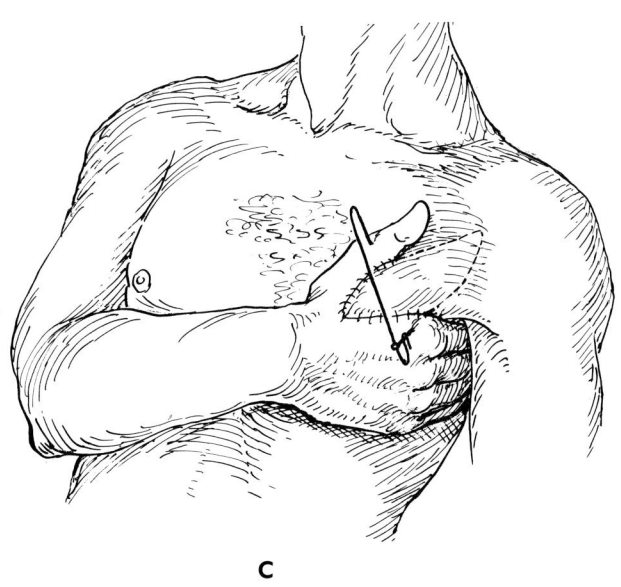

C

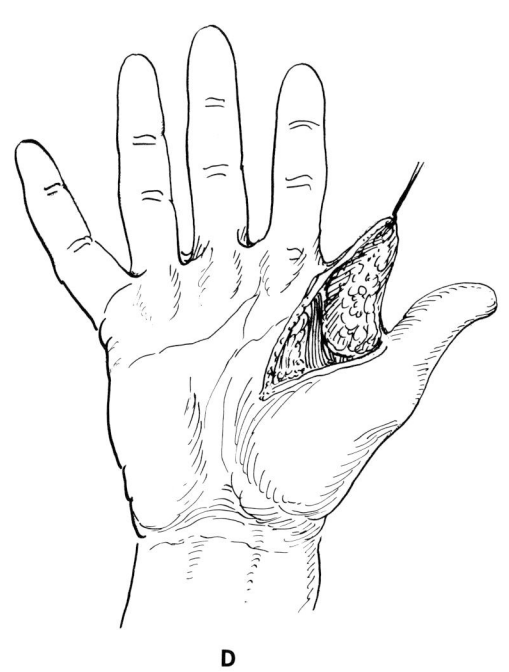

D

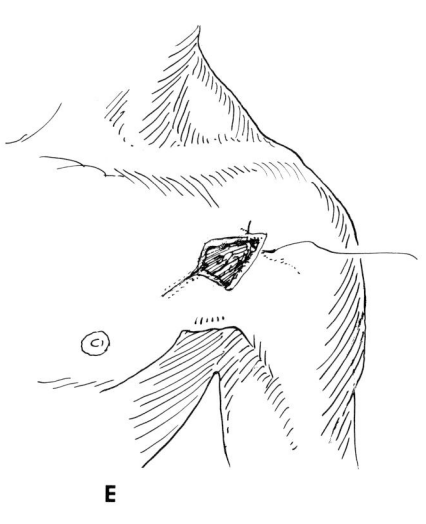

E

141

31
Proper Use and Care of Pedicle Flaps

A pedicle flap that looks beautiful at the operating table may turn out to be a disaster for the patient unless some basic principles are adhered to.

Principles: 1. Indication

There must be a clear indication for a pedicle flap. This rather complex, staged, and patient-trying procedure should always be reserved for circumstances in which no other simpler procedure will suffice. All too frequently pedicle flap procedures are done which are superfluous if one studies their purpose, what is salvaged by them, and what alternative techniques were available.

To use a pedicle flap to save a part of the hand which is superfluous is poor judgment.

Example: Misuse of a Pedicle Flap

A 22-year-old male patient sustained an avulsion amputation of the thumb tip, the index, long, and ring fingers at the metacarpophalangeal joint and the little finger at the proximal interphalangeal joint. The distal one third of the second, third, and fourth metacarpals was denuded of soft tissue in the injury.

The primary surgeon applied an abdominal pedicle flap to cover the distal ends of the exposed metacarpals. (**A, B,** and **C**) This was *inappropriate* since these metacarpal ends add nothing to hand function and they were not needed as a source of usable parts.

Thoughtful evaluation at the time of injury would have resulted in a conclusion that the functional value of the non-amputated hand would be pinch between the residual thumb stump and the foreshortened little finger. To augment this, amputation of the distal parts of the intervening metacarpals would be required. Should this have been done primarily, the pedicle flap would have been unnecessary. The pedicle flap was used to salvage *useless* parts.

Subsequent elective amputation of the index metacarpal at its proximal one third and revision and rotation by osteotomy of the fourth and fifth (**D, E** and **F**) markedly improved hand function and all but eliminated the pedicle flap soft tissue so tediously applied at the time of injury. (**G, H** and **I**)

Skin and Soft Tissue Losses

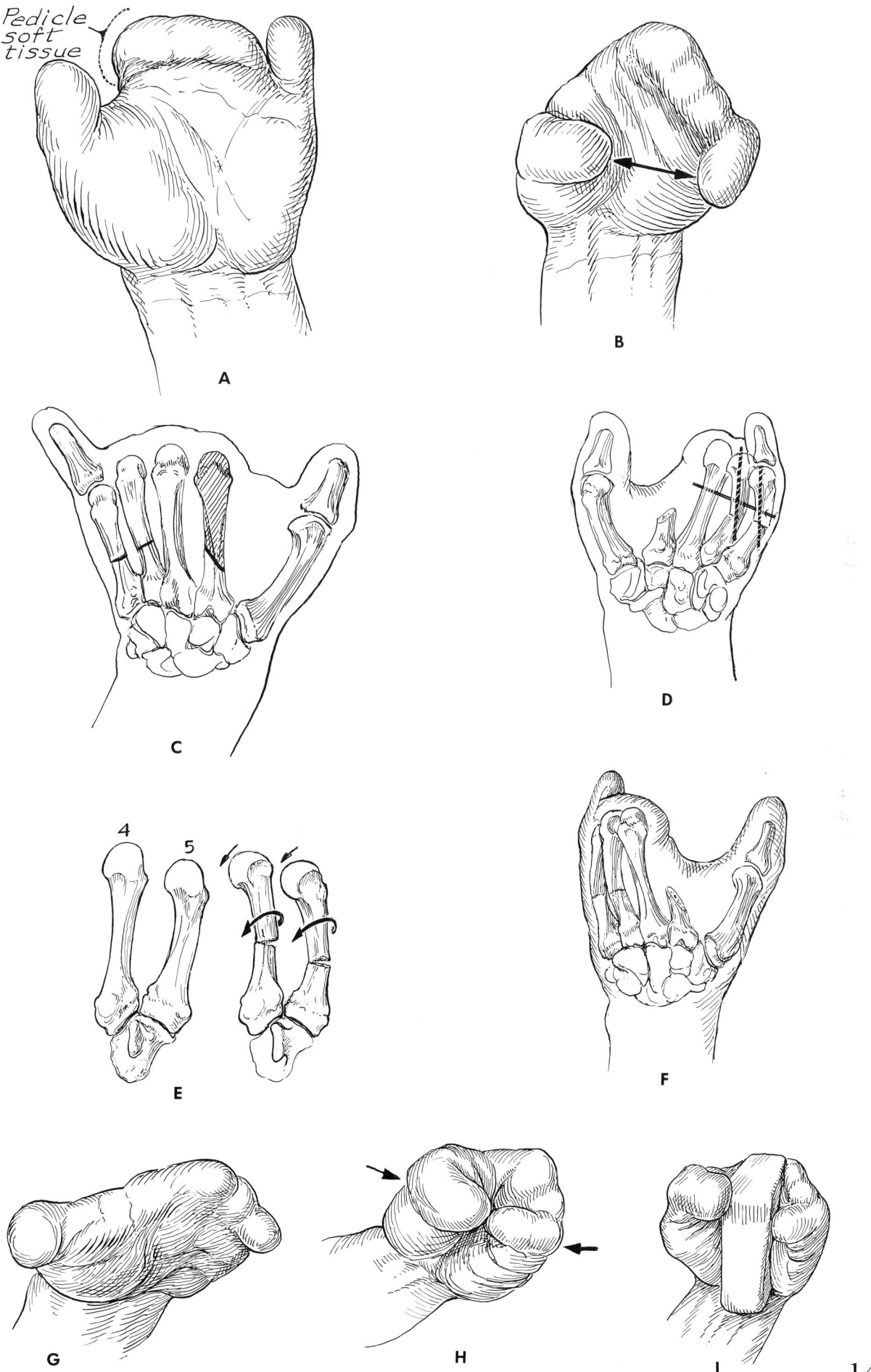

143

31 — Proper Use and Care of Pedicle Flaps

2. Attention to the Pedicle

The lifeline of the tissue being transferred as a flap is the base pedicle. Anything which interferes with flow of blood through this pedicle must be avoided. The pedicle itself may be too long to carry nourishment to the extreme end of the flap. There is no fixed ratio of length to width upon which one may rely since a great deal depends upon the care with which one bases the flap on known vessels. Carried to its extreme, a flap may be transferred on a pedicle consisting solely of such vessels (See Section 15, Island Pedicle Flap for Fingertip Loss). Experience in human beings with pedicle flaps to the hand from the abdomen or chest suggests, however, that a wide-based flap whose pedicle does not cross the midline or a previous scar is most reliable. Any fiddling with the pedicle itself such as tubing it, turning or folding it, or lining it with a skin graft must be done with great care. An otherwise perfect pedicle flap can be ruined by tubing the pedicle tightly without defatting it. Edema collecting in such a tight tube soon results in block of venous outflow and flap gangrene. Removal of tubing sutures at the first sign of compromise of flap circulation may save a flap.

A long flap may be ruined by the position in which the hand is immobilized against the trunk or by a shift in that position which may occur as the patient changes his body position. (**A**) Angulation or compression of the pedicule as a result of hand position must be avoided. Constant attention to the pedicle and the flap in the first day or two may avoid a great deal of grief that comes with flap gangrene.

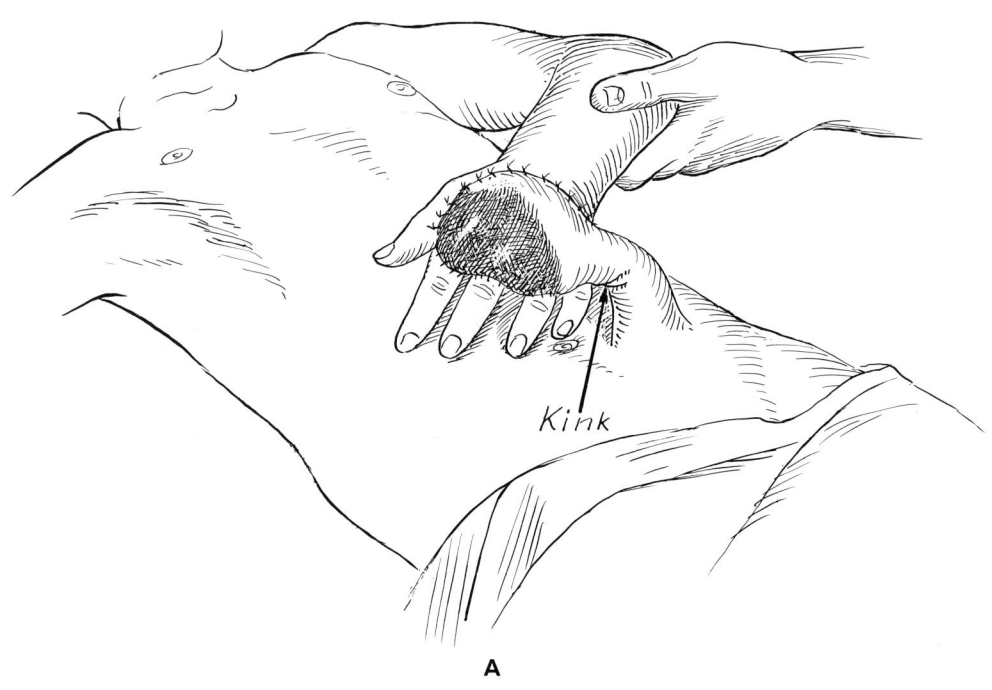

A

Skin and Soft Tissue Losses

3. Placement Anatomically

A pedicle flap must be carefully planned to take advantage of normal skin blood supply. It should be elevated from a donor area comfortably reached by the recipient hand and where the position favors venous return through the pedicle from the flap. In the upright position, venous return is generally better in flaps from the upper half of the trunk but the abdomen and lower trunk can have equally good venous return if the patient is placed in a recumbent position. When possible, the flap should come from an area where the pedicle *does not cross the midline* and where the pedicle has not been previously violated by surgery or trauma. (**B**)

The donor area also is best when the hand can assume a position of function during the period of flap attachment. The contralateral anterior axillary area serves admirably for thumb and dorsal pedicle flaps since the hand assumes the position comfortably; the fingers flex around the pectoral fold; the skin is thin and well endowed with blood vessels; the hand is elevated for good venous return from the hand; and the pedicle venous return is good in the upright as well as the supine position.

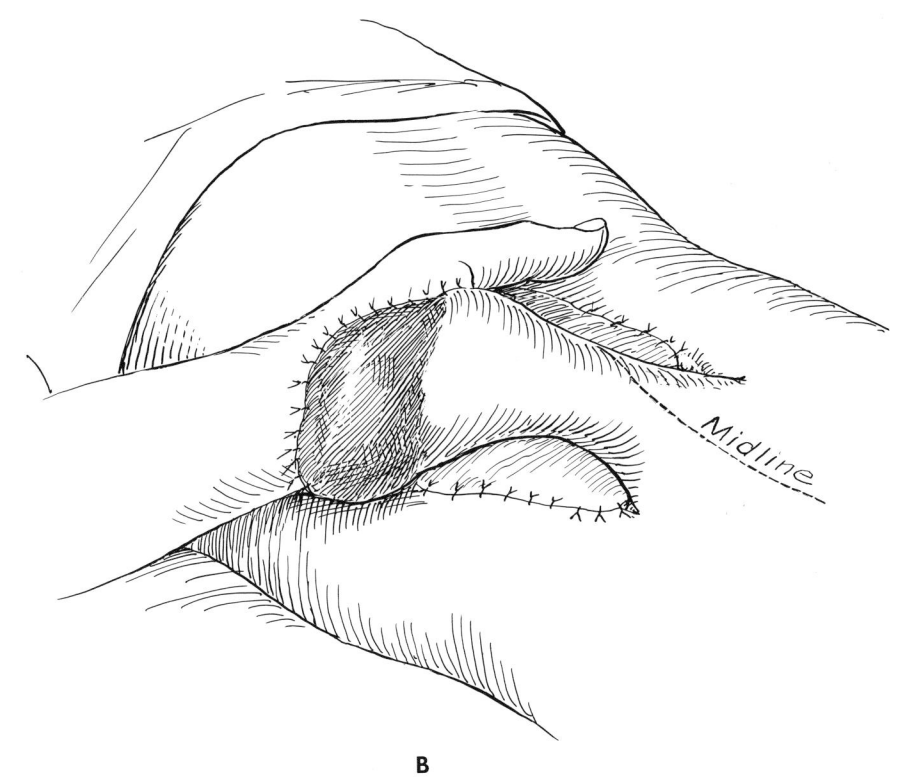

B

4. Delay

After a pedicle flap is planned and marked out on the donor site one may choose to make the incision as planned, then partially or completely dissect the flap from its bed only to then replace it and suture the wound. This delay or first stage of the pedicle flap procedure is best done three or four weeks prior to the actual flap transfer to the recipient site.

When there is serious question as to whether a pedicle flap may survive or not, a delay procedure serves two useful purposes. The delay does result in development of open collateral blood vessels in the pedicle; and if the flap is elevated, precisely as it will be used, it tests the competence of the pedicle to nourish it. A third probable advantage is that the wound edge transferred 3 or 4 weeks after the incision for delay is made is the equivalent of a secondary wound. This is even more advantageous if the recipient area is outlined by an incision at the time of the delay as well. Tensile strength develops rapidly in such a wound and the stage is set for rapid vascularization across the donor site–recipient site wound.

The disadvantage of the delay procedure in addition to an extra operative stage is the production of a flap that is less pliable and adaptable to the recipient site. Thus the delay procedure has not and should not become routine.

When a pedicle flap is to be used to cover an area where vascularized soft tissue is essential, a delay to test the pedicle's competence is clearly indicated. For example, if the dissection will leave exposed bone, or an open joint, the flap used to cover the defect must be reliable or the total reconstructive effort may be jeopardized.

Amputations

32

Single Digit Amputation

Principles

The principles to be adhered to in *solitary* digital injuries are not applicable when multiple digits are injured. The therapeutic principles for single digit amputation are as follows:

1. *The thumb* is the most important single digit in the hand. When traumatic amputation occurs at any level, the surgeon's objective is to salvage all possible skeletal length. (**A**) This may be achieved by simple local wound closure, a local or cross finger flap, an island pedicle flap, or a distant pedicle flap. Length preservation in the thumb is so important that one should not hesitate to use the complicated transfer of vascularized soft tissue to achieve this. (See Sections 14, 15, 22, 27, and page 176.)

2. Injury limited to the *index finger* which results in partial loss of the finger logically is treated on the basis of the level of amputation. The most important function of the index finger is pulp-to-pulp pinch and manipulation of objects with the thumb. The index finger retains this function as long as it retains length beyond the proximal interphalangeal joint. Once the finger is amputated proximal to the proximal interphalangeal joint, it relinquishes its prime function with the thumb to the long finger. If amputation occurs distal to this critical level, substantial therapeutic effort should be made to salvage length. (**B**) This may require simple closure or free grafting, but when more complex vascularized pedicle flaps, either local (cross finger or island pedicle) or distant (trunk or contralateral arm), are required, these procedures are warranted. When amputation is sustained proximal to this critical level, additional shortening of the bone to achieve primary closure is appropriate. Ray amputation of the index finger and metacarpal is frequently a reasonable ultimate restorative measure for such an amputation. (See Section 33, Index Ray Amputation.) On rare occasions ray amputation is indicated at the time of initial therapy.

3. The *little finger* shortened by amputation is best managed initially by simple closure with local tissue even if this requires some bone shortening. If the residual nub is so short that it contributes little to hand function and gives the hand an unsightly appearance, it is best managed by ray amputation (See Section 34, Fifth Ray Amputation). (**C**)

4. The *long and ring fingers* are central in the hand and neither has any generally unique or exclusive function of its own except in certain specific activities (musical, typing, surgical, etc.). Under most circumstances primary therapy for amputations of these fingers is to gain local soft tissue closure even if it requires surgical shortening of bone. The critical amputation level is through the proximal phalanx distal to the metacarpophalangeal joint. (**D**) To remove the whole proximal phalanx of a central finger results in an open space when the hand is cupped, with a result that small objects may unavoidably fall through. Should amputation result in such incontinence of the palmar cup, secondary metacarpal amputation and transfer of the adjacent peripheral ray may be used to narrow the space and restore function and a symmetrical, more normal appearance. (See Section 40, Metacarpal Transfer.)

Amputations

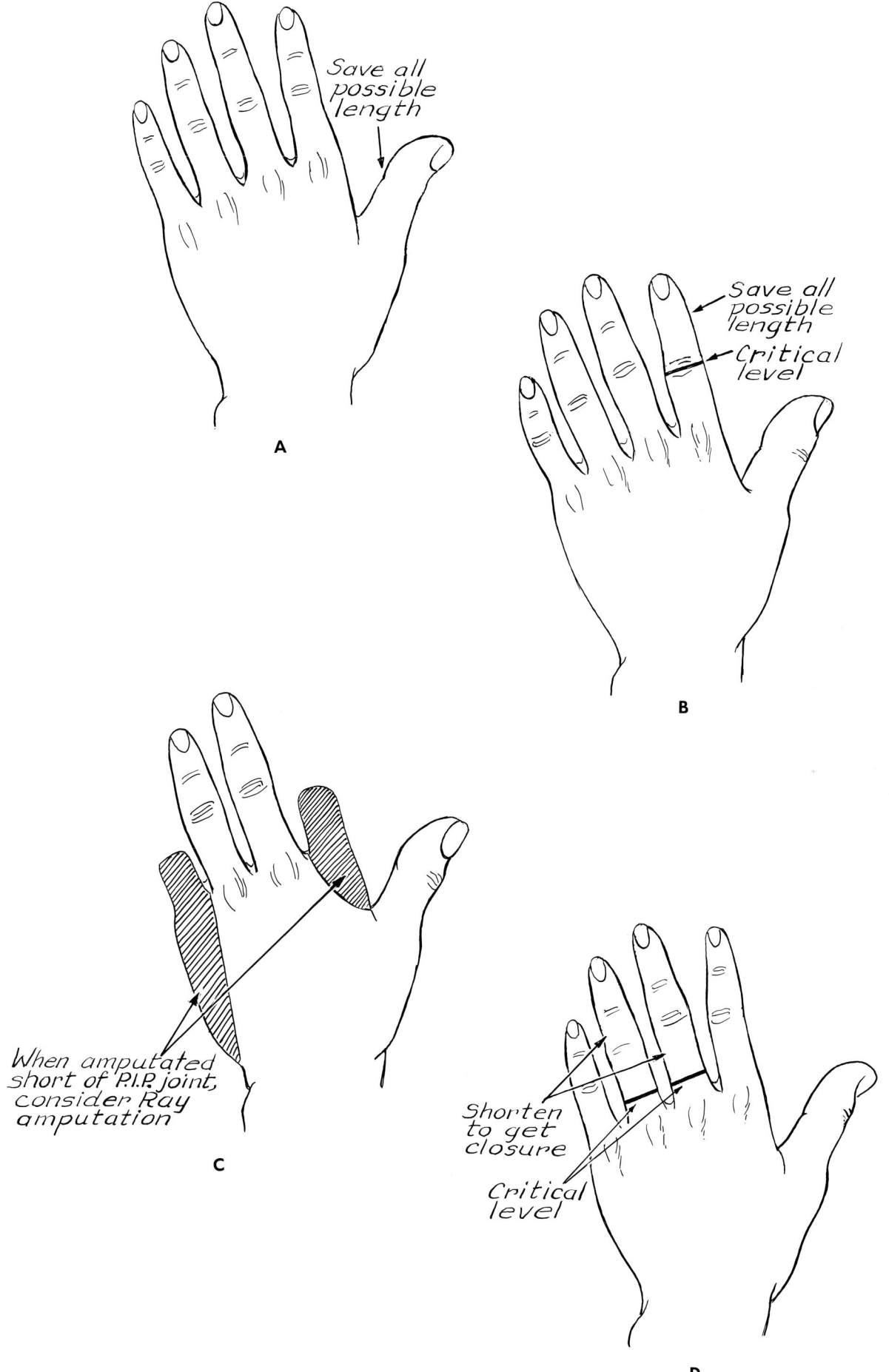

32 — Single Digit Amputation

Index Finger Amputation

The index finger has as its primary function pulp-to-pulp pinch with the thumb. (**E**) It manipulates objects together with the thumb and has greater independent action capabilities than any of the other fingers. When the index finger is shortened by amputation, it may lose this prime function.

As long as a segment of the middle phalanx remains, the index unit will continue to function as an effective pincher. This is particularly true if proximal interphalangeal joint function is retained. (**F**)

If the level of amputation is proximal to the proximal interphalangeal joint, the finger loses its thumb-index manipulative capability. The long finger is promoted, to become the primary pulp-to-pulp pincher with the thumb. The index nub is extended, to remove it from action. (**G**) Under these circumstances, the index finger nub may become a significant deficit by acting as an impinging occupant in the web space between the thumb and long finger. Even when it is extended, the head of the second metacarpal protrudes into the web area preventing proper seating of large objects grasped by the thumb and remaining fingers.

Appearance of the hand is improved and its function may be enhanced by a well executed ray amputation at a proximal level through the metacarpal. (**H**)

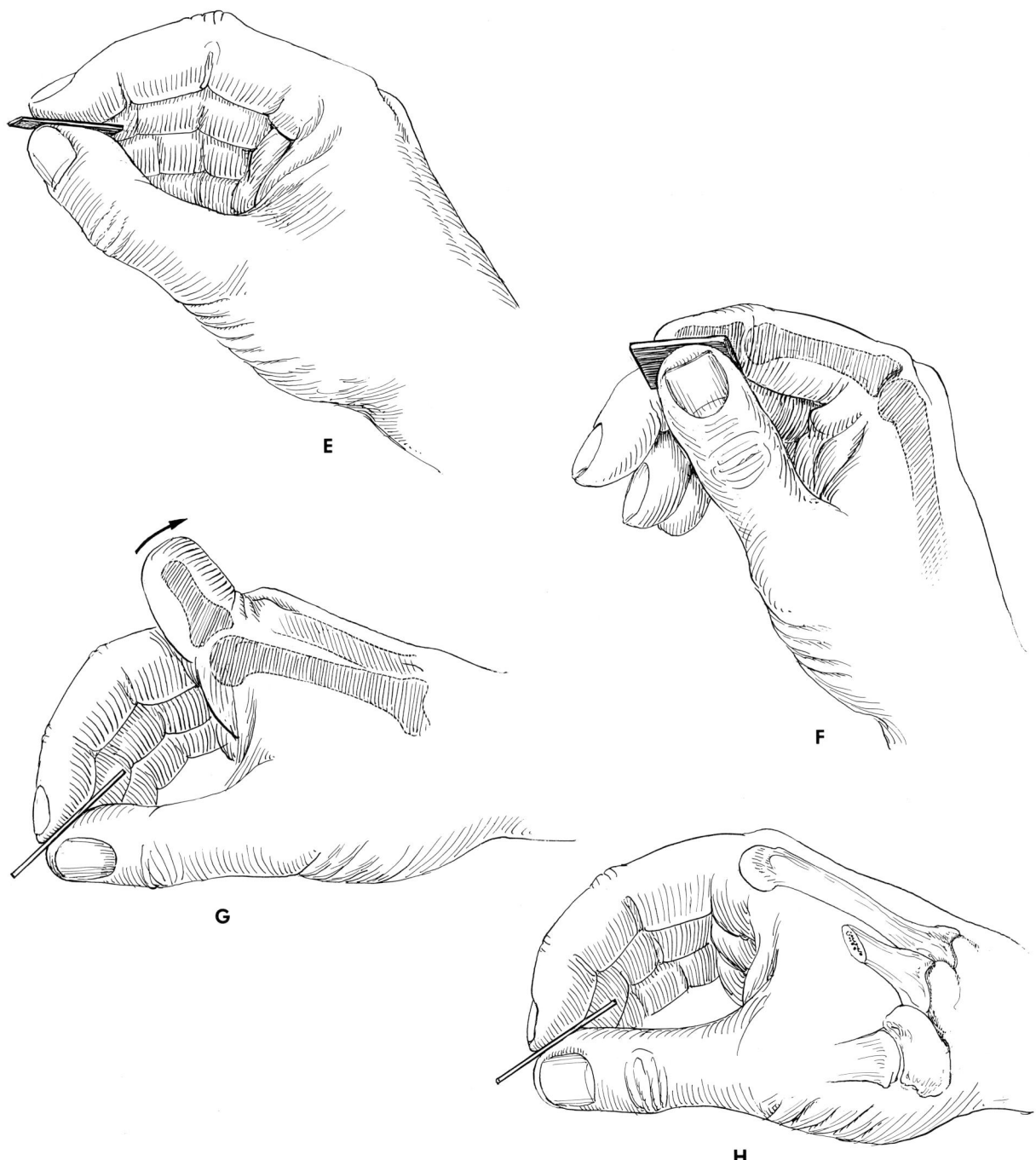

33

Index Ray Amputation

Index ray (digit and metacarpal) amputation should be planned to leave the patient with a smooth web space between the thumb and long finger. Skin incisions are planned in such a way that no scar will violate the contoured first web.

Example

A patient presented with a short painful nub from an amputation at the level of the mid proximal phalanx. (**A**) Ray amputation was elected as appropriate treatment. The incision between the index nub and long finger was planned to be carried to the side of the base of the long finger so as to place the healed wound out of the soft mobile web space. (**B**) A similar point on the radial side of the deformed index finger was chosen so that, after removal of the nub and metacarpal, the skin would fall against the long finger base. (**C**) Curved incisions were planned to expose the proximal portion of the second metacarpal and to allow removal of the superfluous skin and soft tissue. (**D**)

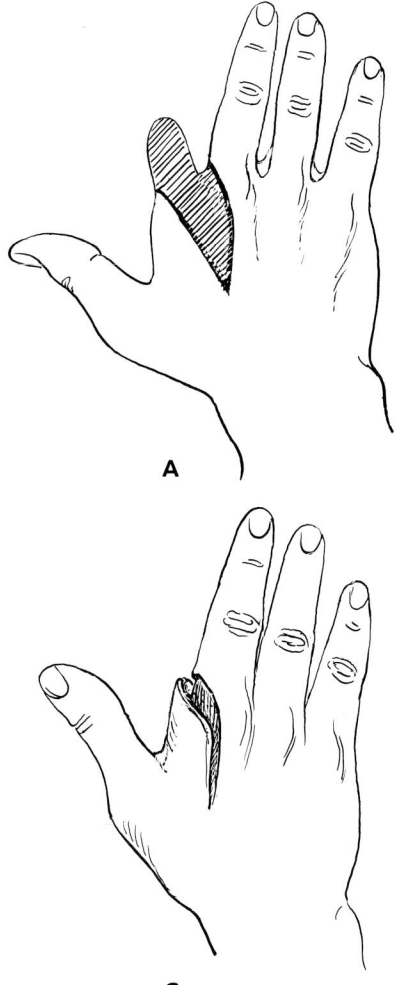
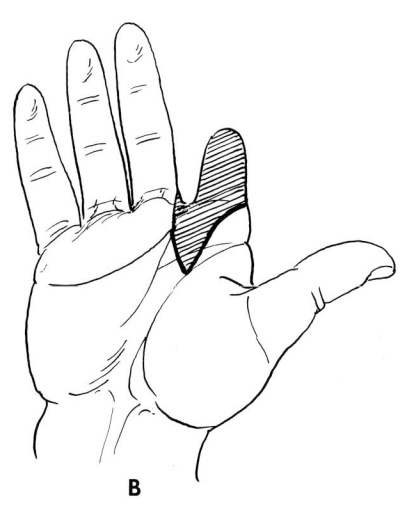
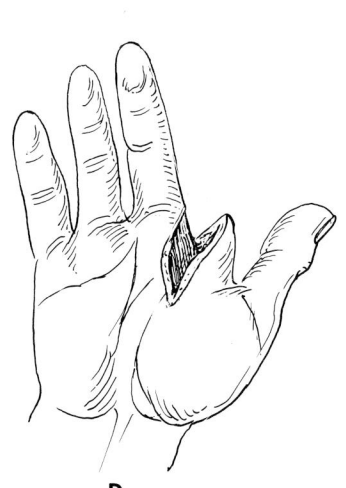

33 – Index Ray Amputation

The index nub to be amputated was held with a towel clip to steady and manipulate it during the procedure. The dorsal incisions were made first. (**E**)

The web space flap was dissected from the underlying first dorsal interosseous muscle in the areolar plane just superficial to its fascia. The extensor tendons and the second dorsal interosseous muscle were exposed. An incision was made through the metacarpal periosteum in preparation for osteotomy. (**F**)

The metacarpal periosteum was elevated with a Joseph periosteal elevator, exposing the proximal half of the metacarpal shaft. The extensor indicis was identified and cut at its incorporation into the dorsal hood at the metacarpophalangeal joint level. It was preserved for transfer to the long finger extensor mechanism. The extensor digitorum slip to the index finger was pulled distally, cut short at the proximal wound edge, and was allowed to retract proximally. (**G**)

Osteotomy was planned across the proximal quarter of the metacarpal. It was designed with a bevel to prevent it from protruding into the web space. (**H**)

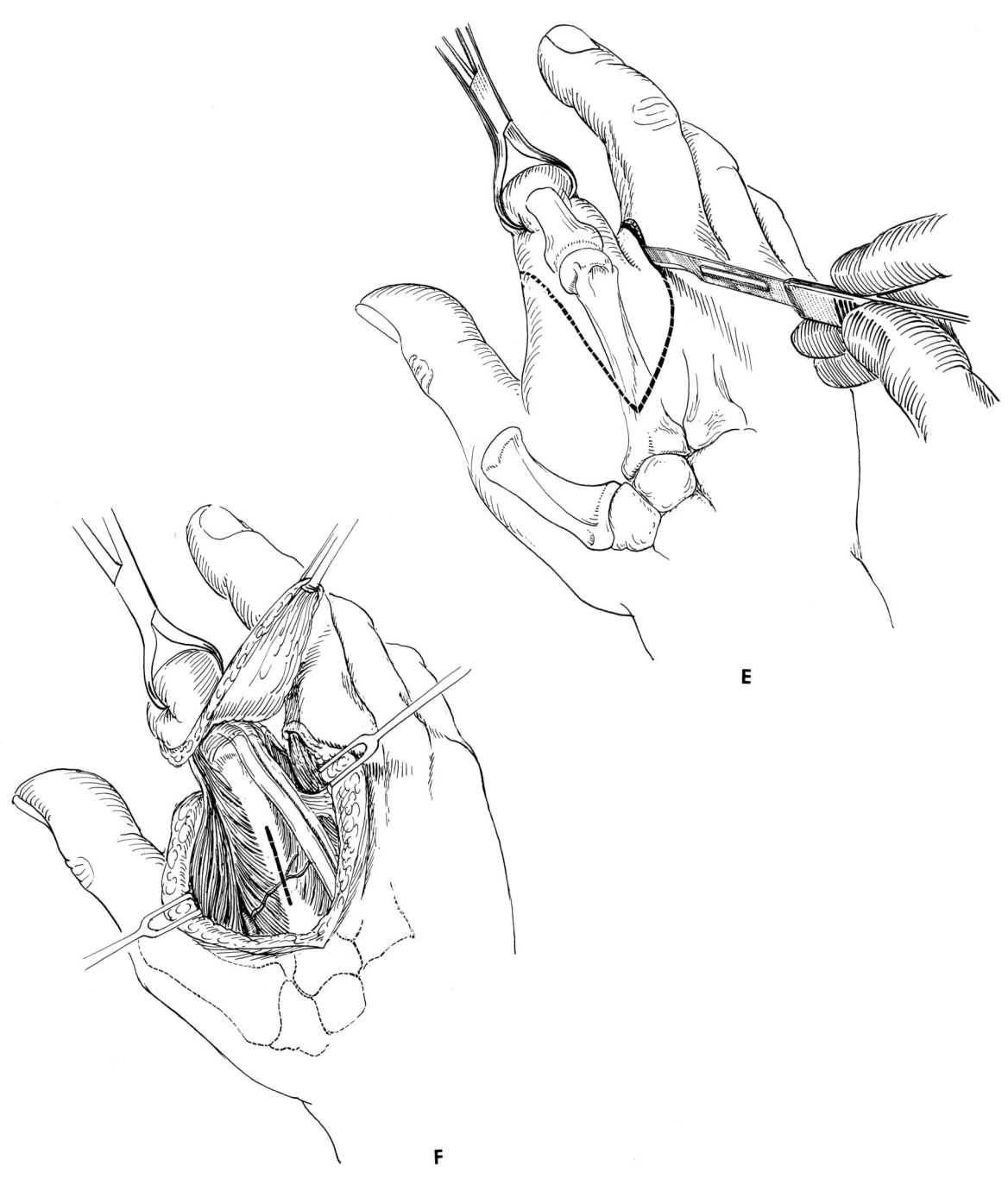

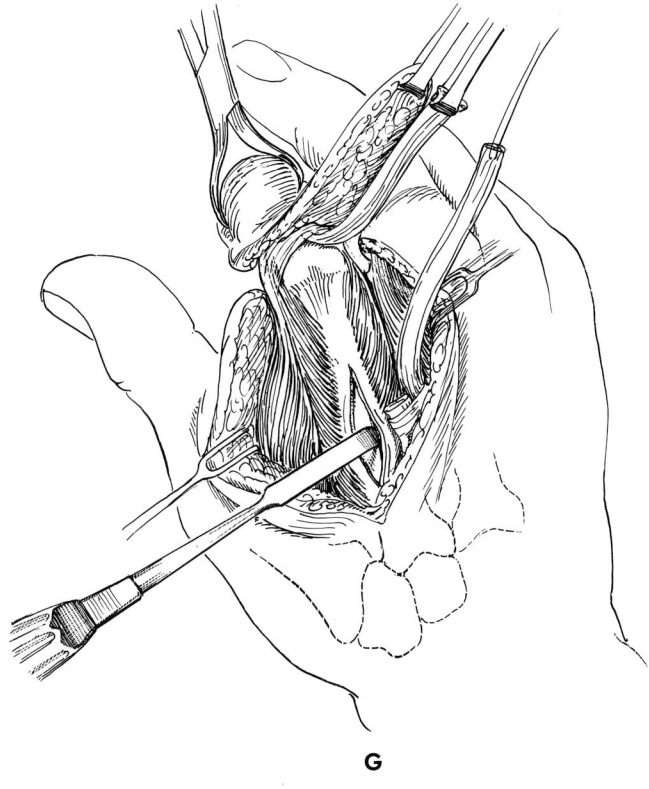

G

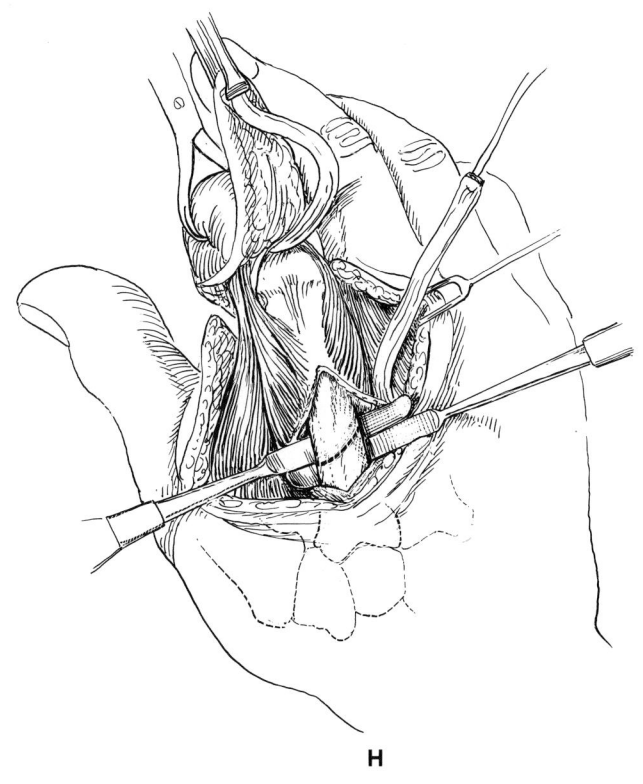

H

33 – Index Ray Amputation

The oblique osteotomy was made with an oscillating bone saw in such a manner that it created the least possible impingement on the normal smooth contour of the web space. (**I**) A small part of the proximal end of the metacarpal was preserved as a buttress for adjacent bones and to retain the insertion of the extensor carpi radialis longus.

The osteotomy was completed and, after release of the first dorsal interosseous at its insertion, the distal metacarpal segment was retracted and rotated in an ulnar direction. The palmar structures were visualized and dissected free. The digital blood vessels were ligated short and transected but the digital nerves were left long for reflection into the interosseous space. The flexor tendons were individually pulled distally and cut short. (**J**) The first palmar interosseous was left *in situ* (it may be excised, depending on the bulk needed in the web space). The extensor indicis was dissected free from the dorsal hood and cut long for transfer to the long finger extensor. The volar plate was removed with the amputation specimen as the tough ligaments between the index and long finger volar plate were sharply transected.

Amputation consisted of removal of the second metacarpal and finger nub, together with the flexor tendon mechanism and the extensor digitorum. Branches of the dorsal branch of the radial nerve covering to the dorsum of the long finger were preserved as the branches to the index nub were cut proximal and away from the incision site. The interosseous muscles and extensor indicis were preserved. The digital vessels were ligated short but the digital nerves were left long for transfer into the depths of the interosseous space for protection of the inevitable neuromas. The tendon of the first dorsal interosseous muscle was transferred to the radial lateral band of the long finger. This may augment abduction of the long finger in pinch and it assures a smooth, contoured first web space between the thumb and long finger. (**K**)

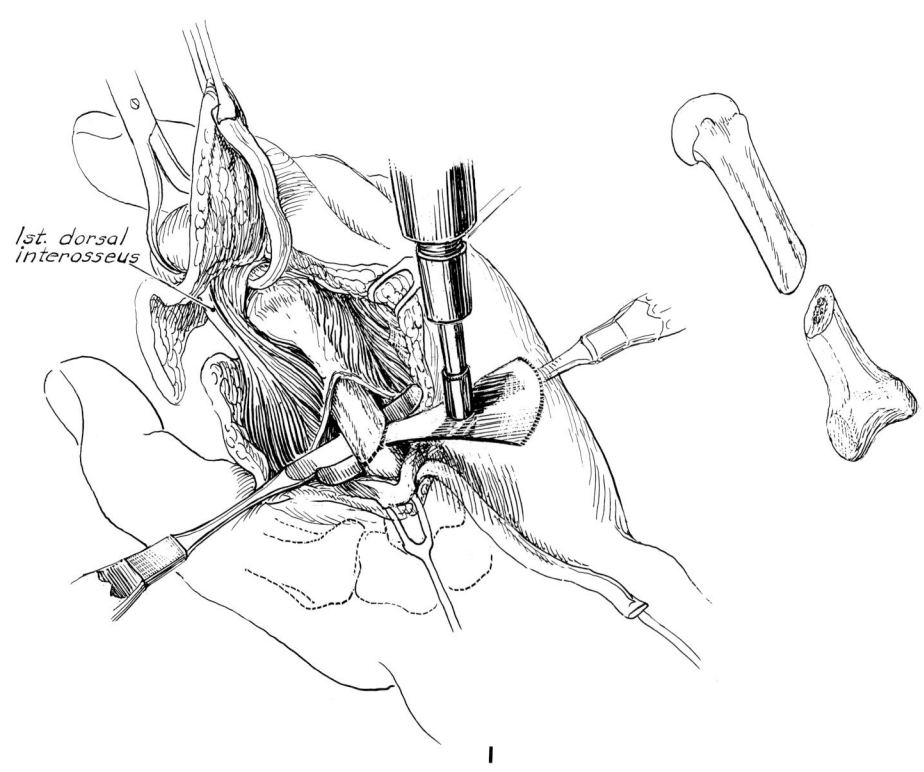

I

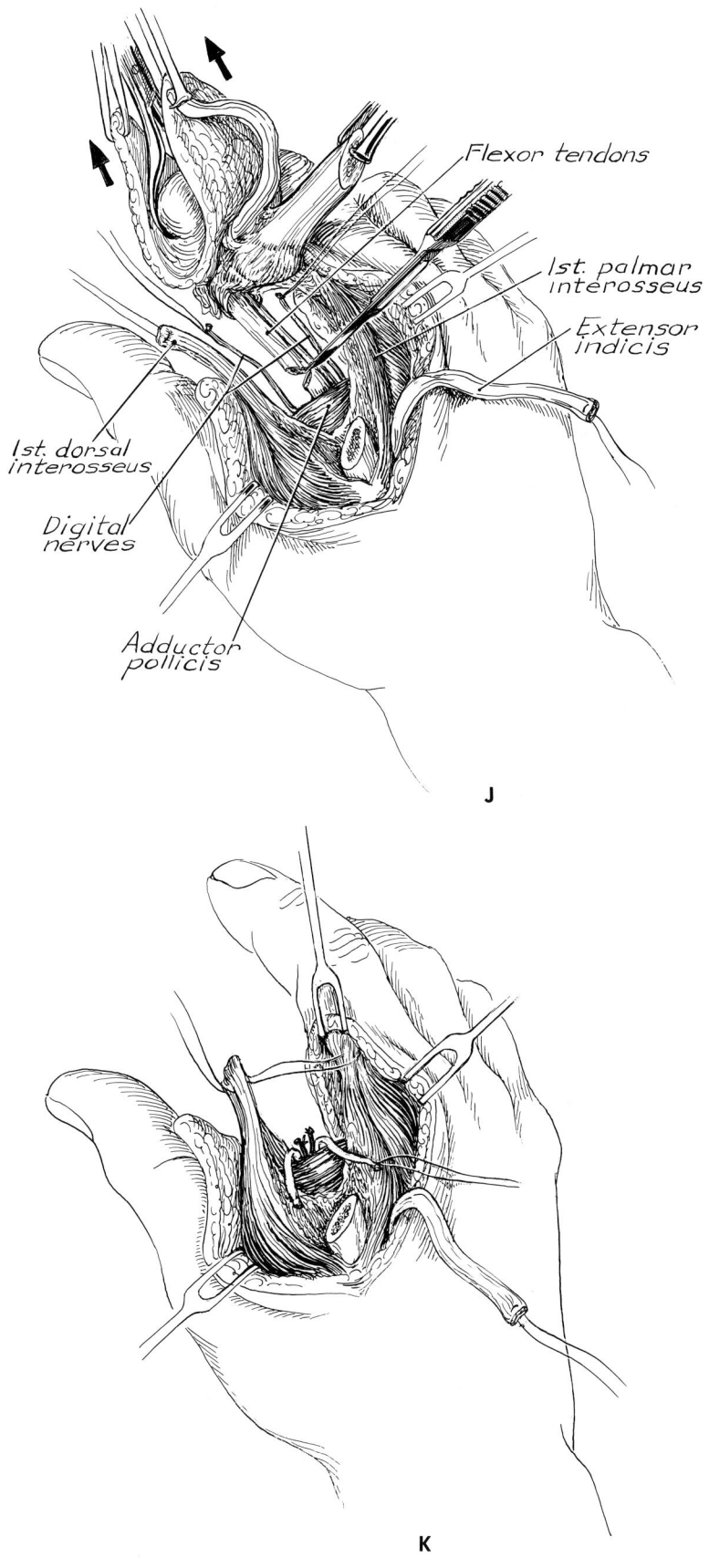

33 – Index Ray Amputation

The independently functional extensor indicis was sutured side to side to the extrinsic extensor of the long finger to give it more independent extension in its new role as primary pincher and manipulator. (**L**)

Skin closure was achieved by starting the suture line on the palmar aspect of the web space flap. This allowed tailoring and adjustment of the skin over the dorsum of the hand where the skin was loose, thin and adjustable. (**M**).

The residual "dog ear" was readily managed by extension of the dorsal incision and adjustment using appropriate wound geometry principles. The smooth web space gave the hand a near normal appearance. (**N**)

The metacarpal amputation level is such that a small segment remains, preserving the insertion of the extensor carpi radialis longus. (**O**)

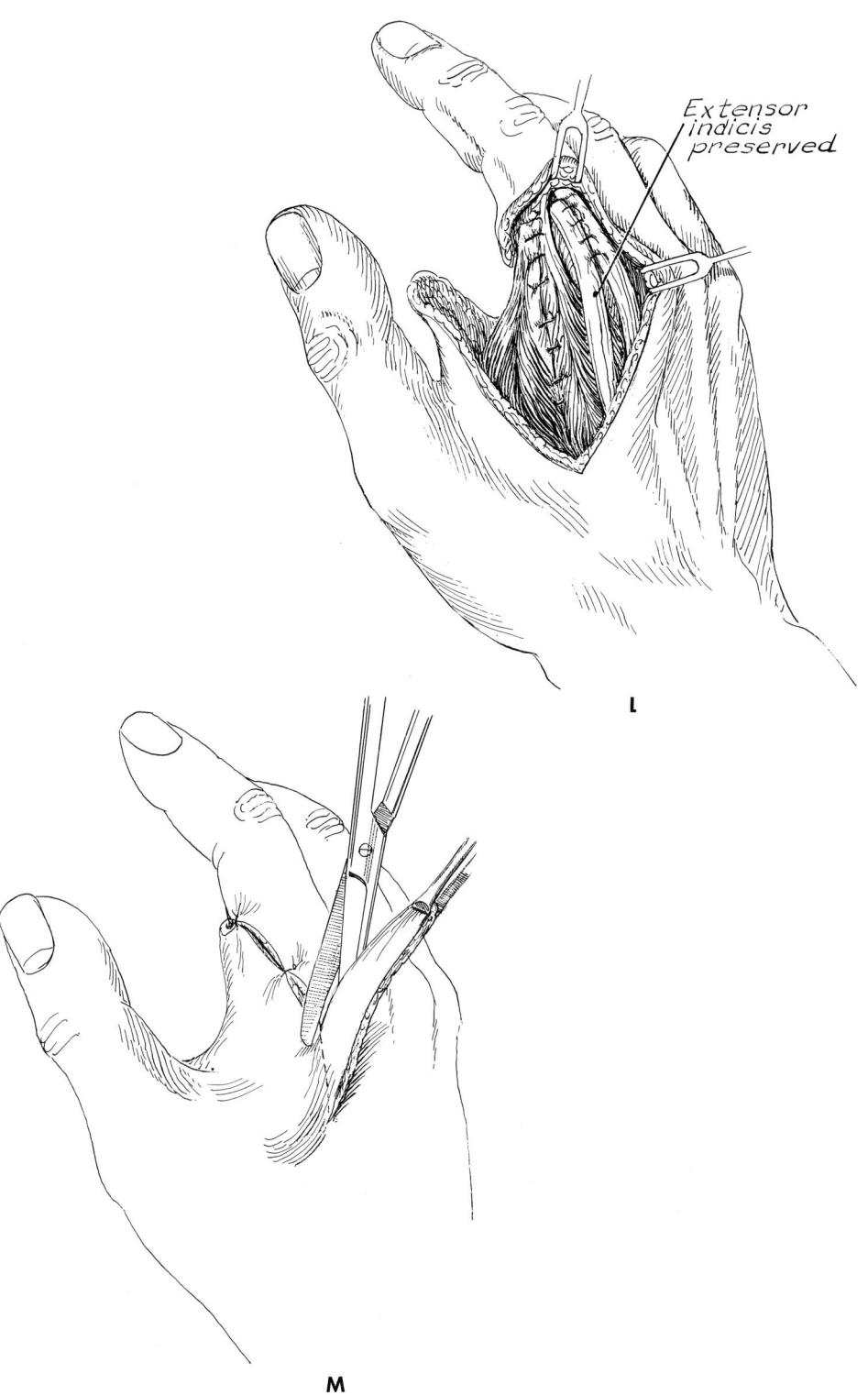

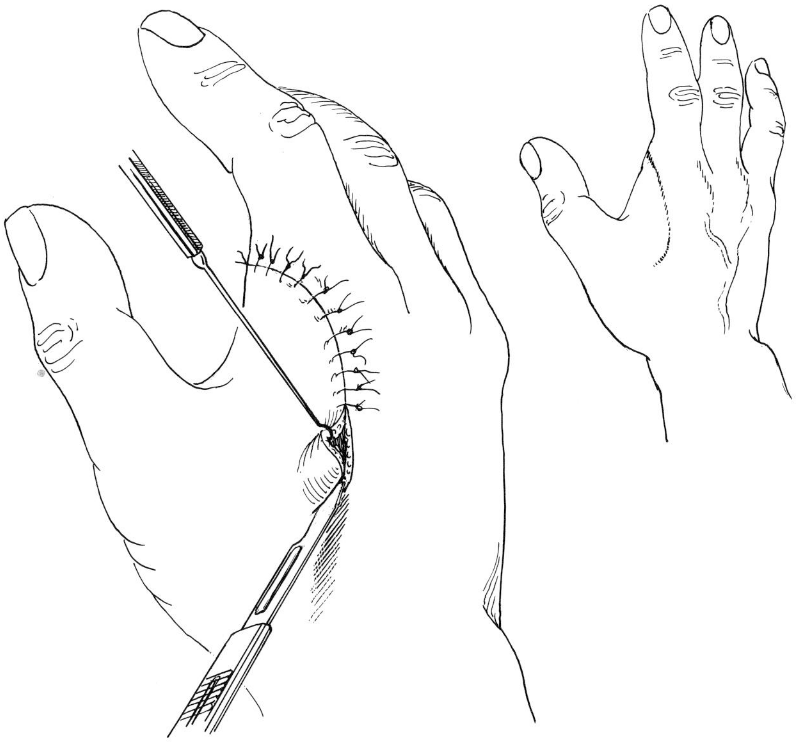

Amputations

N

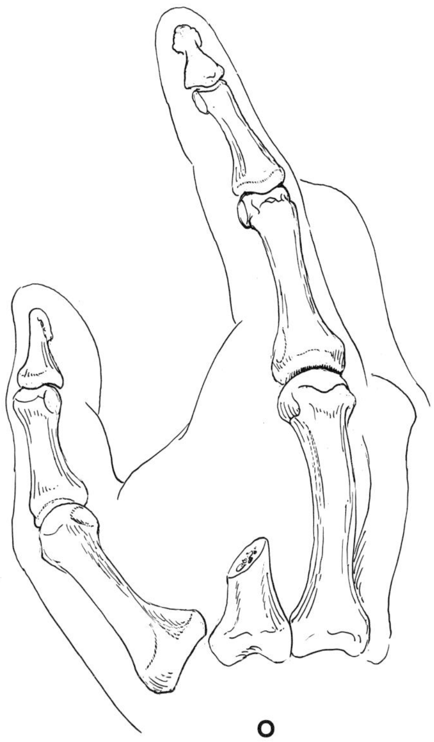

O

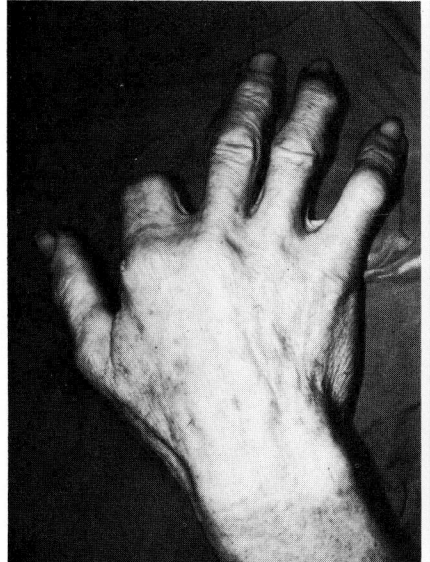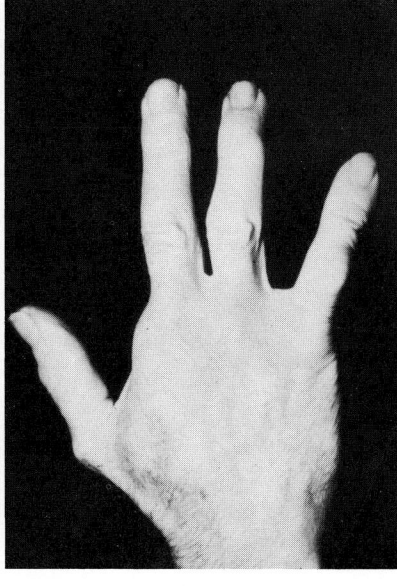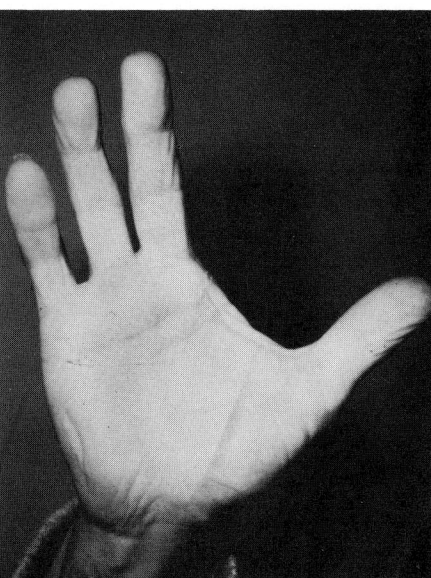

157

34

Fifth Ray Amputation

Principles

The principles of technique outlined for amputation of the index ray apply to amputation of the other peripheral hand ray—the fifth. The little finger is essentially useless when it is lost through the proximal phalanx. As an unsightly nub on the ulnar side of the hand, it has a tendency to catch on pockets, table tops, drawers, and implements. The appearance of the hand is improved by metacarpal amputation when the finger is irreversibly deformed or amputated at a critical level.

Example

A child sustained a traumatic amputation of the little finger through the proximal phalanx and was left with a useless tender nub which drifted ulnarward. Fifth ray amputation was decided upon. The incision was planned to remove the fourth web space by starting it at the base of the ring finger on the ulnar side. The point on the ulnar side of the little finger which would shift to the side of the ring finger after removal of the nub and metacarpal was identified. Curved incisions on the dorsum of the hand adequate in length to expose the proximal portion of the fifth metacarpal were marked out. A similar incision on the palm was planned. (**A**)

The dorsal branch of the ulnar nerve was identified during dissection so that branches to the ring finger could be preserved to avoid anesthesia over the residual peripheral ulnar side of the hand. (**B**)

Elevation of the triangular dorsal flap exposed the dorsal interossei and the subcutaneous portion of the fifth metacarpal. The periosteum was incised and elevated from the proximal half of the metacarpal. An oblique osteotomy was done in such a way that the bone end would fit the new hand contour after amputation. (**C**)

The extensor digiti minimi tendons were cut by retracting them distally and cutting them well proximal. The extensor digitorum slip to the little finger frequently crosses from the extensor to the ring finger just proximal to the metacarpophalangeal joint. The surgeon must be careful not to injure the extensor to the ring finger as he cuts the segment passing to the little finger. The intrinsic muscles were preserved.

Amputations

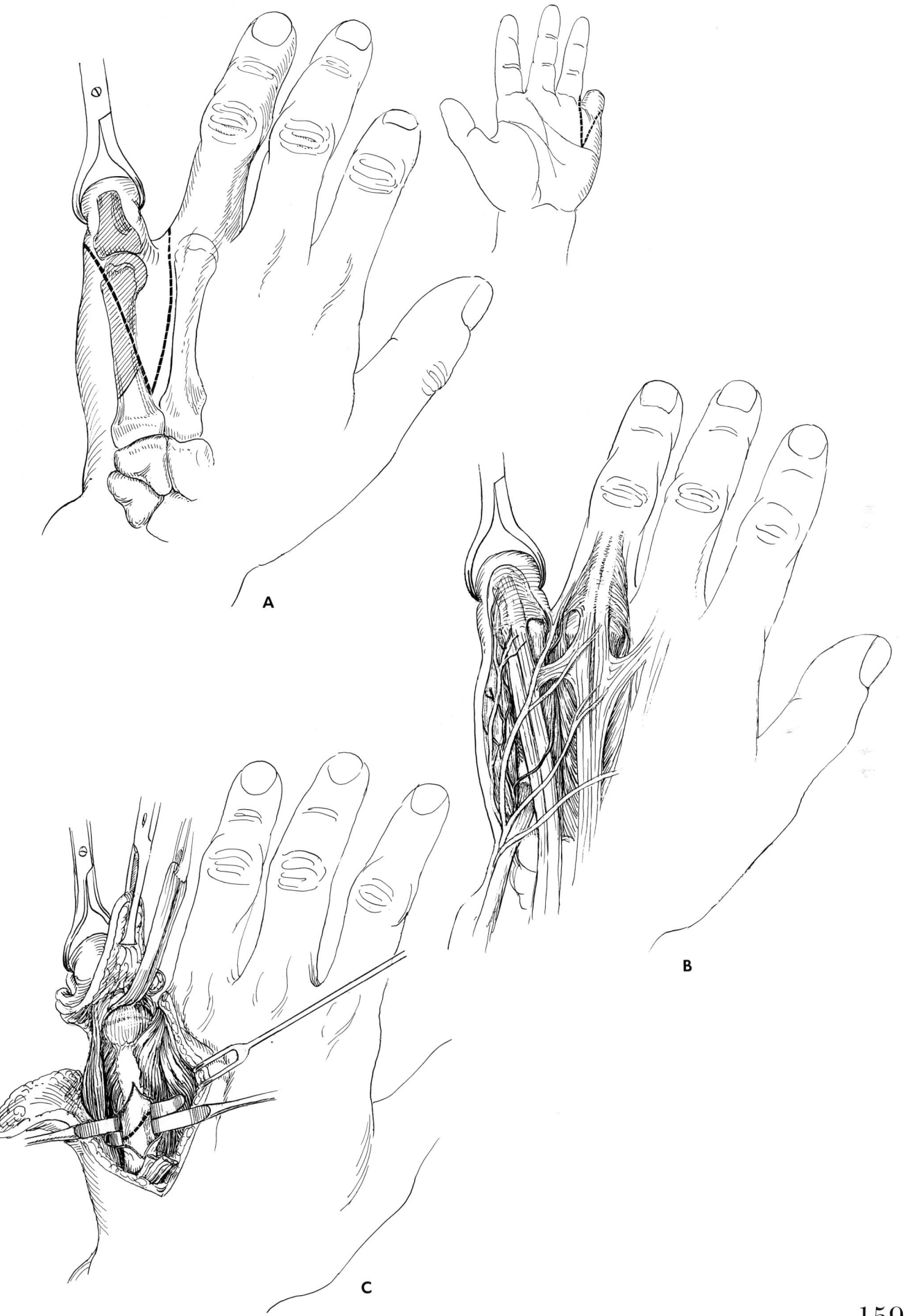

A

B

C

159

34 — Fifth Ray Amputation

The insertion of the abductor digiti minimi into the lateral band and proximal phalanx of the little finger was cut sharply and preserved for transfer to the ulnar lateral band of the ring finger. The digital vessels were ligated short and cut, but the digital nerves were left long so they could be placed deep in the interosseous space to avoid exposed neuroma problems. The flexor tendons were individually pulled distally, cut short and allowed to retract. (**D**)

A knowledge of the anatomy of the hypothenar area of the palm is essential for the precise dissection necessary in this amputation. (**E**)

The abductor digiti minimi tendon was sutured to the lateral band on the ulnar side of the ring finger. Closure of the space left by removal of the metacarpal and metacarpophalangeal joint was achieved by shifting the abductor digiti minimi radially and suturing it to the fourth dorsal interosseous. (**F**)

Adjustment of the skin edges is best achieved by starting the suture closure on the palmar aspect and progressing around to the dorsum. (**G**) The mobile, thin dorsal skin can be tailored to assure smooth closure.

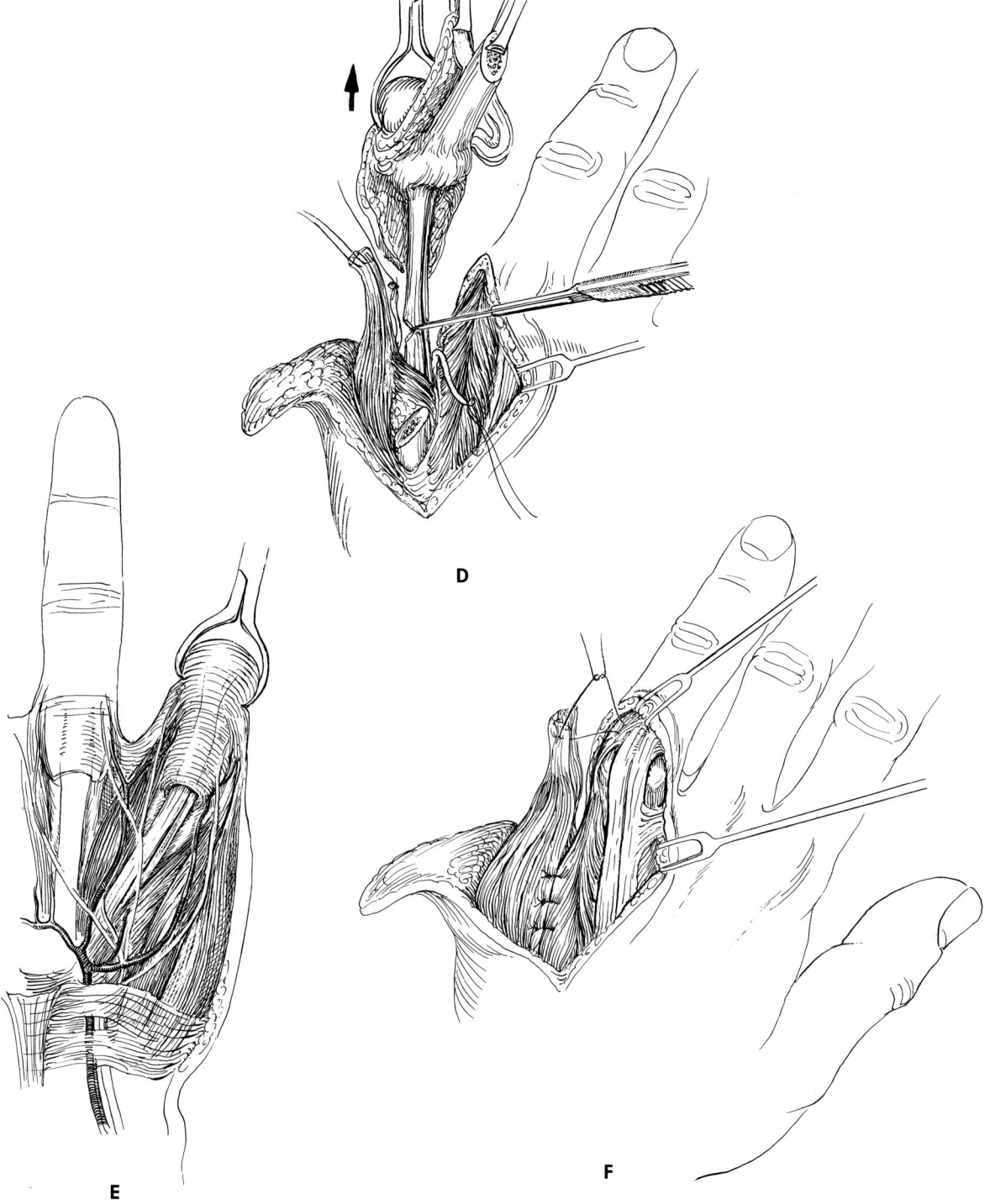

D

E

F

160

Amputations

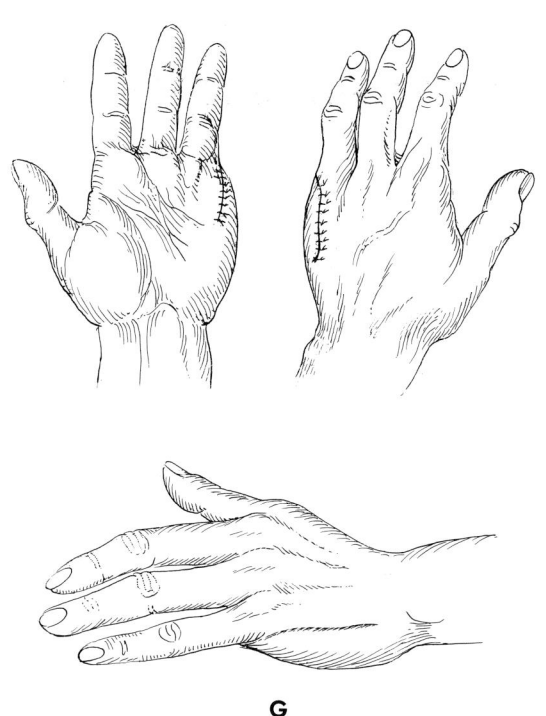

G

A CASE OF PRIMARY FIFTH RAY AMPUTATION

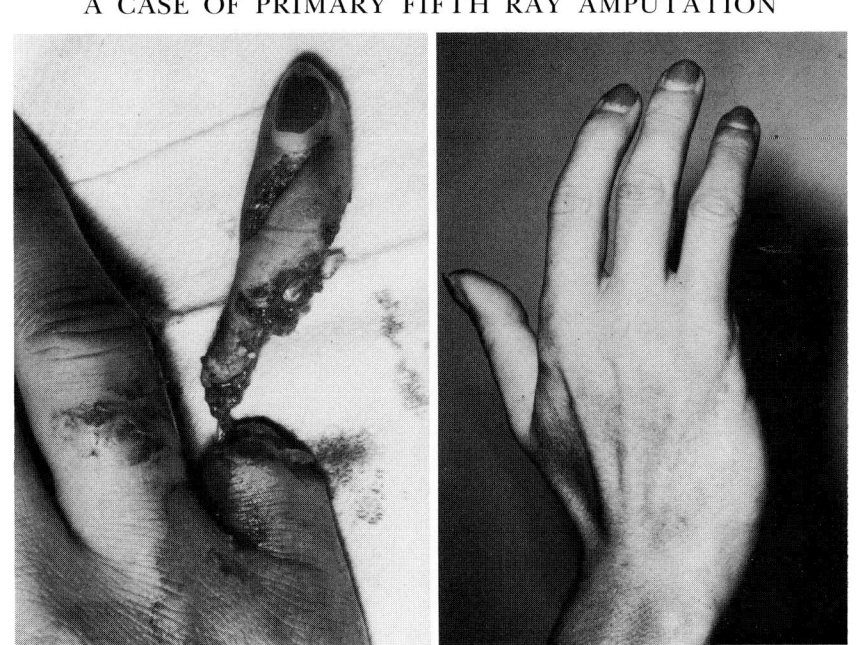

161

35

Salvage of Usable Parts in Severe Hand Injuries

Principles

The rules for treatment of solitary digit injuries are changed when several digits are involved. A digit irreversibly damaged and destined for amputation should be carefully inventoried for parts which may be usable in reconstructing other injured parts. The surgeon should not use distant donor sites for the elements necessary for reconstruction until the possibility of local available parts has been studied. It may be good judgment where a mutilating multidigital injury exists to salvage all parts not stripped of blood supply even when some digits are injured beyond possible functional restoration. Such digits, useless in their own right, may be considered donors for autogenous parts in overall reconstruction of the hand.

Examples of parts that may be utilized either primarily or in secondary reconstruction are suggested by the illustration. (**A**)

Skin. Skin as a free full thickness or partial thickness graft and skin with its subcutaneous tissue on a vascular pedicle is frequently available at the time a digit is amputated. (See Sections 23, 24, 25, 26, 37, and 38.)

Tendon. Tendon from a digit to be amputated or tendon which is useless by virtue of joint fusion is available either as a free tendon graft or as a motorized tendon transfer to restore a lost motor unit. (See Section 25.)

Nerve. The nerves rendered superfluous by digit amputation may serve as nerve transfers to another area of the hand or they may be used as free autogenous nerve grafts if substance has been lost in nerves elsewhere. (See Section 37.)

Bone. Bone for grafting to areas of missing bone substance or for use as pegs in osteotomy or joint fusion sites is very conveniently obtained when a digit is amputated. (See Sections 38, 39 and 40.)

Joint. Joints may be shifted as vascularized composite units to replace irreversibly damaged joints. This may be done as part of a whole neurovascular digit or metacarpal shift or as a joint alone, carried on blood supply left intact as a pedicle. (See Section 41.)

Intrinsic Muscles. Intrinsic muscles, particularly the abductor digiti minimi, may be useful in redistributing motor power in the hand. Such shifts of muscle preserve the intrinsic nerve and blood supply. (See Section 90, page 424.)

Fingernail. The nailbed will survive as a free graft and in unusual circumstances such a graft may be warranted as part of the amputation of the donor digit. (See page 132.)

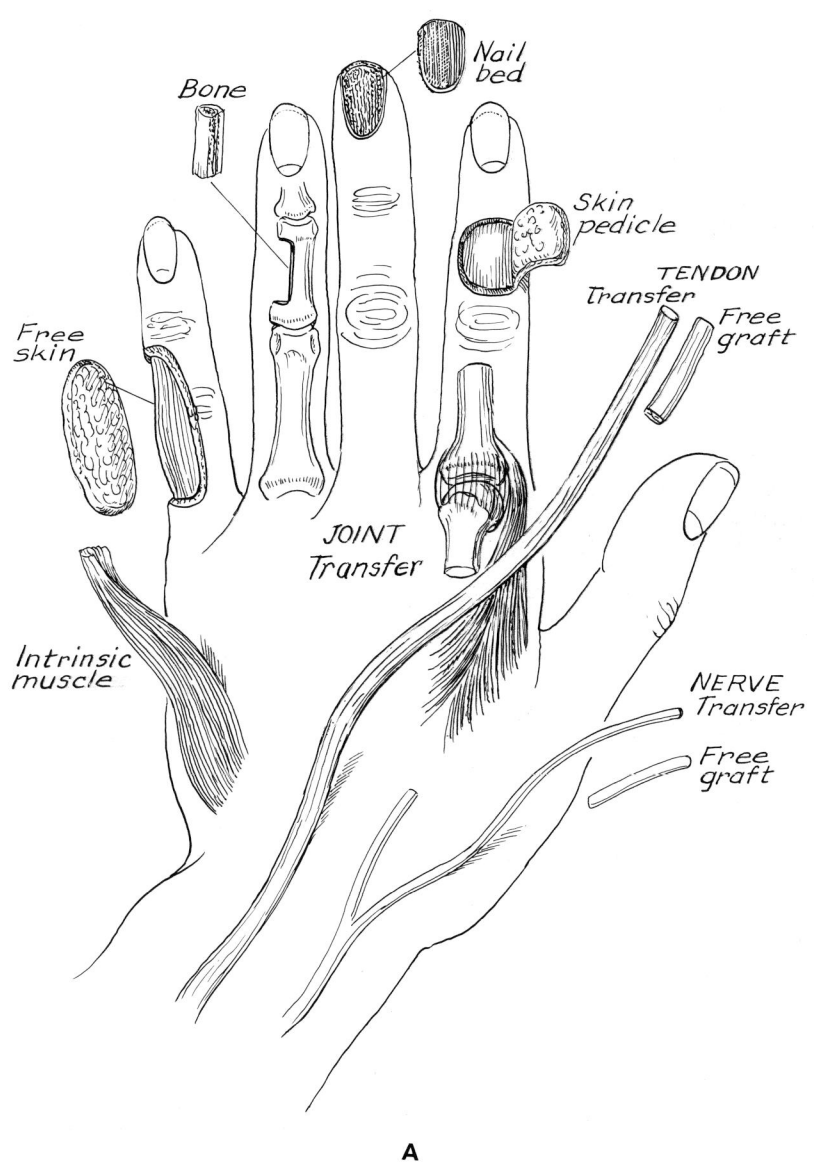

A

36
Use of Damaged Digits as Composite Transfers

Principle

A finger which has been damaged extensively may not serve a useful function of its own. Such a shortened or damaged digit may be transferred as a composite unit to enhance function of another finger or even more frequently of a shortened or totally amputated thumb. Such a composite transfer must be carried on intact blood vessels as a biological transfer.

Example

A young girl sustained traumatic amputation of the thumb through its metacarpal, the index finger at the metacarpophalangeal joint level, and the long finger through the proximal phalanx. (**A**)

An attempt to replant the long finger was unsuccessful and the replanted part failed to regain circulation. (**B**)

The patient was left with a long-finger nub which was useless in its own right. The long-finger nub and its metacarpal were thought to be appropriate for transfer to the thumb position to regain prehensile function. After amputation of the index metacarpal, the long finger ray was transferred to the first metacarpal. (**C**) This was done by preserving the palmar neurovascular bundles and shifting the nub and metacarpal as a composite unit including long flexor and extensor tendons, as well as skin and soft tissues to the thumb position. The unit was rotated into position for opposition with the ring and little fingers.

The patient gained prehensile pinch and grasp function and had a reconstructed thumb with full sensibility, sudomotor function, and permanently transferred blood supply. There were flexion and extension at the metacarpophalangeal joint since the long flexors and extensors of the long finger were preserved. Adequate thenar positioning muscles were left to allow functional positioning of the reconstructed thumb. (**D**)

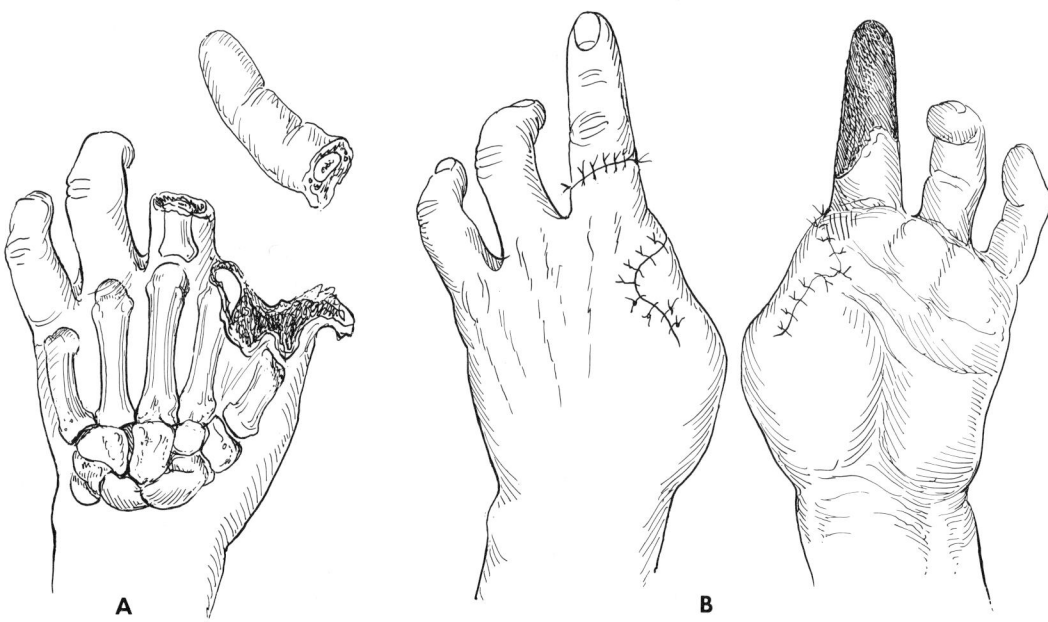

Amputations

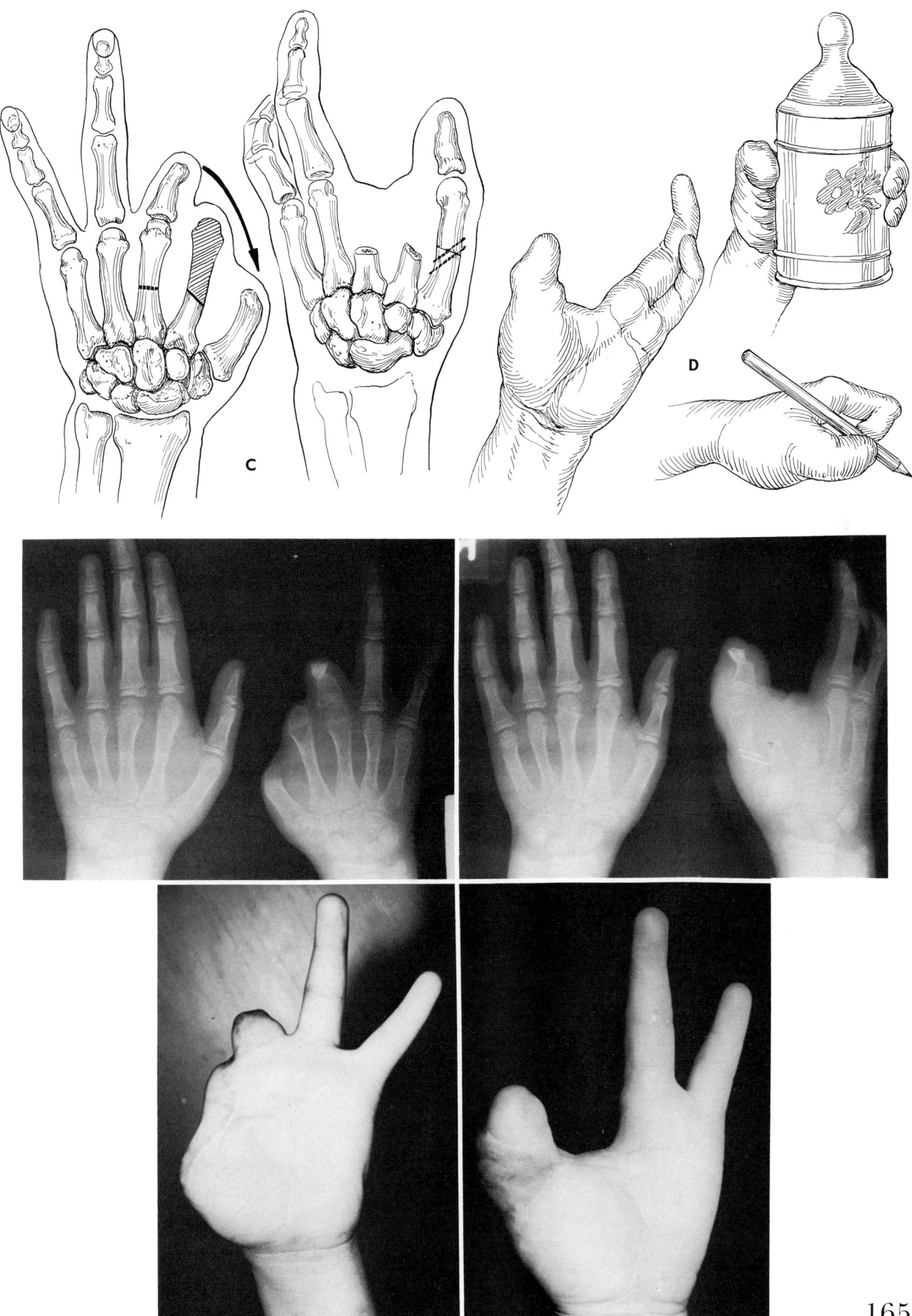

37

Use of Amputated Parts as a Source of Free Grafts of Skin and Nerves

Principle

Several examples of use of bone from amputated hand elements are demonstrated in this volume. Free skin, particularly from the dorsum of amputated parts, and free autogenous nerve grafts have a place in the hand surgeon's armamentarium.

Example

A blast injury in a child resulted in irreversible loss of the thumb tip, the entire index finger, the entire long finger, and soft tissue and neurovascular apparatus on the radial side of the ring finger. (**A**)

The basic requirements for immediate treatment consist of completion amputation of the index and long fingers, closure of the thumb tip injury without sacrifice of length, and careful attention to salvage of the ring finger, which by virtue of amputation of the index and long fingers had been promoted to a finger of prime importance.

The loss of sensibility in the working side of the finger could conceivably be diminished if the digital nerve was restored by grafting. Autogenous digital nerves were immediately available because of the amputation of the index and long fingers. A segment of one such nerve was removed and placed as a free graft by suturing it to the cut ends of the lost digital nerve of the ring finger. (**B**)

It was possible to cover the nerve graft with intact palm skin. The residual skin loss on the radial aspect of the ring finger was covered with split thickness skin from the dorsum of the amputated portion of the hand. (**C** and **D**)

The wounds healed well and the patient has had a slow return of useful, protective sensibility in the radial side of the ring finger. (**E**) Whether this is attributable to the nerve graft per se, spontaneous recovery, or cross over from the ulnar side is impossible to state with conviction.

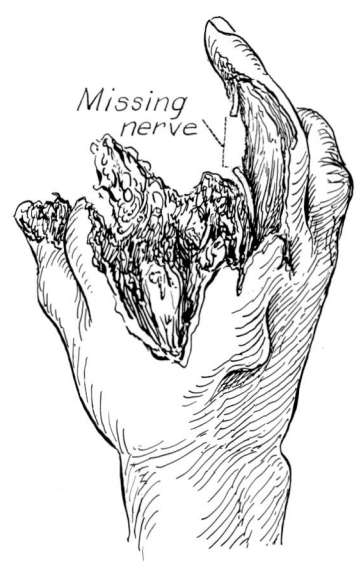

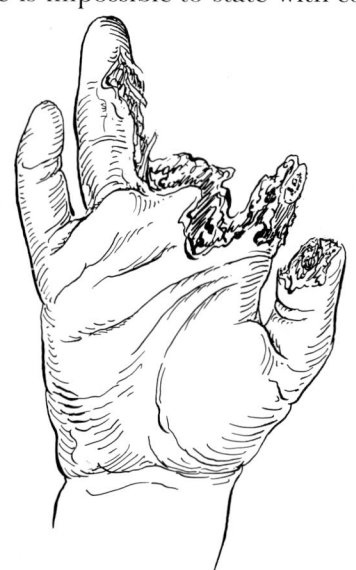

A

Nerve graft
Graft

B

C

Skin graft
Normal residual skin covers nerve graft

D

E

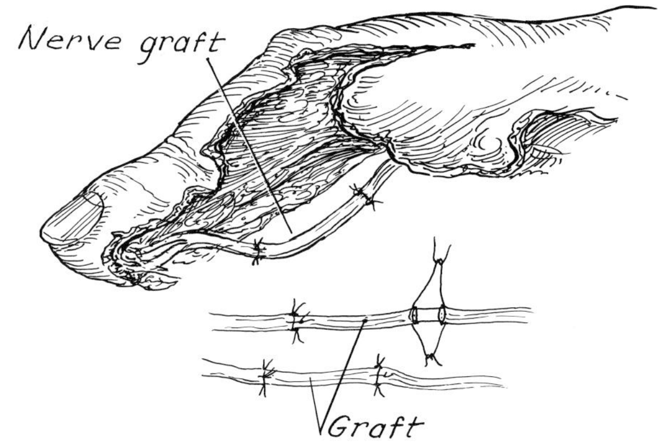

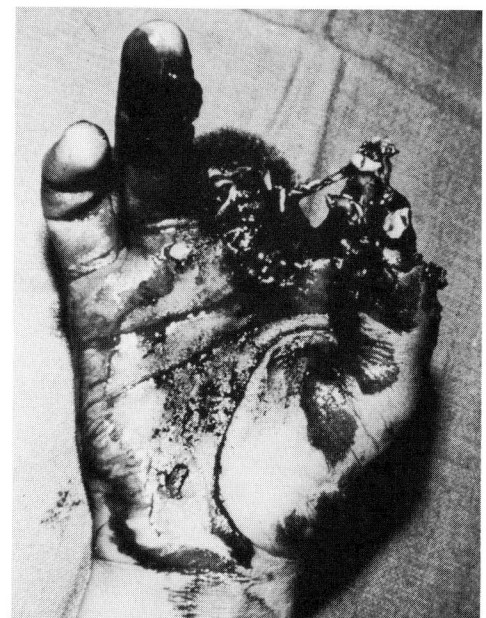

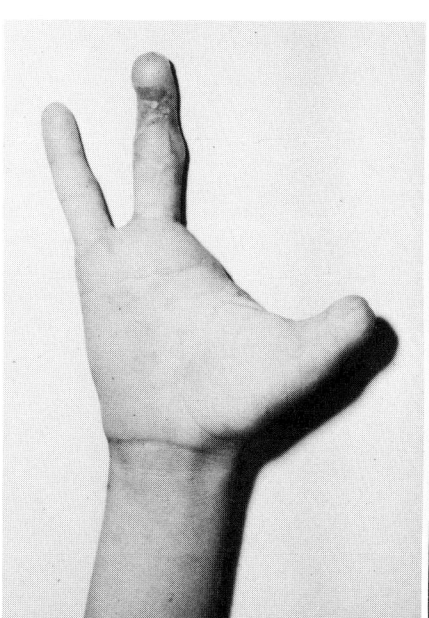

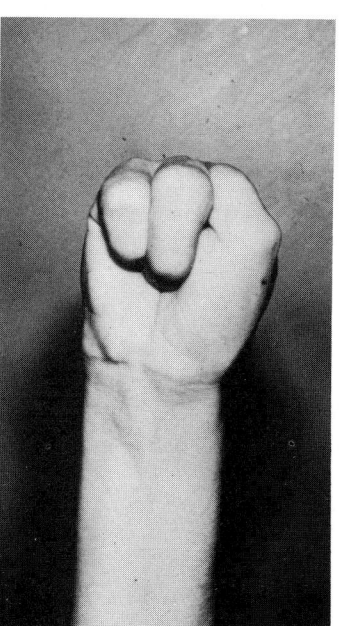

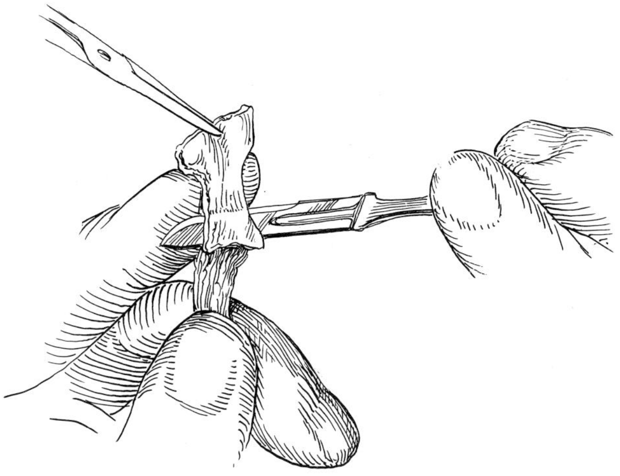

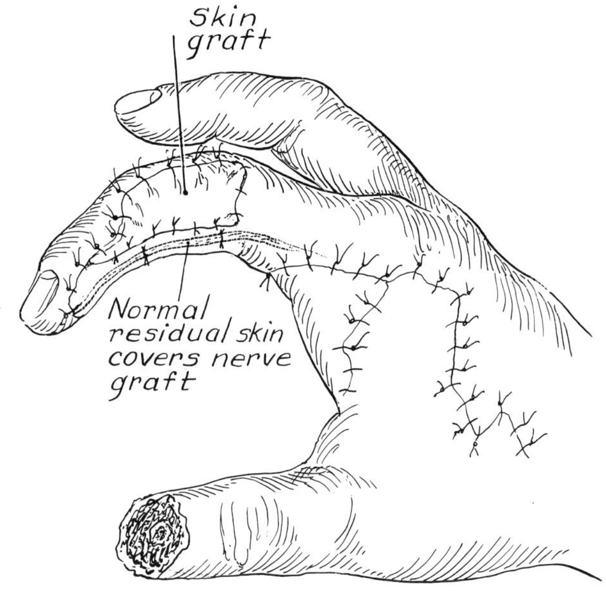

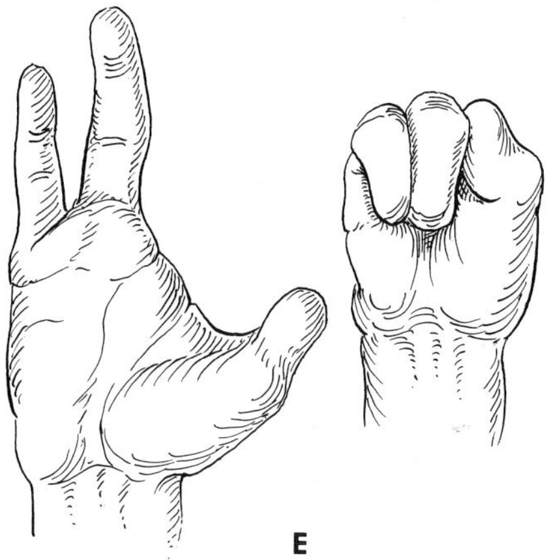

38

Double Use of a Finger Fated for Amputation

Principle

A finger destined for amputation may contribute a number of usable elements simultaneously or in stages.

Example

A patient suffered a power saw injury which amputated his thumb through the proximal phalanx and all but amputated the index and long fingers through the proximal phalanges.

The index and long fingers barely survived on the residual dorsal skin flaps. The neurovascular bundles, flexor tendons, and all except a narrow isthmus of the skin and dorsal cortex of the phalanges were traumatically transected. The atrophic, anesthetic index finger became rigidly fixed at the interphalangeal joints and reconstruction seemed senseless. The long finger retained some passive motion at the proximal interphalangeal joint but it suffered skin loss adjacent to the joint which hampered attempts to increase its range of motion. (**A** and **B**)

The ring and little fingers were uninjured. The disadvantage of a shortened thumb was amplified because the only remaining functional fingers were on the ulnar aspect of the hand.

An index ray amputation under these circumstances would contribute significantly to functional and cosmetic restoration. The digit, however, possessed parts which would further improve function. The skin and soft tissue could contribute to improved functional range of motion and protective cover if it were transferred to the skin-deficient area over the proximal interphangeal joint of the long finger. The remaining index nub of proximal phalanx proximal to the site of injury and, therefore, fully innervated and vascularized would be useful as a composite island transfer to regain length in the thumb.

The skin from the index finger was filleted from the tendinous and skeletal elements of the index finger through a mid-palmar incision. The middle phalanx and digit tip were amputated. (**C**)

A vascularized flap of tissue thus created was used as a cross finger flap to resurface the skin-deficient area on the long finger. (**D, E,** and **F**)

Three weeks later the flap was released and the amputation of the index digit was completed to the site of the original saw cut injury.

Subsequently, at a third stage, the fully innervated index nub was transferred to the thumb amputation site to augment its length.

An incision circumscribing the nub at the level of the metacarpophalangeal joint was outlined. The continuation of the incision was planned to carry out an index metacarpal (ray) amputation and to create a continuous curved line across the first web space and up the thumb to the site of the traumatic amputation. (**G**)

Amputations

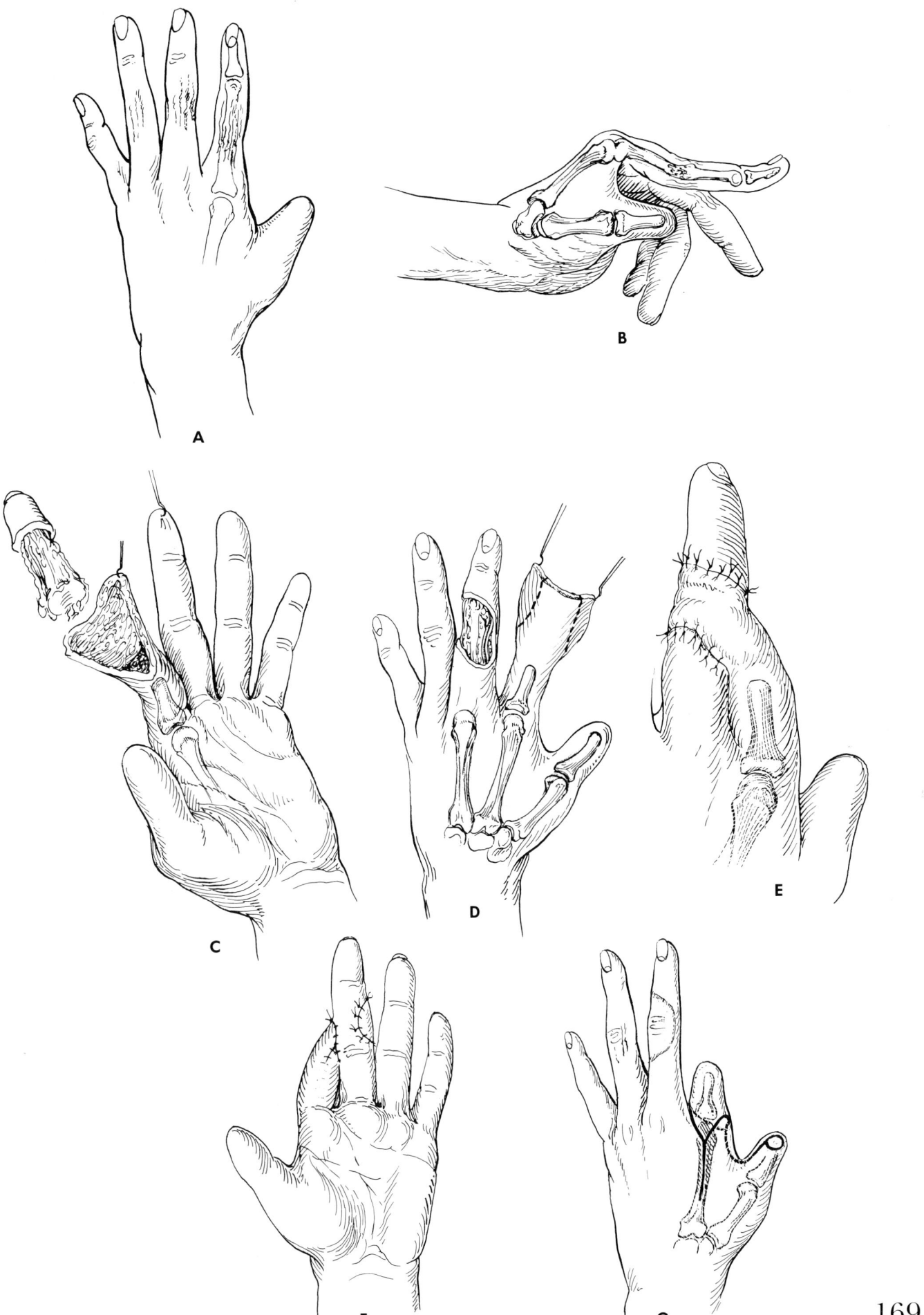

169

38 – Double Use of a Finger Fated for Amputation

The two palmar neurovascular bundles to the nub were isolated and protected as was a single dorsal vein. The metacarpal and long flexor and extensor tendons were removed. The metacarpal was saved as a source of bone for construction of a bone peg. The first dorsal and palmar interossei were sectioned at their musculo-aponeurotic area leaving the nub hanging only by the neurovascular structures and one dorsal vein. (**H**)

A medullary bone peg was made from cortical bone fashioned from the amputated metacarpal. (**I**) The thumb amputation site was circumscribed and excised. The end of the proximal phalanx of the thumb was freshened and the bone peg was driven into its medullary cavity leaving 1 cm. protruding to receive the proximal phalanx of the index finger, which remained a part of the composite nub. The proximal end of this phalanx was freshened and the medullary cavity was prepared to receive the bone peg. (**J**)

Transfer was accomplished and the proximal phalanges of the thumb and index nub were solidly fixed by the intramedullary bone graft and an obliquely placed single Kirschner wire.

The ray amputation was completed by smoothing and angling the proximal end of the index metacarpal, shifting the first dorsal interosseous, and appropriately tailoring the overlying skin. (**K**)

The first web space was closed by interdigitating the flaps which had been elevated to allow transfer of the composite unit. (**L**)

The additional 1.5 to 2.0 cm. of length acquired by the thumb allowed it comfortably and efficiently to manipulate in opposition to the ring and little fingers. (**M**)

The ultimate fate of the long finger will depend on the result of additional reconstructive efforts.

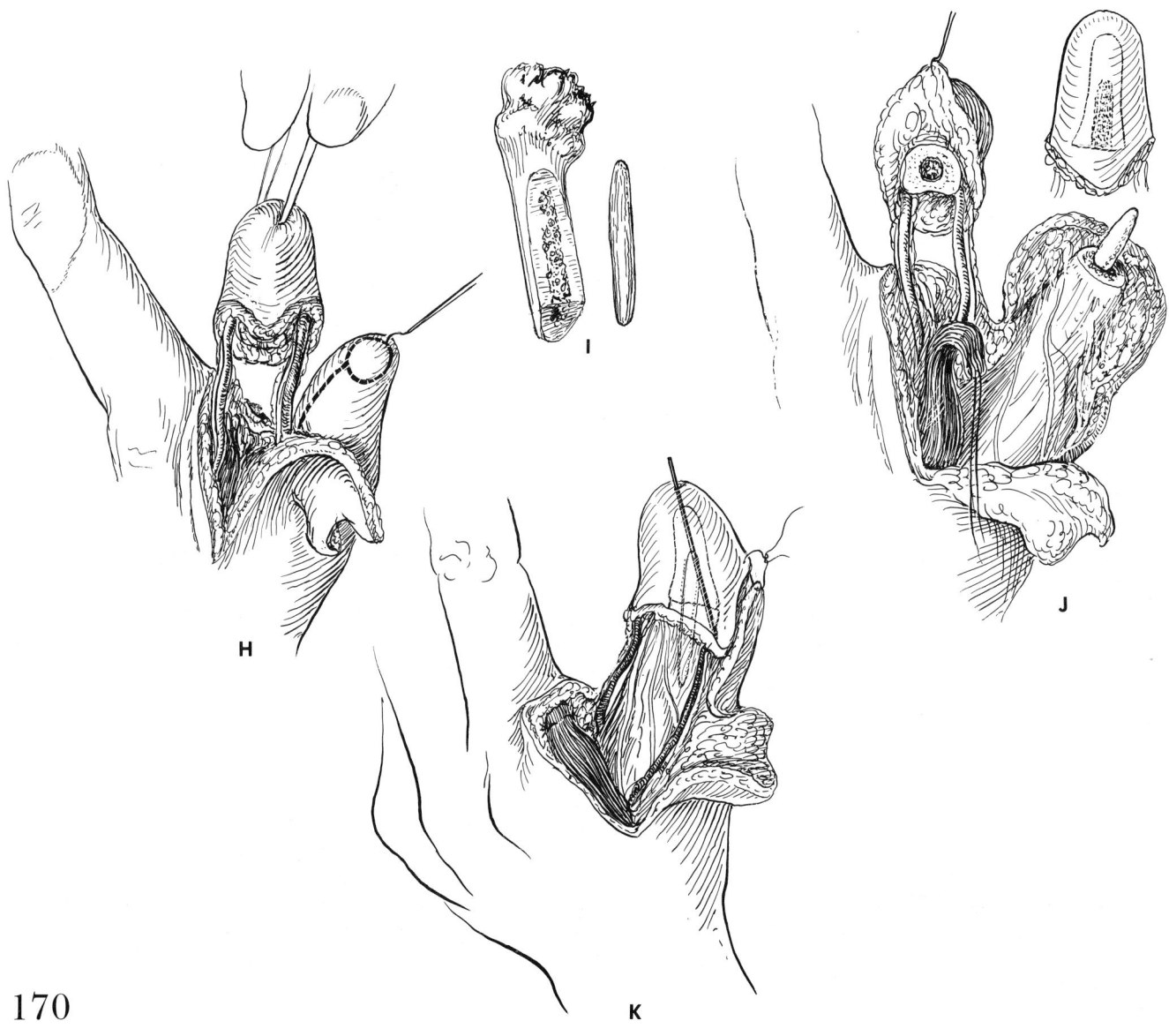

Amputations

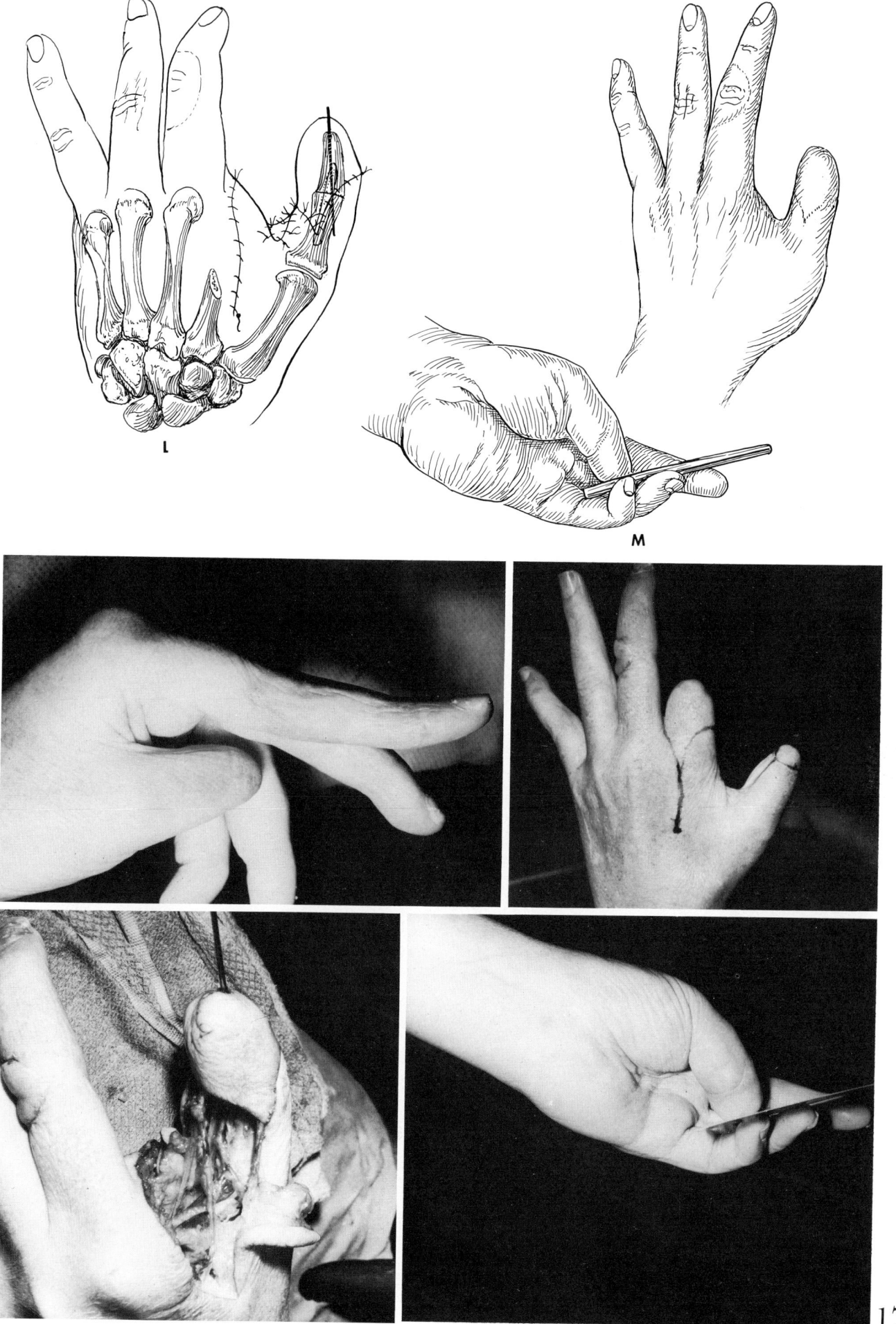

171

39
The Primary Island Pedicle Flap for Salvage After Trauma

Principle

The island pedicle flap contributes skin and soft tissue with sensibility to a deficient recipient area. A very important addition is the permanent new blood supply introduced by the flap. In acute injuries a new blood supply may mean the difference between salvage and loss by amputation. When distal vessels have been destroyed or removed by the injury while important devascularized components of the digit remain, immediate restoration of blood supply using a vascularized island pedicle flap may save the parts in jeopardy. Any severe injury of the index finger or thumb may warrant treatment by immediate transfer of an island pedicle flap.

Avulsion or blast injury of the index finger may result in loss of important palmar skin and soft tissue, exposing underlying bone or tendon which is devoid of blood supply and soft tissue protection. To salvage such a finger one must obtain skin and soft tissue coverage with intrinsic blood supply. A distant pedicle flap would serve this need but would leave the important index finger forever without full sensibility and with less adequate blood supply than could be acquired permanently by island pedicle transfer. Since full reconstruction of the index finger with sensibility would ultimately require an island pedicle transfer, it seems logical to consider it primarily under proper conditions.

Example: Index Avulsion

A young man sustained a grinding avulsion injury to the palmar aspect of his left index finger. The distal phalanx was exposed and its periosteum was abraded off in the injury. (**A**)

After careful cleansing and debridement of the injured index finger, careful measurement of the extent of soft tissue loss was made. An island pedicle flap from the ulnar side of the long finger was outlined after the surgeon assured himself that there had been no injury which would compromise the blood supply to the long finger. (**B**)

The island pedicle flap was elevated from the finger by the technique described elsewhere. (See page 78.) The pedicle flap was sutured in place and the donor area was covered with a free skin graft, with proper side cuts to avoid a straight midline palmar scar in the finger. (**C**)

The hand was carefully dressed and, aside from a wound check and examination of the free skin graft in five days, the hand was kept dressed for ten days. Early motion was instituted once the soft tissues had healed sufficiently. Prompt healing followed and full function was restored to the index finger in four weeks. (**D**)

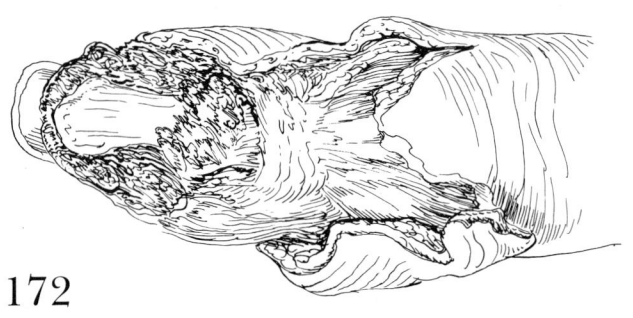 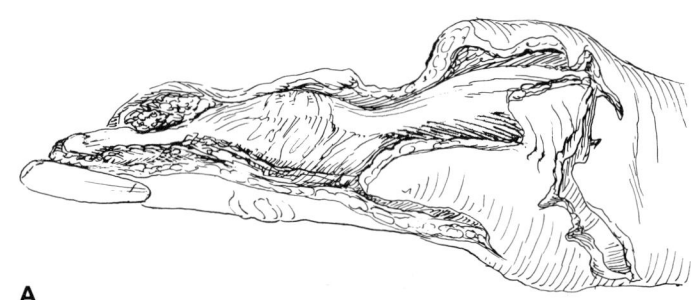

A

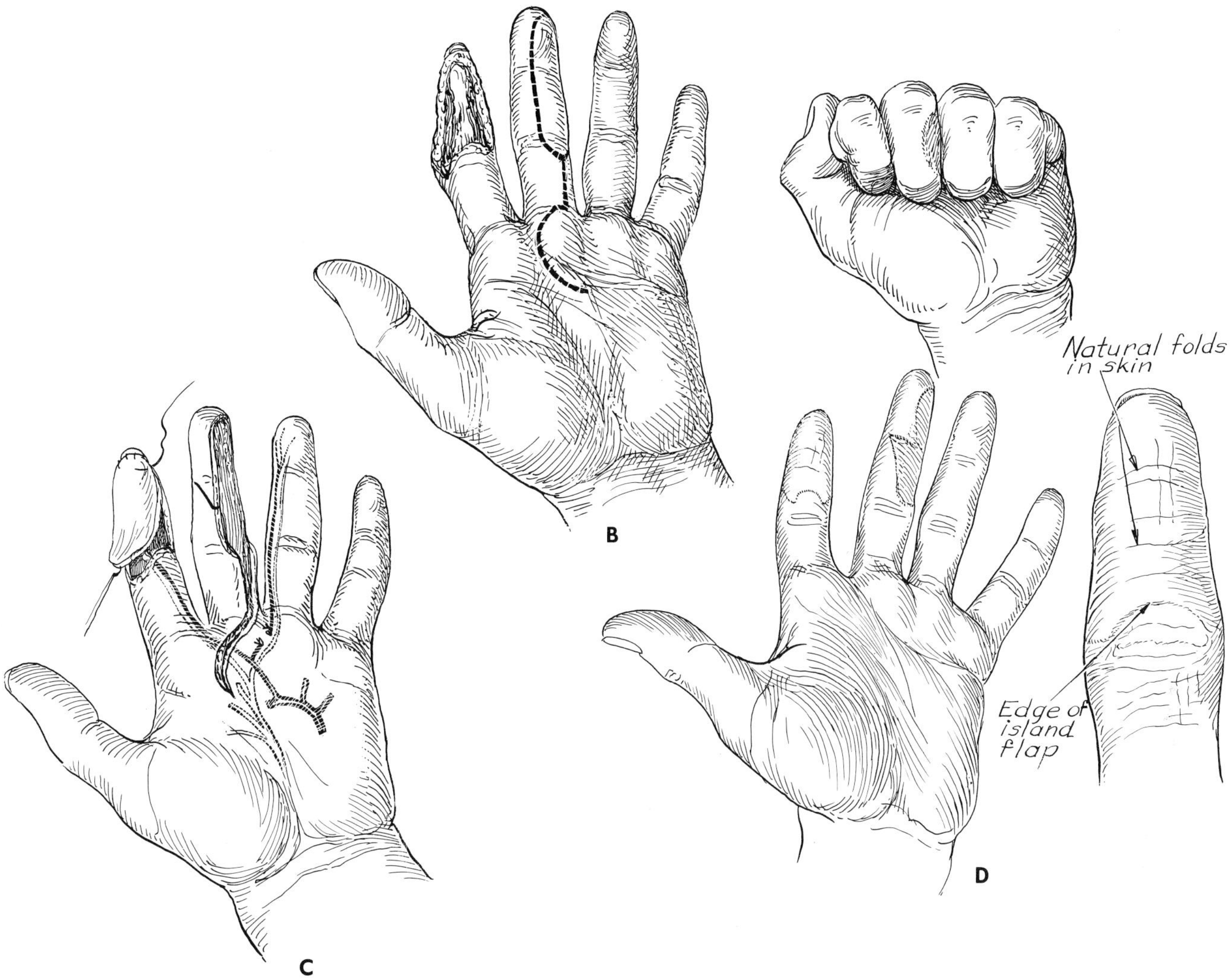

Amputations

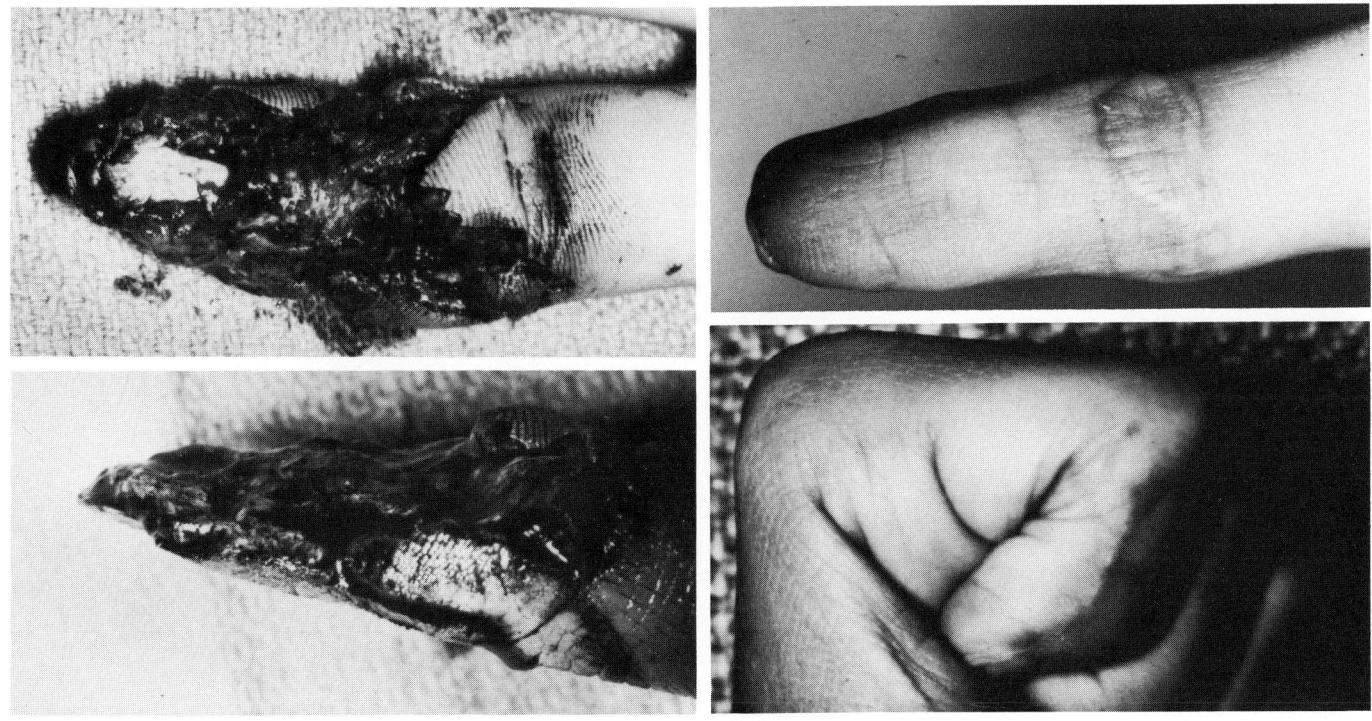

Natural folds in skin

Edge of island flap

B

C

D

173

39 – The Primary Island Pedicle Flap for Salvage After Trauma

Example: Ring Avulsion

A left hand ring avulsion injury was sustained by a 12-year-old boy whose career objective required use of all his fingers. Lost in the avulsion were the skin and subcutaneous tissue beyond the mid proximal phalanx and the entire finger distal to the distal interphalangeal joint. (**E**)

To gain immediate vascularized and fully sensitive skin and soft tissue over the denuded functional residual finger, an island pedicle flap was planned. The flap was outlined on the adjacent side of the long finger to carry nearly the entire side of the long finger to the ring finger. (**F**)

The island of skin and subcutaneous tissue was dissected, preserving the proper digital vessels and nerve. It was passed to the ring finger deep to the palmar fascia. An incision was marked across the straight palmar incision on the donor finger to receive a dart of skin graft to be used to resurface the donor site. (**G**)

The island of skin and subcutaneous tissue was draped over the ring finger after the condyle of the disarticulated end of the proximal phalanx was rongeured back to give the finger proper contour. The residual raw area on the dorsum of the hand was resurfaced with a free full thickness skin graft. The donor site on the long finger was also resurfaced, using a free full thickness skin graft with a dart to break up the palmar midline incision. (**H**) As soon as healing was complete, the "dog ear" folds where the island flap folded on itself were removed. (**I**)

Function was restored early after operation and the ring finger, now shortened by the length of the distal phalanx, functions well. (**J**)

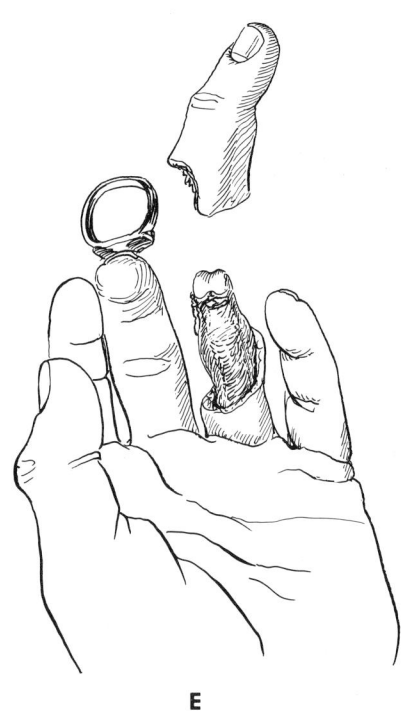

E

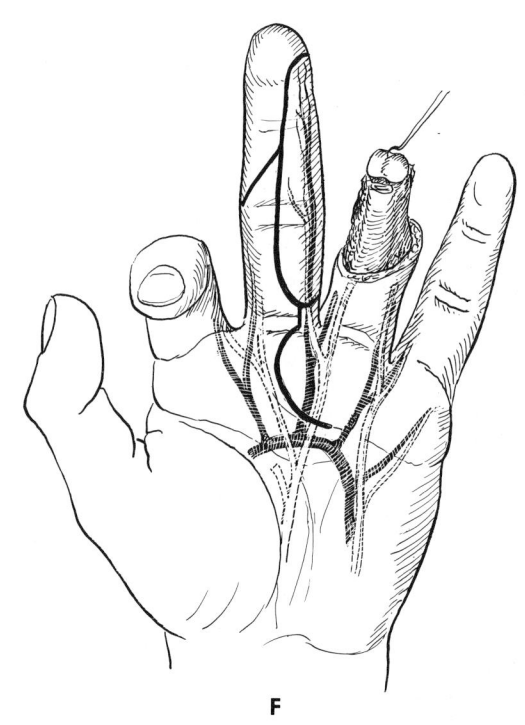

F

Amputations

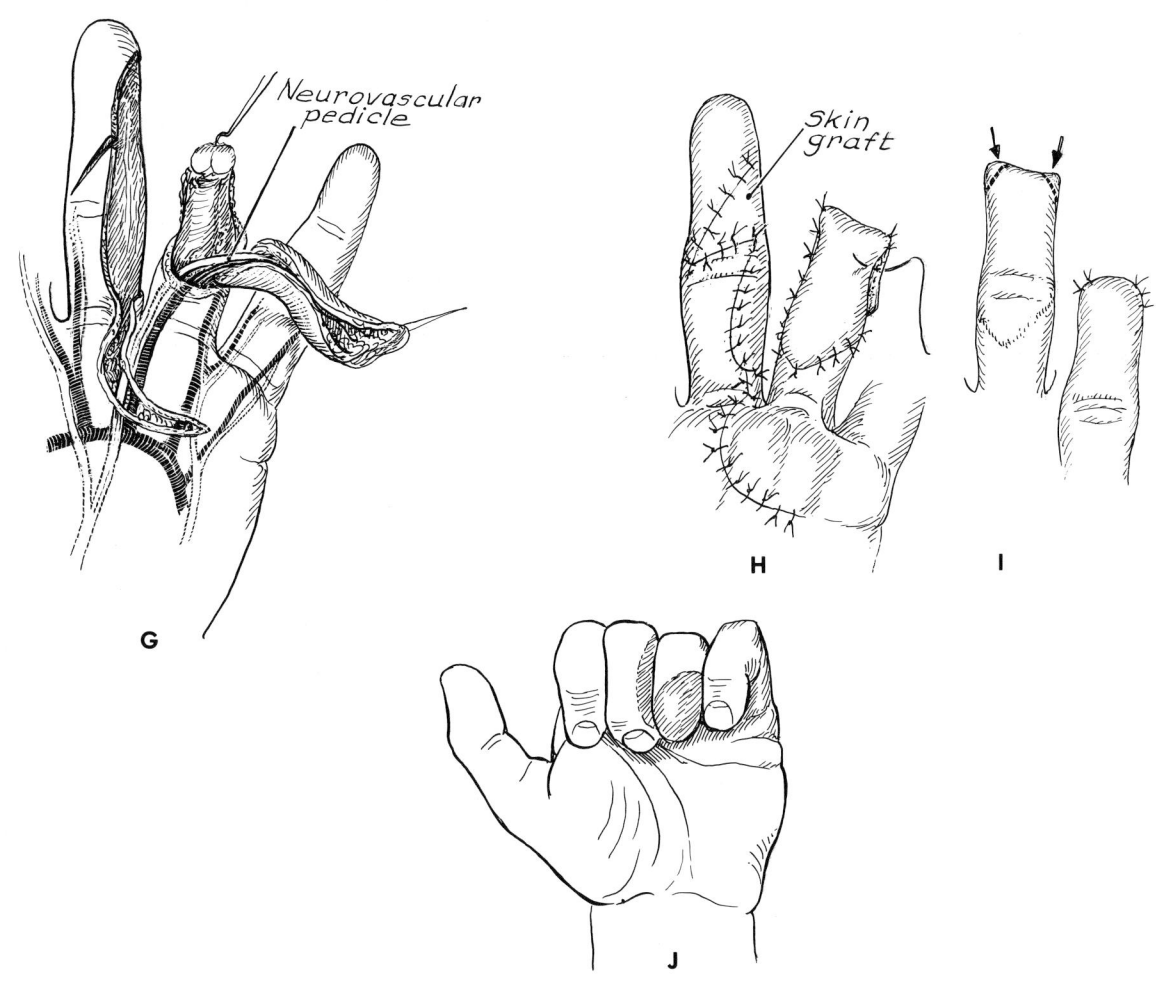

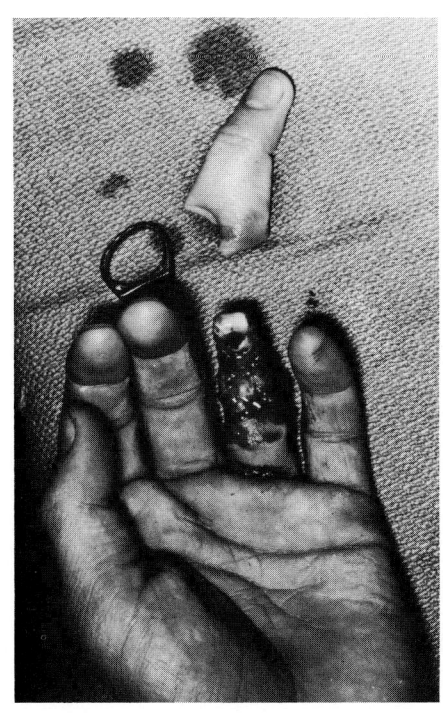
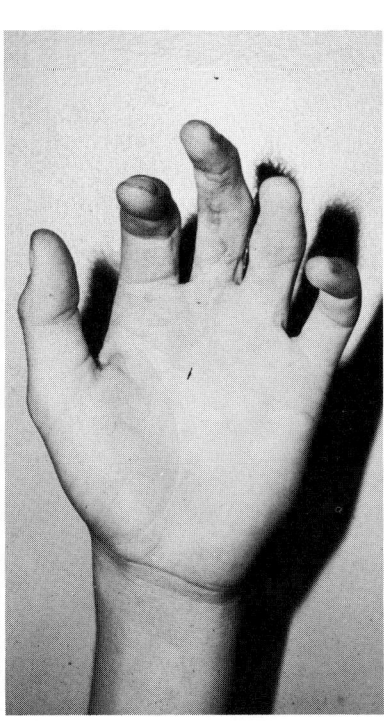
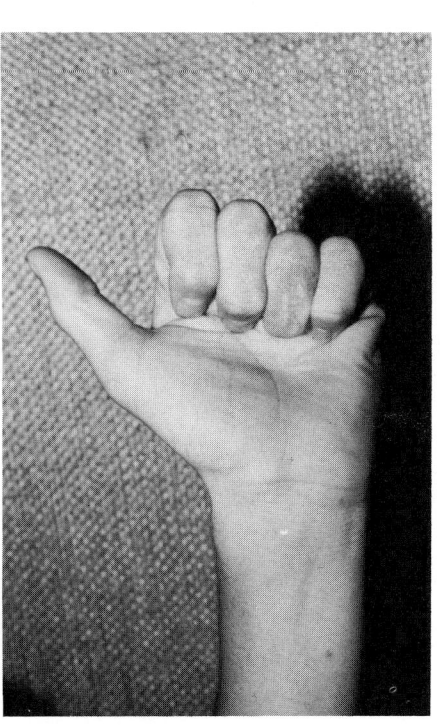

175

39 – The Primary Island Pedicle Flap for Salvage After Trauma

Example: Thumb Avulsion

A total avulsion of the soft tissues and the distal phalanx of the thumb occurred in a female secretary when the thumb was caught in a moving cable. The flexor pollicis longus and the extensor pollicis longus tendons ruptured at the musculotendinous junctures high in the forearm. They were extracted with the avulsion amputation. The residual thumb proximal phalanx was devoid of soft tissue cover. (**K**) Salvage by immediate reconstruction using a primary island pedicle flap was decided upon.

A long island-pedicle flap from the ulnar side of the long finger seemed appropriate for such a reconstruction. (**L**)

After careful debridement of the thumb avulsion site, an island pedicle flap of maximum size was elevated from the ulnar side of the long finger using the technique described on page 78. The pedicle flap was of sufficient length to gain coverage not only of the proximal phalanx but of a part of the distal phalanx, which was replanted as a free bone graft. The distal phalanx was filleted from the amputated part. Its joint surface and the joint surface of the proximal phalanx were removed by osteotome and rongeur, and the distal phalanx was replaced using a single Kirschner wire. The pedicle flap was used to resurface the entire palmar aspect of the thumb and it was turned over the tip of the thumb to cover the bone graft. The remaining portion of the dorsal aspect of the proximal phalanx was resurfaced with a free skin graft. This skin graft was taken as part of the skin graft removed for resurfacing the donor finger. (**M**)

Such a patient with an avulsion injury of the prime finger in the hand has a mandatory indication for immediate pedicle flap coverage for salvage. Although a distant pedicle flap could serve this purpose maximum benefit from surgery would then have required a subsequent addition of an island pedicle flap to supply sensibility. The superior quality and permanence of new thumb blood supply furnished by a primary island pedicle flap together with immediate protective sensibility allowed confident replacement of the totally devascularized distal phalanx as a free bone graft. The time saved by elimination of staged reconstruction was an additional benefit of the immediate island pedicle flap method for salvage of the devascularized residual thumb skeleton. The patient quickly gained use of the salvaged thumb. (**N**)

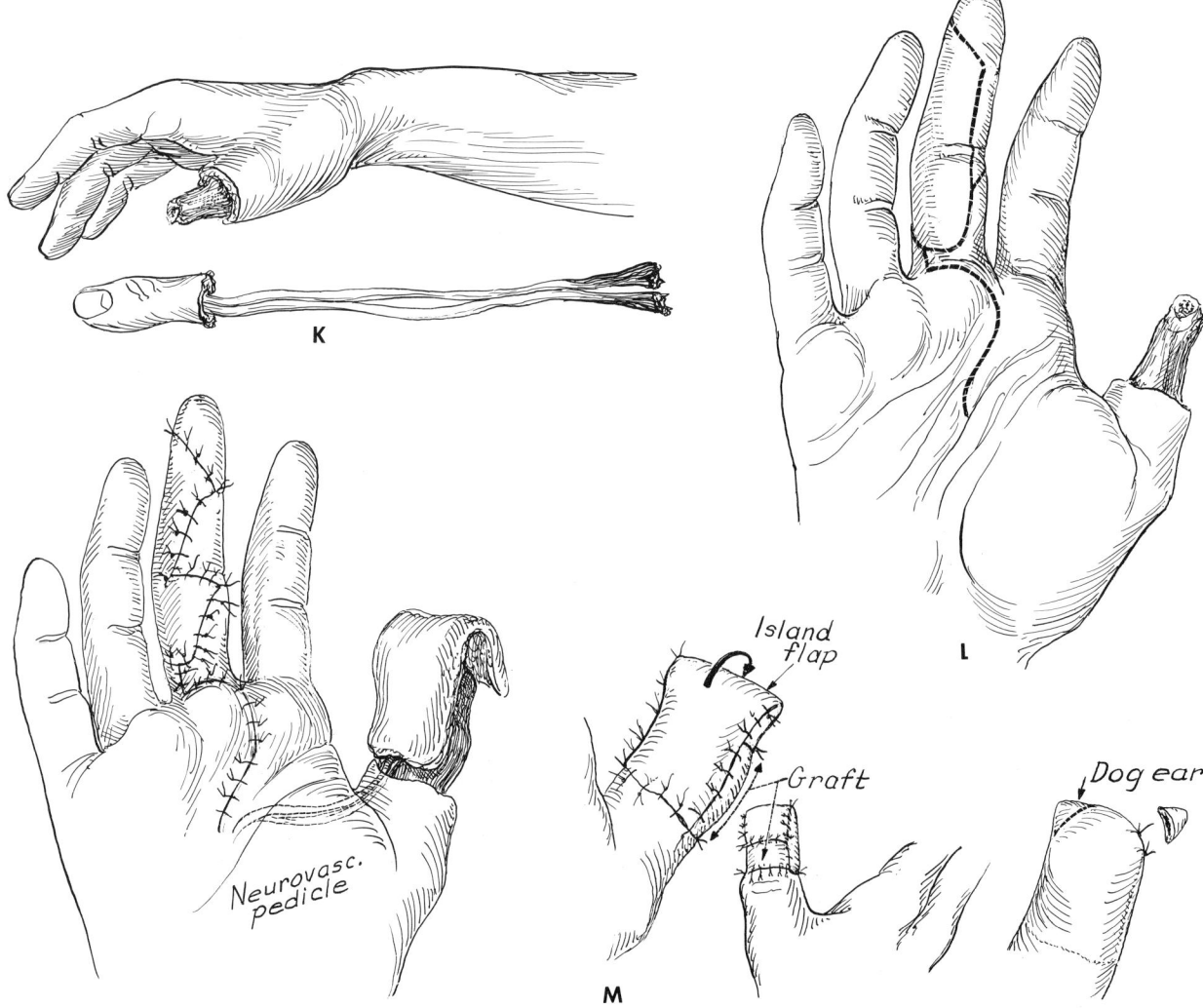

Amputations

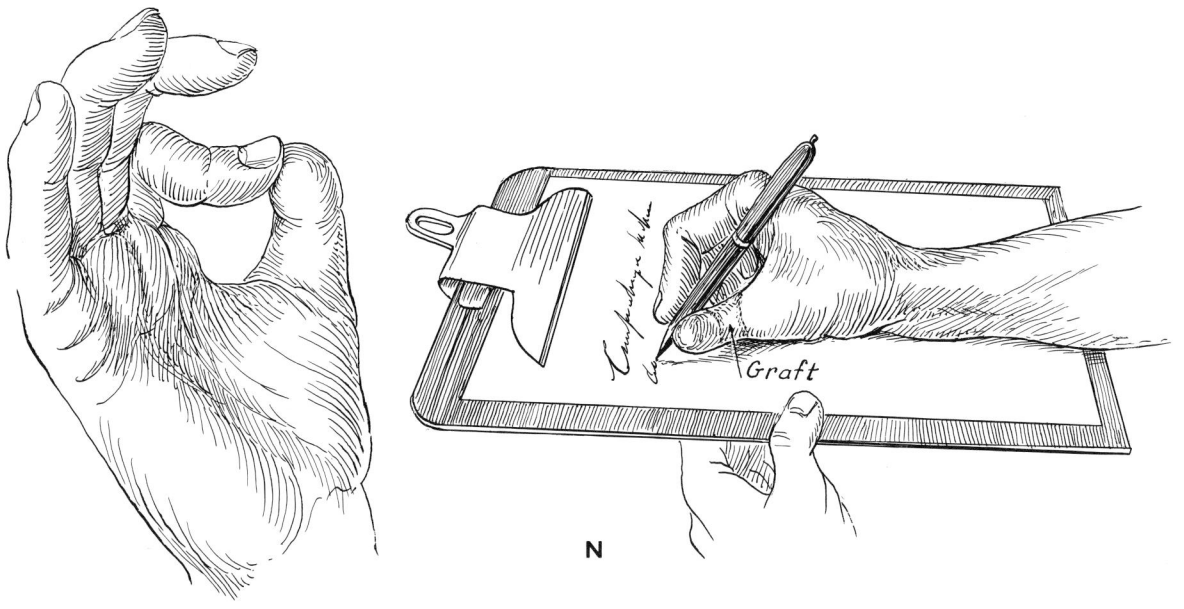

N

INJURY

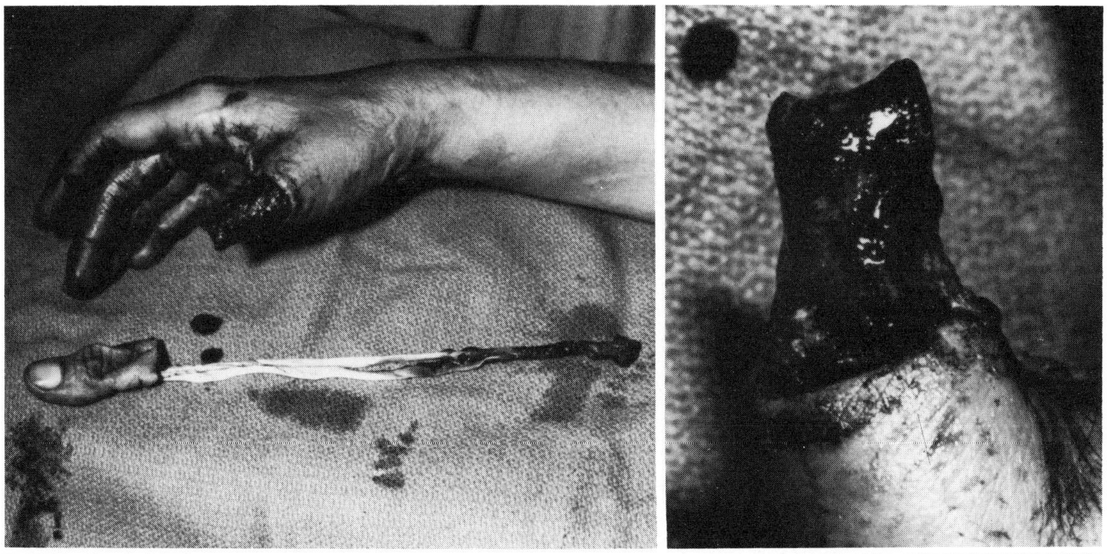

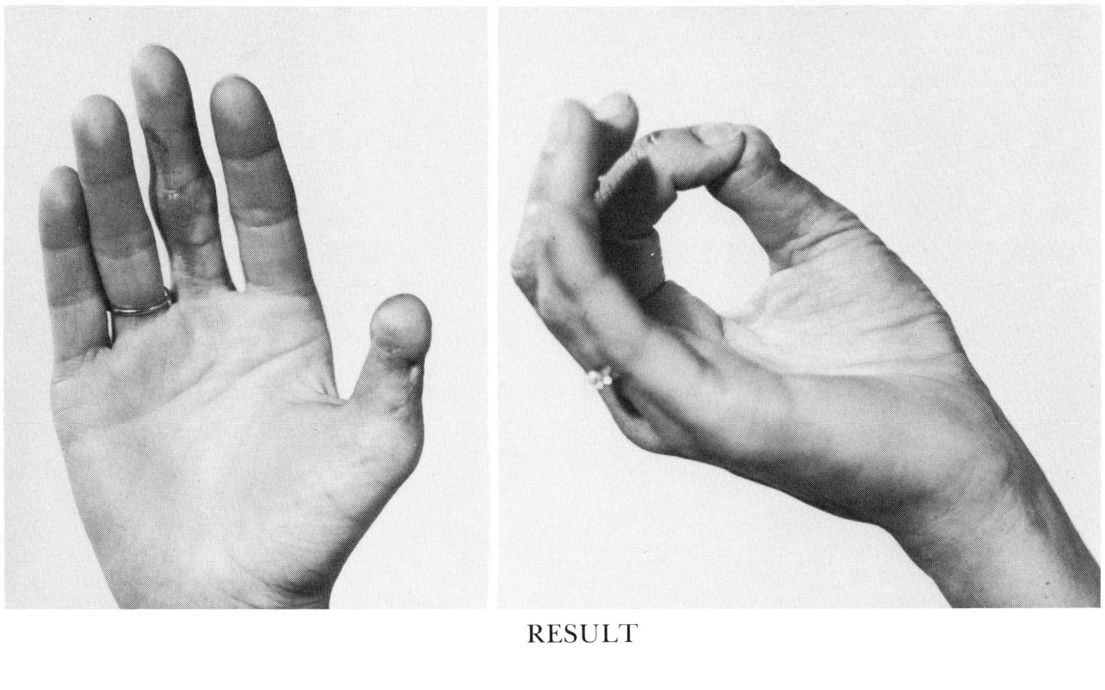

RESULT

177

COMBINED DISTANT PEDICLE FLAP AND SECONDARY LOCAL ISLAND PEDICLE FLAP

Example

A misfire explosion of a homemade bomb resulted in amputation of the thumb and lacerations of the index, long, and ring fingers of a high school boy. (**A**)

The wounds were debrided carefully and no tendon or nerve injury was found in the fingers. To salvage as much length as possible in the thumb, the distal phalanx was replaced in normal position and fixed with a single Kirschner wire. The reconstructed thumb skeleton was devoid of intrinsic blood supply; therefore, to secure skin and soft tissue coverage with blood supply was mandatory. (**B**)

A pedicle flap was elevated and tubed by making parallel incisions in the contralateral infraclavicular area. The hand was brought to the chest wall and the exposed thumb skeleton was covered by suturing the tubed pedicle flap over it. (**C**)

Three weeks later the tubed pedicle flap was cut free from the chest wall and fashioned to proper contour as a thumb tip. (**D**)

In order to restore sensibility, sudomotor function, and improved intrinsic blood supply to the reconstructed thumb, an island pedicle flap from the ulnar side of the long finger was planned. (**E**) The technique for island pedicle transfer was described on page 78.

The working surface of the reconstructed thumb was surgically denuded of epithelium leaving deep dermis intact. (**F**)

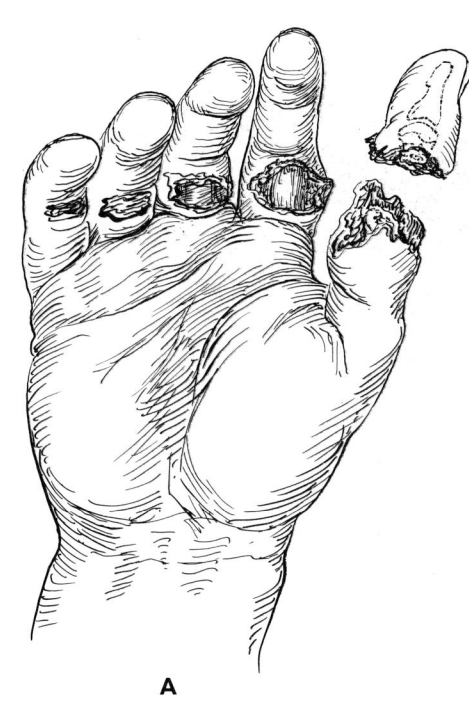

A

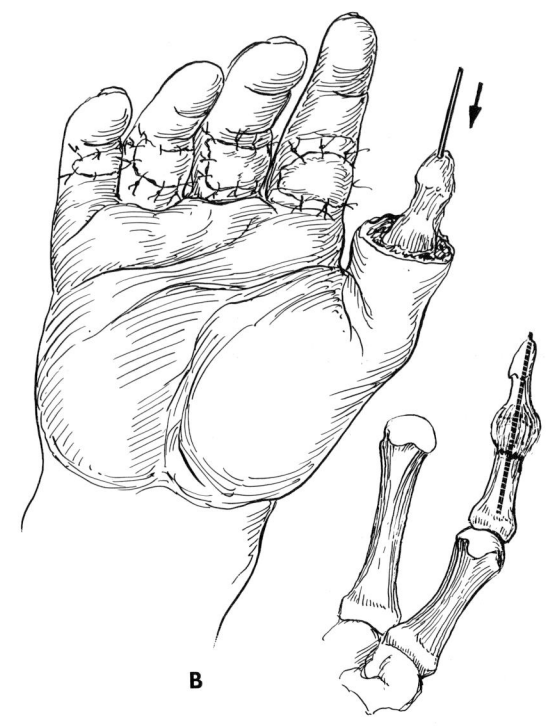

B

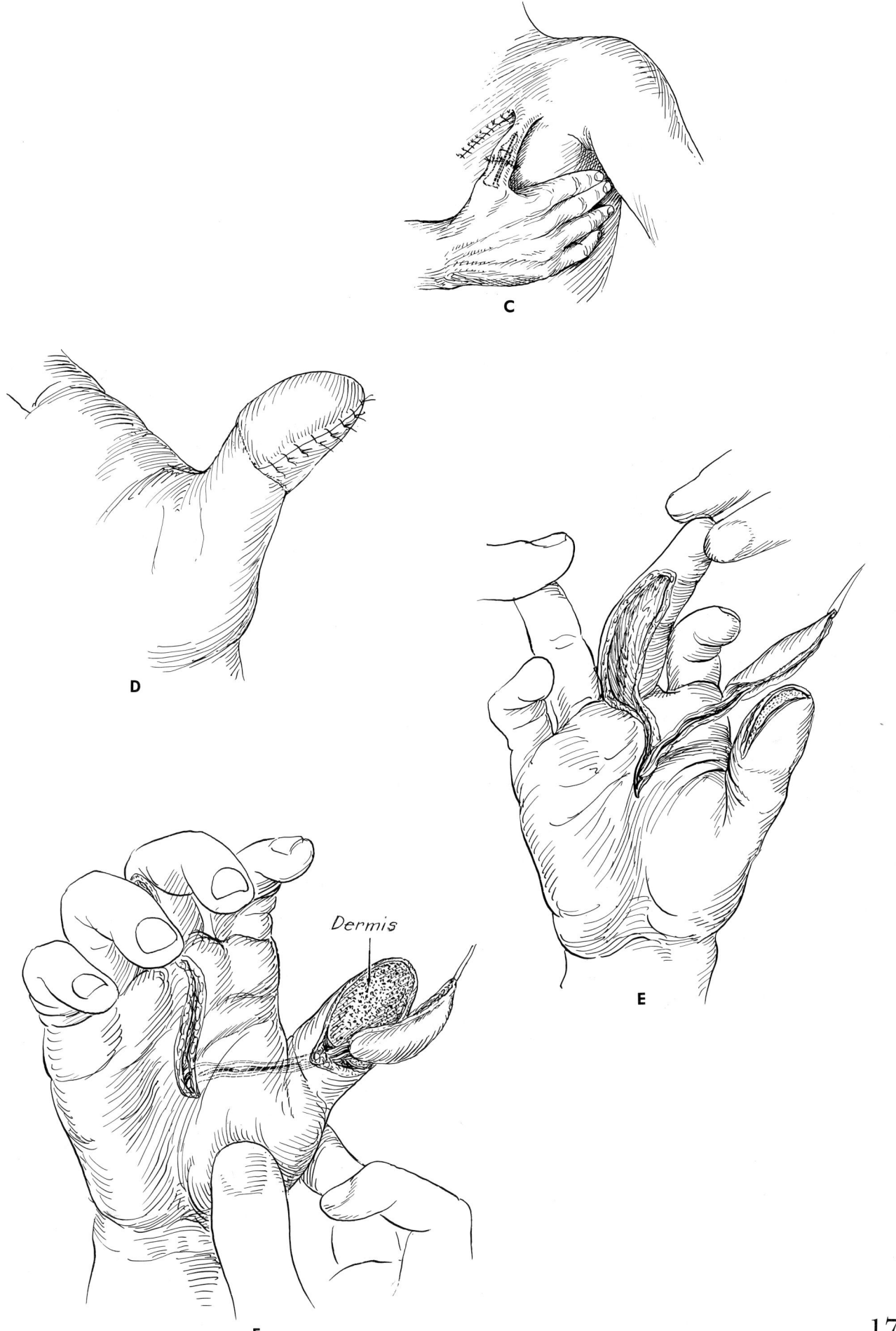

179

39 – The Primary Island Pedicle Flap for Salvage After Trauma

The island pedicle flap was draped over this and sutured in place. (**G**) The donor site on the long finger was resurfaced with a free full thickness skin graft. The midline incision on the palmar surface of the donor finger was broken up by a transverse incision and insertion of a dart of the free skin graft. (**H**)

After healing the reconstructed thumb had restored sensibility and sudomotor function. The patient used the thumb well, and regularly used the reconstituted sensory surface for manipulation and pinching. The permanently transferred intrinsic blood supply added vascular competence to the thumb. (**I**)

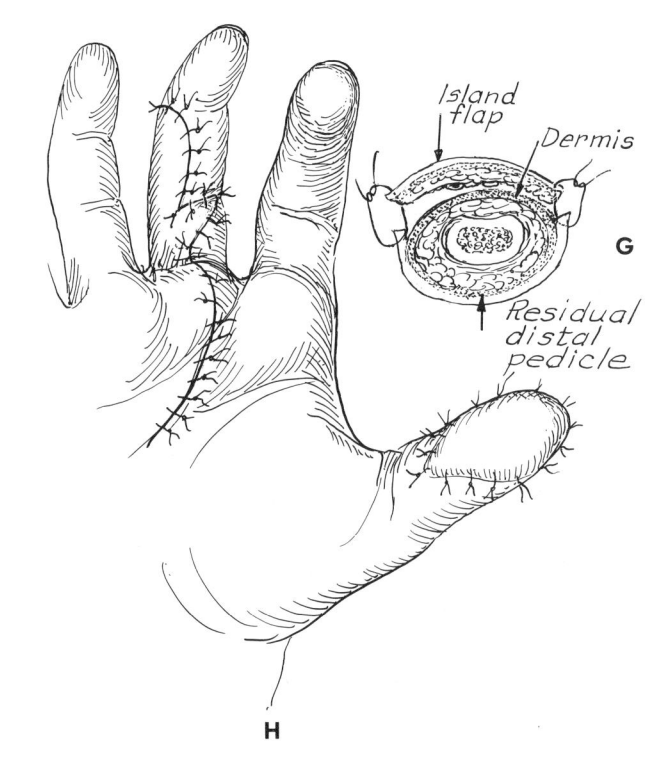

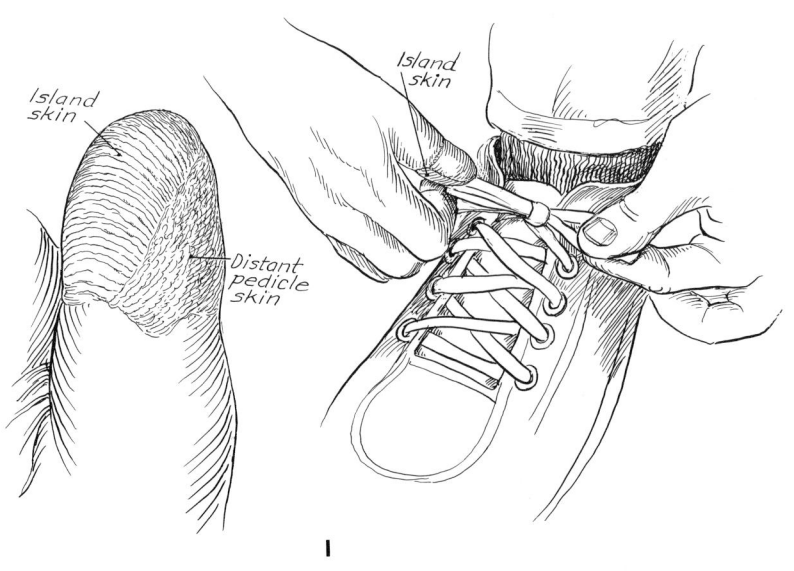

Amputations

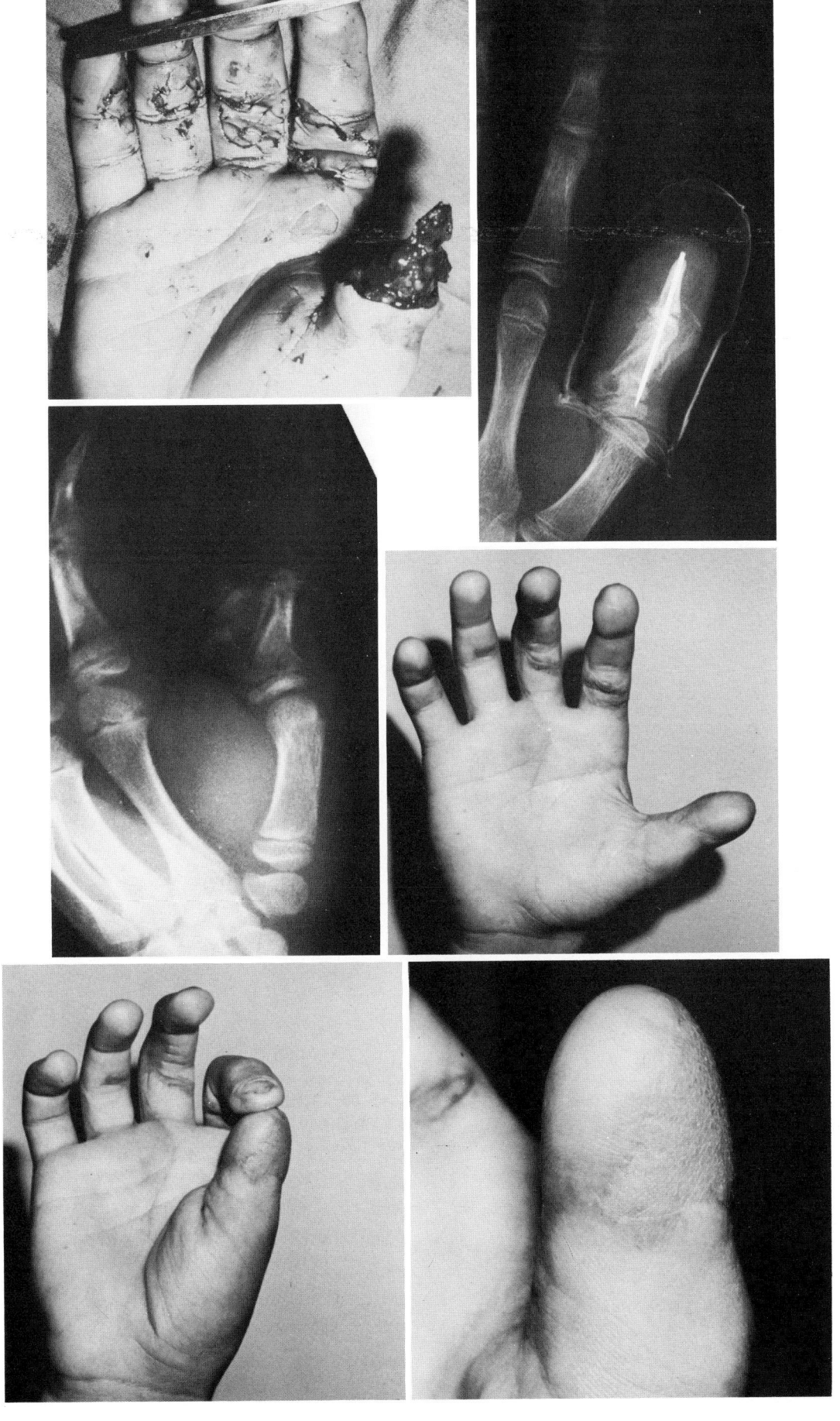

181

40

Metacarpal Transfer

Principle

When amputation of either the long or ring fingers occurs at or proximal to the metacarpophalangeal joint, an incompetent palmar cup results. When one tries to cup small objects in the hand, the objects are prone to fall through the space left by the loss of the central finger. (**A**)

In addition, some patients object to the appearance of a hand with either a central nub if amputation occurs through the proximal phalanx or the space described above. Although it is not commonly indicated, the space may be closed by metacarpal amputation and transfer of the adjacent peripheral ray to the base of the amputated metacarpal. Some acceptable results have been achieved by metacarpal amputation alone, but commonly such an attempt to narrow the hand without metacarpal shift of the adjacent peripheral ray results in malrotation of the ulnar finger or fingers. Flexion of the malrotated digits results in crossing of them with remaining fingers. When the ring finger is lost, the little finger ray is shifted and when the long finger is lost, the index ray is shifted if the operation is indicated at all.

Amputations

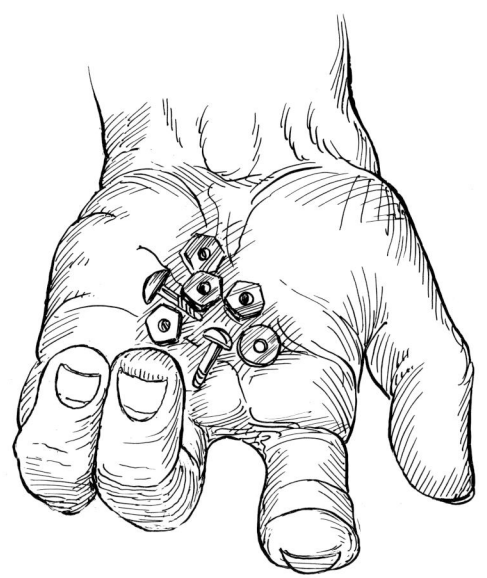

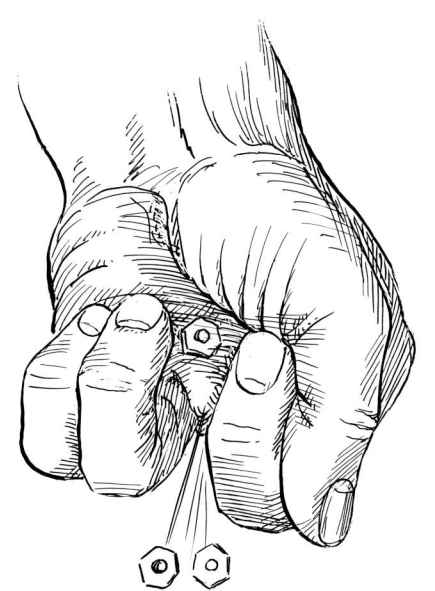

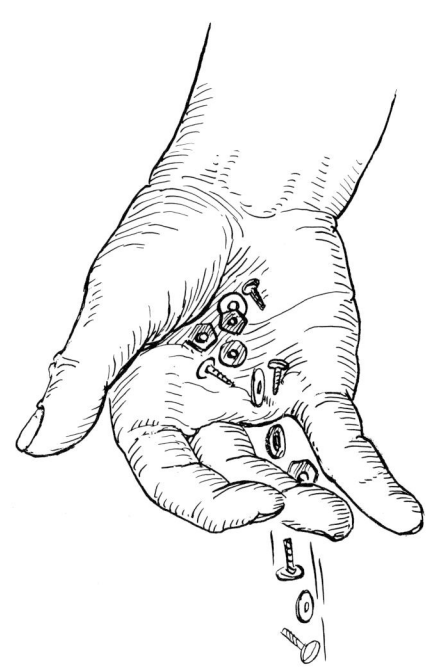

A

183

40 — Metacarpal Transfer

INDEX METACARPAL TRANSFER

If amputation of the long finger ray is done, the best method to avoid the problem of rotation of the ring and little fingers so that they cross the index finger in flexion is by a shift of the index ray to the base of the long finger metacarpal.

Example

A female adult patient sustained a traumatic amputation of the long finger at the metacarpophalangeal joint. In her work she handled small objects and the space in her hand left her unable to cup them in her hand. She was also bothered by the appearance of a space in her hand at the amputation site. A metacarpal transfer of the index ray together with an amputation of the residual long finger metacarpal was decided upon.

An incision for the procedure was planned to preserve the normal web space between the index and long fingers as the index is shifted one digit space ulnarward. (**A**) The web space skin was preserved as a unit and the incision on the radial side of the ring finger was placed precisely to receive the index web flap. Sufficient skin was preserved in the wide web space to serve as web skin when the space was narrowed to normal. The skin was left attached to the ulnar base of the index finger and its free edge carried to the base of the ring finger. Extension of the incisions was planned to remove the intervening skin and to allow exposure of the long finger metacarpal and the proximal part of the index metacarpal. A dot placed on the skin between the two metacarpals at their proximal one-third marked the point at which the dorsal incisions would meet for excision of the intervening skin. (**B**) The palmar incisions were designed to meet distal to the distal palmar crease, excising a triangle of palmar skin to achieve smooth closure with the metacarpal shift.

The plan was to excise the distal two thirds of the long finger metacarpal together with the bulk of the second dorsal interosseous muscle, the extensor tendons and the flexor tendons leaving the third dorsal interosseous long, cutting it at the insertion into the dorsal hood or its equivalent. (**C**)

After the incisions were made, the long finger metacarpal was exposed dorsally and it was cut sharply and squarely at the junction of the proximal and middle one-third of its length. The extensor tendon was cut short and the metacarpal, together with the extensor tendon and skin, was dissected up to expose the intermetacarpal ligaments. The palmar incisions were deepened, exposing the neurovascular bundles to the long finger. The vessels were ligated and cut and the nerves were left long to be placed back in the protected intermetacarpal space. The intermetacarpal ligaments were sharply cut close to the long finger metacarpophalangeal joint leaving available edges of the ligament on the index metacarpophalangeal and ring metacarpophalangeal for later juncture. The flexor tendons were individually pulled distally, cut short, and allowed to retract into the palm and wrist. The skeletal ray and its tendons and skin were removed and kept sterile as a source for a medullary bone peg.

The index metacarpal was then exposed and subperiosteally dissected at the junction of its proximal and middle one-thirds. It was cut sharply and squarely across, leaving the same length of metacarpal between the osteotomy and the metacarpophalangeal joint as that in the long finger metacarpal just amputated. (**D**)

Amputations

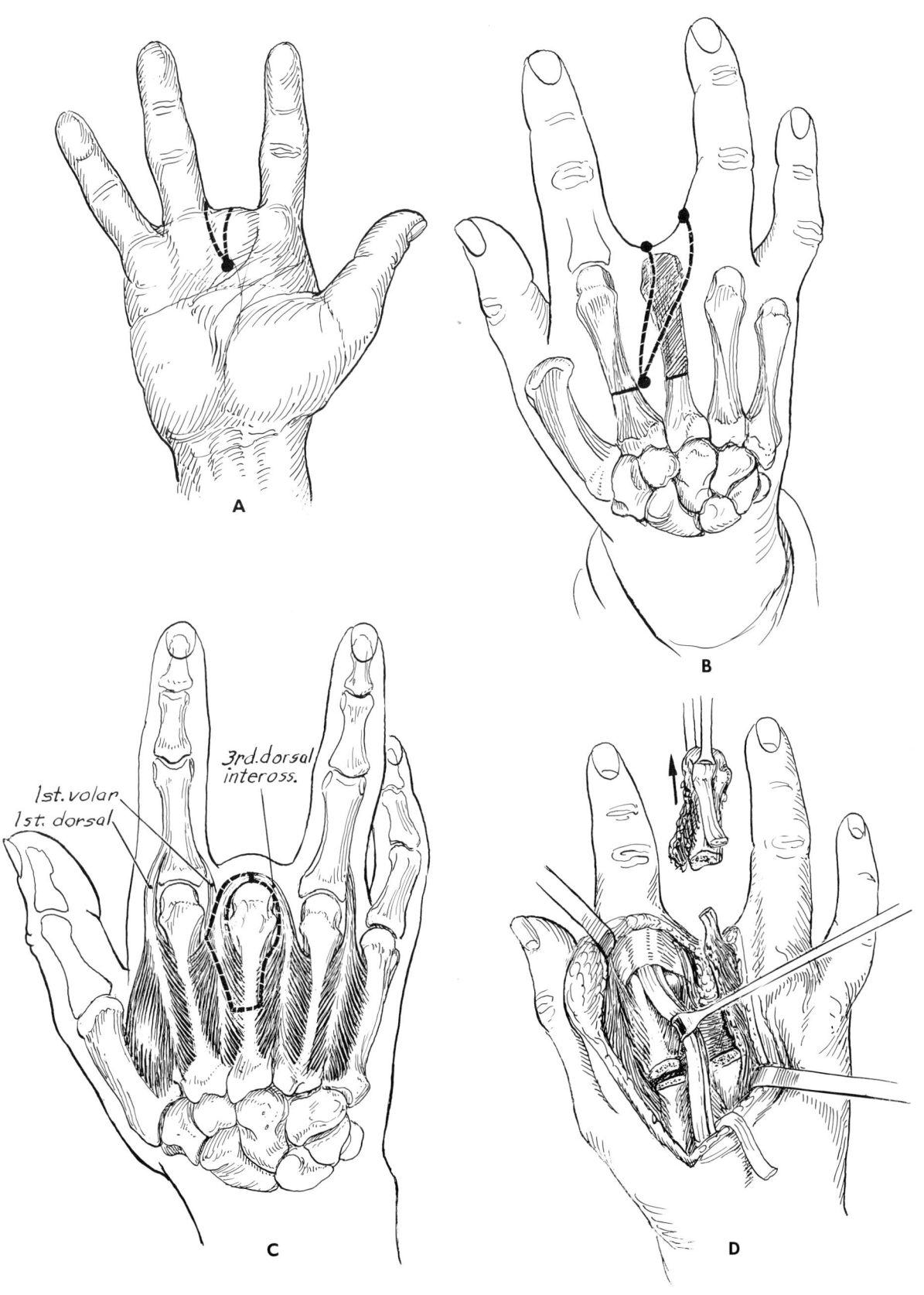

185

40 – Metacarpal Transfer

A bone peg was fashioned from the amputated metacarpal. It was inserted into the medullary cavity of the proximal cut end of the central metacarpal. The index ray was shifted to the position previously occupied by the long finger ray and seated over the bone peg which was inserted into the index metacarpal medullary canal. (**E**) The third dorsal interosseous added just enough bulk to avoid any dead space after the metacarpal shift. (If the interosseous muscles, the second and third dorsal, previously inserted on the long finger interfere with the shift by occupying too much space, one or both may be excised).

A suture or two joining the intermetacarpal ligaments on the adjacent side of the index and ring finger volar plates helped to stabilize the ring finger.

A longitudinal Kirschner wire was passed through the medullary cavity (as described for an open metacarpal fracture; see page 250) to lend stability at the osteotomy site.

After rotation was precisely corrected for proper relationship with the ring and little fingers on flexion, a Kirschner wire was passed transversely from the index to the ring finger metacarpals. (**F** and **G**)

The skin was appropriately trimmed to avoid irregularities or "dog ears" at the incision extremes and the wounds were closed. (**H**)

An immobilizing plaster cast was applied and the hand was kept splinted for about eight weeks.

The Kirschner wires were left in for 12 weeks. (Occasionally, the wires threaten to protrude or work out spontaneously and must be removed earlier.) Active exercise was started after removal of the cast with the Kirschner wires still in place. A symmetrical three-fingered hand without amputation stumps or an abnormal space was the result. (**I**)

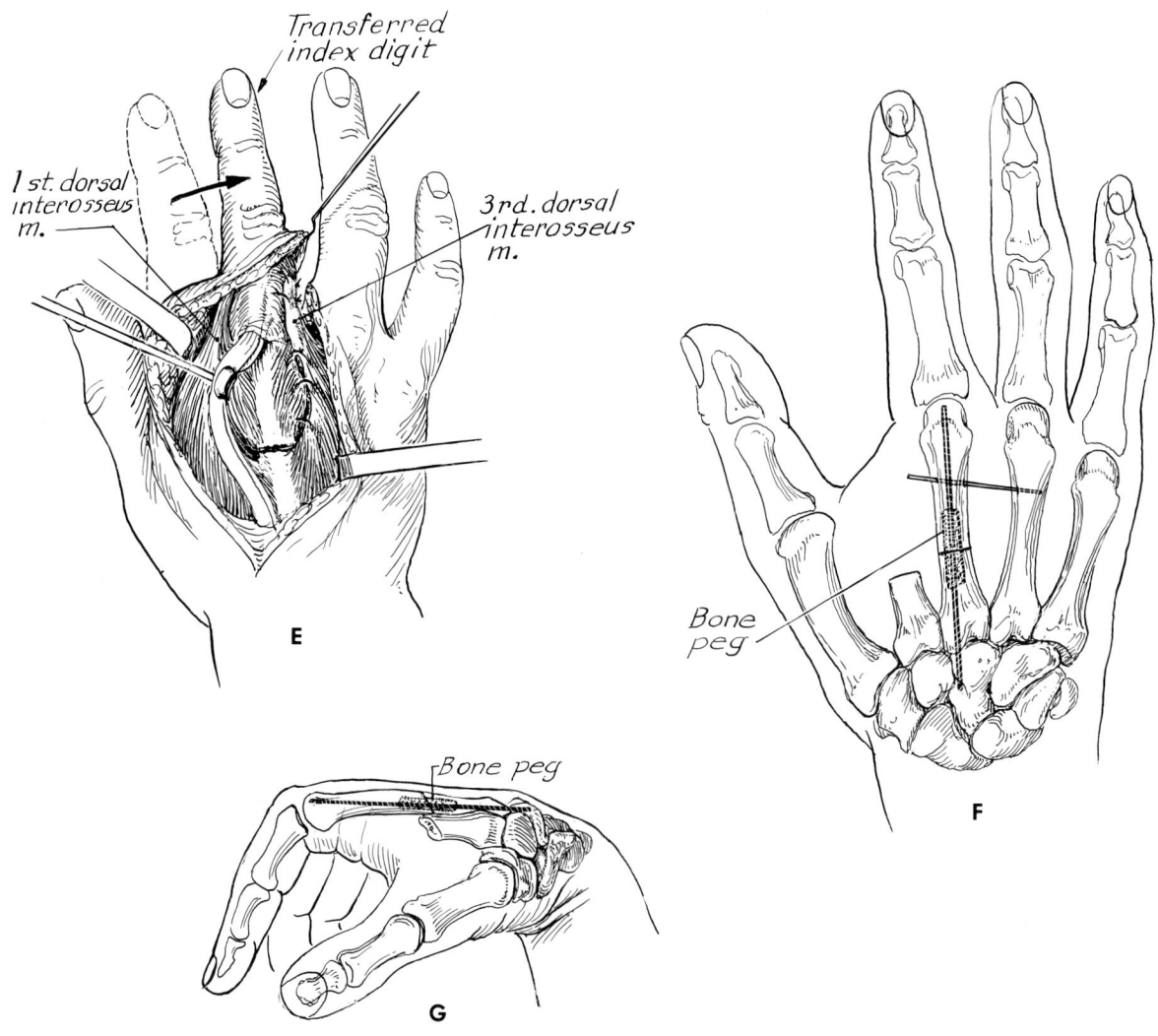

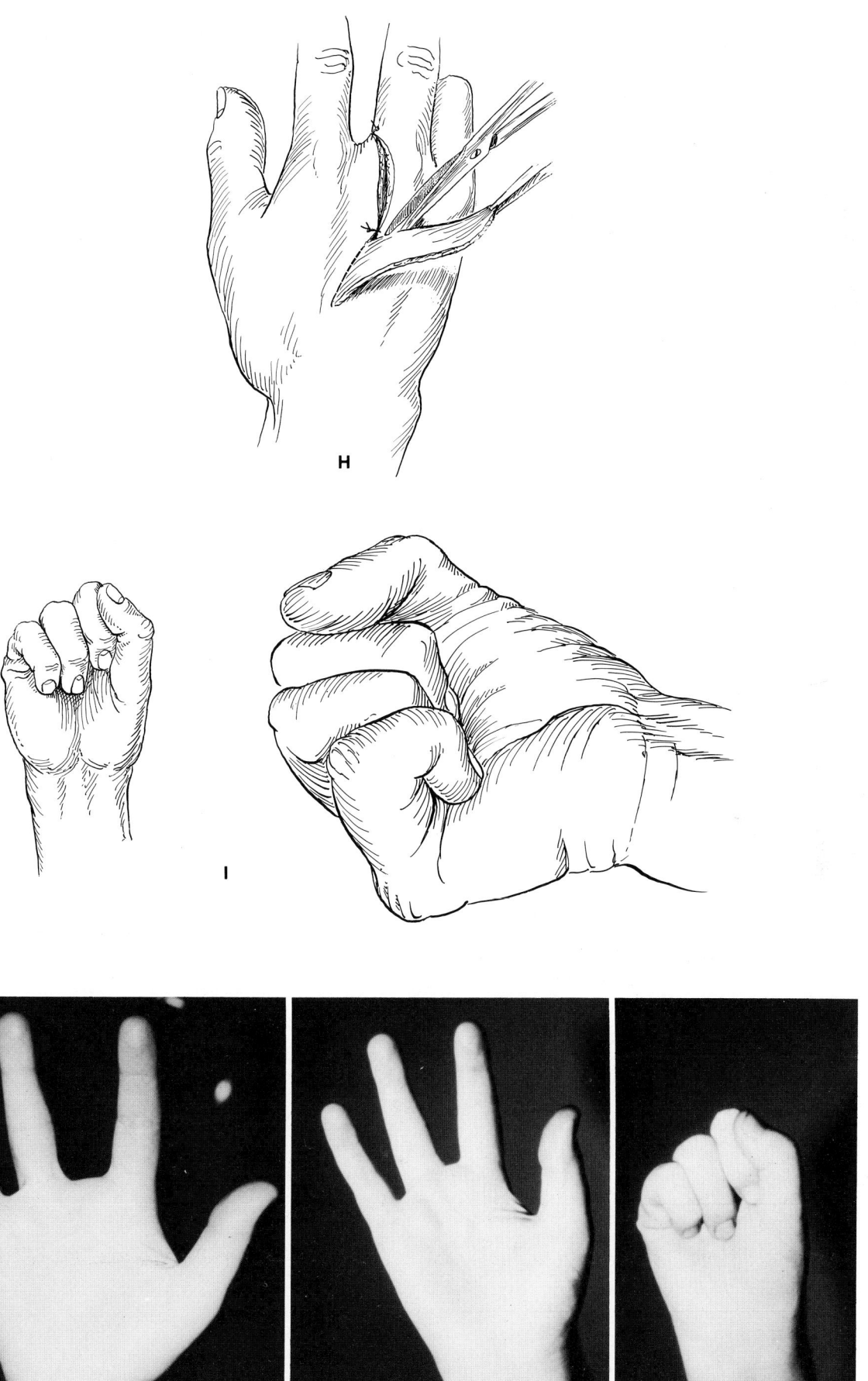

PREOPERATIVE   POSTOPERATIVE

LITTLE FINGER METACARPAL TRANSFER

This procedure is used when indicated in a patient undergoing ring finger metacarpal amputation. The principles of the procedure are the same as for index metacarpal transfer.

Example

A severe ring avulsion injury resulted in amputation of the left ring finger at the metacarpophalangeal joint. To eliminate the wide space between the long finger and little finger for functional and cosmetic improvement an amputation of the ring finger metacarpal and transfer of the whole little finger ray to the base of the ring metacarpal was elected. The incision was planned in such a way that the web skin between the little finger and ring nub was preserved. Since the little finger metacarpal head falls proximal to that of the ring finger, it is wise to remember that the web skin will fall more proximal on the ulnar side of the long finger than does the normal ring finger web. Extra skin was preserved on the ulnar side of the long finger in the web space to avoid a skin deficit after the shift was made. The proximal mark on the dorsum of the hand was made between the ring and little finger metacarpals at the junction of their proximal and middle thirds. (**A**) A palm incision was planned in the same manner as that described for the index metacarpal transfer.

The procedure for removal of the metacarpal, skin, flexors, extensors, and stump is the same as that described for the index metacarpal transfer. The second palmar and fourth dorsal interossei may be removed or left *in situ* as necessary for space filler.

The length of little finger metacarpal left cannot be sufficient to shift the metacarpophalangeal joint to the position previously occupied by the ring metacarpophalangeal joint. (**B**) The increase in length would cause too much tightness in the digital motors. The little finger ray can be stretched a half centimeter or so to create a symmetrical looking hand. (**C**) If after transfer of the little finger ray the extensor mechanism appears too tight, more metacarpal should be removed. The metacarpal shift is done in the manner described above for the index metacarpal transfer.

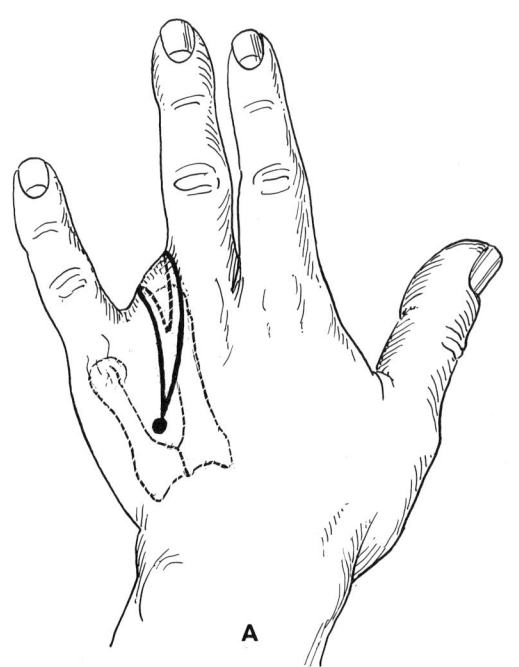
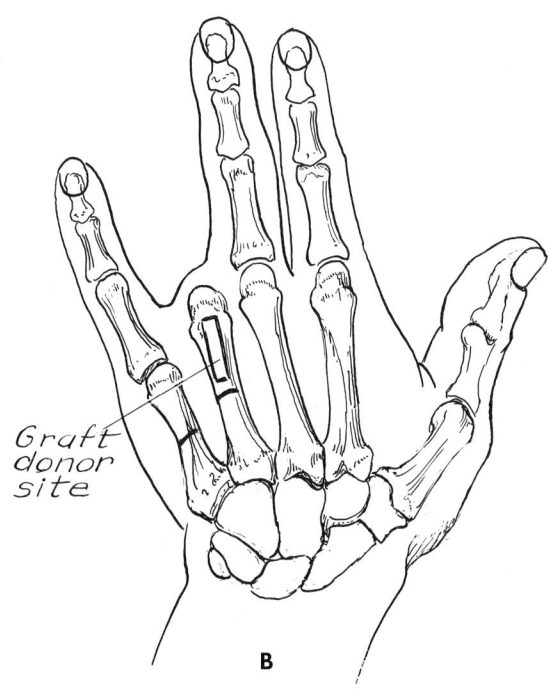

Amputations

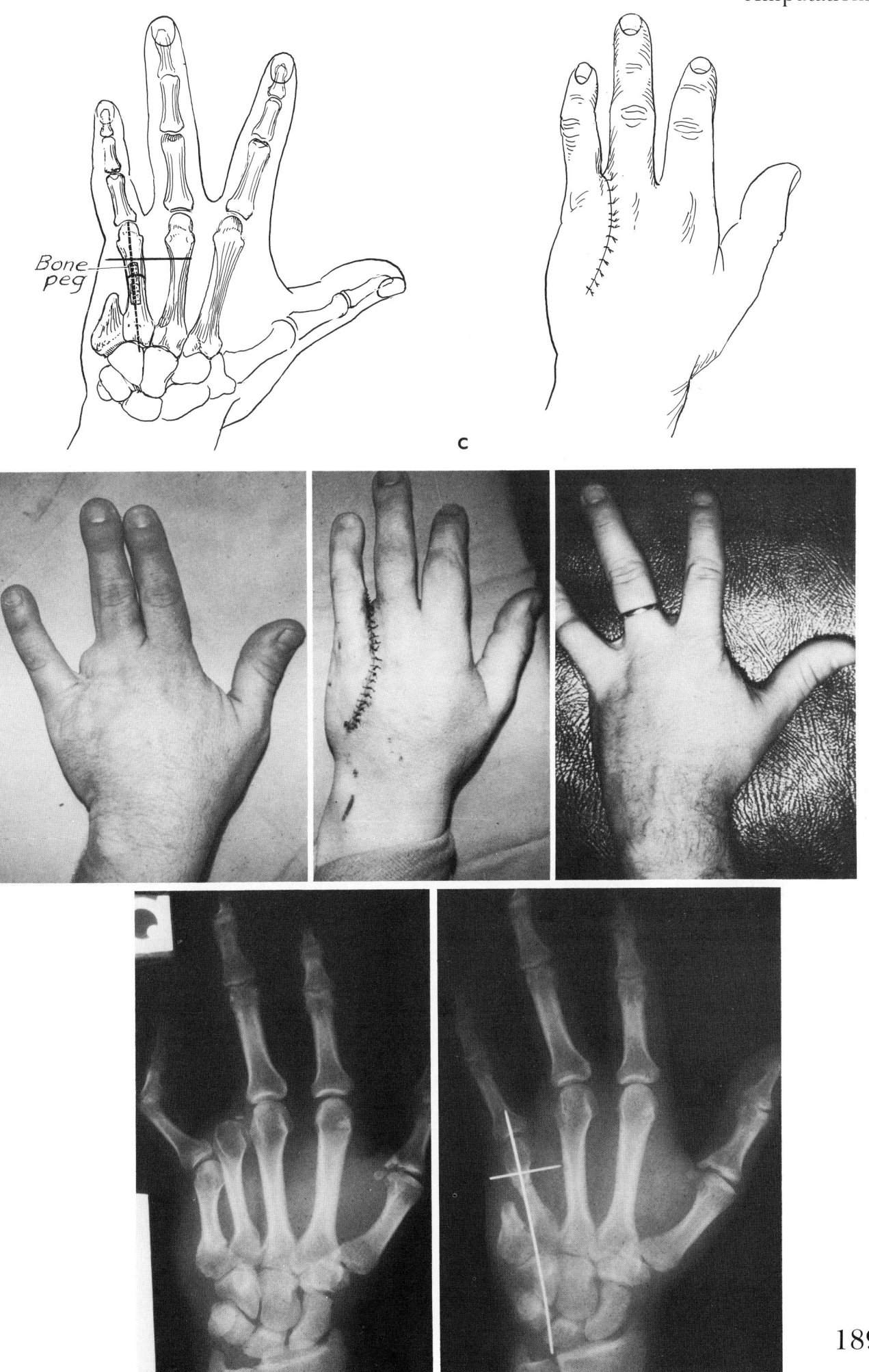

c

41

Composite Transfer of a Joint

Principle

Although free transplantation of whole joints is not a reliable procedure the transfer of a whole joint *with blood supply* may be very useful.

Example

A laboring man sustained a crushing, tearing cable injury which amputated the index finger through the middle phalanx and severely disrupted the metacarpophalangeal joint of the long finger. After initial care and healing of the wounds he was left with an exquisitely tender index finger stump with poor skin coverage back to the proximal interphalangeal joint. The proximal interphalangeal joint was stiff but the index metacarpophalangeal joint was normal. The long finger had normal interphalangeal joints and was functionally intact except for the metacarpophalangeal joint which had only ten degrees of motion. The finger was ulnar deviated because of destruction at the metacarpophalangeal joint. In essence, the patient had a poor index finger with a good metacarpophalangeal joint and a normal long finger with a destroyed metacarpophalangeal joint. (**A**) A combination of these components logically could produce a good finger with a normal metacarpophalangeal joint.

Composite transfer of the index metacarpophalangeal joint, long extensor tendons and dorsal hood having the first dorsal interosseous intact was decided upon.

The incision was planned as one would design it for an index ray amputation. (**B**)

Osteotomies were planned to preserve the proximal third of the proximal phalanx and the distal half of the metacarpal in the index ray. Osteotomies were planned at the same level in the long finger and its metacarpal in preparation for removal of the metacarpophalangeal joint. (**C**)

The extensor mechanism of the index finger was sectioned over the proximal phalanx and the index nub was amputated. (**D**) The long flexor tendons of the index finger were pulled distally, cut short, and allowed to retract. The extensor mechanism of the long finger was sectioned at about the same level and the finger was reflected ulnarward in preparation for amputation of the metacarpophalangeal joint together with the second dorsal interosseous muscle. The proximal extensor was left long.

The metacarpophalangeal joint was dissected from the flexor tendon mechanism and removed with the second dorsal interosseous. (**E**) The adductor pollicis was preserved by leaving the periosteum of the metacarpal intact.

The index metacarpal osteotomy allowed shift of the index metacarpophalangeal joint with the extensor mechanism and first dorsal interosseous to the base of the long finger metacarpal.

Amputations

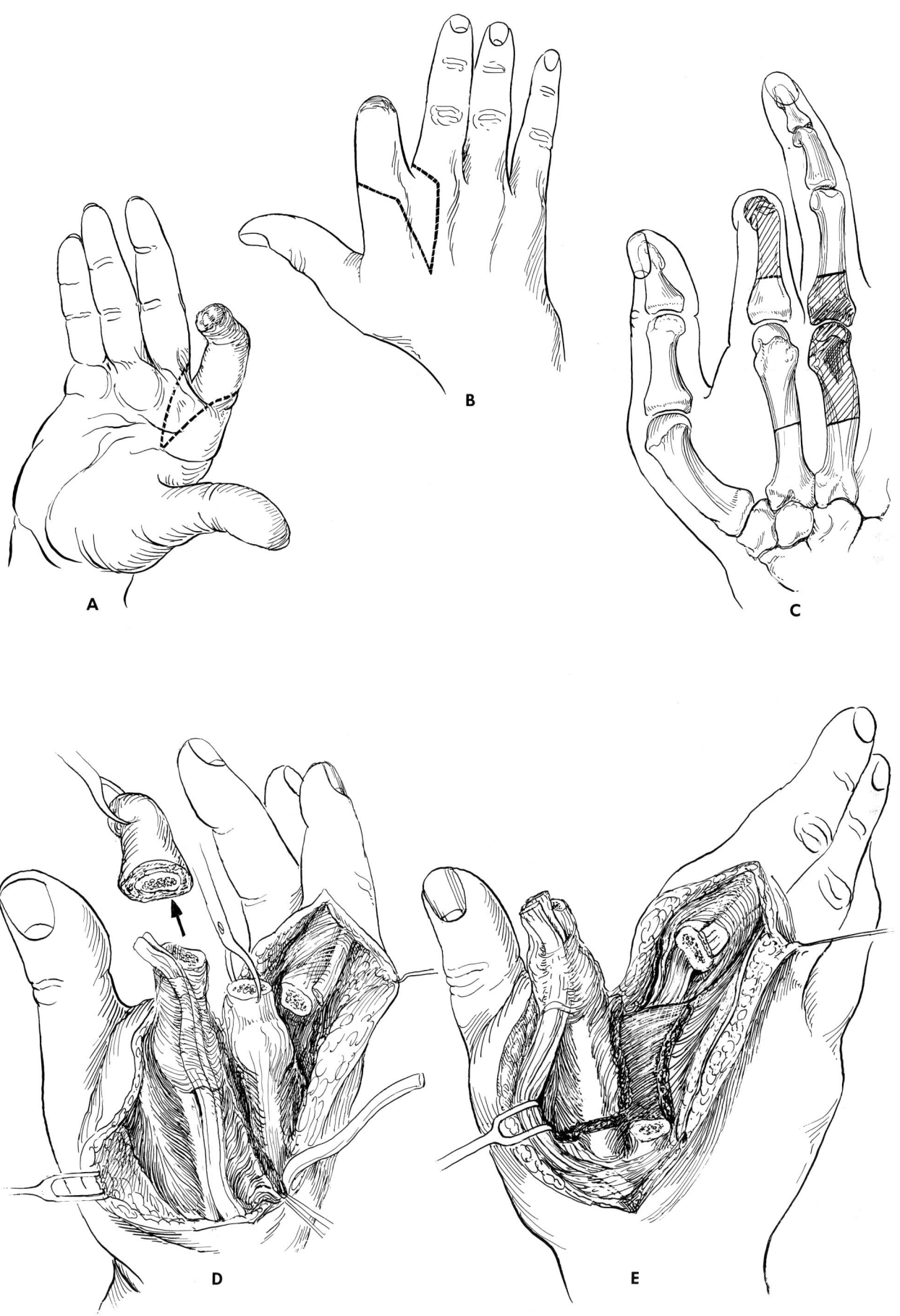

191

41 — Composite Transfer of a Joint

Bone pegs were fashioned from the amputated long finger metacarpal. These were used for intrameduallary fixation at the distal and proximal osteotomy sites. (**F**) Single Kirschner wires were inserted for additional stabilization.

The extensor mechanism of the index finger was fixed to the extensor of the long finger at the level of the proximal phalanx. (**G**) The first palmar interosseous insertion was reinforced with sutures and the extensor digitorum to the long finger was sutured side to side to the extensor digitorum to the index finger as an intertendinous bridge. (**H**)

The skin incisions were closed like those in a ray amputation. (**I**)

After ten weeks of immobilization the patient was allowed to exercise the parts. After several months the patient regained nearly full range of motion in the restored finger. (**J**)

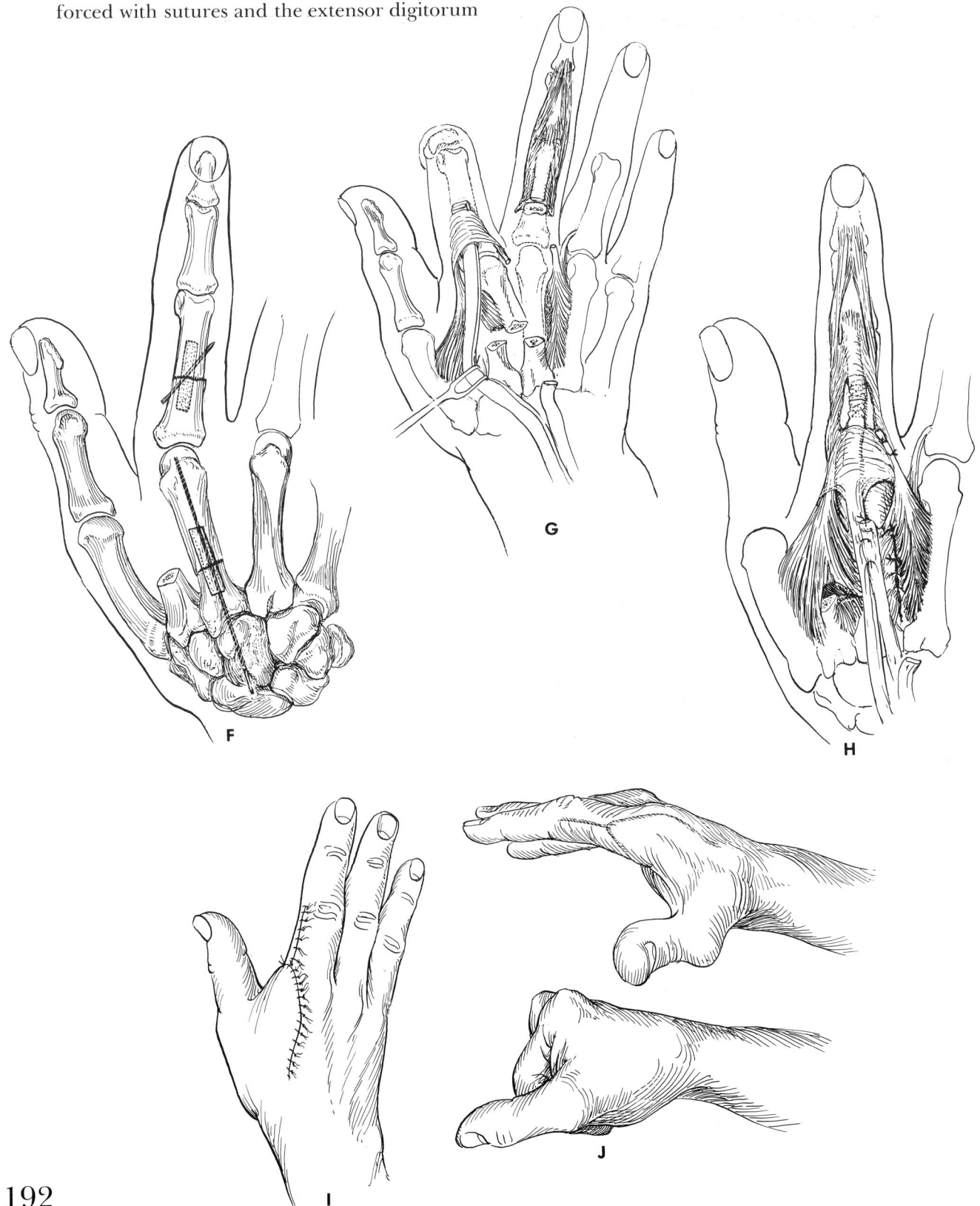

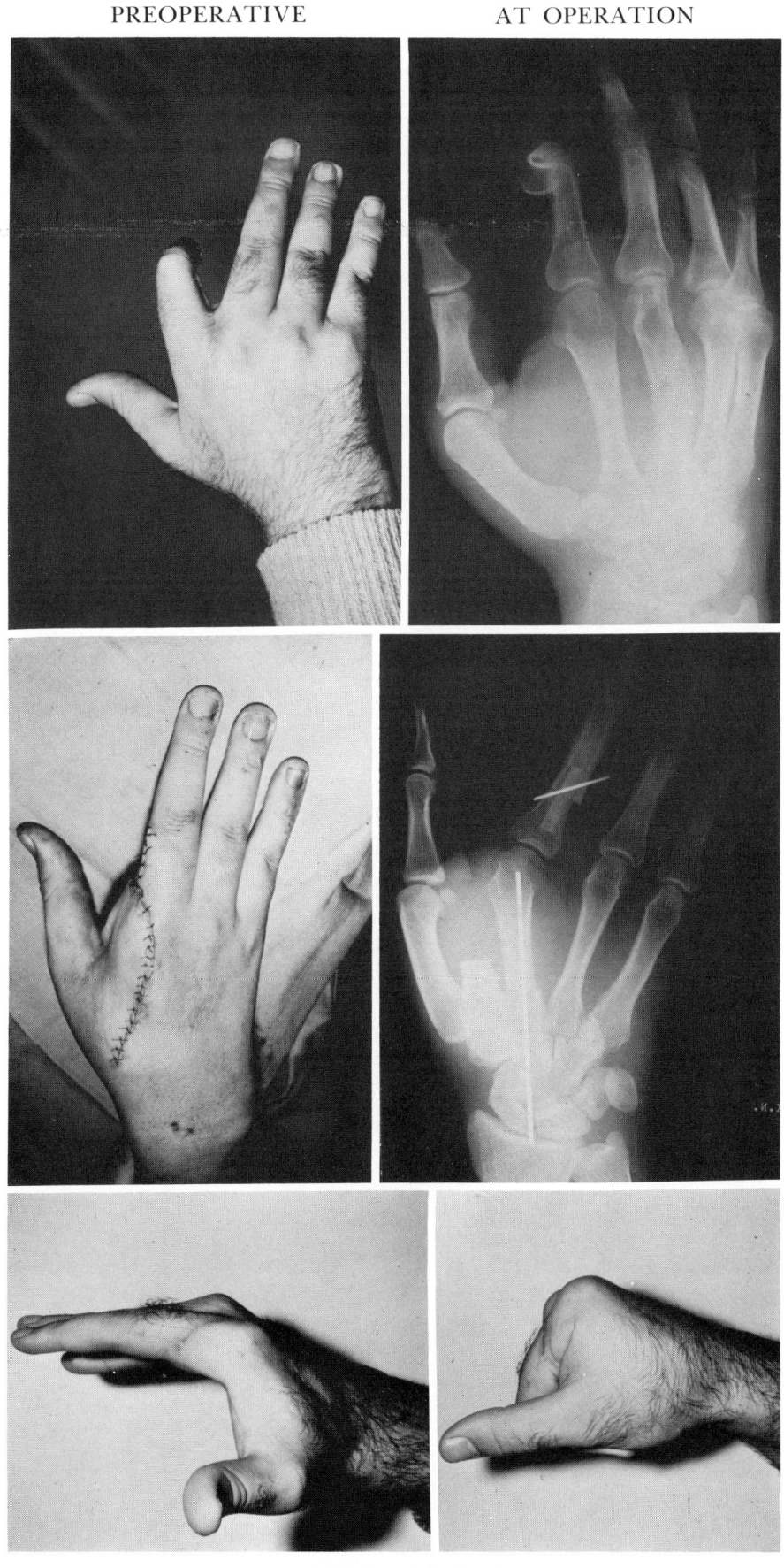

PREOPERATIVE AT OPERATION

POSTOPERATIVE

Vascular Reconstruction

42
Allen's Test

This simple test may be used to assess the competence of the major arterial contributors to blood supply in the hand and the functional efficiency of the vascular arches in the hand. (**A**)

Palpate the radial and ulnar pulses at the wrist and prepare to compress these arteries. (**B**) Have the patient make a very tight fist. (**C**)

Compress the arteries and ask the patient to extend the digits. The hand will be blanched white. (**D**)

Release pressure on one of the arteries and observe the return of a red flush on the hand. (**E**)

Normally, the flush is immediate and progresses across the whole hand without delay. This confirms the patency of the artery and the competence of circulatory collaterals through the vascular arches. The test may be done to assure oneself of competence of each of the two major arteries prior to surgery or as a test of competence after repair, thrombectomy, other manipulation, or injury.

The Allen test principle may be used in clinically assessing the competence of the two proper digital arteries in the finger. It may be done by observing return of color after compression of both arteries and release of one or a cutaneous electronic pulse meter (used by anesthesiologists) may be applied to the digit tip. Compress one artery, the other, then both to see the individual proper artery contribution to cutaneous blood supply. The technique may be useful and less trying and dangerous than angiography when one is planning an island pedicle flap from a donor finger whose digital artery may have been damaged by an injury proximal to the finger.

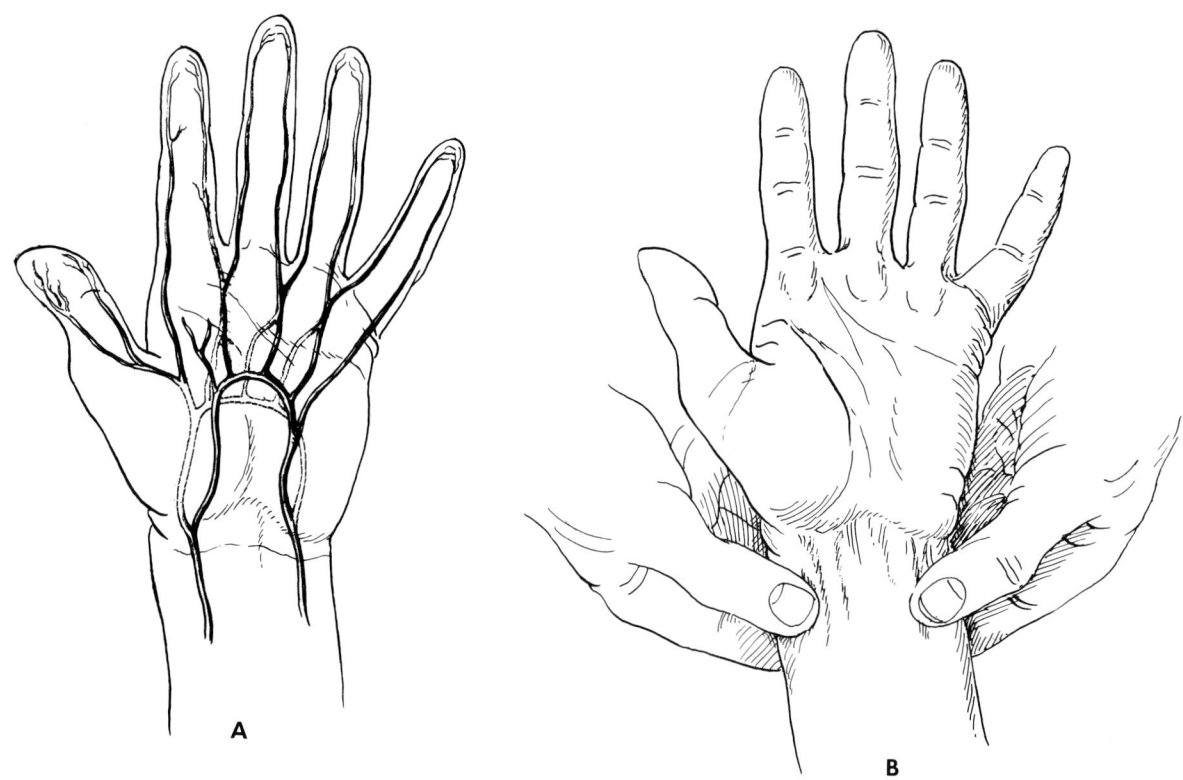

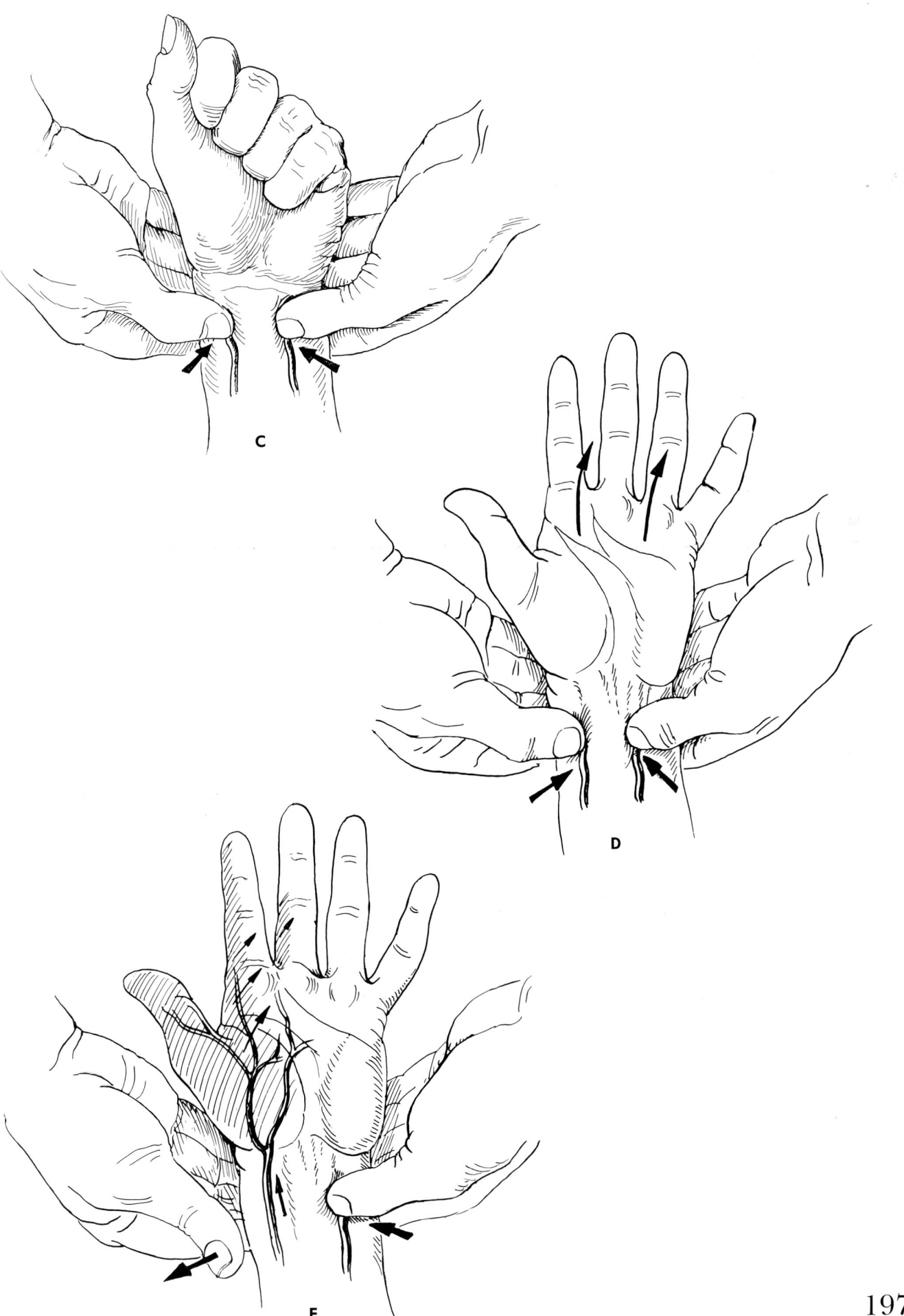

197

43

Vascular Reconstruction

Principles

Although any single artery in the upper extremity may be sacrificed without significant chance of gangrene there is ample evidence that diminished arterial blood supply from such a loss may result in symptomatic even disabling ischemia with use or positioning. Multiple arterial injuries are not uncommon in severe upper extremity injuries. High priority must be assigned to vascular repair under these circumstances.

Advances in microsurgery allow reliable repair of vessels a millimeter in diameter. (**A**) This has made it possible to repair even the small vessels within the hand and proximal part of the finger.

The technique for repair of blood vessels is the same in principle whether one is dealing with large or small vessels and whether they be arteries or veins. Gaps in arteries may be overcome by inserting vein grafts.

The ends of vessels to be anastomosed must be cleanly cut either straight across or at an angle which is matched by an angle cut in the end of the vessel to be matched. Key stitches are placed through the vessel wall after stripping it of superfluous soft tissue and adventitia. (**B**) The first stitch is tied down and the second is placed diametrically opposite in each vessel end. (**C**) Using the key stitches as guy wires, additional sutures are placed through the vessels, being careful not to pick up the back wall of the vessels. (**D**) By switching the guide sutures, the vessel is turned over to complete the back wall anastomosis. Distal then proximal clamps are removed and only if serious persistent leakage occurs are more sutures recommended.

Example

REPLANTATION

A 45-year-old male patient sustained a complete traumatic amputation of the left thumb, index, long, and ring fingers through the metacarpals in a power saw accident. The amputated ring finger was badly mutilated but the remaining fingers were intact as a unit consisting of thumb, index finger and long finger including the distal portion of the corresponding metacarpals. (**E**)

The amputated parts were placed in ice by the patient's co-workers and he was transferred to the hospital. When replantation was decided upon, the amputated part was perfused with heparinized dextran prior to replantation. After preparation and debridement of the amputated unit, it was replanted using microvascular techniques by Dr. Stephen Cary of Santa Rosa, California. The radial artery in the first web space and the common digital artery to the adjacent sides of the index and long fingers and a single dorsal vein were repaired. Skeletal fixation was achieved with Kirschner wires. The patient received 20 million units of penicillin, 500 mg. of streptomycin, and 200 mg. of heparin in divided doses during the surgical procedure. The patient was transferred to Stanford University Hospital immediately after operation. The patient had some extravasation of blood at venipuncture sites and continuous oozing of blood from his wound. Intravenous heparin, 50 mg. every 4 hours, was continued and he received transfusions to maintain his blood volume. This required 8 units of blood in the first 48 hours. In addition, 500 ml. of low molecular weight dextran was given every 12 hours and streptomycin and penicillin were continued. The replanted fingers were dusky but there was evidence of capillary filling.

The long finger demarcated developing dry gangrene of all except the proximal dorsal skin. (**F**) It was amputated using the surviving dorsal flap to cover a small palmar area which was devoid of soft tissue. This revisional surgery was carried out 5 weeks after replantation.

Vascular Reconstruction

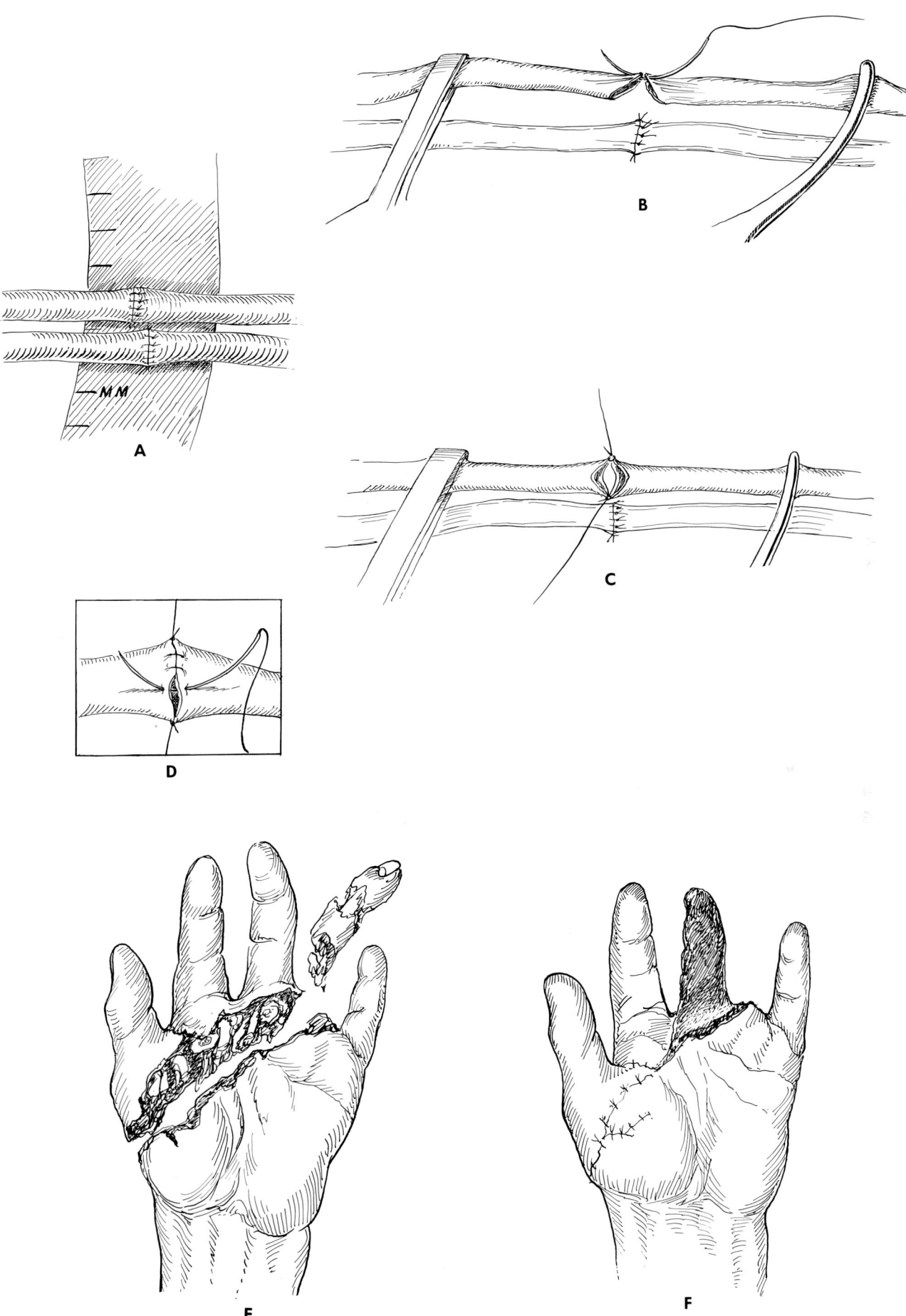

199

43 — Vascular Reconstruction

The thumb and index finger survived and have regained usable protective sensibility. After several small revisional amputation procedures and repair of the index flexor tendons, a rotational osteotomy of the index metacarpal, and finally an extensor tendon reconstruction, the patient has been left with useful replanted parts.

Three years after replantation of the index finger and thumb, they have regained important functional usefulness. (**G**) The patient builds models in his trade as a designer. He requires prehensile capability in his left hand and sensibility is very important in the opposable parts.

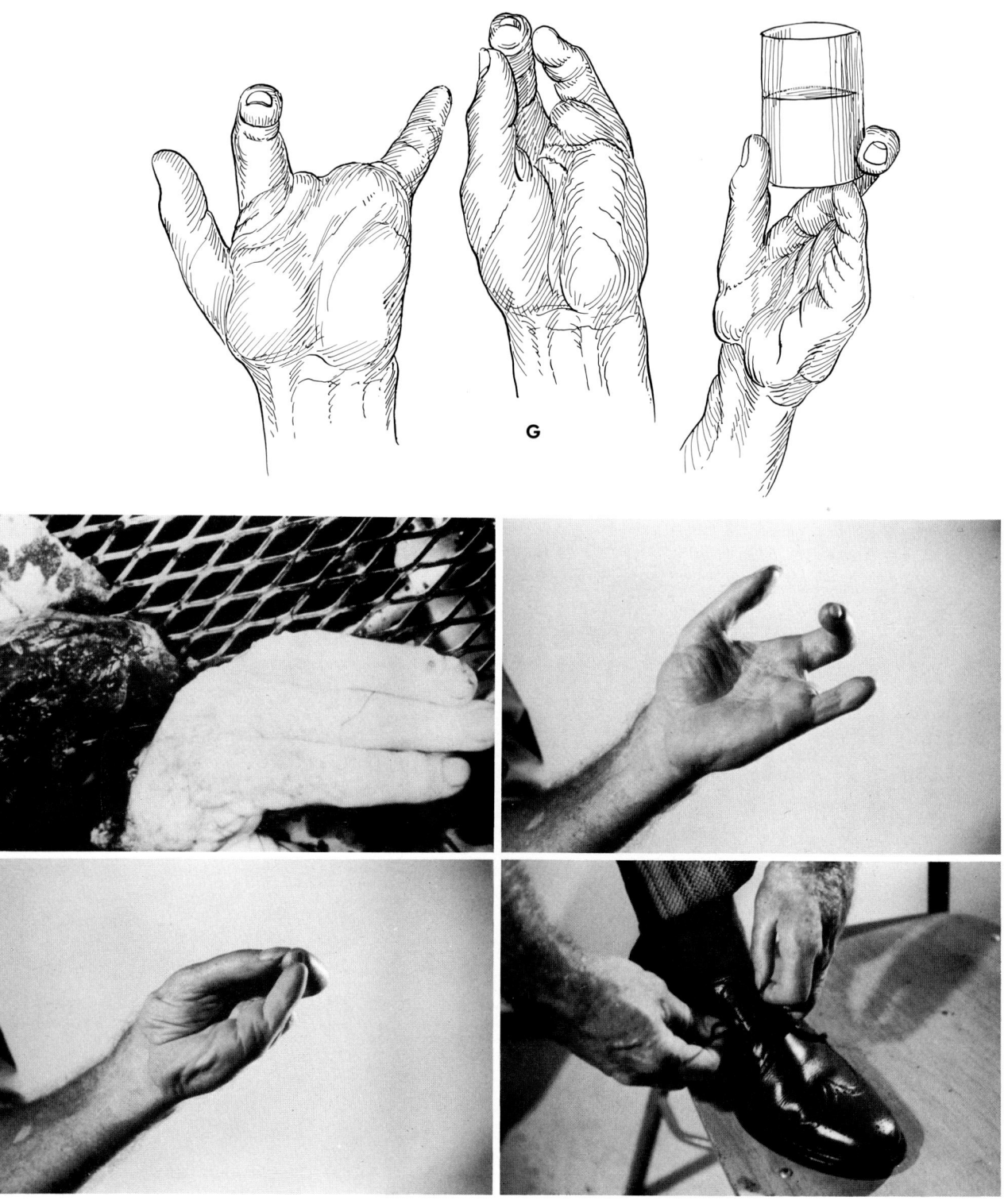

G

Nerve Surgery

Sensory and Motor Deficits in Acute Median Nerve Injury at the Wrist

Median Nerve Injury at the Wrist

The median nerve is most commonly injured at the wrist level where it is the most superficial structure to pass through the carpal tunnel. It lies just beneath the palmaris longus and the deep investing fascia of the forearm at the level of the palmar wrist creases. At the level of the proximal flexion crease at the wrist the median nerve lies to the ulnar side of the flexor carpi radialis and superficial to the flexor superficialis to the index digit.

One should suspect a median nerve injury with any laceration across the palmar aspect at the wrist level.

Median Nerve Sensory Pattern

The median nerve supplies sensibility to the important digits which man generally uses to assess his environment by tactile gnosis. The palmar aspects of the thumb, index, long and radial half of the ring finger, and the radial side of the palm are median-innervated. (**A**) There is extension to the dorsum over the tips of the above digits from the palmar digital nerves.

Median Nerve Motor Innervation in the Hand

By its recurrent motor branches in the palm the median nerve innervates all the intrinsic muscles which lie radial to the flexor pollicis longus. (**B**) There are two and one-half such muscles and their prime function is to position the thumb in palmar abduction on opposition. They form the thenar eminence and consist of the abductor pollicis brevis, opponens pollicis, and the superficial head of the flexor pollicis brevis. The lumbricals to the index and long fingers are also innervated by the median nerve through tiny branches from palmar common digital nerves. (See Anatomy, Section 1.)

The easily detectable findings immediately after median nerve transection at the wrist are:

1. Anesthesia and loss of sudomotor function (sweating) over the palmar aspect of the thumb, index, long and radial half of the ring fingers.

2. Lack of active ability to palmar abduct the thumb to position it for pulp-to-pulp opposition with the fingers.

There may be anatomical variations in the patterns of sensory loss but one must be prepared to differentiate partial nerve injury from complete transection with part of the area classically innervated by the median nerve innervated by the ulnar. The differentiation can readily be made before exploration of the wound by anesthetic block of the ulnar nerve.

In an unconscious patient, an uncooperative patient, or a child where the measurement of sensibility depends on the patient's subjective response, assessment of sudomotor (sweating) function may be very useful. Observation with a magnifying lens or ophthalmoscope or fingerprinting using the Moberg ninhydrin test is helpful in this situation. (**C**)

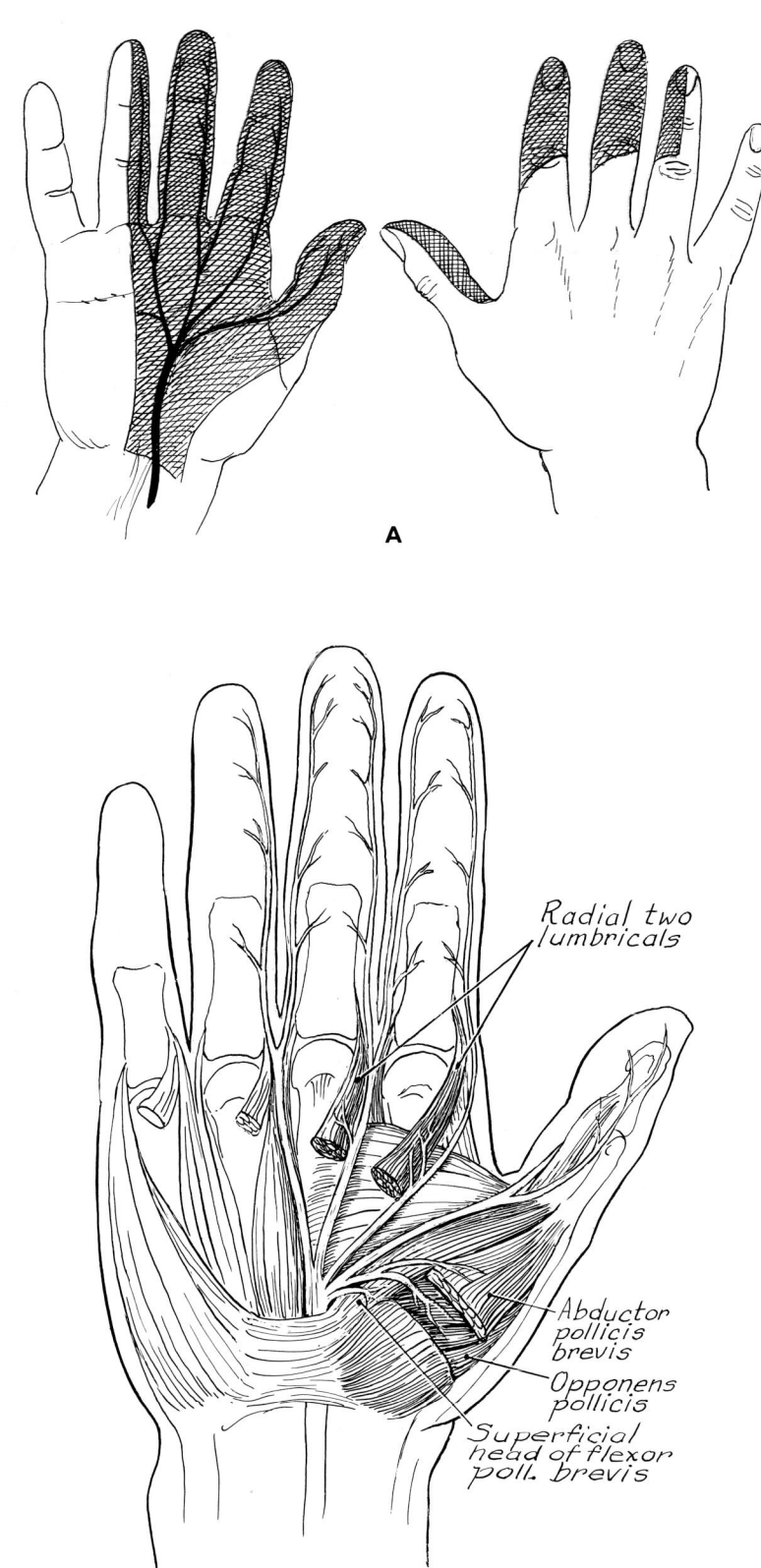

203

The Moberg test consists of taking fingerprints from all fingers of the hand on paper uncontaminated by handling. The paper is dipped in ninhydrin solution in acetone or the paper is sprayed with ninhydrin solution and heated gently over a warm light bulb. A ninhydrin spray used by criminologists is handy in an emergency suite. It can be obtained from criminology laboratories. Ninhydrin stains purple the amino acids excreted in sweat, and prints made of fingers with normal sweating stand out boldly after staining while those of fingers without sudomotor function produce little or no stain.

Motor power loss must be specifically tested for since there is no atrophy immediately after injury and muscle tone still exists in the denervated muscles. Testing palmar abduction of the thumb against gravity and against resistance, comparing it with the uninjured side, is most important in assessing motor loss after median nerve injury. Occasionally all of the thenar muscles will be innervated by the ulnar nerve (ulnar nerve hand) and palmar abduction of the thumb will be normal. If one wishes to be sure that this is the case and that he is not dealing with a partial median nerve injury sparing the motor nerves, an ulnar nerve block or electrical stimulation over the ulnar nerve will answer the question. The variations in innervation of the thumb intrinsic muscles are detailed in Section 1.

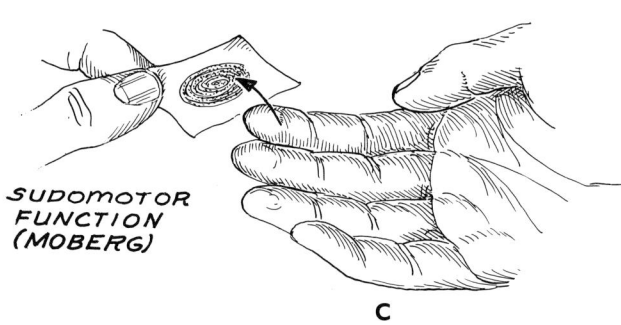

SUDOMOTOR FUNCTION (MOBERG)

C

45

Primary Nerve Repair

Principle

A clean, sharp transection of a peripheral nerve should be managed by primary reconstruction if the wound surgeon is versed in the proper technique for repair. Identification of nerve ends is crucial. Differentiation from adjacent lacerated tendons is elementary. The nerve has a dull, cream-colored appearance when compared with the glistening white tendon. There is universally at least one identifiable surface blood vessel on the nerve, and the cut end has bulging nerve funiculi.

Example

MEDIAN NERVE TRANSECTION AT THE WRIST

If the nerve has been sharply cut, it may be repaired straight away. If ragged ends are left by laceration, the nerve ends should be recut sharply.

SQUARE TRANSECTION OF PERIPHERAL NERVE ENDS

When ragged, lacerated nerve ends are found in treating an acute injury, the nerve ends must be sharply and squarely recut in preparation for accurate repair. When the surgeon repairs a nerve secondarily, the neuroma must be resected sharply and squarely from the proximal nerve end and the distal healed cut end must be sharply and squarely freshened. Precise section through the nerve is aided by wrapping the nerve in a piece of plastic material such as Vi-Drape to make it tense like a link sausage. (**A**) A single cut through the turgid nerve and plastic results in a sharp clean transection with sheath and axones cut at the same level. (**B** and **C**)

As an alternative, one may render the nerve turgid by injecting normal saline within the sheath and then sectioning it with a single cut with a sharp blade. (**D**)

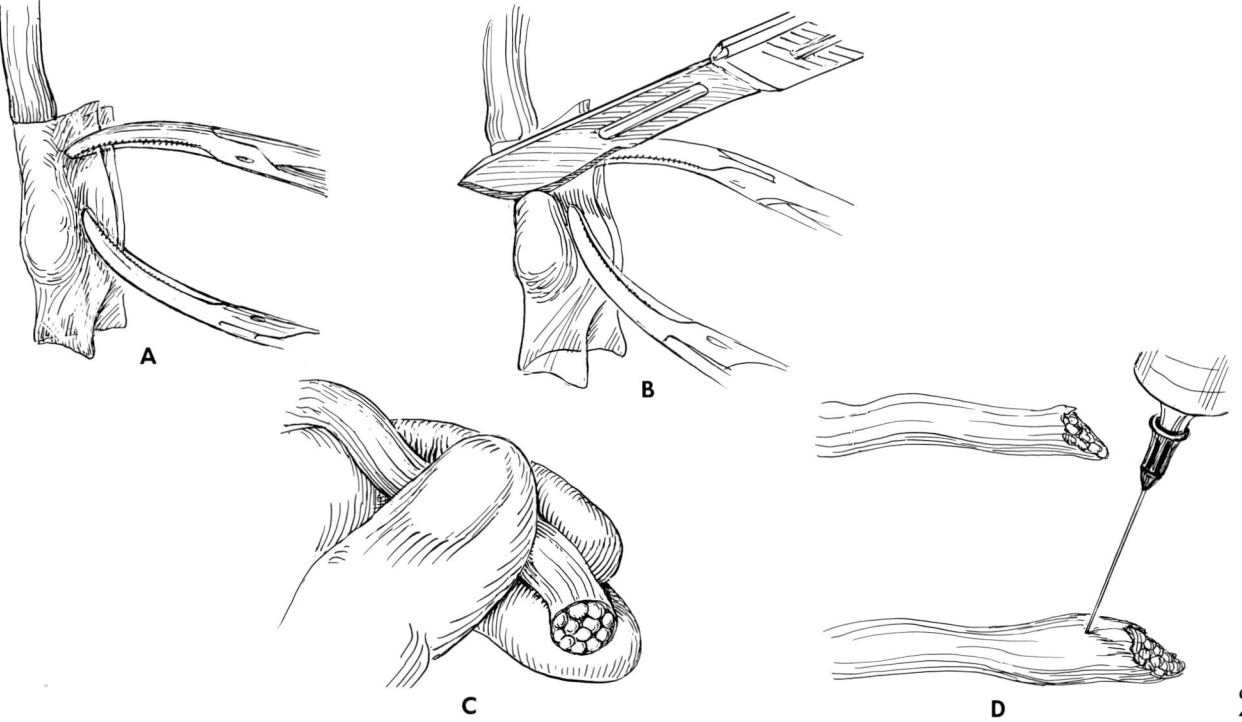

205

45 — Primary Nerve Repair

Fine (6-0 to 8-0) vascular silk swaged on a curved needle is used for the repair. A preliminary pass or two of the silk through local fat will lubricate it in preparation for nerve sheath repair. (**E**)

The first suture is passed through the sheath at the proximal and distal cut ends of the nerve at some identifiable point such as that marked by a longitudinal surface blood vessel. (**F** and **G**) The second suture is placed precisely opposite the first in the circumference of each nerve end. (**H**)

By gentle traction on these sutures, the task of placing additional sutures is simplified. (**I**) Once the surgeon is satisfied that an adequate number of sutures has been placed between the tethering threads on one side, the whole nerve may be turned over by switching the guy sutures. (**J**) Sutures are placed close enough together in the sheath to keep the tiny funiculi inside the repaired nerve sheath. Alignment of the surface blood vessel or the major funiculi assures the surgeon that there is proper coaptation of the nerve ends without major axial malrotation. (**K**) The repaired nerve is placed in loose areolar tissue and is covered with vascularized fat whenever possible. (**L**) Direct adjacent tendon repair may result in scar callus incarceration of the nerve repair and therefore should be avoided if possible.

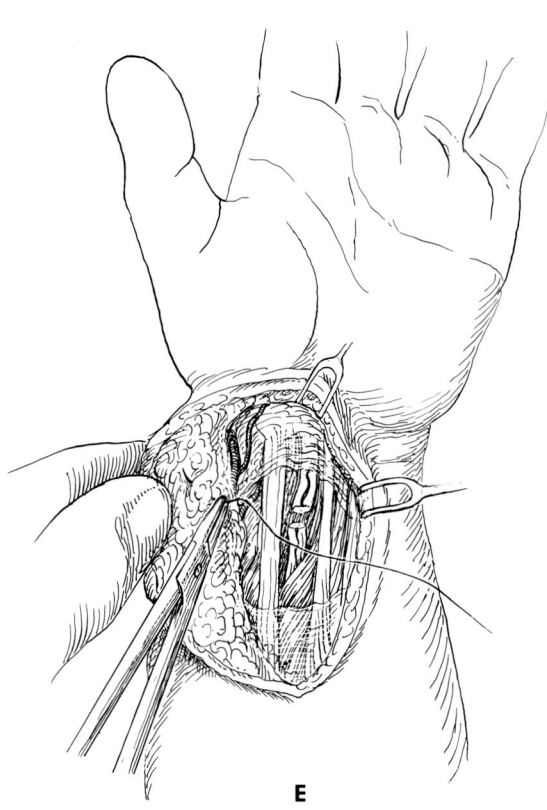

E

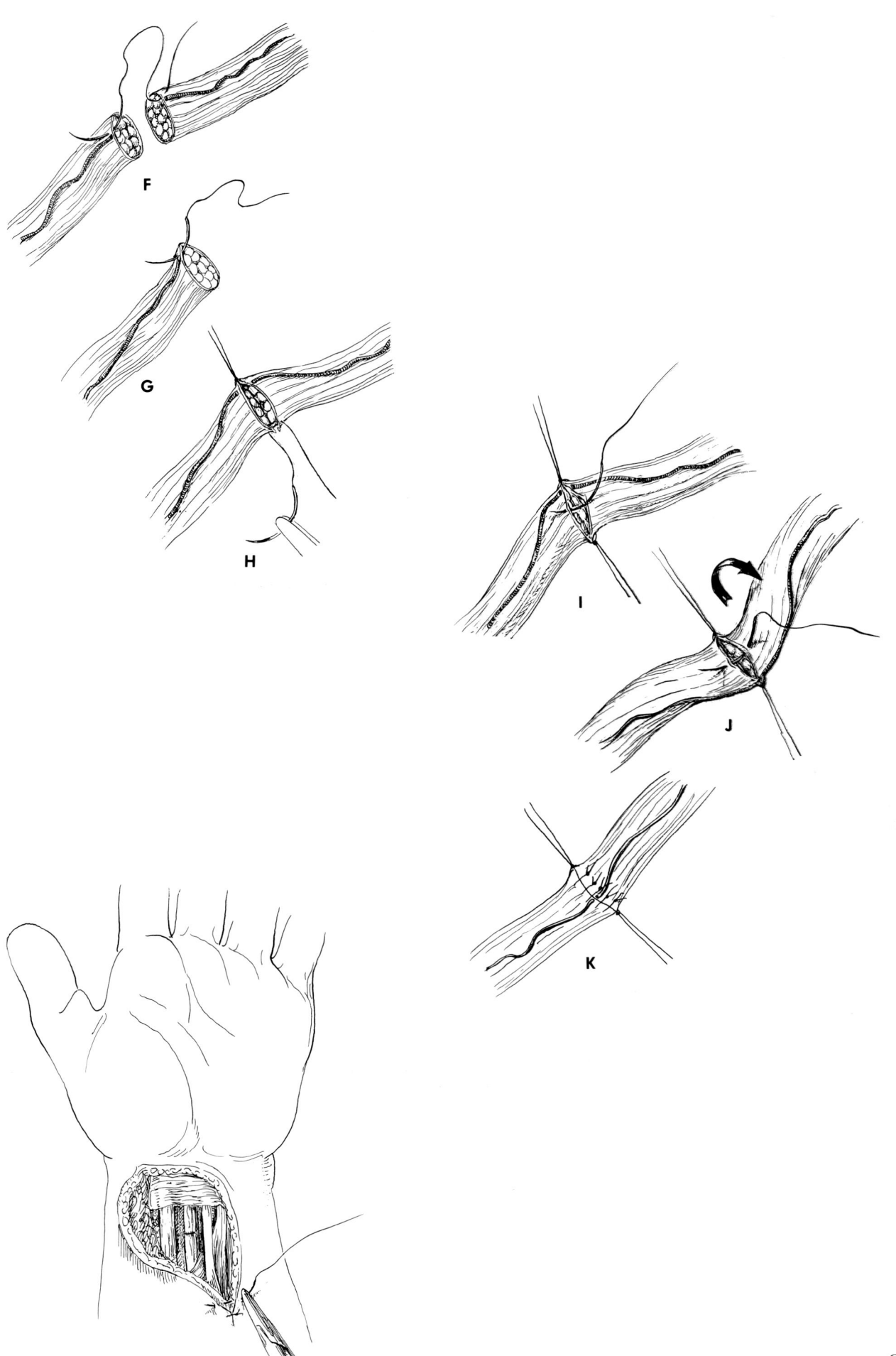

46

Findings and Treatment Late After Median Nerve Injury at the Wrist

SIMULTANEOUS NERVE REPAIR AND OPPONENS TRANSFER LATE AFTER MEDIAN NERVE INJURY AT THE WRIST

Principles

Following nerve transection, Wallerian degeneration of the nerve occurs distal to the transection. Atrophy of denervated muscles develops and the other changes ensue.

EXAMINATION LATE AFTER MEDIAN NERVE INJURY AT THE WRIST

Changes which follow low median nerve injury and are detectable after a few weeks are:

1. Anesthesia over the palmar aspect and dorsal tips of the thumb, index, long and radial half of the ring finger. A variable part of the radial two-thirds of the palm of the hand is also anesthetic.

2. Dryness and atrophy of skin over the same distribution. The fingerprint ridges are less prominent and the skin may be dry with desquamating scales of dry keratin. The skin appears thin making the underlying blood vessels more visible than on the normal hand.

3. Ulcers and scars over the anesthetic area from lack of protective sensibility. Cigarette burns, hot stove or dish burns, abraded areas and self-inflicted ulcers are most common.

4. Paralysis of the thenar thumb positioning for pulp-to-pulp opposition with the fingers. (See variation in innervation, page 221.)

5. Atrophy of the thenar muscles resulting in a flat or scooped out thenar area particularly detectable by comparing it with the uninjured hand.

6. Painful neuroma with electric shocklike tenderness at the site of laceration at the wrist.

7. Sympathetic dystrophy with burning pain and even full-blown causalgia may be evident. It is more frequent after injuries of the median nerve and medial cord of the brachial plexus than after injuries to the other peripheral nerves. This is perhaps because these nerves carry a quantitatively larger proportion of sympathetic and sensory nerves than other nerves.

Principles

The denervation atrophy of the small intrinsic muscles is reversible for several months after denervation if reinnervation is achieved. Failure to achieve reinnervation results in development of irreversible denervation atrophy after a variable period of time. It is essentially hopeless to expect to achieve functional reinnervation of these small muscles if they have been denervated for a year.

The distal nerve sheath remains intact after Wallerian degeneration of the axonal nerve component but it slowly becomes less and less receptive to ingrowth of new axons as time passes. The restoration of sensibility by nerve repair is clinically nearly as good with a repair done at 3 or 4 months as that done one month after injury. The restoration of sensibility becomes less and less reliable if repair is done after six or eight months; nevertheless, useful sensibility has been reported after nerve repair as long as seven years after injury.

One should attempt nerve repair even late after injury to try to restore protective sensibility. Since it is unlikely that useful intrinsic motor power will be restored by reinnervation, it is proper to carry out nerve repair and an appropriate tendon transfer simultaneously.

Example

Laceration of the median nerve occurred one year prior to surgery, and anesthesia over the thumb, index, long, and half of the ring finger persisted. Complete atrophy of the thenar muscles with loss of active opposition capability was evident. A positive Tinel's sign was elicited at the laceration scar but none distal to that point. (**A**)

Exploration revealed an unrepaired median nerve transection and a neuroma at the proximal cut end. (**B**)

After resection of the neuroma and distal nerve scar, the median nerve was repaired using the technique described in Section 45. A classical opponens transfer using the ring finger superficialis was performed at the same time. (**C**) The technique is described in Section 90.

A simple procedure thus simultaneously may restore protective sensibility and generate substitute opponens function.

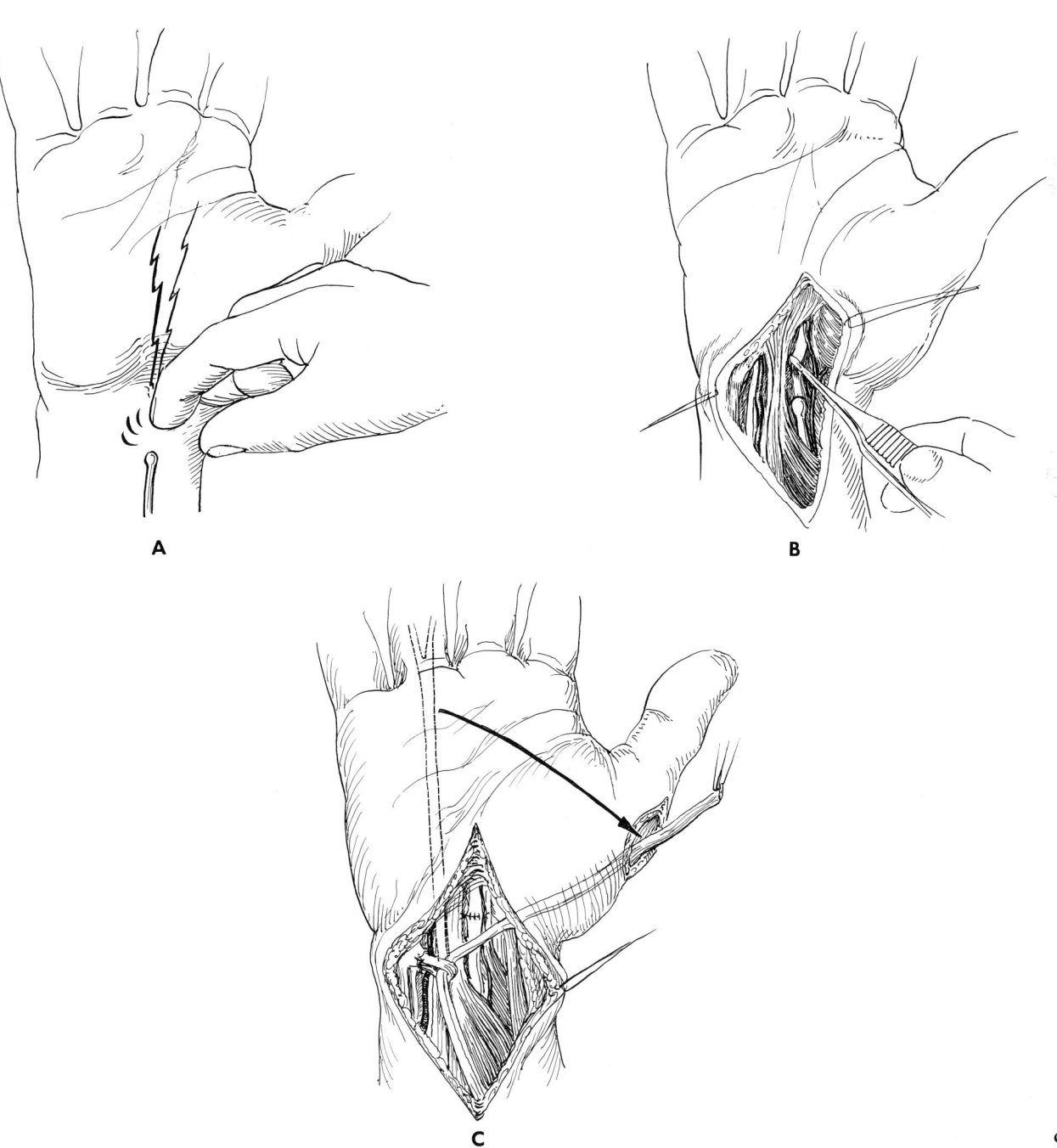

47

Acute Ulnar Nerve Transection at the Wrist

The ulnar nerve is vulnerable at the wrist level. It is protected by the flexor carpi ulnaris, which lies superficial to it through the whole forearm. At the wrist the ulnar neurovascular bundle, including the ulnar artery, vein, and nerve, becomes superficial and passes into the hand outside the carpal tunnel. It courses adjacent and radial to the prominent pisiform bone which protects it once it reaches the distal palmar wrist crease. In the interval proximal to the pisiform where the ulnar nerve becomes superficial, it is particularly subject to injury. The flexor carpi ulnaris is nearly always injured in ulnar nerve transections just proximal to the wrist.

Ulnar Nerve Sensory Pattern

The ulnar nerve through its palmar sensory branches supplies sensibility to the palmar aspect of the little finger and ulnar half of the ring finger. It is not an unusual variation for the adjacent sides of the ring and long fingers to receive sensibility from the ulnar nerve. This anatomical variation is shown as oblique line shading. (**A**)

The dorsal sensory branch is responsible for sensibility over the dorsal ulnar aspect of the hand on the little and ulnar half of the ring finger. (**B**) The rest of the dorsal skin is innervated by the dorsal branch of the radial nerve. (**C**) The dorsal branch of the ulnar nerve emerges from the main nerve trunk above the wrist at variable levels in the distal one-third of the forearm. Thus an injury to the trunk of the ulnar nerve at the wrist will *not* cause anesthesia over the dorsal aspect of the ulnar fingers.

Ulnar Nerve Motor Innervation in the Hand

The ulnar nerve is responsible for innervation of all intrinsic muscles in the hand except for the two and one-half muscles radial to the flexor pollicis longus which make up the thenar eminence and the lumbricals to the index and long fingers. The hypothenar muscles receive innervation from the superficial branch of the ulnar nerve and from the deep or motor branch as it passes through these muscles to plunge into the deep palm. All of the interossei, the lumbricals to the ring and little fingers, the thumb adductor and deep head of the flexor pollicis brevis receive innervation from the deep motor branch. (**D**) (See Variation in Intrinsic Muscle Innervation Patterns, Section 51.)

Findings Immediately After Ulnar Nerve Injury at the Wrist

1. Loss of sensibility and sudomotor function (sweating) over the palmar aspect of the little finger and ulnar half of the ring finger and a variable portion of the ulnar side of the palm of the hand proximal to these fingers.

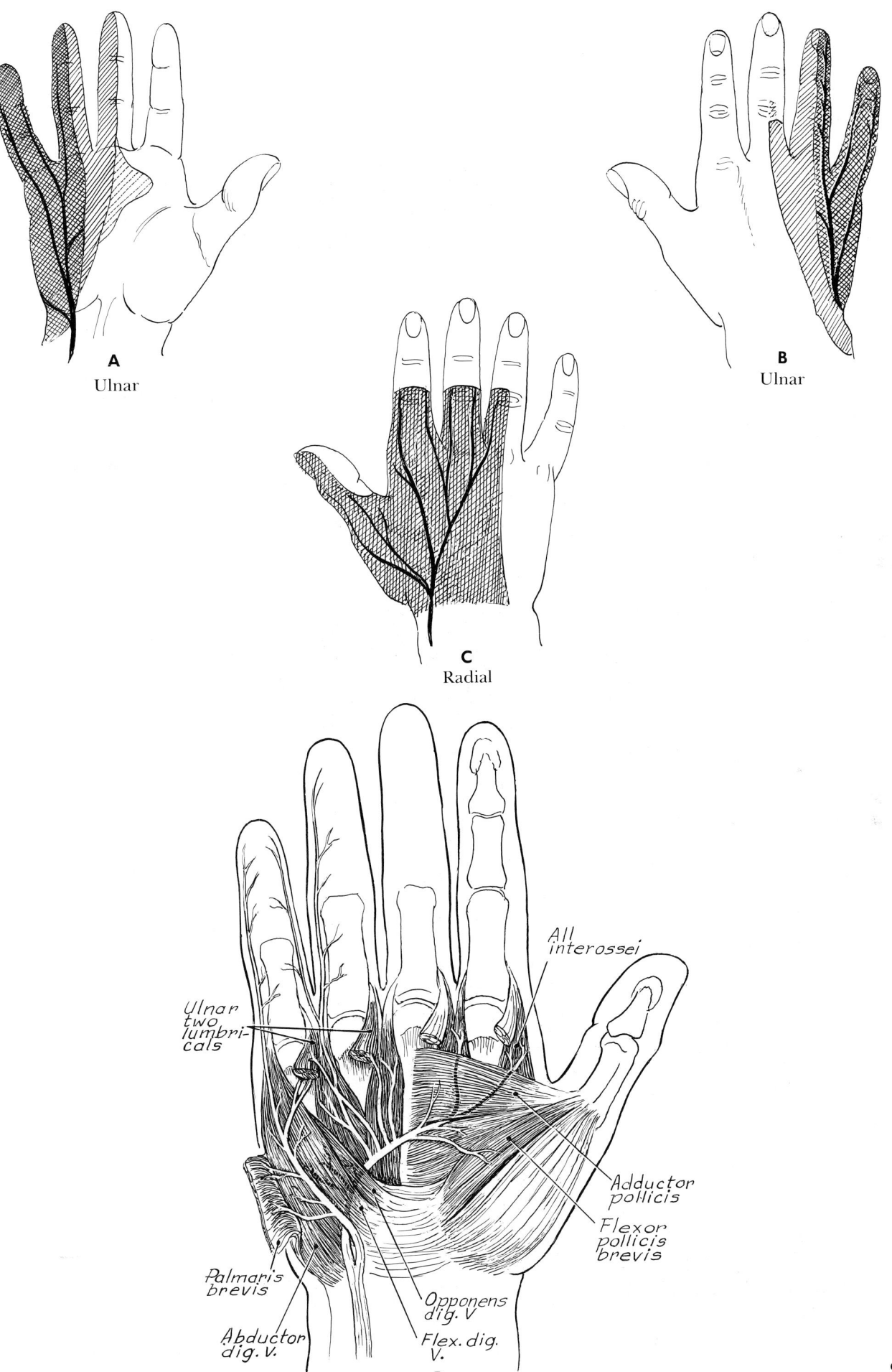

2. Loss of motor function in all of the hypothenar muscles, all interossei and the adductor to the thumb. It is difficult to specifically assess clinically the loss of lumbricals of the ring and little fingers and the deep head of the flexor pollicis brevis. The patient will be unable to abduct and adduct his fingers in the extended position. Hyperextension of the metacarpophalangeal joints with flexion of the interphalangeal joints (clawing) of the fingers may be evident early but it is more reliable to test actively the finger intrinsic muscles. He will be unable to assume the "intrinsic plus" position (see pages 18 and 19), with the metacarpophalangeal joints in flexion and the interphalangeal joints in extension.

Adduction of the thumb will be weakened so that the patient will be unable to squeeze an object held between the metacarpal heads of the thumb and index finger in the first web space. An attempt to pinch pulp of thumb to pulp of index finger, forming a circle with the two digits, (**E**) frequently results in collapse of the thumb metacarpophalangeal joint into recurvatum (Froment's sign). (**F**)

Atrophy of intrinsic muscles and changes in the skin are not evident early.

Progressive Changes After Ulnar Nerve Injury at the Wrist

Changes which follow low ulnar nerve injury detectable after a few weeks are:

1. Anesthesia over the palmar and dorsal tips of the little finger and ulnar half of the ring finger. The palm of the hand over the hypothenar area and for a variable distance across the palm is also anesthetic.

2. Dryness and atrophy of the skin over the same distribution. Fingerprint ridges on the little finger are less prominent and the thinning of the skin makes underlying blood vessels more visible than normal.

3. Ulcers and scars over the anesthetic area from chronic lack of protective sensibility.

4. Ulnar claw hand position with variable degree of fixed deformity of the semiflexed interphalangeal joints. This deformity, consisting of hyperextension of the metacarpophalangeal joints and flexion of the interphalangeal joints, may only be evident in the ring and little fingers. It is always most severe in these two fingers even if it does appear in the index and long fingers. Paralysis of all intrinsic muscles in the hand except those on the radial side of the long flexor to the thumb (abductor pollicis brevis, opponens pollicis, and superficial head of the flexor pollicis brevis) and the lumbricals to the index and long fingers which are innervated by the median nerve.

Inability actively to assume the intrinsic plus hand attitude with the metacarpophalangeal joints flexed and the interphalangeal joints extended. Inability to adduct the thumb to pinch an object placed in the first web space between the heads of the thumb and index metacarpals. A positive Froment's sign with inability to avoid recurvatum deformity of the thumb metacarpophalangeal joint on forceful pinch between the thumb and index pulps. This is the equivalent of claw deformity in the fingers.

5. Atrophy of the ulnar innervated intrinsic muscles. This is most clearly evident in the hypothenar muscles on the palm and in the first web space over the first dorsal interosseous muscle on the dorsum. Atrophy of all the interossei may be visible when one compares the two hands. The hollow interosseous spaces between the extensor tendons can be seen. Prominence of the long flexors to the fingers, particularly the long and little fingers, is notable on comparison. The shrunken lumbricals to the ring and little fingers and the atrophic palmar interossei account for this and the general flat thin appearance of the whole body of the hand.

6. Painful and/or tender neuroma at the wrist. Percussion at the site of suspected injury results in paresthesias which are referred to the ring and little fingers.

7. Sympathetic dystrophy. This is less common in pure ulnar nerve injuries than in median nerve injuries but is not rare.

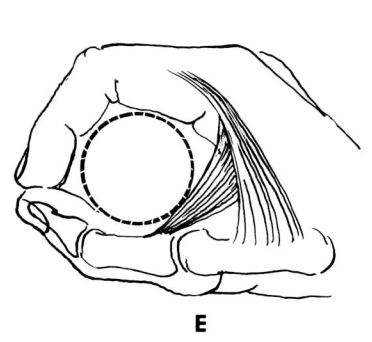
E

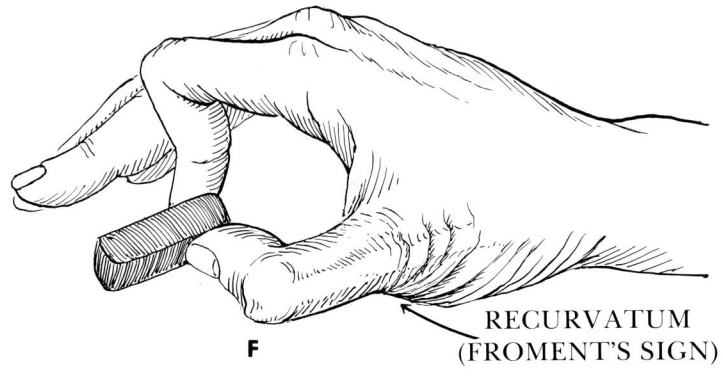
F RECURVATUM (FROMENT'S SIGN)

Acute Injury of the Motor Branch of the Ulnar Nerve

Principles

Stab wounds in the palm may sever the important motor branch of the ulnar nerve as it crosses the palm with the deep vascular arch deep to all the long flexor tendons. (**A**)

The rather subtle changes in hand function that result immediately after injury might be missed by casual examination. With normal sensibility in the ulnar innervated fingers and with persistent function in the hypothenar muscles, the only subjective tipoff the patient may give is that his hand feels clumsy or generally weak. One must test for active function of the interossei and thumb adductor to make the proper diagnosis.

In the event that the motor branch of the ulnar nerve has been transected in the palm, it should be repaired. If proper coaptation of the cut nerve ends can be achieved, the prognosis is good for adequate though reduced intrinsic muscular function. The relatively distal site of transection and the fact that one is repairing a pure motor nerve militates in favor of a good functional result.

The deep branch (motor) of the nerve is readily found by locating the deep palmar vascular arch by separating the long flexor tendons in the palm. Generally adequate length of nerve for repair without tension can be acquired by dissecting the nerve from surrounding structures over a short distance both proximal and distal to the transection site. If one cannot get the nerve ends together without tension, the motor branch can be dissected from the superficial part of the ulnar nerve to a level above the wrist. If the nerve still fails to reach the distal cut end, the nerve may be rerouted through the carpal tunnel more directly to the distal cut end. (See page 214.)

The nerve is repaired in standard fashion. Magnification may help a great deal in achieving a precision repair. If the motor branch of the ulnar nerve is not repaired, paralysis of the interossei, lumbricals to the ring and little fingers, and the thumb adductor creates significant disability. Atrophy of these intrinsic muscles and weakness in the absence of any sensory deficit are classical findings in late ulnar motor branch palsy. (**B**)

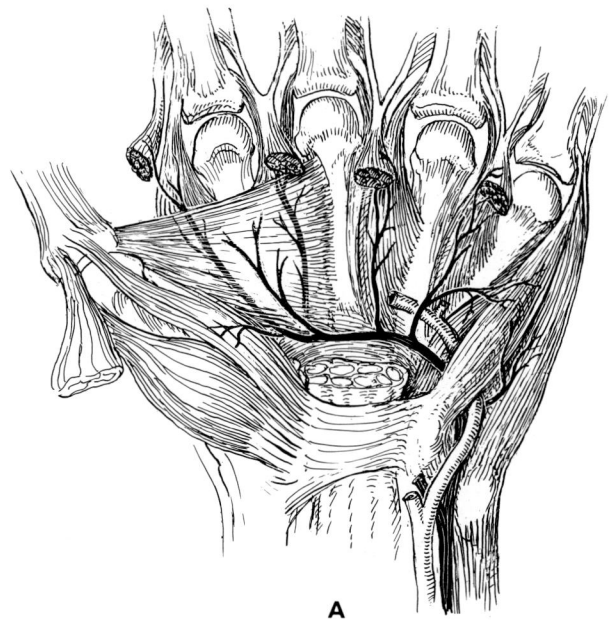

A

48 — Acute Injury of the Motor Branch of the Ulnar Nerve

Example: No Nerve Loss

Transection of the motor branch of the ulnar nerve occurred six months prior to surgery when the patient sustained a stab wound over the heel of the hand from broken glass.

Secondary or delayed repair was warranted and was carried out. Since the patient was seen within one year from the date of injury, an incision over the heel of the hand distal to the pisiform prominence allowed exposure of the deep branch of the ulnar nerve as it plunged into the hypothenar muscles. (**C** & **D**)

The muscles were transected over the nerve to follow its course into the deep palm. (**E**)

It was followed to the site of transection which was obvious because of the neuroma which had formed at the cut nerve end. (**F**)

Resection of the neuroma and of the scar at the distal cut end of the nerve prepared the nerve for repair. After repair the patient had nearly full recovery of function in one year. The prognosis for recovery of motor function after repair of the deep motor branch of the ulnar nerve in the first six months after injury is good. The fact that one is repairing a pure motor nerve a short distance from the muscles it innervates accounts for the probability of success.

Principle

If loss of substance in the motor branch of the ulnar nerve exists, it may be overcome by rerouting the nerve through the carpal tunnel. This may be useful at the time of injury or at the time secondary surgery is done.

Example: Loss of Nerve Substance

A crush laceration injury resulted in transection of the motor branch of the ulnar nerve in the hypothenar area. Part of the nerve was debrided at the initial operation. Two months after soft tissue healing, an elective rerouting and repair of the motor branch of the ulnar nerve was done. A curvilinear incision was planned which simultaneously would expose the ulnar nerve at the wrist and the carpal tunnel. (**G**)

The ulnar tunnel beneath palmar fascia was opened and the deep motor branch injury was located. (**H**)

The distal end was dissected free and the carpal tunnel was opened by incising the flexor retinaculum at the wrist. (**I**)

The nerve was transposed through the carpal tunnel to gain length and a nerve repair was completed after resection of the neuroma proximally and the scar distally. (**J** and **K**)

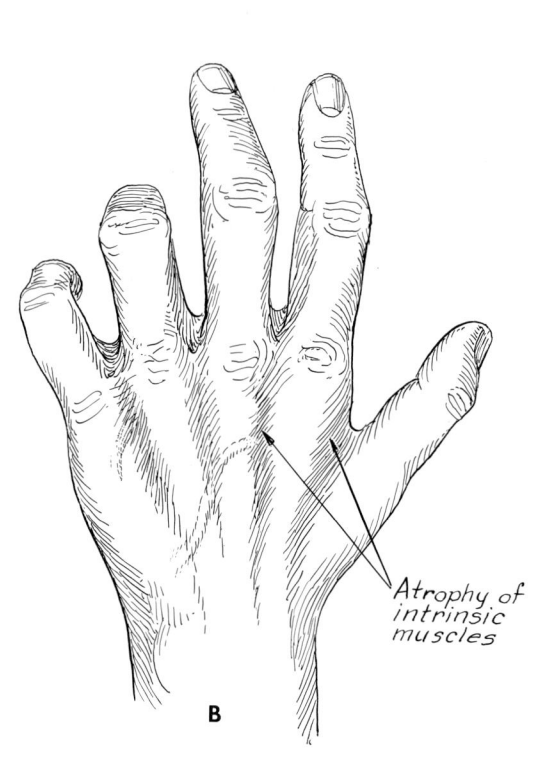

B

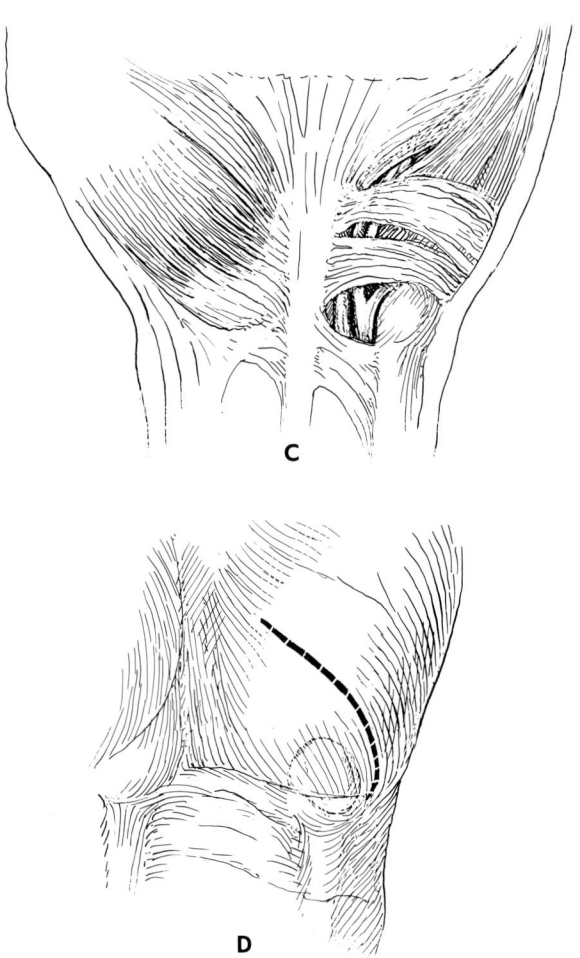

C

D

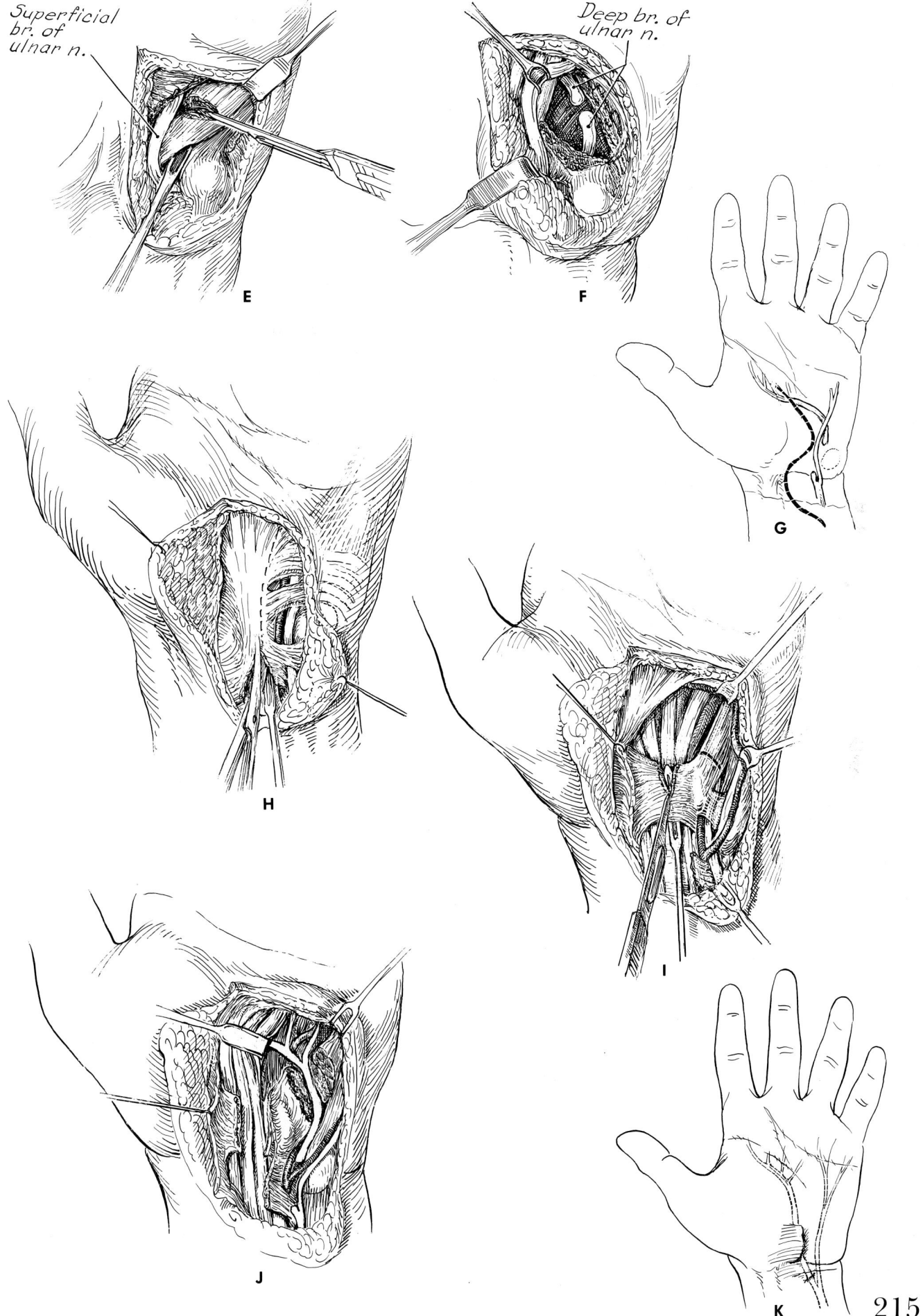

Digital Nerve Repair

Digital nerve repair after complete laceration is a worthwhile procedure for numerous reasons:

1. It is successful in restoring useful sensibility if end-to-end coaptation can be achieved. The result is optimized because it is a pure sensory nerve.
2. It diminishes the atrophy of a digit which occurs after denervation. This is particularly true when both proper digital nerves have been cut.
3. It diminishes the problem of painful neuroma by redirecting axonal sprouts distally to reinnervate specialized end organs.

A digital nerve can be repaired successfully as far distal as the middle of the middle phalanx. (**A**) Beyond this level arborization is so extensive that a single trunk for repair is not present. Furthermore, after healing of lacerations distal to this, the nerve sprouts from the large number of tiny end branches seem clinically to reinnervate the tip pulp sufficiently to result in adequate sensibility.

Once the diagnosis is established and the indication for repair is determined, the technique is straightforward. The nerve ends are identified and dissected separate from the vessels over sufficient length to achieve loose end-to-end coaptation allowing for nerve end resection.

Attached soft tissues are removed leaving a clean nerve sheath for sutures. The separated vessels should be ligated. The nerve ends usually must be recut by a single swipe of a sharp razor blade. This is best done using a piece of sterile tongue depressor beneath the nerve as a cutting board. (**B**)

Sutures of 7-0 silk with swaged on round needles are appropriate for nerve sheath coaptation. The suture material should be passed forward and back through local fat to lubricate it before using it in the nerve sheath. (**C**) The surface tension on silk sutures may otherwise pull through the sheath with resistance which frays the sharply cut sheath.

For improved precision an ophthalmologist's loupe is helpful and for even greater accuracy of closure, the operating microscope may be used. If the microscope is used, a few more sutures of 10-0 monofilament suture may be used. Without handling the nerve with instruments, the first suture is passed through its sheath at one cut nerve end and then through the other in such a way that the knot will be on the outside of the nerve.

After the first suture is tied, it is used as a retractor to identify the opposite side of the nerve circumference both proximal and distal, for precise placement of the second suture.

With the nerve ends held by the first two sutures, a third and fourth or even more may be accurately placed to achieve the best possible end-on coaptation. (**D**)

All sutures are then cut short and the finger is placed in enough flexion to take tension off the repair and the skin is closed. (**E**)

After a latent interval of two or three weeks regeneration should result in progression of Tinel's sign down the finger from site of repair to tip at a rate of about one finger phalanx length per month. (**F**)

The initial return of feeling is described as hypersensitivity which is not unlike the sensitivity of an epithelially denuded wound. As time passes, the hypersensitivity gives way to more normal sensibility.

Nerve Surgery

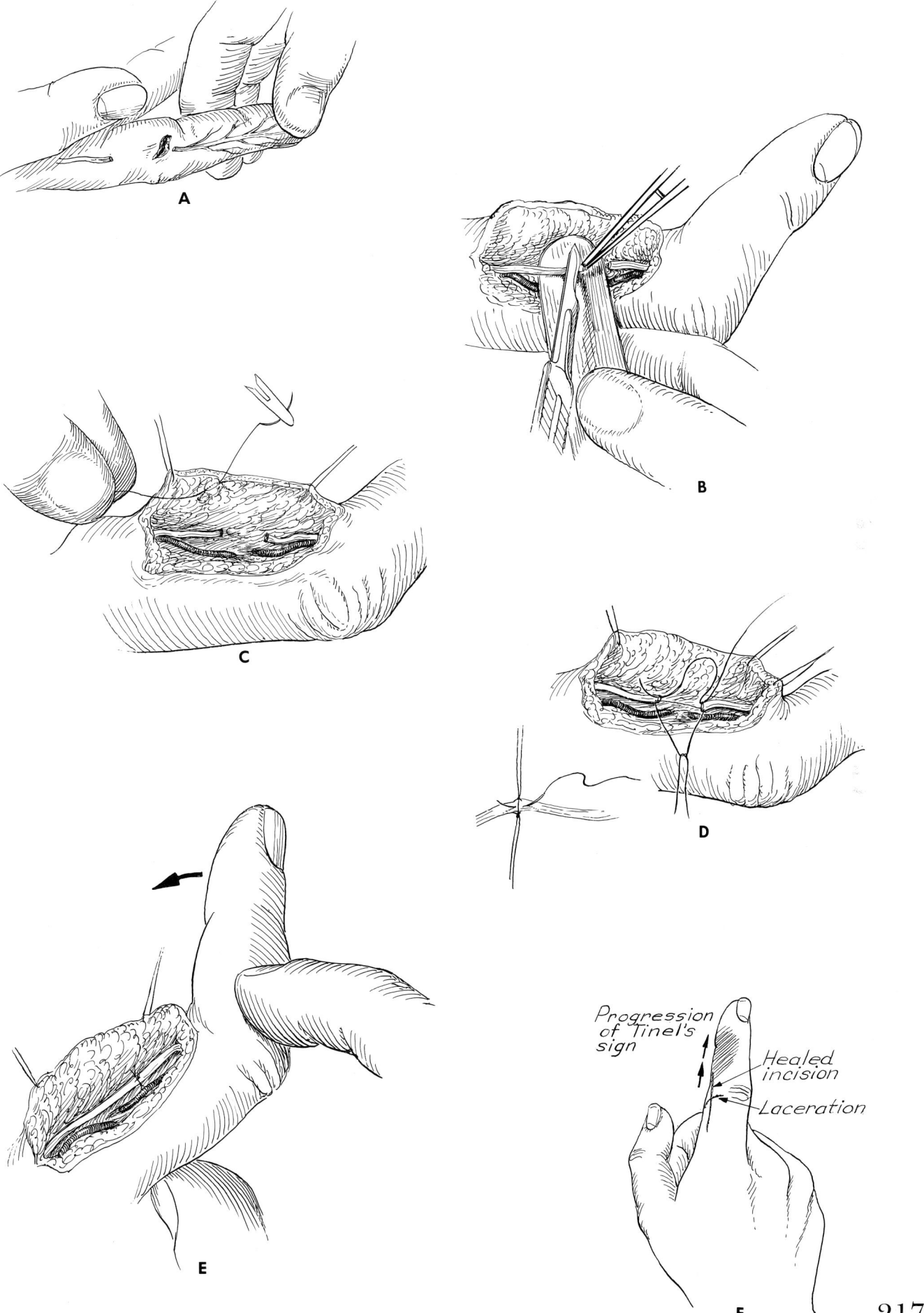

50
Small Superficial Sensory Nerve Branches

Injuries to small superficial sensory nerves to the skin surface of the hand may be troublesome if they go unrecognized. A knowledge of the anatomical location of these nerves is important for nerve block anesthesia and to avoid surgical injury to them. (**A**)

The Dorsal Branch of the Radial Nerve

The dorsal or superficial branch of the radial nerve courses through the forearm in relationship to the brachioradialis muscle on the radial side of the arm.

The nerve crosses the "anatomical snuff box" between the extensor pollicis brevis and the extensor pollicis longus in the loose subcutaneous tissue. It divides into multiple branches which give sensibility to the dorsum of the hand over the radial two-thirds, the dorsum of the thumb, index, long, and half of the ring finger proximal to the distal interphalangeal joint. (**B**)

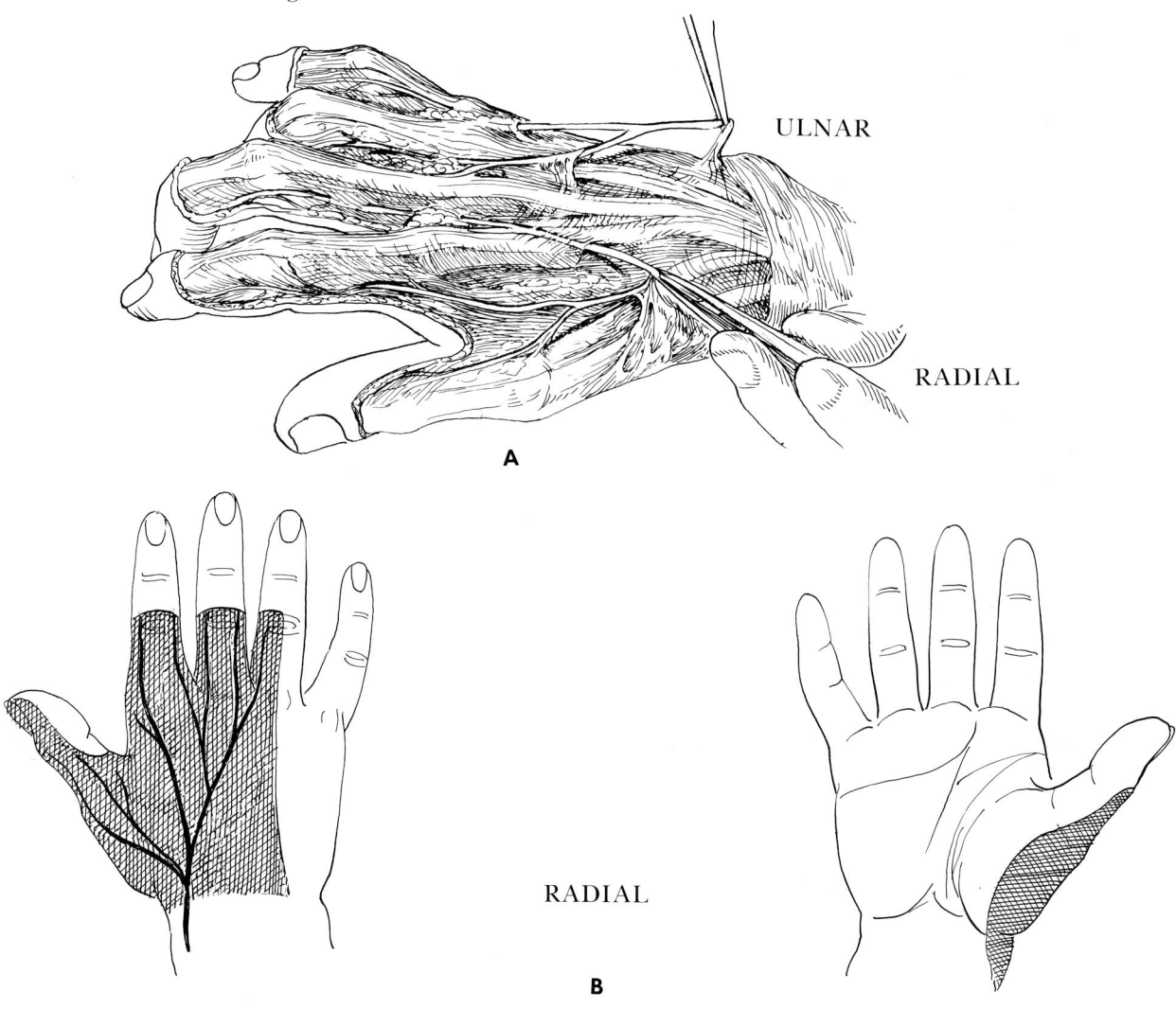

The nerve is superficial and subject to injury particularly in the distal forearm and over the "anatomical snuff box" at the wrist.

Surgery in the snuff box area for such things as De Quervain's tenosynovitis, fusion of the thumb carpometacarpal joint, repair of the extensor pollicis longus, and wrist surgery requires careful attention to the nerve to avoid injury.

Division of the nerve at the wrist results in anesthesia over the area described above. In itself this may not cause major difficulty except for the fact that unrecognized injury or self-induced injury in the anesthetic area may initiate and sustain *ulceration of the dorsal skin*. (**C**)

After a few weeks a tender neuroma at the site of nerve transection is the rule. This may be very troublesome and may be a compelling reason for immediate repair of a recognized transection of the nerve or a secondary repair. (**D**)

The Dorsal Branch of the Ulnar Nerve

The dorsal branch of the ulnar nerve leaves the main trunk and the rest of the ulnar neurovascular bundle at a variable site but usually at about the junction of the middle and distal third of the forearm. From the point of departure beneath the flexor carpi ulnaris it courses dorsally and penetrates the deep fascia to lie in the subcutaneous tissues over the distal forearm. It passes just radial to the palpable prominence of the ulna head at the wrist and divides into branches which give sensory innervation to the dorsum of the hand over the ulnar third and the dorsum of the little finger and the ulnar side of the ring finger proximal to the distal phalanges.

It is well to remember that this nerve is not blocked by an ulnar nerve block at the wrist nor is it injured by a palmar laceration of the ulnar nerve at the wrist.

If the nerve is transected, it should be repaired for the same reasons that the dorsal branch of the radial nerve should be and by the same technique.

Repair of the Dorsal Branch of the Radial Nerve

The dorsal nerves are small but are amenable to repair with fair reliability of success since they are pure sensory nerves. The repair is easier with magnification but may be done with 2 to 4 sutures of 7–0 silk after the silk is lubricated by passing it forward and back several times through some of the fat found in the wound.

Since some dorsal veins are likely to be present in the area, one may choose to sheath the nerve repair in a small vein segment. This is accomplished by passing a small free segment of the *vein over* one end of the nerve prior to nerve repair. After completing the nerve suture, the small vein segment may be slipped over the repair like a protective sleeve. (**E**)

The Palmar Cutaneous Branch of the Median Nerve

The median nerve commonly gives off a small cutaneous branch as it courses superficial at the radial aspect of the flexor digitorum superficialis tendons. This palmar cutaneous nerve pierces the deep fascia to become subcutaneous just above the wrist. It passes to the radial side of the root of the palm and thenar eminence outside the carpal tunnel. It innervates a variable patch of the proximal portion of the radial side of the palm and skin of the thenar eminence.

Transection of the nerve may result in a patch of numbness over the proximal palm. A painful neuroma may develop at the proximal cut end of the nerve. (**F**) There is generally enough crossover from fibers branching from the common digital nerves in the palm so that the anesthetic patch creates only an insignificant functional problem.

If the neuroma is troublesome, it may be managed by *recutting the nerve and placing the proximal end in the deep flexor compartment where it will not be subjected to repeated percussion*. (**G**)

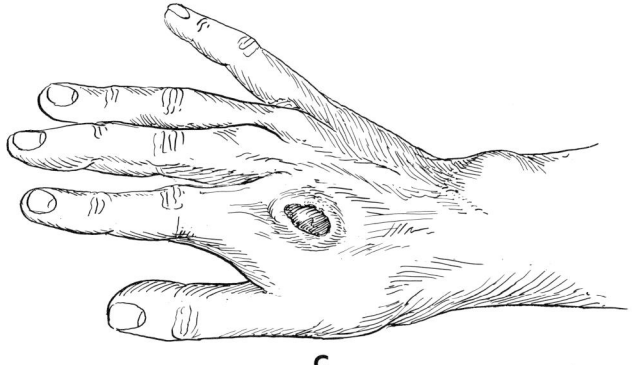

c

50 — Small Superficial Sensory Nerve Branches

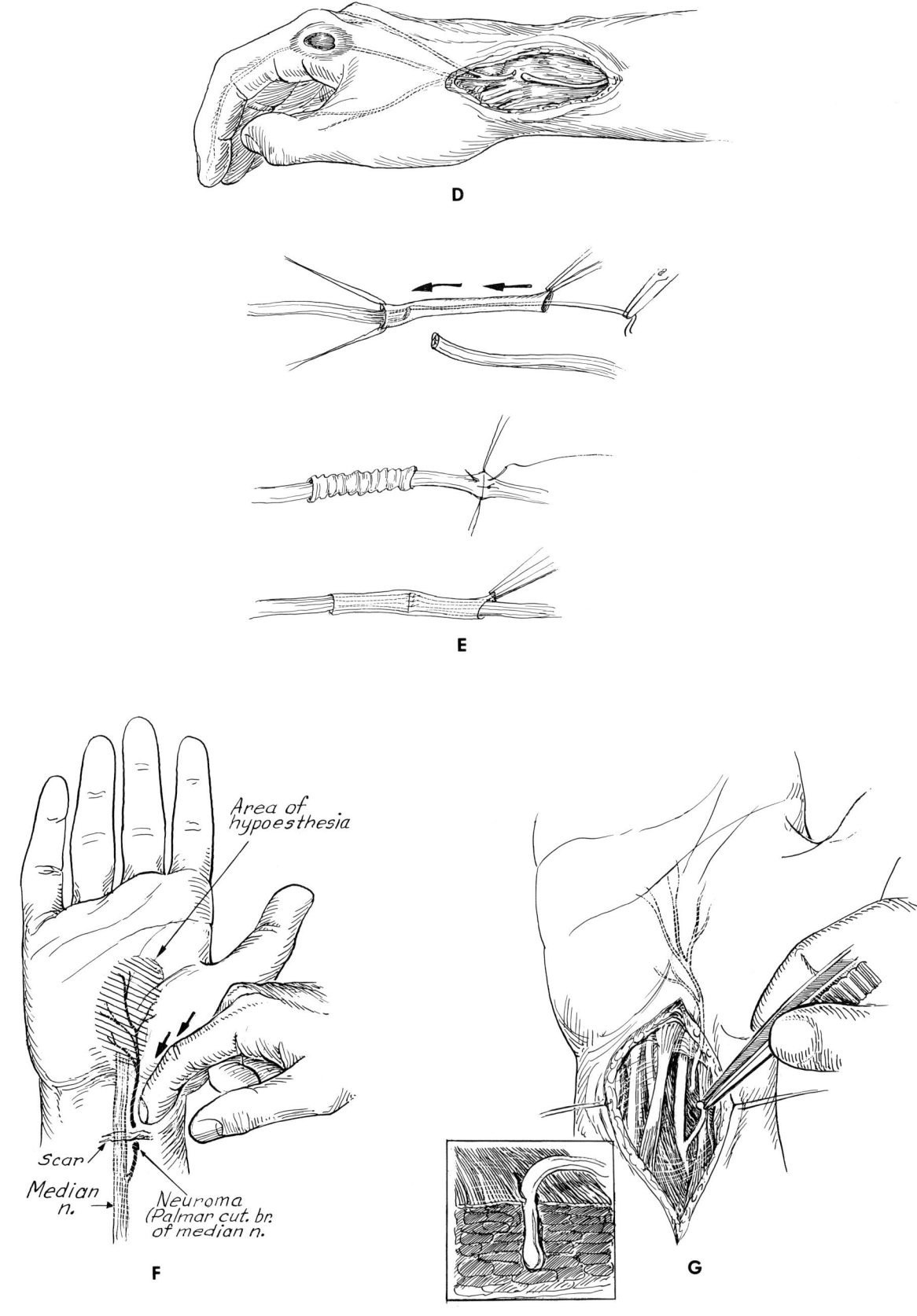

51

Facts Influencing Care of Nerve Injuries at the Wrist

Variation in Intrinsic Muscle Innervation Patterns

The intrinsic muscle innervation divides into median and ulnar at the line where the flexor pollicis longus crosses the thumb intrinsic muscles, since the superficial head of the flexor pollicis brevis lies radial and the deep head lies ulnar to this line. It is also at this area where the crossover of median to ulnar or ulnar to median is most frequent. The reported incidence of innervation of the two heads of the flexor pollicis brevis is as follows:

Innervation*	Superficial Head	Deep Head
Exclusively median	57%	12%
Exclusively ulnar	20%	67%
Dual	23%	21%

In median nerve palsy the superficial head may be adequate to accomplish useful opposition positioning in 20 per cent of cases and possibly even to 43 per cent.

---

*Sunderland, S.: *Nerves and Nerve Injuries.* E. & S. Livingston Ltd., Edinburgh, 1968.

Functionally Important Areas of Sensibility

Whenever sensibility is to be restored to the hand and, particularly, if sensibility is to be transferred from one area of the hand to another by nerve transfer, grafting, or island pedicle techniques, the surgeon must think through the whole issue of what areas are important to the specific patient. This varies considerably according to the patient's needs in his occupation or avocations but some generalizations can be made. The pulps of the opposing surfaces of the digits of manipulation, the thumb, index finger, and long finger are important in perception of texture, temperature and hardness. These areas are the key to man's ability to assess his environment by touch. (**A**)

Peripheral areas in the hand such as the ulnar side must have sensibility to protect the hand from injury. Anesthesia on these areas sets the stage for unrecognized burns and other trauma. (**B**) Preservation of sensibility and restoration of sensibility lost in these areas are considered very important.

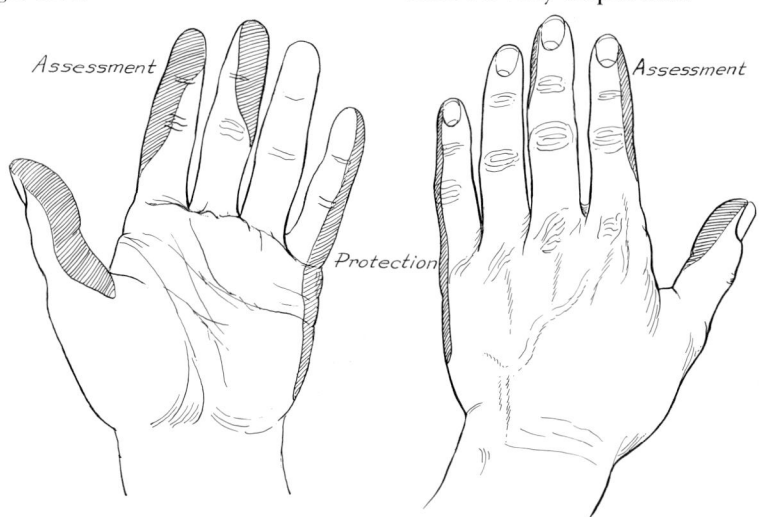

221

52

Injury of the Ulnar Nerve at the Elbow

As the ulnar nerve leaves the arm from its position adjacent to the medial head of the triceps, it becomes superficial to pass into the groove between the medial epicondyle of the humerus and the olecranon. At this point it is covered only by skin and fascia and it is therefore subject to injury when a laceration occurs. (**A**) Transection of the nerve at this level results in all of the findings described for ulnar nerve transection at the wrist but in addition:

1. There is loss of sensibility over the dorsum of the wrist and hand over the ulnar third and the dorsum of the little finger and ulnar half of the ring finger. Anesthesia is complete then over the little finger and ulnar half of the ring finger. Lack of protective sensibility of the little finger sets the stage for commonly occurring unrecognized injury to the finger and chronic ulceration. (**B**)

2. Paralysis of the flexor carpi ulnaris is detectable by specific testing. There is weakness in combined flexion and ulnar deviation of the wrist. Paralysis of the flexor digitorum profundus muscles to the ulnar two or three fingers is also evident. The profundus tendons to the long, ring, and little fingers emerge from a common muscle belly with partial septal separation only. Profundus function in these three fingers is interdependent and weakened in ulnar nerve transection at the elbow. Curiously, the absence of profundus flexion power makes the clawing deformity in high ulnar nerve paralysis less evident clinically than in low ulnar palsy. Total function, however, is more severely compromised.

Repair of the Ulnar Nerve at the Elbow

When the ulnar nerve is injured in close proximity to its passage through the bony groove created by the medial epicondyle, repair generally is best accomplished by relocating the nerve. *Rerouting* the nerve anterior to the medial epicondyle adds needed length to diminish tension on the nerve and it avoids the repeated mandatory stretch tension that occurs with every elbow flexion when the nerve remains *in situ*.

Transection of the ulnar nerve at the elbow level is best treated by primary repair using the technique described for median nerve repair.

Since several months will pass between the time of repair and the regrowth of functional axons to the hand, the surgeon should consider keeping the denervated intrinsic muscles in the most receptive condition for reinnervation. Maintain muscle length by passive range of motion exercises and dynamic splinting. Denervation atrophy may be delayed by electrical stimulation of the intrinsic muscles by therapists or by utilization of a small portable electrical stimulator. (**C**)

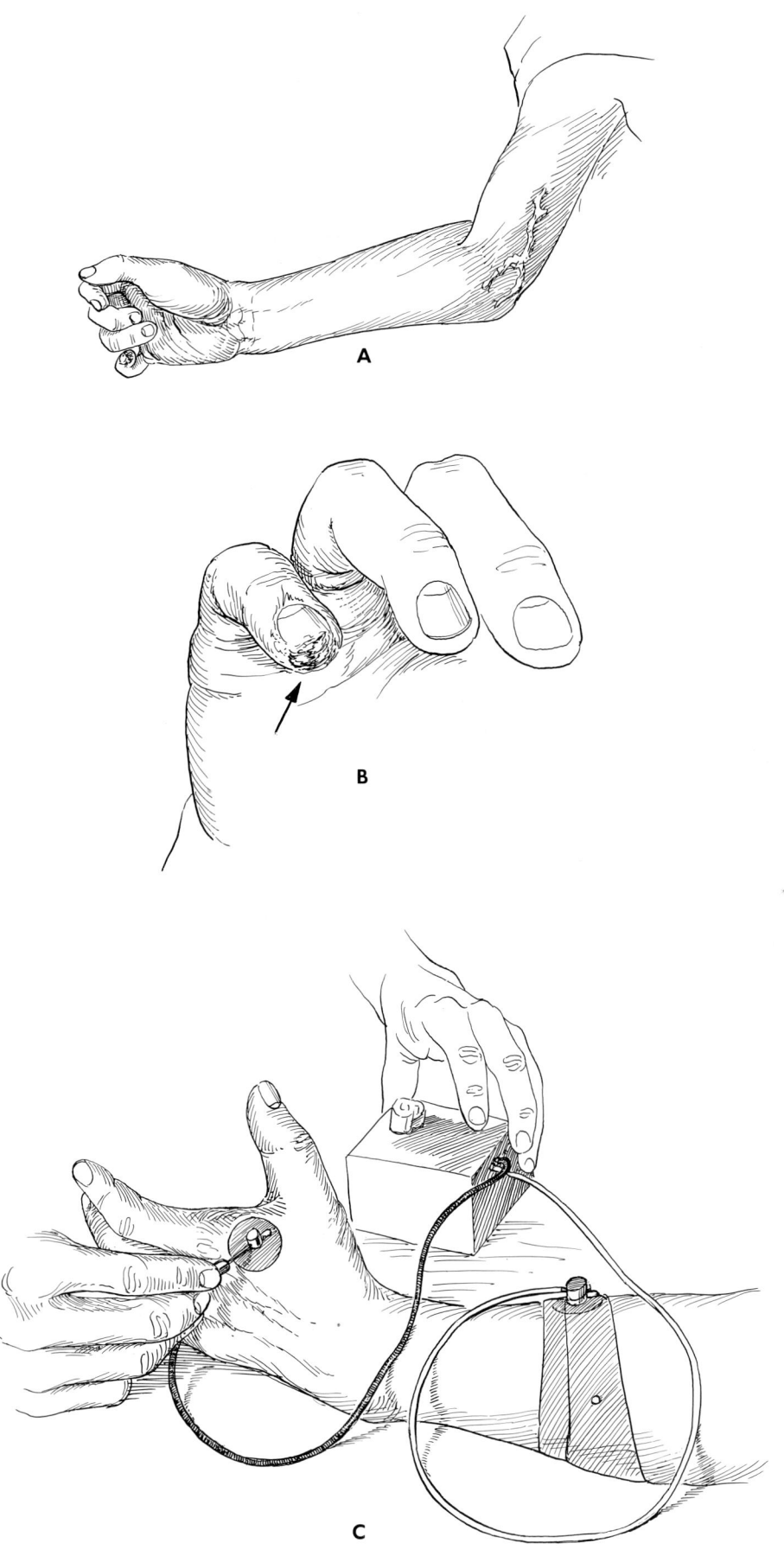

52 — Injury of the Ulnar Nerve at the Elbow

To transpose the nerve anterior to the medial epicondyle one must gain good exposure through a generous curved incision anterior to the epicondyle. (**D**) The fascia overlying the elbow joint and the medial muscles above and below it is elevated as an apron by dissection from the mid-ulnar plane toward the antecubital fossa. (**E**) The proximal and distal nerve ends are exposed and if the nerve has been transected one may dissect the nerve both proximally and distally, rerouting it by passing the distal nerve retrograde *medial to the superficial flexor muscle origins on the medial epicondyle.* The proximal nerve end is brought in front of the epicondyle and suture repair to the distal nerve is accomplished. The apron of fascia is brought over the nerve and sutured back to its original position with care not to angulate or compress the nerve proximally. (**F, G,** and **H**)

If transposition of an intact ulnar nerve at the elbow is indicated for chronic nerve compression or to gain length in the nerve for a repair in the forearm, the procedure is more complex.

The surgeon may choose to cut the origins of the superficial flexor muscles from the medial epicondyle, transfer the nerve anteriorly, and then reattach the muscle origins. Alternatively, the medial epicondyle may be separated by osteotomy, carrying with it the superficial flexor origins. The nerve may then be transposed forward and the medial epicondyle reattached to its previous site.

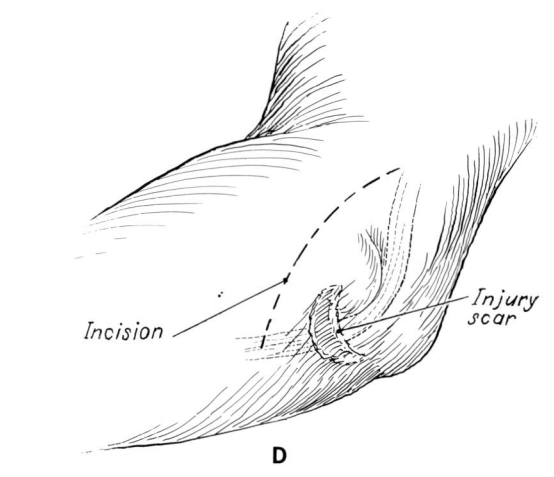

D

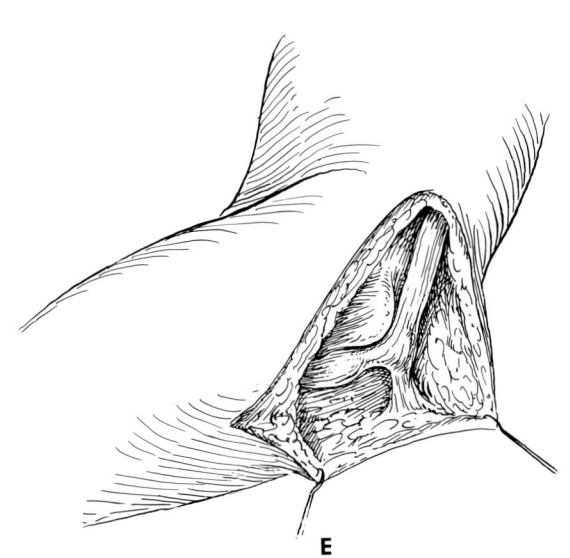

E

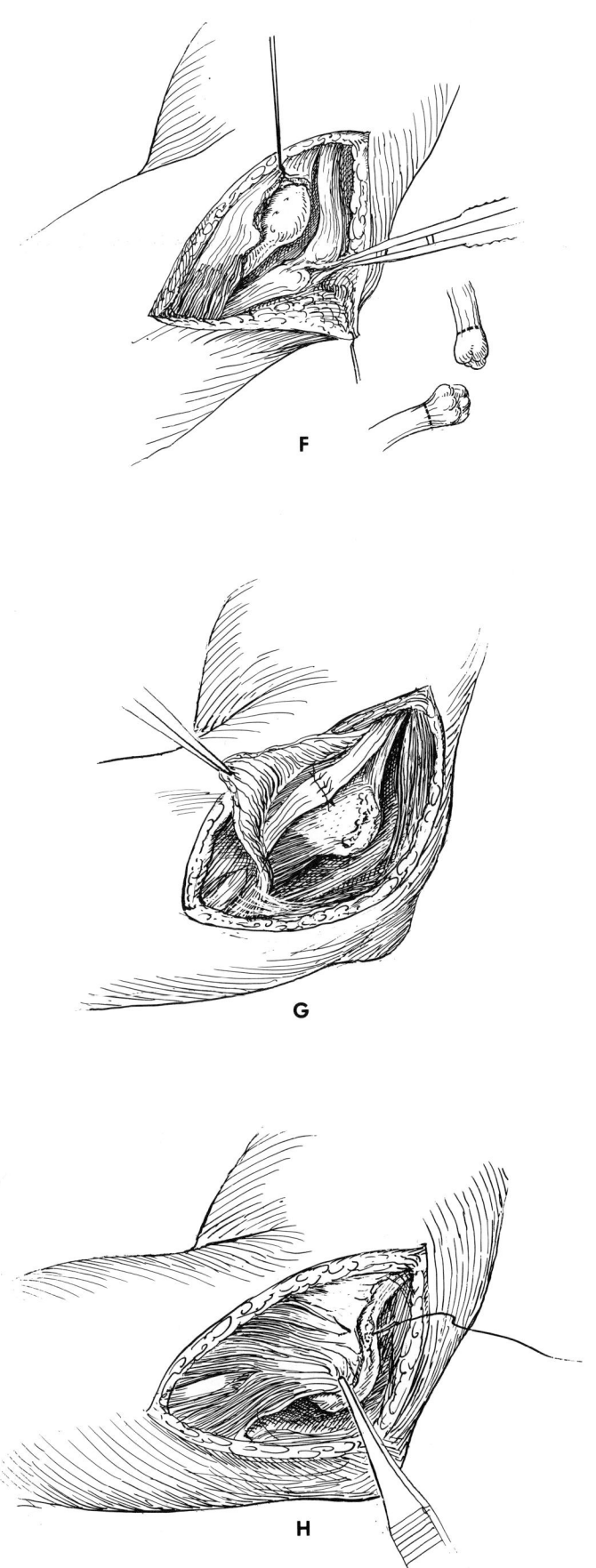

53
Radial Nerve Paralysis

The radial nerve is most commonly injured at the mid-humeral level where it lies in the spiral groove of the humerus. Fractures or severe lacerations may transect the nerve. Even more commonly the nerve is acutely compressed or stretched but remains in continuity in humeral fractures. The early effect is a general paralysis of the primary extensor supinator group of muscles in the forearm and weakness in the elbow extensors. Sensibility is lost over the radiodorsal aspect of the radial two-thirds of the wrist and hand and the dorsum of the thumb, index, long, and radial half of the ring finger proximal to the level of the distal interphalangeal joint.

All of the muscles on the dorsum of the forearm are innervated by the radial nerve. (**A**) These consist of the three muscles in the "mobile wad" which can be picked up by one's opposite thumb and index finger (**B**) and all of the extrinsic extensors of the fingers and the intrinsic abductor and extensors of the thumb. (**C**) The muscles in the "mobile wad" are the brachioradialis and extensor carpi radialis longus and extensor carpi radialis brevis.

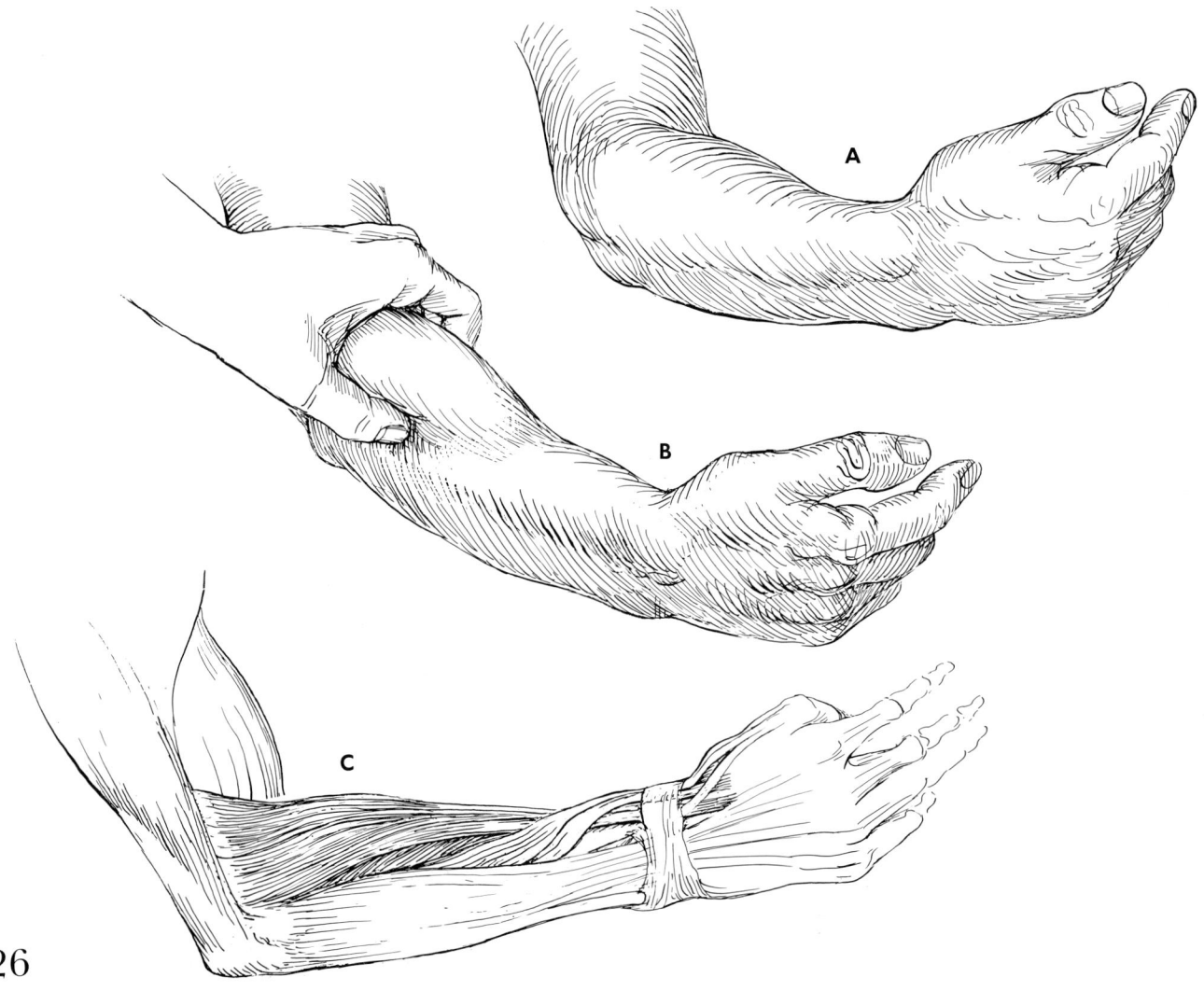

Nerve Surgery

The supinator is radial-nerve innervated as is the small triangular anconeus which is essentially part of the triceps. The part of the triceps below the spiral groove and distal to the site of radial nerve injury is also paralyzed. Clinically, radial nerve palsy patients present a classical "wrist drop." (**D**) The inability to actively extend the wrist robs the patient of power to flex his fingers well with his intact long flexors. (**E**)

On careful clinical analysis one finds "finger drop" at the metacarpophalangeal joint so that when the wrist is supported an attempt to extend the fingers results in flexion of the metacarpophalangeal joints with weak extension of the interphalangeal joints under the influence of the intact innervated intrinsic muscles. (**F**)

If one supports both the wrist and metacarpophalangeal joints in extension, the patient finds it possible to actively extend the interphalangeal joints. (**G**)

With the wrist supported in extension, grip is restored to full power. (**H**)

The thumb is adducted and the patient is unable to extend it at the carpometacarpal and metacarpophalangeal joints. Support of the thumb at the carpometacarpal and metacarpophalangeal joints allows the patient to extend the interphalangeal joint weakly. The power to supinate the forearm is diminished but present unless one robs the biceps of its power to supinate by placing the elbow in extension.

Repair of the radial nerve if it is sectioned at the humeral level is likely to result in useful reinnervation of the various muscle groups if it is done well technically and early after injury. When the nerve is damaged beyond repair, or if the nerve injury is more than a year old, one should consider tendon transfers to substitute for the motor loss.

During paralysis of the radial innervated muscles the wrist and fingers should be kept supple and capable of a full range of motion by physical therapy and dynamic splinting.

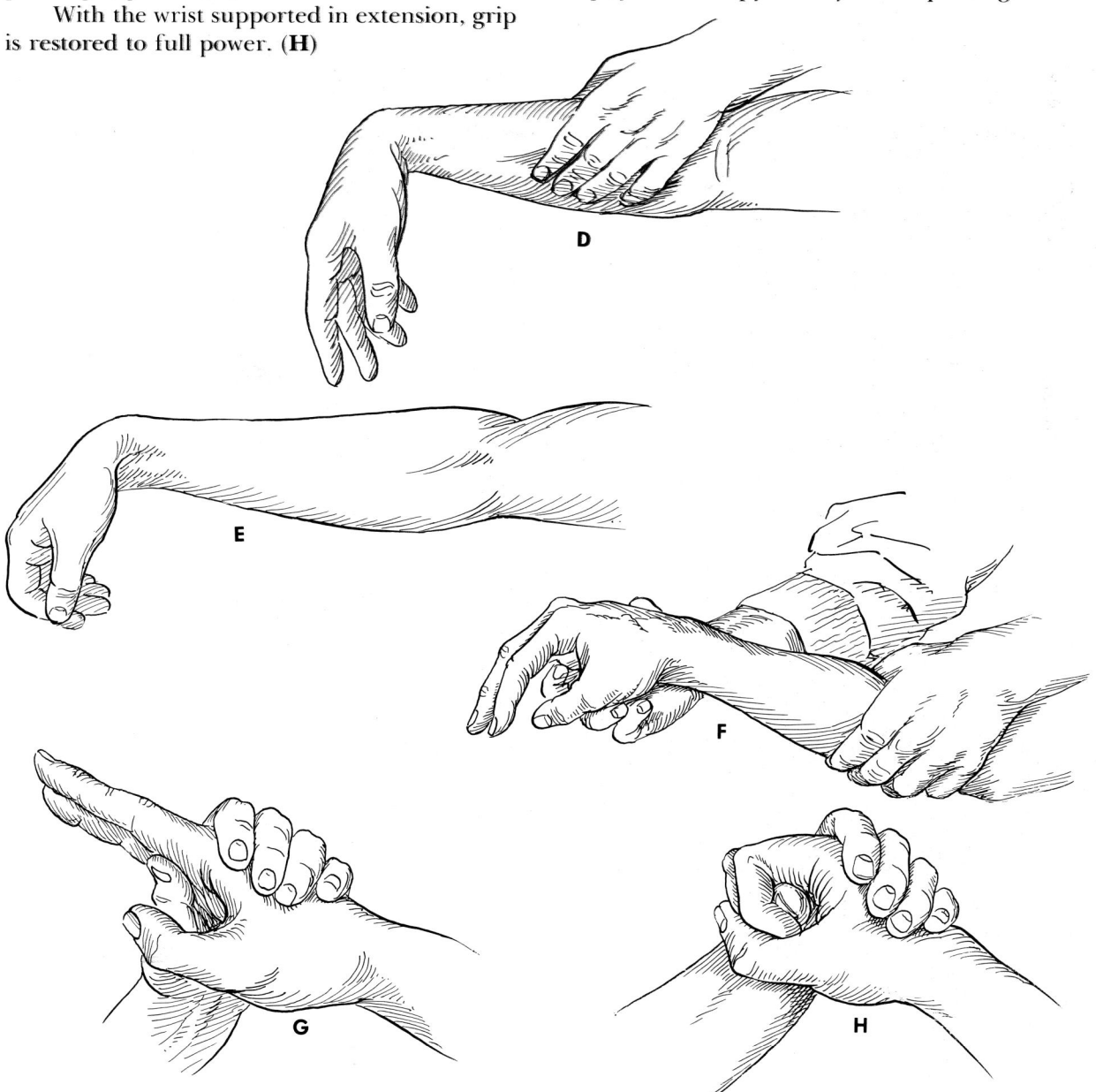

Median Nerve Injury at the Elbow

Classically, the median nerve innervates all of the muscles on the palmar aspect of the forearm except the flexor carpi *ulnaris* and the *ulnar* half or two-thirds of the flexor digitorum profundus which are *ulnar* nerve innervated. The remaining median innervated muscles make up the flexor-pronator group and consist of the pronator teres, pronator quadratus, flexor carpi radialis, palmaris longus, flexor pollicis longus, all of the flexor digitorum superficialis group, and the radial portion of the flexor digitorum profundus (index). High median nerve paralysis results in findings described for median nerve palsy at the wrist plus those resulting from paralysis of the forearm muscles listed above.

1. The patient is unable to flex the distal joint of the thumb although he may weakly flex the metacarpophalangeal joint. The index finger is weak in flexion and has no strength for flexion of the interphalangeal joints. The strength of interphalangeal flexion progresses as one examines the long, the ring, and then the little finger.

2. Specific testing for independent proximal interphalangeal joint flexion will show absence of superficialis function in all four fingers.

3. Wrist flexion is weak and is achieved by contraction of the ulnar innervated profundi and flexor carpi ulnaris. The wrist thus flexes in ulnar deviation.

4. There is loss of forearm pronation against gravity.

Repair of a median nerve transection at the elbow may be aided significantly both by positioning the elbow in 90° of flexion and, when necessary, by rerouting the nerve superficial to the pronator teres. (**A**)

Rerouting of the nerve is done with care to preserve all of the motor branches possible to the muscles in the flexor pronator compartment.

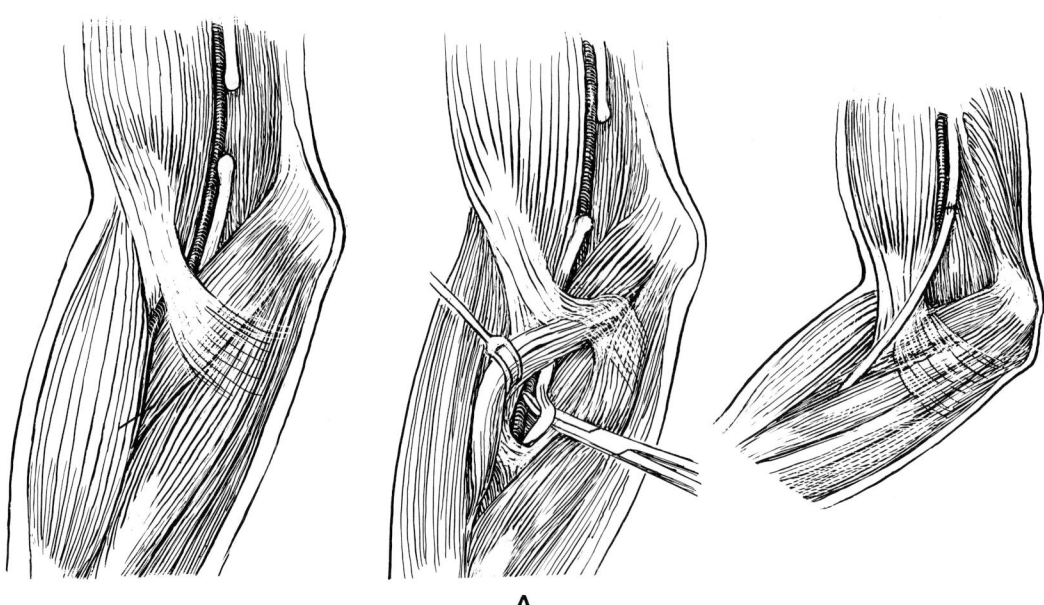

A

Tests to Sharpen Diagnosis Late After Nerve Injury

There are tests of sensibility and motor function to assess the quality of recovery and which help to differentiate the complete nerve injury from one that is partial or incomplete.

Tests of Sensibility

LIGHT TOUCH

Light touch is best evaluated quantitatively using the modern equivalent of von Frey hairs, calibrated monofilament nylon fibers which produce graduated pressures when applied to the hand with the Weinstein-Semmes Pressure Aesthesiometer. Using this technique, progress in return of light touch sensibility can be assessed by reexamination at intervals with confidence that the pressure applied is standard at each examination. Localization of the point being touched by the patient with eyes closed is helpful since misidentification, although it confirms regrowth of axons down a different peripheral channel than before, does absolutely confirm regrowth across the site of nerve juncture. With normal innervation patients feel and localize touch at pressures of about 2.4 to 2.8 mg.

Sensibility is considered protective only at 3.8 mg. and when more than 6 mg. is unrecognized, the part is considered anesthetic.

DEEP SENSIBILITY

Deep sensibility may be tested crudely by evaluating the patient's ability to identify passive positioning of the distal interphalangeal joint without visual aid.

SUDOMOTOR FUNCTION

Evaluation of areas of the hand for sweating may be done by careful visual observation with a magnifying glass or ophthalmoscope. Specific fingerprint testing using the ninhydrin test has been described. (**A**) (See page 204.)

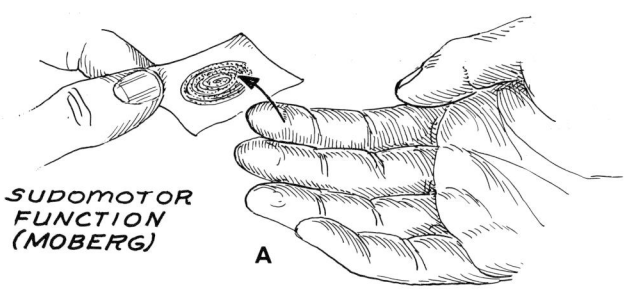

SUDOMOTOR FUNCTION (MOBERG)
A

Tinel's Sign

Percussion over the anatomical region occupied by a peripheral nerve distal to a site of earlier repair will yield an electrical-shocklike sensation that radiates toward the area normally innervated by that nerve if the axons have grown to that point. Tapping should be initiated distally over the area denervated by the injury. As the examiner progresses proximally toward the site of repair, the patient will respond when the site of a positive Tinel sign is reached. (**B**)

Two-Point Discrimination

The skin is touched lightly with two points simultaneously at a measured distance apart and the patient must recognize correctly whether he is being touched by one or two points. (**C**) A Boley gauge is manufactured specifically for this purpose but an eye caliper is perfectly adequate. Normal discriminatory thresholds have been worked out for the hand and are available in chart form. Generally, the fingers have upper limit of normal range of 3 to 7 mm.; the distal palm 5 to 9 mm. and the proximal palm 7 to 10 mm.

Tests of Motor Function

Electromyography

Needle electrodes placed in a muscle denervated by nerve injury may give the physician a great deal of helpful information. (**D**) Over-interpretation of findings must be guarded against. A normally innervated muscle is electrically silent at rest but when it is voluntarily contracted, action potentials are produced. These may be read out on an oscilloscopic screen or be transmitted as sound. Immediately after nerve transection, the muscle is electrically silent and there is no response to voluntary attempts to activate the muscle. Over a two or three week period, electrical silence is replaced by fibrillation potentials in the denervated muscle. This is thought to coincide with development of Wallerian degeneration in the peripheral nerve. Electromyography is electively done at a month or six weeks after injury, at which time fibrillation potentials will be well established. Diminution of fibrillation and action potentials on attempt to voluntarily contract the muscle being tested will precede clinical evidence of return of motor function in the muscle. The quality and quantity of reinnervation are not measurable by electromyography.

Nerve Conduction Time

Measurement of the elapsed time between stimulation of a nerve and response of a muscle innervated by that nerve at a measured distance away is the basis for nerve conduction time analysis. Delayed conduction may occur in any of a number of neuropathies other than nerve injury. Conduction velocity in meters per second calculates out to 45 to 70 in the upper extremity major nerves. Delayed or absent response may point to nerve compression or denervation, respectively.

Nerve Block

Equally useful is a nerve block of the major nerve to the hand other than that which had been injured. This will demonstrate non-standard variants in innervation pattern which may have raised the surgeon's suspicion that the injured nerve was partially injured.

Direct Nerve Stimulation

At the time of surgical exploration of a nerve, a nerve stimulator can be of inestimable value.

Nerve Block

Local anesthetic nerve block is a simple and extremely valuable tool in refining diagnosis of peripheral nerve injuries both primarily and

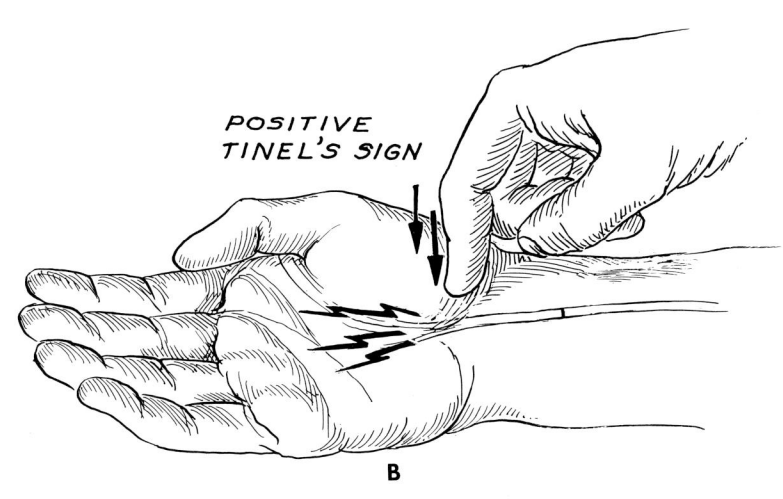

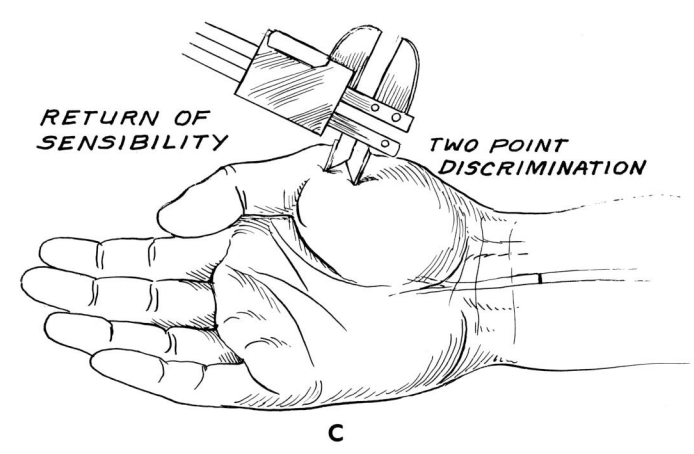

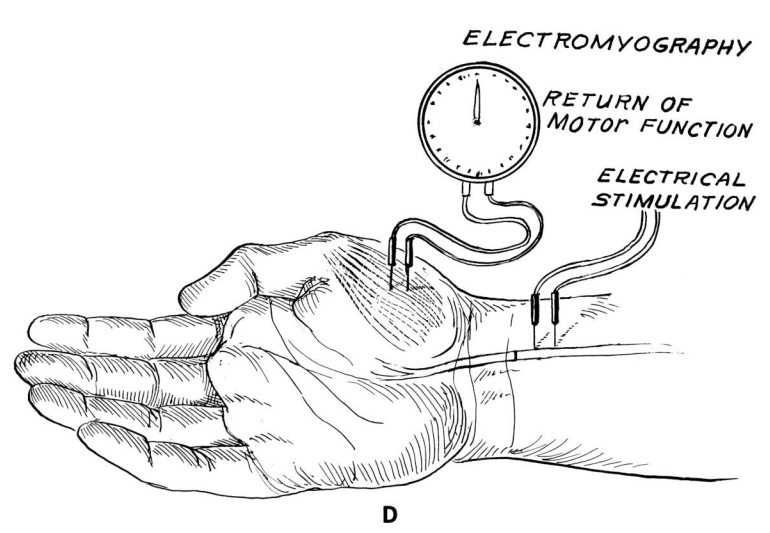

secondarily. (**E**) The procedure need not add to the procedure appropriate to normal surgical care of the patient if it is used as part of the anesthetic for a planned operative procedure. Local anesthetic block of the nerve injured and whose distal function is in question will reap invaluable information and allow the surgeon confidence in designing his surgical approach. The block is done proximal to the site of injury. Following block, any change in motor or sensory capability peripheral to the injury site must be attributable to a part of the nerve that has escaped injury or to possible recovery of function in the case in which the injury occurred several months before.

Example

A patient sustained a laceration injury at the wrist several weeks before examination. (**F**) The wound was healed and there were paresthesias referred to the thumb, index finger, and long finger on percussion over the wound. (**G**)

The thenar muscles were as strong as those on the normal side and appeared opposed normal. Anesthesia was evident over the palmar aspect of the thumb, the index finger, and the *radial half of the long finger*. (**H**) The ulnar half of the long finger and adjacent side of the ring finger had perfect sensibility and sudomotor function. Since this area classically is innervated by the median nerve, the question was whether the median nerve had been partially transected or whether the ulnar nerve was supplying sensibility to the adjacent sides of the long and ring fingers. The functioning oppositional muscles of the thumb raised the same question.

A block of the ulnar nerve at the wrist rendered the little finger and ulnar half of the ring finger anesthetic but sensibility remained in the adjacent halves of the long and ring fingers. (**I**) The power of opposition of the thumb was completely lost with the block.

This simple diagnostic procedure confirmed the diagnosis of partial injury of the median nerve. The funiculi destined to become the common digital nerve to the adjacent sides of the long and ring fingers were intact.

At the time of surgery which was to be done under regional anesthesia, the median nerve alone was blocked above the site of injury. The adjacent sides of the long and ring fingers became anesthetic and there was no detectable change in the quality of function of the thenar muscles.

The wrist could then be explored with confidence that resection of the median nerve could be done without risk of sacrificing intrinsic motor function. Furthermore, the surgeon was cautioned to preserve the uninjured sensory funiculi that diagnostic block had demonstrated were present.

On exploration of what clearly seemed a partial injury of the median nerve, the median nerve was exposed but so also with little extension of the field of exploration was the ulnar nerve.

Stimulation of the ulnar nerve resulted in contraction of the intrinsic muscles in the hand and enough of the thenar muscles to bring the thumb into neutral opposition.

Stimulation of the median nerve above and below the site of injury resulted in no motor response. This lent further assurance that resection and repair of the median nerve was done at no risk of losing intrinsic motor power.

At operation electrical stimulation of the ulnar nerve resulted in contraction of the thenar positioning muscles *normally* innervated by the median nerve. (**J**)

Repair of Partial Nerve Injury by Secondary Surgery

Exploration of the median nerve revealed scar and neuroma at the site of injury. Precision lysis of the scar revealed one funicular portion of the nerve to cross the area uninterrupted. This funiculus was dissected proximal and distal for a distance of 2 cm. and was preserved intact. The neuromatous portion proximally and the scar distally in the remaining bulk of the nerve were resected to show clearly the funicular pattern in cross section. (**K**) By mobilizing the nerve these nerve ends could be approximated and repaired with sheath sutures. The intact funiculus assumed a gentle curved attitude and remained uninterrupted. (**L**)

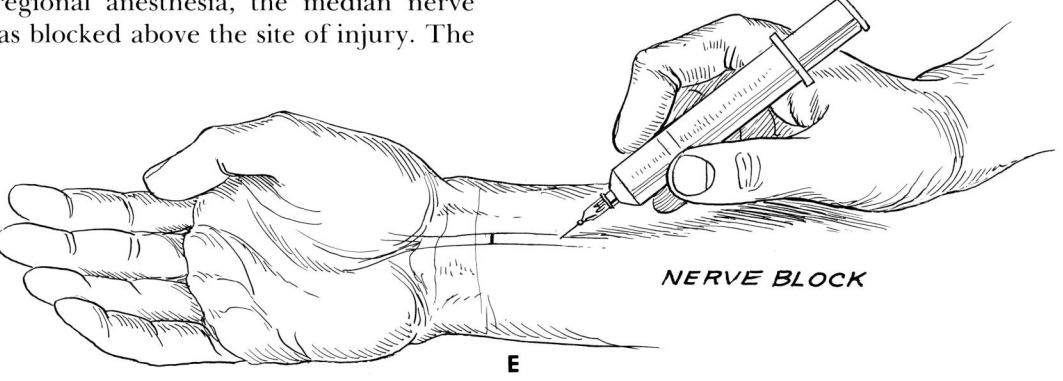

NERVE BLOCK

E

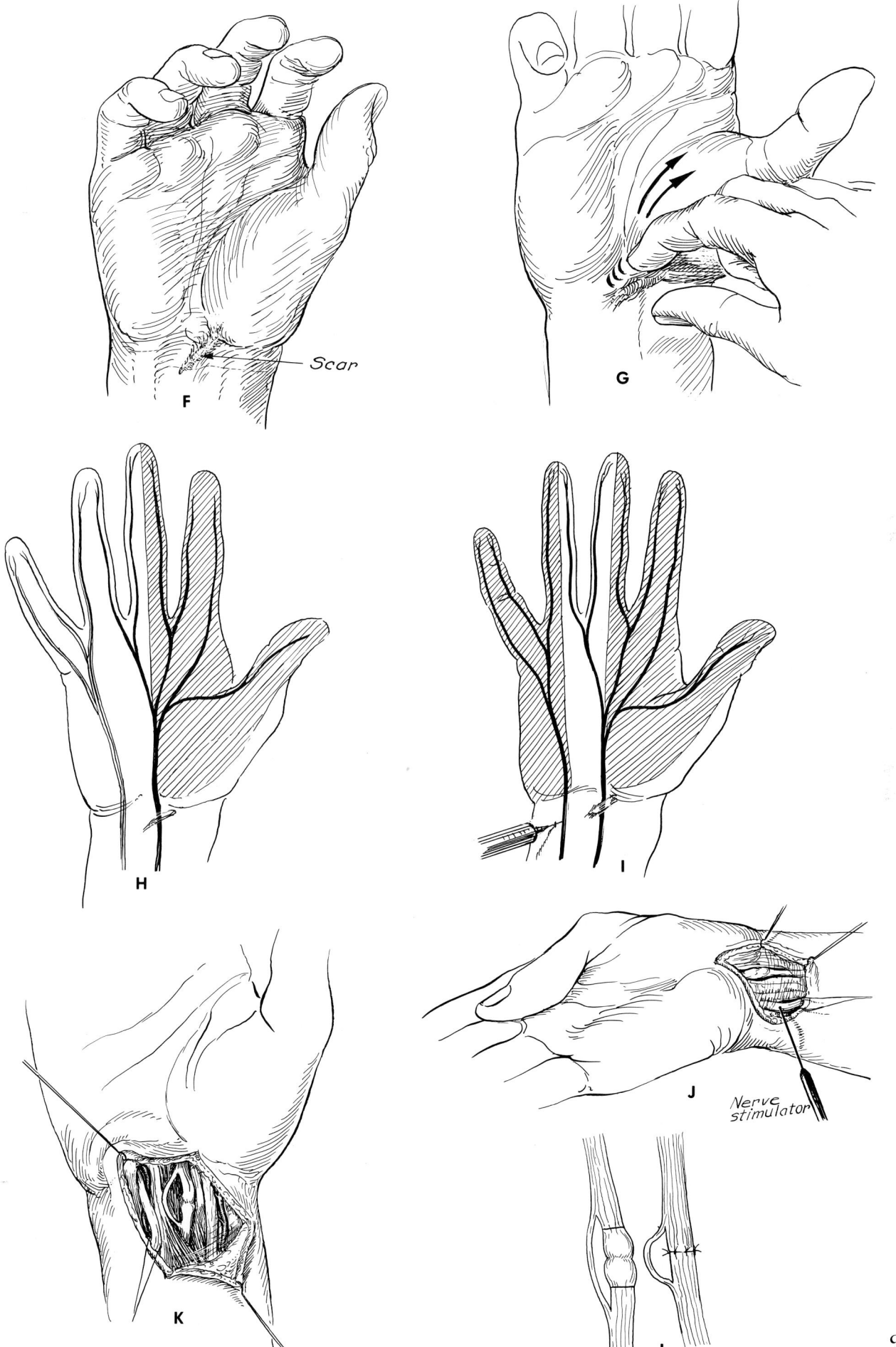

Nerve Surgery

233

56

Nerve Gaps

Small nerve gaps are the rule at the time a nerve is repaired. It is usual that the nerve ends must be recut sharply after a traumatic section or neuroma, and scar must be resected in the case of secondary repair. Where there is little or no loss of nerve substance as a result of injury, the residual nerve gap may be overcome by dissection of the nerve from its fascial attachments both proximal and distal and by gentle traction on the nerve sheath. Blood supply to the major peripheral nerves is such that it may be stripped of all adjacent tissue for several inches without risk of ischemia. Observers have reported bleeding from the cut end of such a nerve after severing all connections over a distance of 20 cm. The ulnar nerve has been mobilized from axilla to wrist without becoming ischemic.

When loss of substance in the nerves becomes more significant, the surgeon may combine a variety of tactics to overcome the gap. Rigorous preservation of blood supply to the nerve by gentle handling and dissection is essential.

In addition to stripping and gentle traction, the following techniques are most useful:

JOINT POSITIONING

Once the nerve is dissected free from tissues which restrain it, additional nerve length to overcome a gap is acquired by optimum joint positioning. (**A** and **B**)

With the exception of the ulnar nerve at the elbow, the major nerves cross the flexor surfaces of the elbow, wrist and digital joints. Clinical experience suggests that maximum fixation in flexion of the elbow should be at 90° for this purpose. Flexion of the wrist should not exceed 40° and the digital joints about 45° each to close nerve gaps.

TRANSPOSITION OF THE NERVE

The ulnar nerve may be transposed out of its position behind the medial epicondyle of the humerus to the flexor side of the elbow joint. (See procedure, page 222.) The median nerve is bound down just distal to the elbow as it passes between the two heads of the pronator teres. Rerouting it superficial to this muscle shortens its course. The motor or deep branch of the ulnar nerve in the hand may be transposed to a position through the carpal tunnel to gain length. (See procedure, page 214.)

NERVE CROSSOVER

If parallel peripheral nerves are injured at different levels, one may suture the long proximal end of one to the long distal end of the other. This may be particularly helpful in the case of digital nerves where a nerve from a finger destined for amputation is used to suture to the distal end of another digital nerve. (**C**) This is particularly useful since digital nerves are pure sensory nerves.

The median and ulnar nerves have been crossed (advertently as well as inadvertently) with recovery of sensibility and some motor power.

SHORTENING OF THE EXTREMITY

Restoration of nerve function in an extremity is sometimes so important that surgeons have shortened the extremity by planned osteotomy to overcome the nerve gap. The procedure has limited usefulness and perhaps is indicated occasionally at the humeral level. Up to three inches of the humerus can be removed without loss of significant function from the shortening per se.

Nerve Surgery

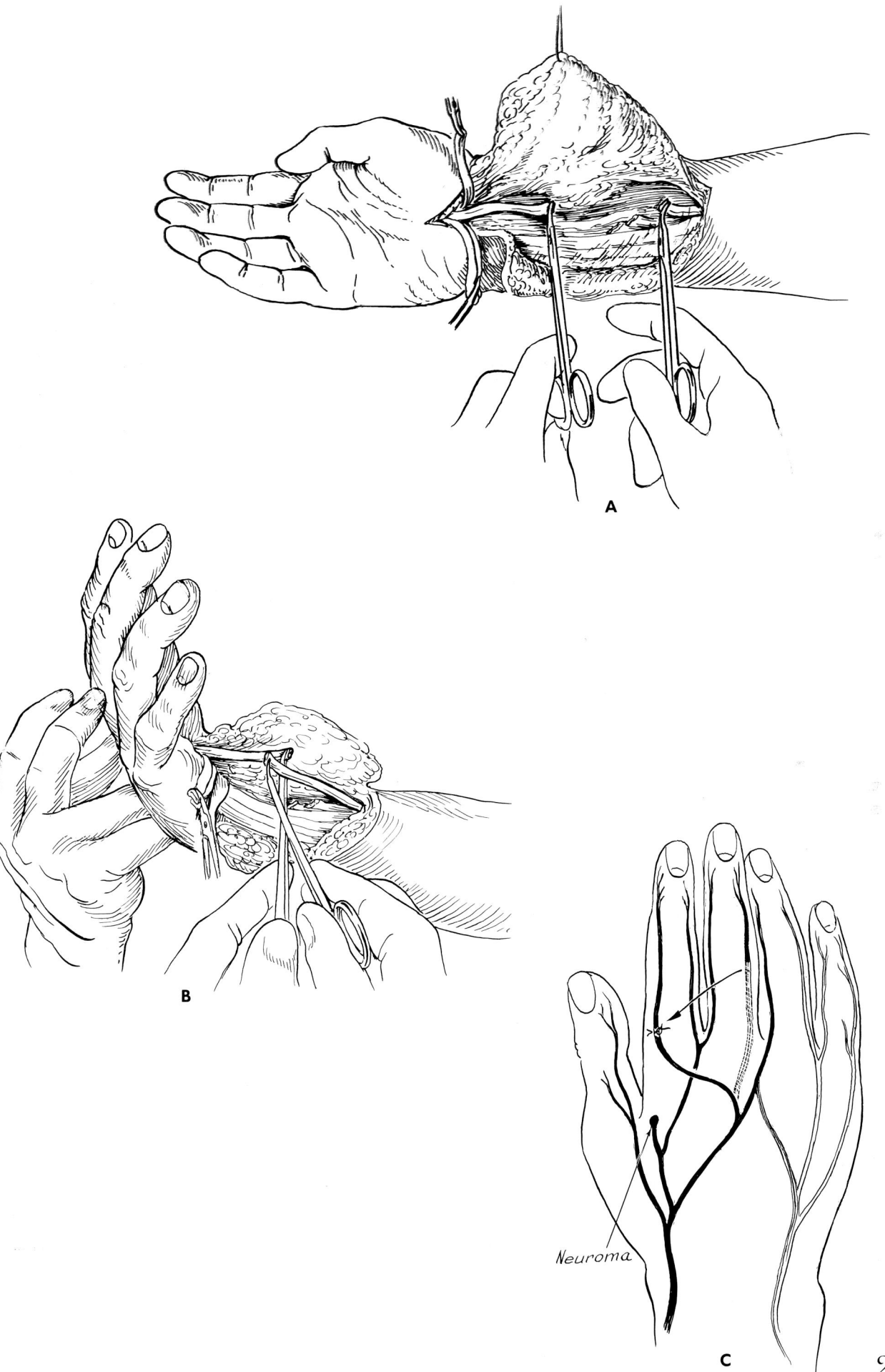

235

56 — Nerve Gaps

Nerve Grafting

Autogenous nerve grafts remain the only clinically reliable grafts at present. Homografts and heterografts of nerve remain experimental but it seems certain that they will become more dependable in the years ahead.

Some disability will result from removal of any intact autogenous nerve to use as a graft. The commonly chosen donor nerves are the dorsal branch of the radial nerve; the sural nerve; the cutaneous nerves of the arm and forearm; and the cutaneous nerves of the thigh and leg. These small nerves must be assembled into a cable configuration for use in bridging gaps of major nerves. (**D**)

One may wish to use a nerve graft consisting of a part of the injured nerve itself by splitting it. Other nerves irreparably damaged in the same traumatic incident should be considered as an appropriate source of nerve for grafting.

Pedicle nerve grafts in the forearm using modifications of the Strange-Seddon procedure are more reliable than are free grafts. The classical Strange-Seddon procedure is used to overcome a gap in the median nerve in the forearm where there is also a gap in the adjacent ulnar nerve. (**E**)

At the first procedure the two cut proximal nerve ends are sutured to one another and the ulnar nerve is crushed or cut at a level to allow enough length to swing down into the flap at a second stage. (**F**)

At the second stage several months later the ulnar nerve segment is swung down and a distal juncture is created to the distal cut end of the median nerve or to both median and ulnar nerves. (**G**)

As a modification of the procedure, one may cut the ulnar nerve proximally and create a juncture between the proximal cut end of the median nerve and the distal new cut end of the ulnar nerve, creating an **S**-shaped median to ulnar configuration. (**H** and **I**)

At a second stage several months later, the **S**-curved median nerve and ulnar graft are straightened and a juncture at the distal end of the graft to the old distal cut ends of median and ulnar nerves is created. (**J**)

Combining the Techniques in Specific Nerve Gaps

It is well to be aware of some general principles which may affect the choice of specific procedures as well as the choice to abandon attempts to overcome the nerve gap by direct suture of the nerve end to end.

The average critical gap length beyond which one might best abandon the attempt averages somewhere between 5 and 12 cm.

When transposing a nerve or positioning a joint to gain additional length in a nerve, it is best judgment to choose a joint away from the site of injury and projected repair. The choice of manipulation at the elbow when the injury is at the wrist and vice versa will avoid direct local stretching of the suture line after early healing as the joint is brought back to a full range of motion in stages.

Using the various techniques singly or in combination one may gain approximately the following lengths in the major nerves. (Tables are modified from Grantham, E. G., Pollard, C., Jr., and Brabson, J. A.: Peripheral nerve surgery: Repair of nerve defects. Ann. Surg. 127:696, 1948.

MEDIAN NERVE

Site of Lesion	Usual Defect Repaired With Ease (in centimeters)	Maximum Defect Which Can Be Repaired (in centimeters)
Arm and elbow area	6	8
Elbow with transposition	10	12
Upper forearm	4.5	6
After transposition	5.5	8
Distal forearm	4	5
Wrist	1.8	2.5

ULNAR NERVE

Site of Lesion	Usual Defect Repaired With Ease (in centimeters)	Maximum Defect Which Can Be Repaired (in centimeters)
Arm	2	3
After Transposition	6	10
Elbow after Transposition	5.2	9
Distal Forearm after Transposition	6.5	10

RADIAL NERVE

Site of Lesion	Usual Defect Repaired With Ease (in centimeters)	Maximum Defect Which Can Be Repaired (in centimeters)
Axilla	2.3	2.5
Arm	6.2	8.0
Elbow	3.4	5.0
Posterior Interosseous	1.0	1.5

Nerve Surgery

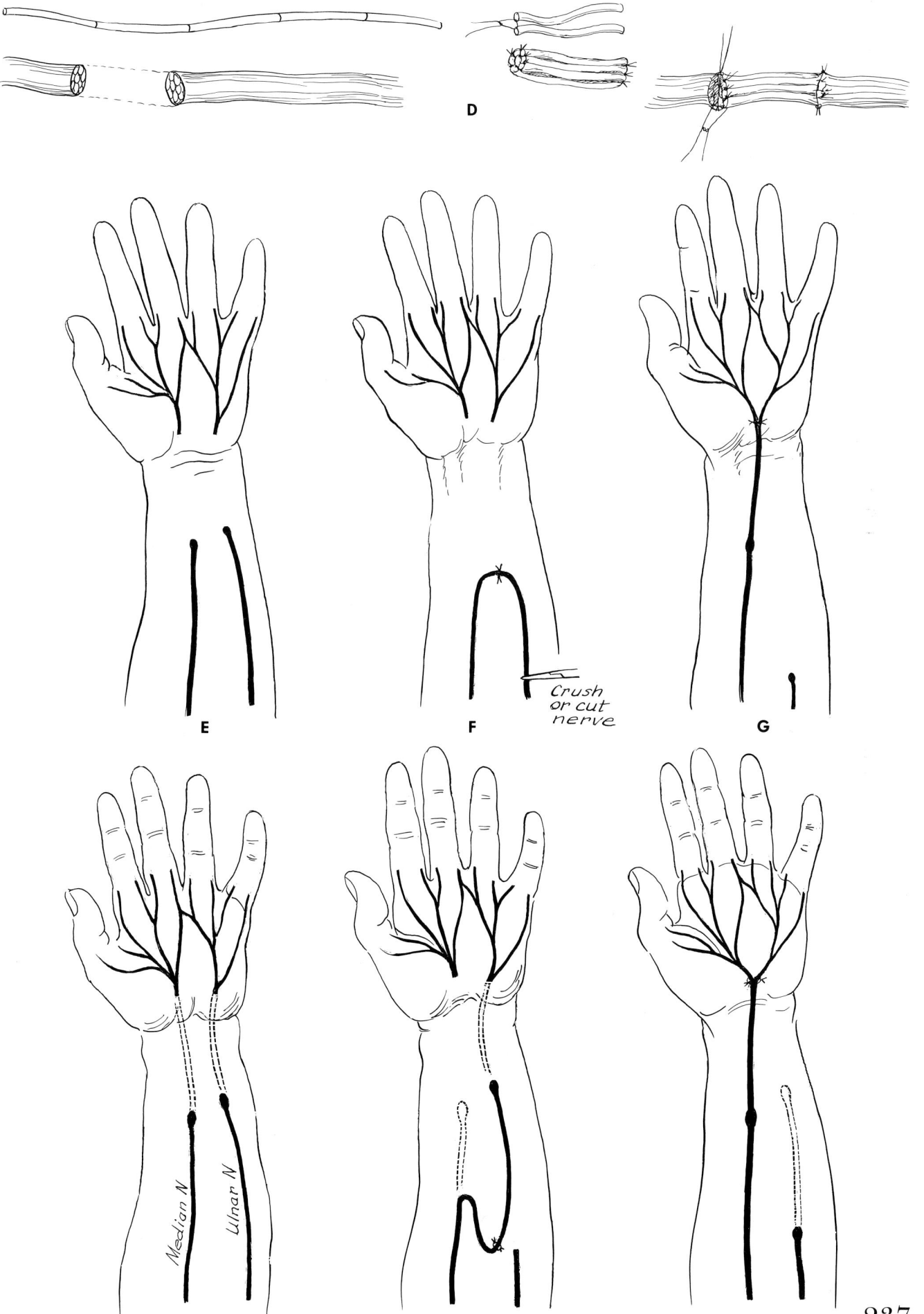

237

57
The Island Pedicle Technique

Transfer of a digital nerve with innervated skin within the hand is a proper means of transferring sensibility to an area of critical importance from an area of less functional value. The biological pedicle technique consists of transferring skin and soft tissue on intact arteries, veins, and nerves to provide both full thickness surface coverage and full sensibility and sudomotor function. The technique was described for use in providing contour and sensory resurfacing of the thumb tip on page 78. The technique is also useful where lack of sensibility in a critical area is the only deficit.

Example

A patient with an uncorrectable nerve gap in the median nerve from above the wrist to the palm and an intact ulnar nerve presented with problems in manipulating objects with the prime digits, the thumb, and the index finger because of lack of sensibility and sudomotor function. There was no skin or circulatory deficit. It seemed logical to transfer sensibility from the ulnar side of the ring finger to the important radial side of the index finger. An island pedicle flap from the ring finger was designed, taking the skin and soft tissue from the entire ulnar side of the ring finger. (**A**)

Since no circulatory problems existed, it seemed reasonable to shift the anesthetic soft tissue from the recipient index finger as a vascularized island flap to the ring finger donor area in exchange. Such an area was outlined on the recipient area of the index finger. (**B**)

The ring finger island pedicle flap was dissected from the finger, carefully preserving the proper digital artery, veins and nerve in the palm. (**C**)

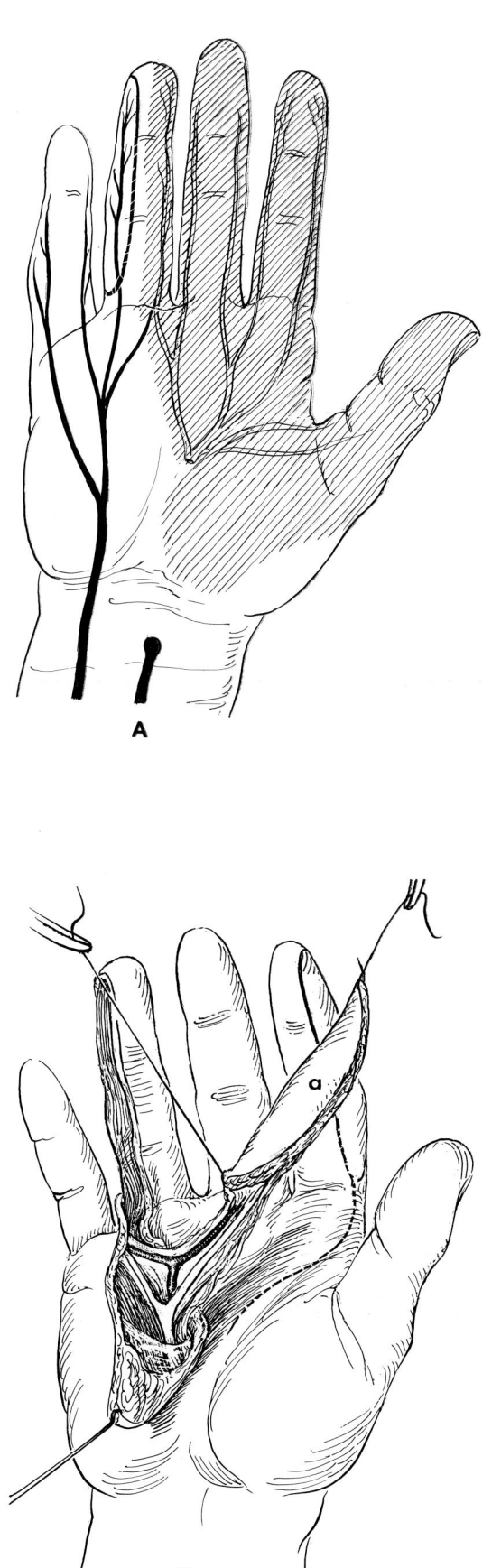
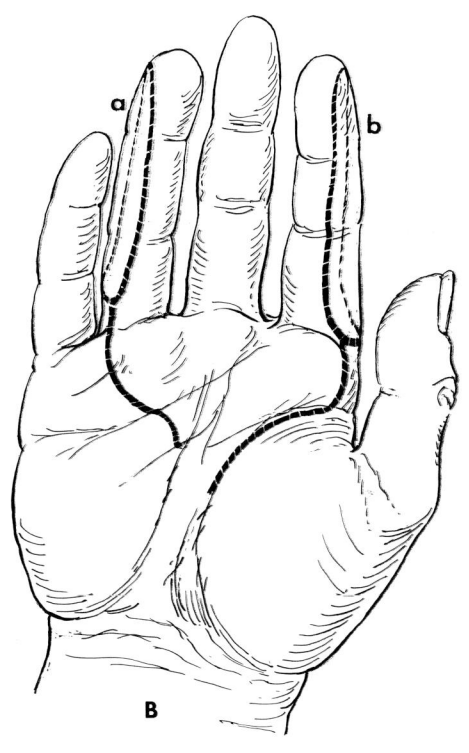

57 – The Island Pedicle Technique

Ligation and transection of the proper digital artery and veins to the radial side of the little finger close to its origin from the common digital artery to the adjacent sides of the ring and little fingers was essential to get adequate vascular bundle length to the island. The common digital nerve was split far enough proximally to allow transfer of the island without tension while preserving sensibility to both the island and the radial side of the little finger. Dissection of the recipient site island flap was then completed, preserving the proper digital neurovascular bundle to it. (**D**)

The innervated island pedicle flap from the ring finger was passed beneath the palmar fascia to the index finger and incisions were planned to create two Z-plasties on the palmar side of the finger. (**E**)

The anesthetic but vascularized flap from the index finger was switched beneath the palmar fascia to the donor site on the ulnar side of the ring finger and after similar Z-plasty incisions were made on the palmar surface, both islands were precisely sutured in place. (**F**)

The working surface of the prime manipulating finger, the index, was thus restored to a finger of full sensibility and sudomotor function. The island exchange obviated the need for any free graft and resurfaced the sensory donor finger with full thickness hand skin with subcutaneous tissue.

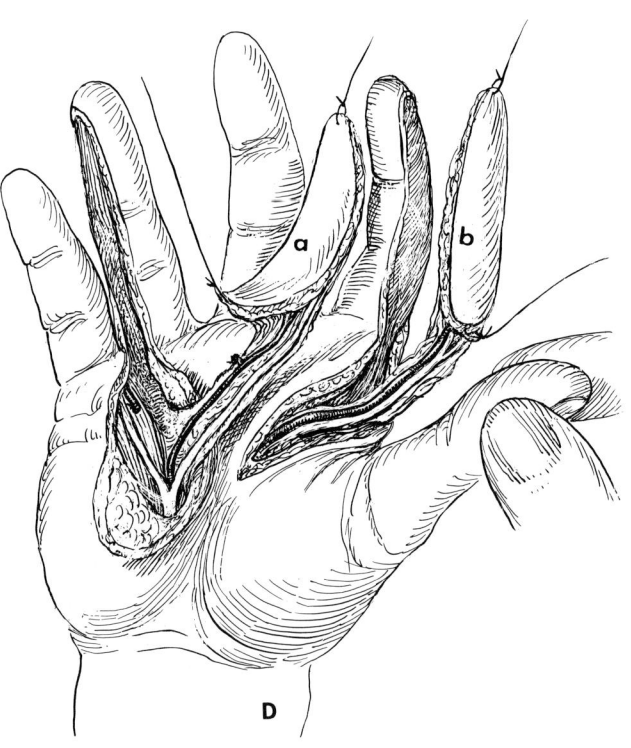

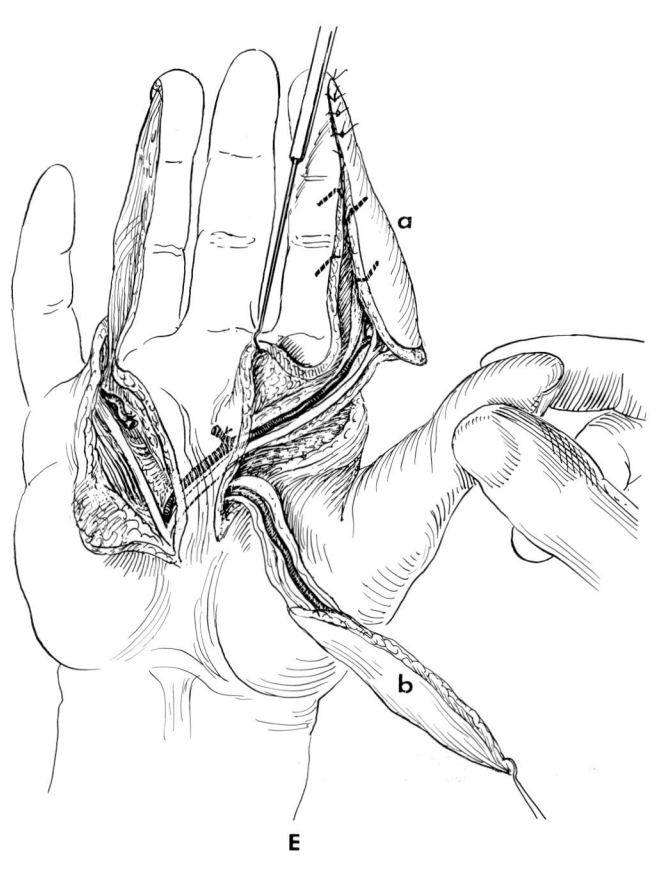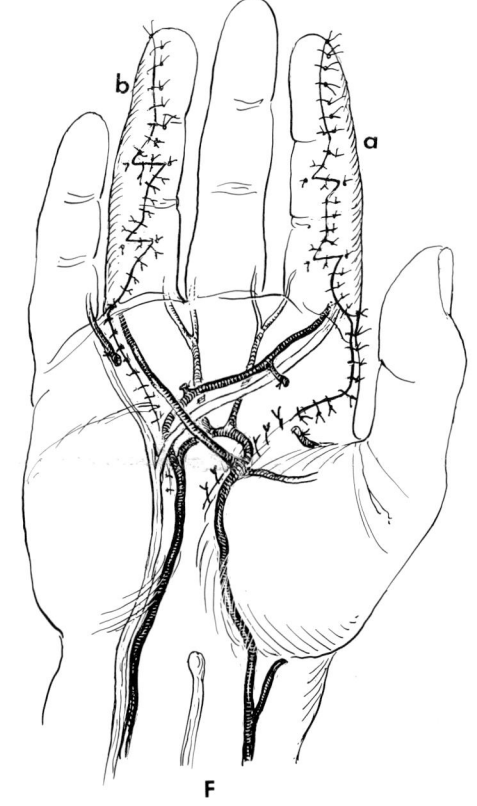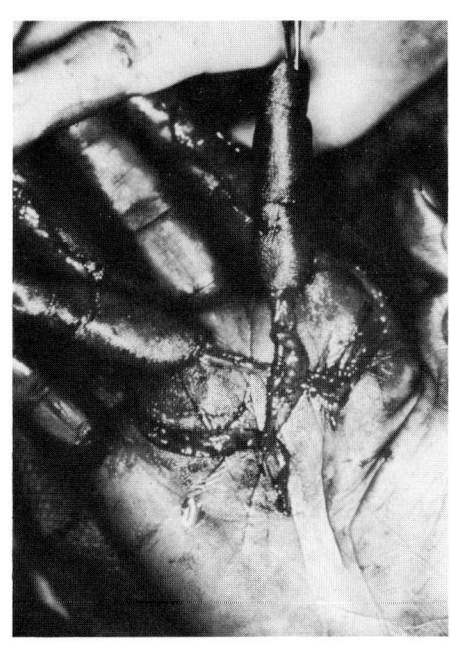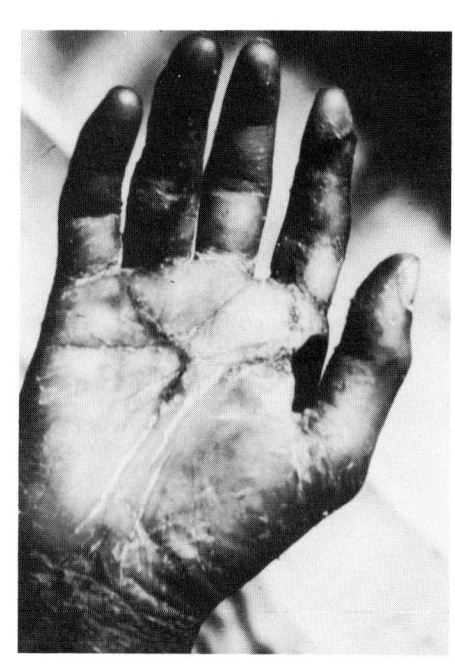

58
Combined Island Pedicle and Nerve Transfer

In situations in which a deficit of soft tissue and uncorrectable nerve gap exists over the proximal part of a prime digit, one might consider combining the techniques of nerve crossover transfer and the island pedicle technique.

Example

Following an avulsion injury over the proximal phalangeal level of the palmar surface of the thumb, the patient was left with a skin deficit over the proximal thumb and an anesthetic but fully viable thumb tip. Flexion contracture resulted with healing and an unstable scar existed over the proximal palmar aspect of the thumb. **(A)**

Surgical release of the scar allowed full extension of the thumb and revealed the cut distal end of the proper digital nerve to the radial side of the thumb tip. An island pedicle flap was planned from the ulnar side of the long finger. It was taken proximal enough so that there would be a substantial remaining digital nerve at the distal end of the flap. **(B)**

As the skin and soft tissue flap was elevated, the proximal vessels and nerve were preserved and the digital nerve at the peripheral end of the flap was identified and cut long. **(C)** The proper digital artery to the adjacent ring finger was ligated and cut and the proper digital nerve in the palm was split to allow full mobility of the island pedicle flap without tension on the nerves. **(D)**

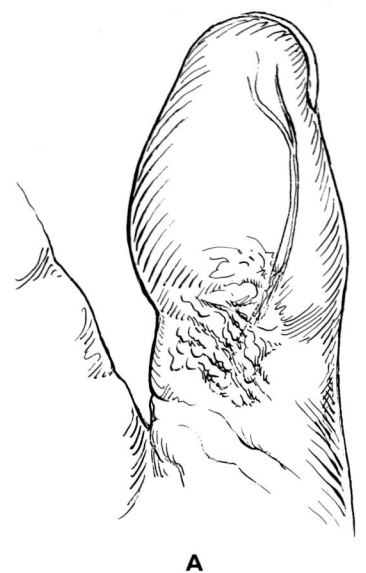

A

Nerve Surgery

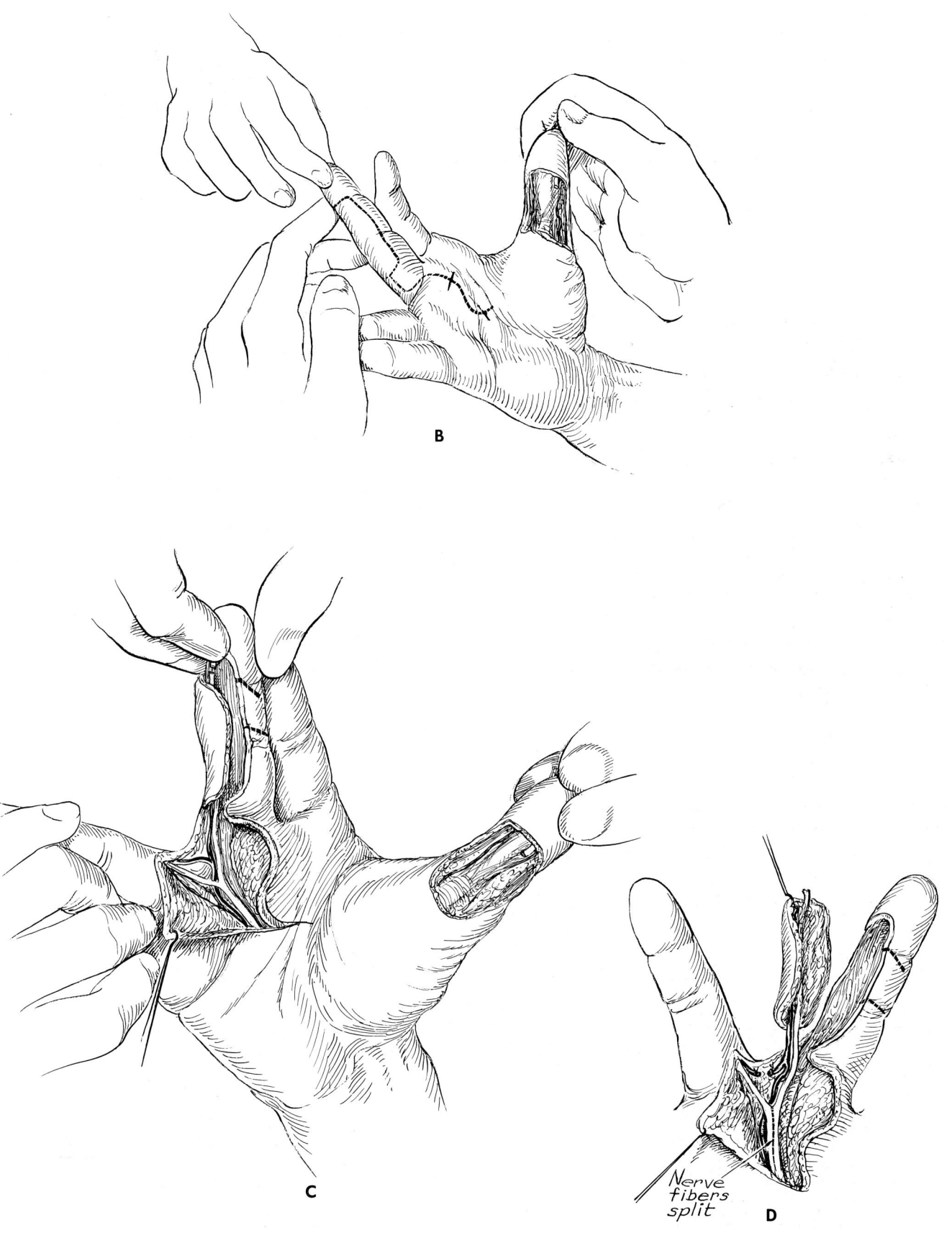

243

58 — Combined Island Pedicle and Nerve Transfer

The island pedicle flap was carried beneath the palmar fascia to the thumb base and laid in position. The digital nerve protruding from the end of the island flap was sutured according to the technique described for digital nerve repair (Section 50) to the cut nerve end to the thumb tip and the island flap was sutured in place.

A free full thickness skin graft was placed over the donor site and the straight midpalmar incision was broken up by making incisions across it and inserting angular tongue extensions of the skin graft. (**E**)

After healing, the patient had full functional restoration. Sensibility was immediately intact in the island flap and after a few months adequate sensibility appeared in the thumb tip. The patient misidentified it as sensibility in the long finger but used the restored thumb well.

PREOPERATIVE

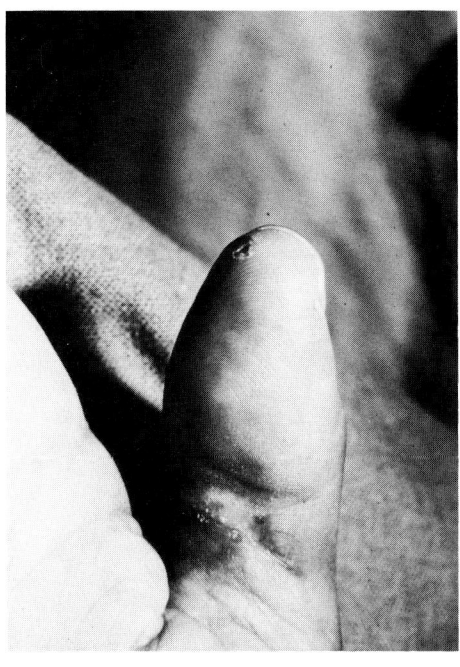

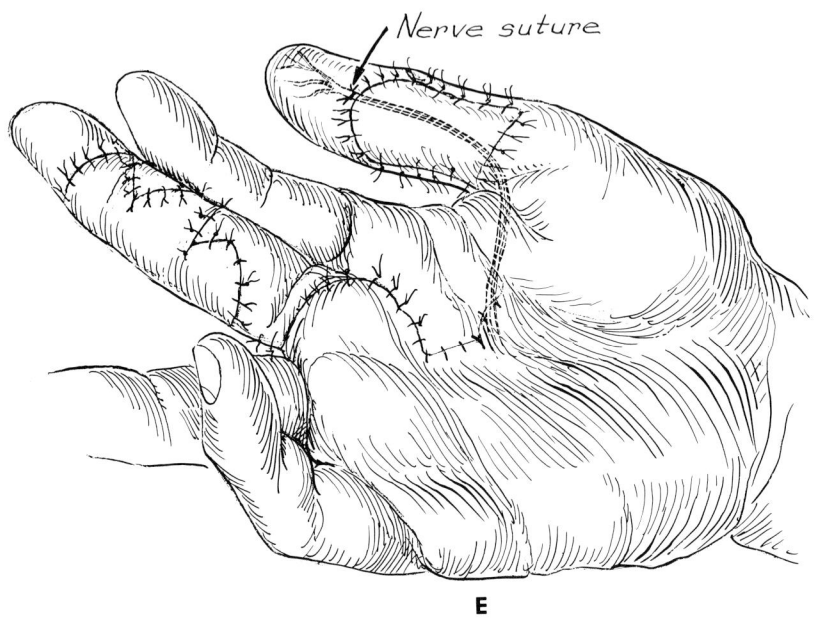

E

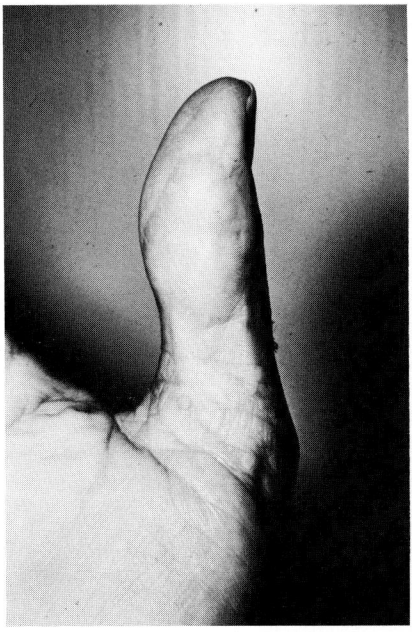
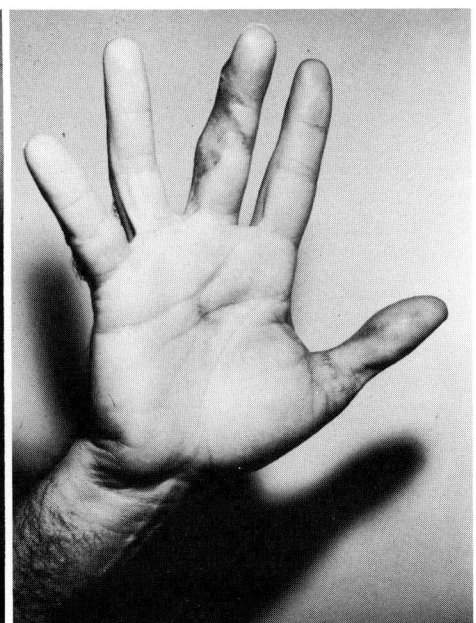

POSTOPERATIVE RESULT

Bone and Joint Reconstruction

Fractures in the Hand

Principles

1. Unless there is a need, by specific positioning, to temporarily relax a tendon or nerve which has just been repaired or transferred, the injured hand is best managed by immobilizing it in the "position of function." The position of function is assumed by the hand when all muscles are in relaxed balance with the wrist in a position so that the first metacarpal is in line with the radius. (**A**)

In the uninjured hand, relaxed muscle tone brings the fingers into a natural posture in which the pulps of the digits lie at equidistant radii from the pulp of the thumb. (**B**) The degree of flexion of the interphalangeal joints increases from the index finger to the little finger.

2. If a single digit is immobilized, it should be placed in the position it would assume if the whole hand were in the functional position. (**C**)

3. No joint should be immobilized which does not require immobilization to achieve stability at the site of fracture. Generally, immobilization of the joint proximal and the joint distal to the fracture is mandatory. In the hand additional immobilization may be essential when changes of position of that joint may cause tenodesis-like forces which will stress the fracture site or influence the reduction.

4. Internal fixation with devices such as Kirschner wires must be done in such a way that the immobilizing device does not create distraction rather than compression coaptation at the fracture site.

5. Small autogenous bone pegs are very useful in treatment of unstable fractures in the hand skeleton.

6. Callus at fracture sites (particularly in metacarpals) may not show by x-ray until long after clinical stability is present. After immobilization for six or eight weeks, one should judge continuing need for immobilization on clinical stability supplemented by x-ray evidence of healing. X-ray evidence of complications and non-healing with resorption, sequestration, and mal-reduction establishes the need for films.

7. Normally, when fingers are flexed *individually* into the palm, the tip of the finger in each case points to the tubercle of the carpal scaphoid. This fact and observation of the nail bed plane in relationship to other fingers help one to judge angulation and rotation in metacarpal and phalanx fractures. (**D**)

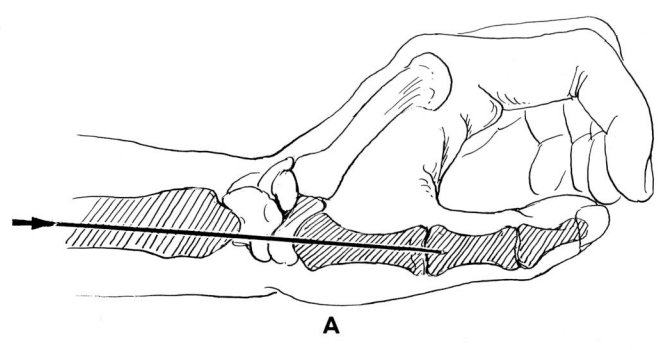

A

Bone and Joint Reconstruction

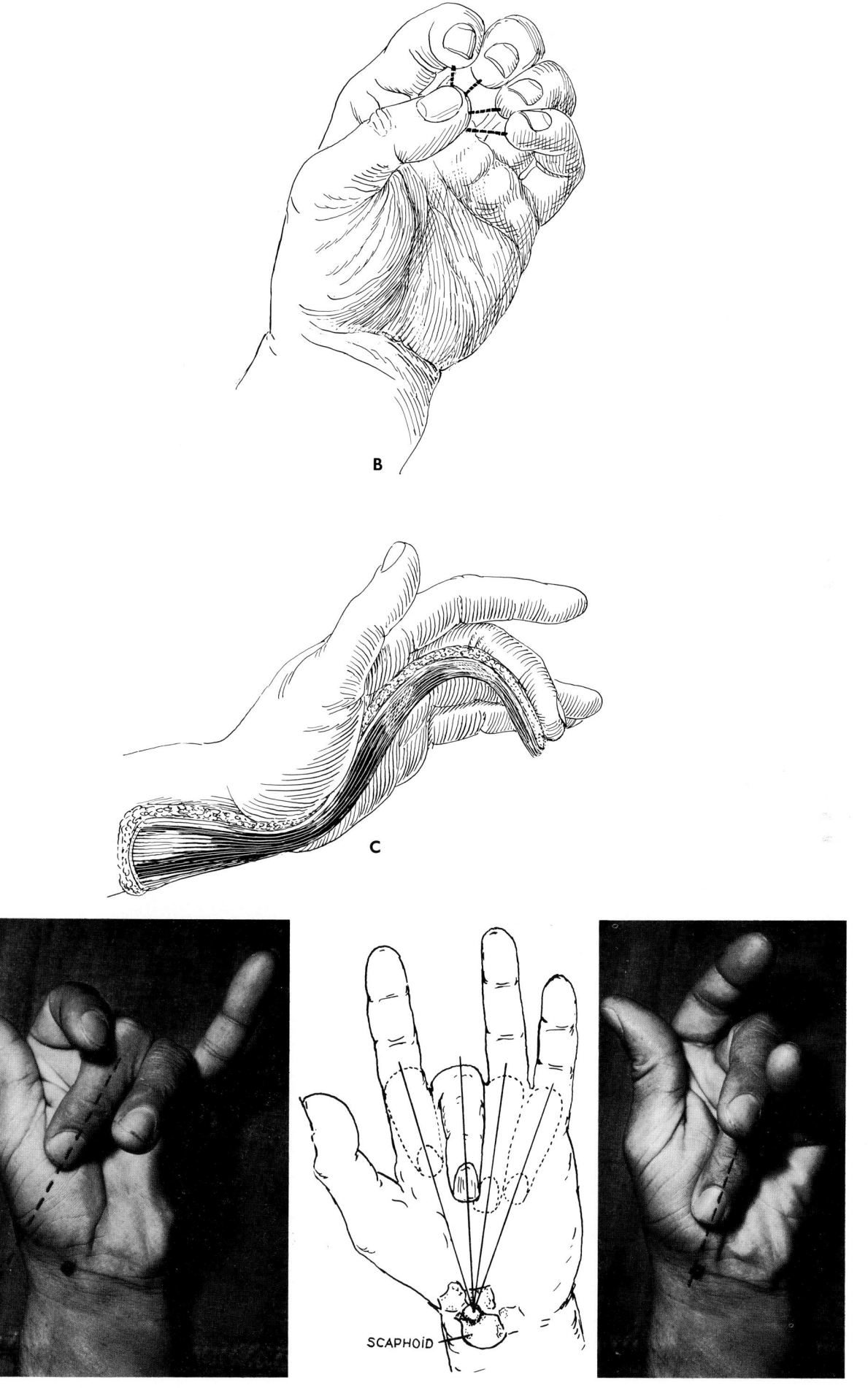

59 — Fractures in the Hand

UNSTABLE CLOSED METACARPAL FRACTURE

Example

A direct blow to the hand of an adult male resulted in a transverse fracture of the long finger metacarpal at its midshaft. Dorsal angulation at the site of fracture resulted. (**A**) (Dorsal angulation at the fracture site is usual because of the pull of both the intrinsic muscles and the powerful long flexors.) Closed reduction of this unstable metacarpal fracture with Kirschner wire fixation was achieved by the following technique. Reduction was achieved by dorsal pressure over the fracture site and a dorsal push on the metacarpal head using the flexed digit. (**B**)

With the fracture palpably reduced, a Kirschner wire was inserted into the metacarpal head through the metacarpophalangeal joint which was held in full flexion. Once the wire was in the distal fragment it was very helpful in gaining proper reduction of the unstable metacarpal fracture. (**C**)

When the Kirschner wire was well across the fracture site, the wrist was flexed and the wire insertion continued until the wire made its exit dorsally distal to the wrist. (**D**)

The Kirschner wire was then extracted proximally until its distal end was out of the metacarpophalangeal joint. (**E**) When the joint could be put through a full range of motion, confirming the withdrawal of the wire, the wire was withdrawn another centimeter and then cut short at the proximal end. The end of the wire was eased beneath the skin by advancing the puncture site over it, using skin hooks.

With the longitudinal wire in place, further stability was achieved by inserting a transverse Kirschner wire across the distal metacarpal fragment to an adjacent metacarpal. (**F**) Proper rotational position was determined in relationship to the other fingers by flexing the finger to see that it pointed to the palpable carpal scaphoid tubercle. (See illustration under Principles in this Section.)

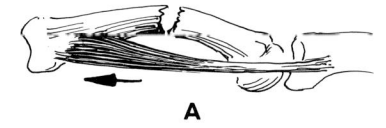

A

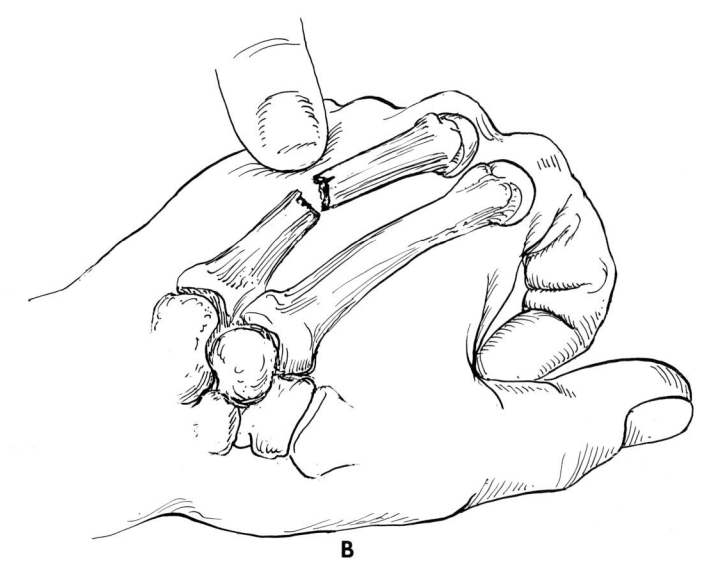

B

Bone and Joint Reconstruction

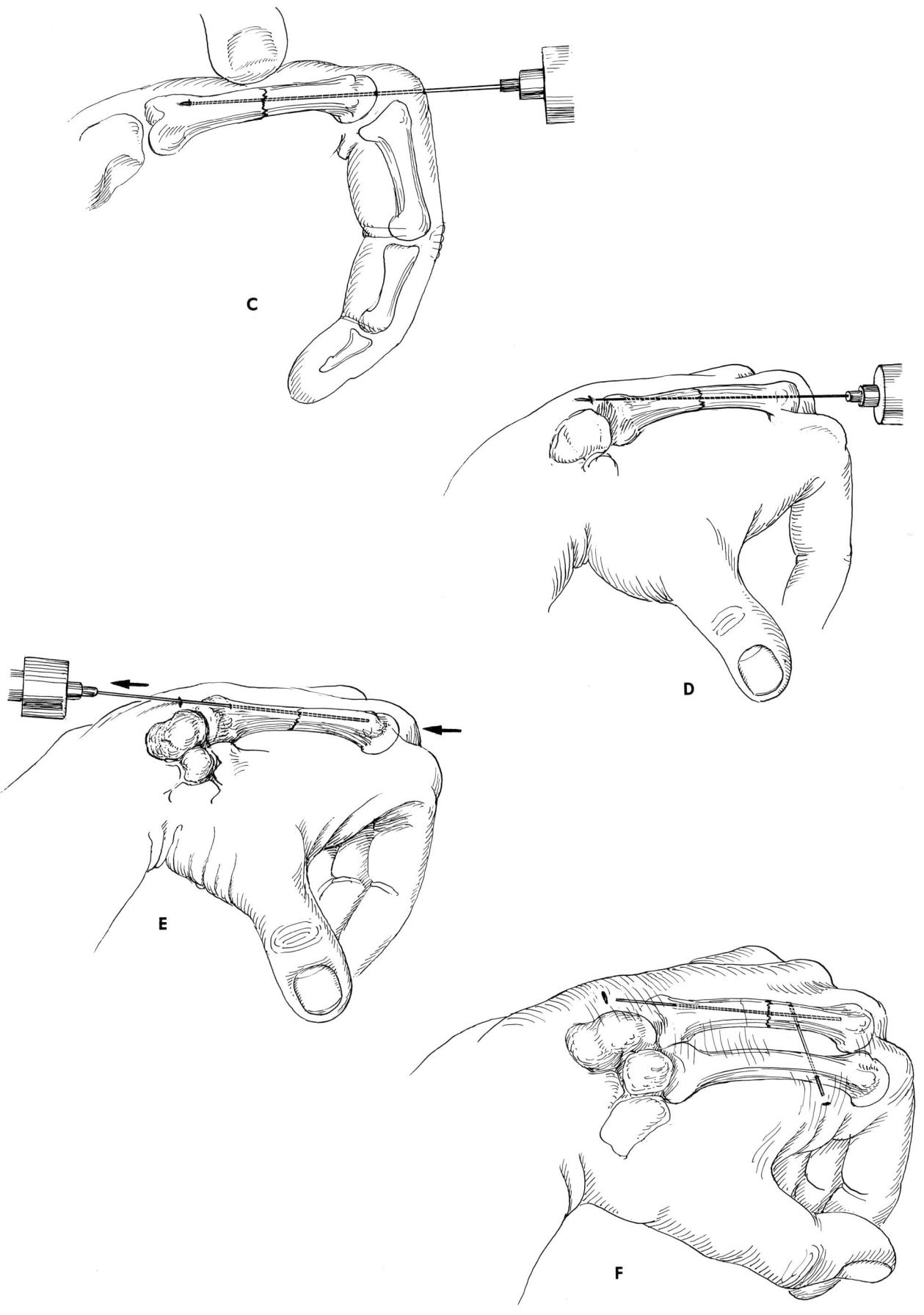

59 – Fractures in the Hand

OPEN METACARPAL FRACTURE

Example

A dorsal crush laceration occurred over the mid index finger metacarpal level in a young laboring man. He sustained a metacarpal fracture and laceration of the index digit extensor tendons. Reduction of the unstable metacarpal fracture required Kirschner wire fixation. Fixation of the metacarpal at the site of metacarpal fracture when there is an open wound gives one the opportunity to center the Kirschner wire quite precisely. A sharpened wire was inserted backwards from the site of metacarpal disruption into the distal fragment. With the metacarpophalangeal joint flexed, the wire was advanced through it and the overlying extensor tendon and skin. (**A**)

The Kirschner wire was then retracted retrogradely until it just disappeared from the fracture site. (**B**)

After reduction of the fracture under direct vision, the Kirschner wire was advanced across the fracture site into the proximal segment of the metacarpal. Advancement then continued with the wrist flexed until the wire made its exit from the dorsal proximal metacarpal edge to protrude through the skin distal to the wrist. (**C**)

The Kirschner wire was then pulled out until free motion was possible in the metacarpophalangeal joint. (**D**) A transmetacarpal wire was used to control rotation as shown in the closed reduction (Pg. 249 F).

Both wires were cut short so they disappeared beneath the skin. The extensor tendons were repaired and the skin laceration was sutured closed. (**E**) The wires were removed under local anesthesia when healing was secure at eight weeks.

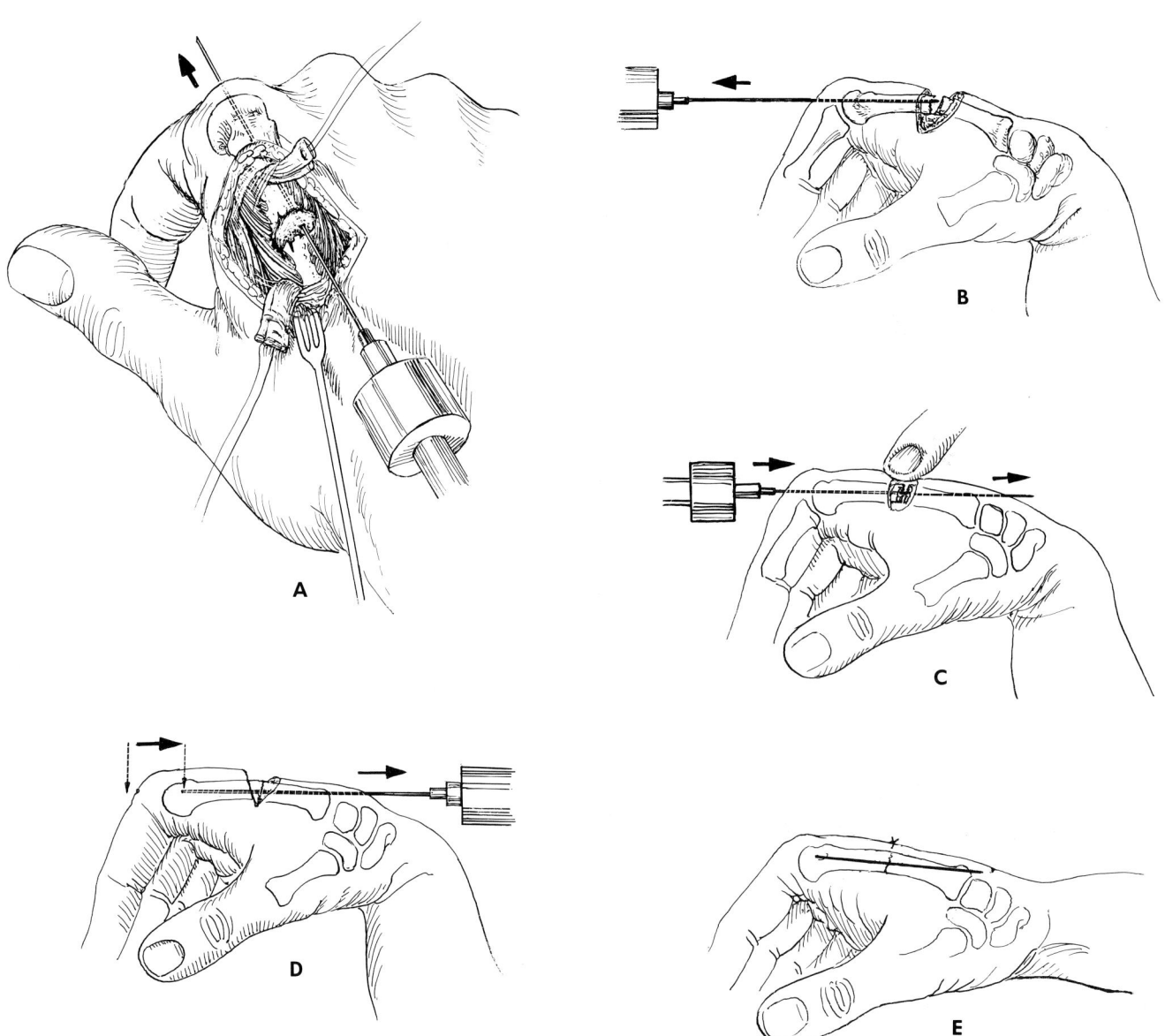

Bone and Joint Reconstruction

FRACTURES OF THE DISTAL PHALANX

Principles

Closed fractures of the distal phalanx are best treated by molding the fracture parts and immobilizing the distal interphalangeal joint with a palmar splint. If the fracture is coupled with avulsion of the extensor or flexor mechanism, more extensive immobilization and sometimes open reduction is required. (See Tendon Injuries.)

Open fractures and, particularly, near-complete amputation may be handled best by Kirschner wire fixation.

Example

A young adult sustained near amputation of his ring finger from an accidental injury with a hatchet. A very small pedicle of skin remained, bridging the radial side of the injury. (**A**) Precise replacement was achieved by inserting a short Kirschner wire retrogradely through the distal fragment of the distal phalanx and tip skin. (**B**)

The wire was extracted retrogradely to allow precise open reduction of the fracture. (**C**) The wire was advanced across the fracture site. (**D**)

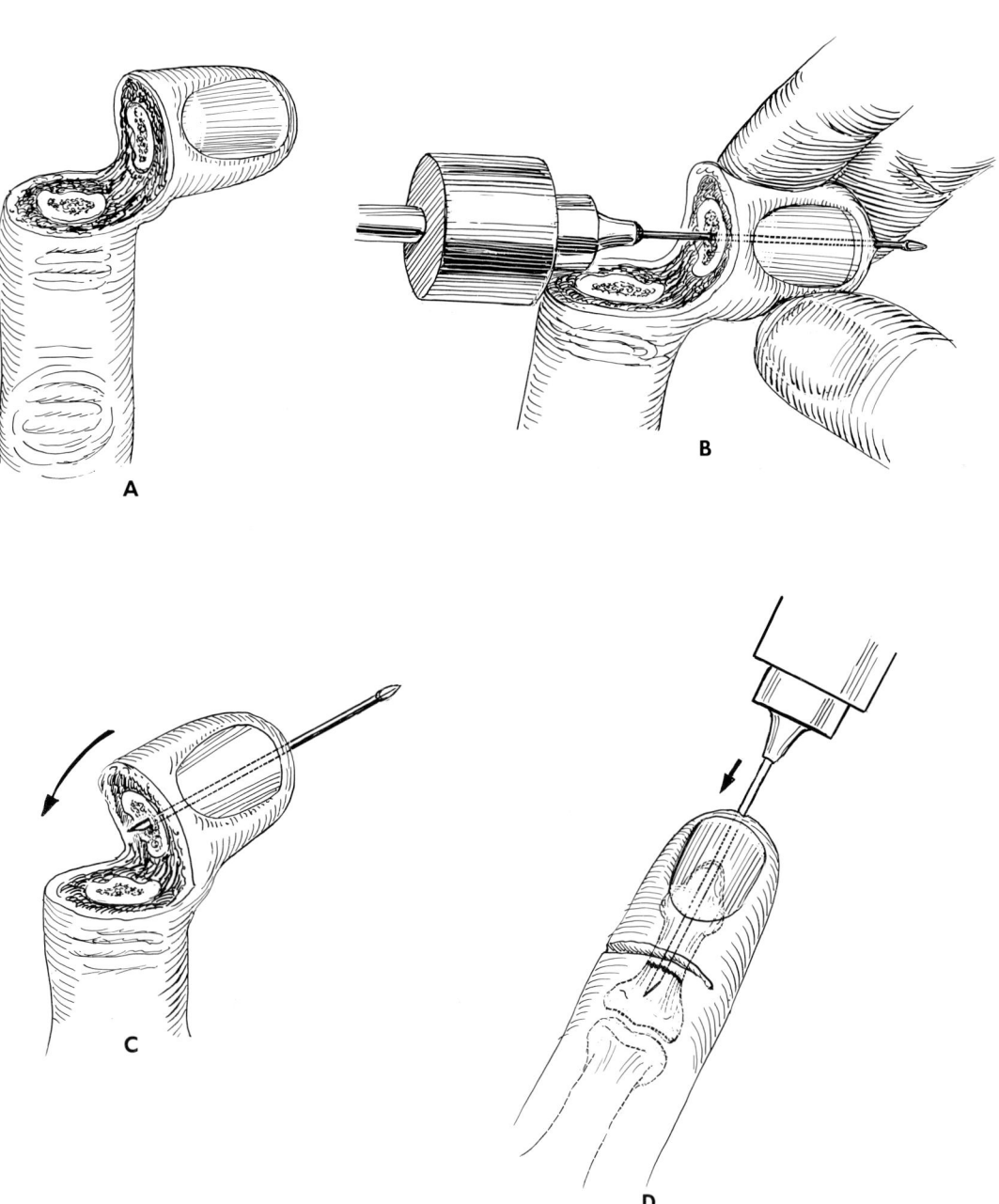

59 — Fractures in the Hand

The wire was cut short at the skin level, and careful skin closure was achieved. (**E** and **F**)

The finger tip survived after a period of circulatory deficiency, and the patient was left with no loss of finger length. The Kirschner wire was removed in five weeks when soft tissue healing was well advanced.

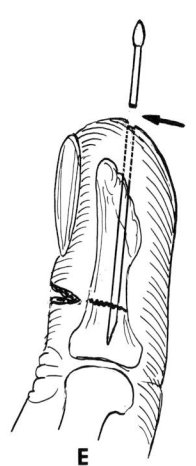

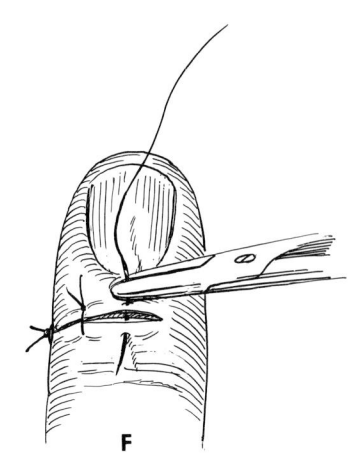

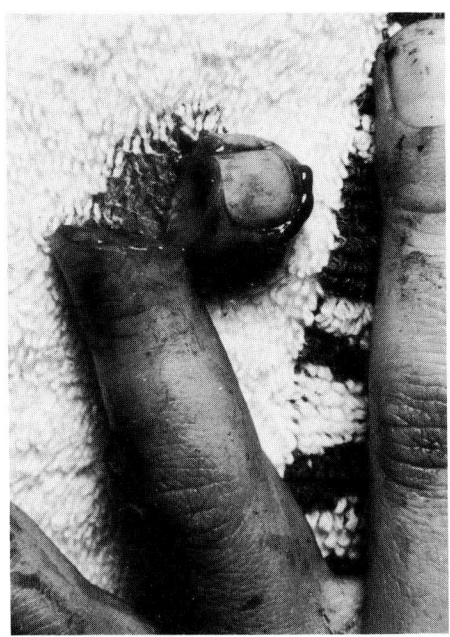

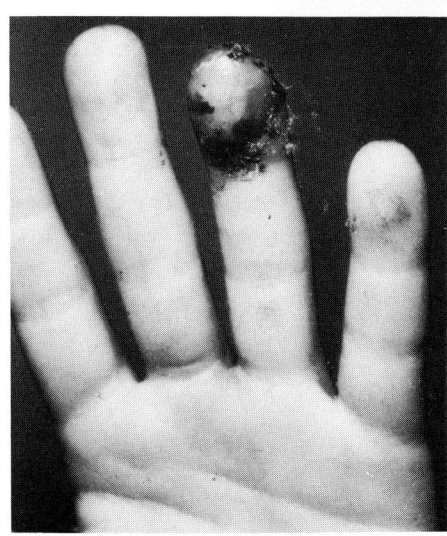

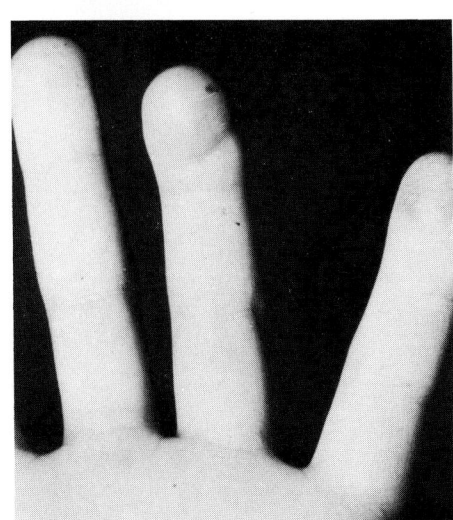

BENNETT'S FRACTURE

Principle

Bennett's fracture at the proximal end of the first metacarpal is generally unstable. It is difficult to immobilize in a way that assures maintenance of reduction without surgical fixation.

Example

A skier sustained a classical Bennett's fracture when he fell with his right thumb outstretched. Dislocation of the thumb carpometacarpal joint coupled with fracture of the proximal metacarpal lip which attaches to joint capsule resulted. (**A**)

The fracture dislocation could be reduced by traction on the thumb and pressure on the radiodorsal aspect of the metacarpal, but it was very difficult to sustain. Closed Kirschner wire fixation was chosen as appropriate treatment.

While the metacarpal was held in reduction, a single Kirschner wire was inserted across the base of the metacarpal and fracture into the carpus. A second wire across the first and second metacarpals was inserted for added security of fixation. (**B**)

The wire kept the base of the metacarpal from slipping off the greater multangular. This, together with a fitted plaster cast with the thumb extended and in radial abduction, obviated the need for open reduction.

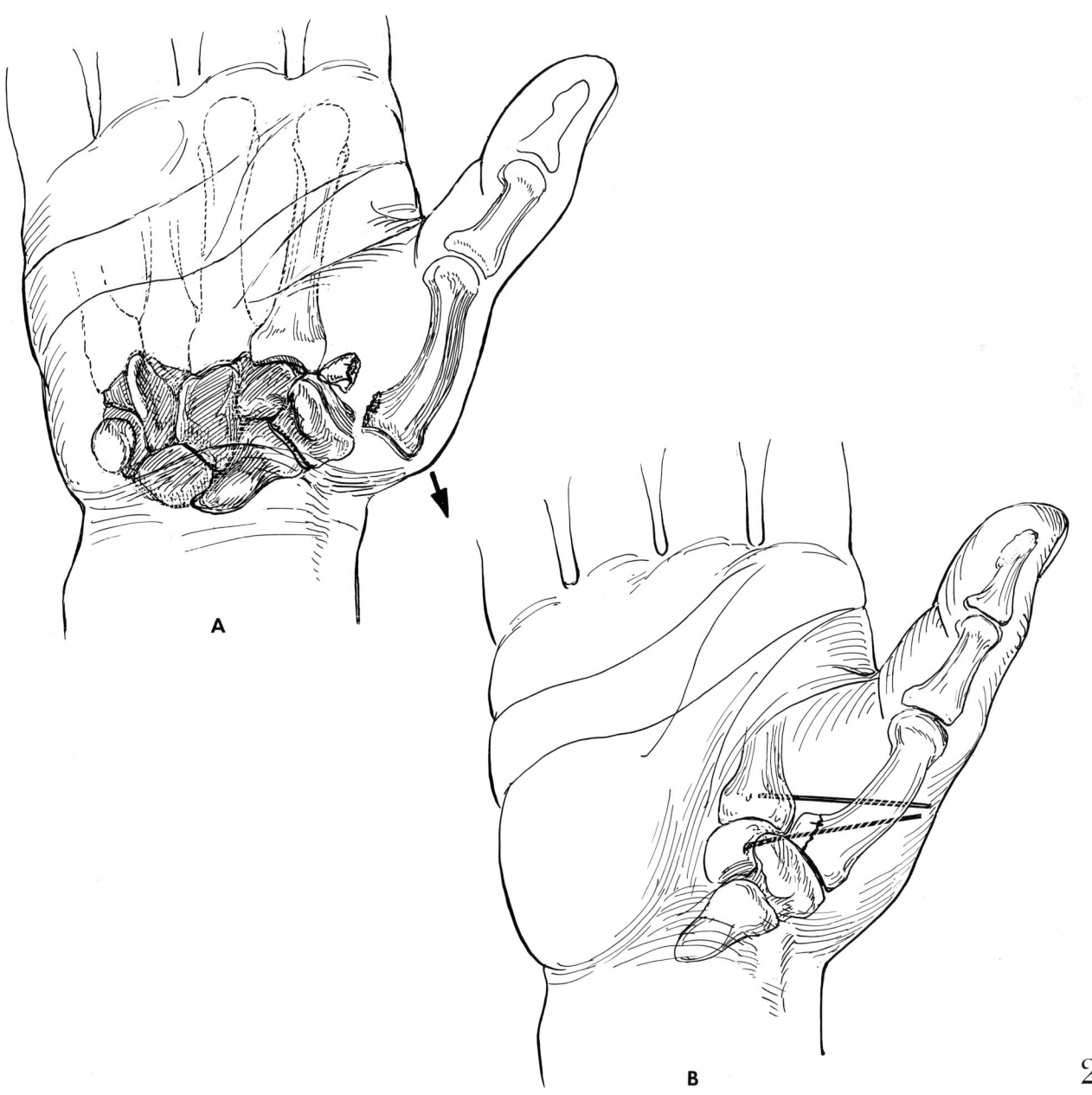

Stiff Proximal Interphalangeal Joints

The small size and precision fitting of the surfaces of the finger joints make them subject to stiffness after minor anatomical physical alterations. Until recently, surgeons have been reluctant to attempt reconstruction with the aim of restoring function to the proximal interphalangeal joints. Fusion seemed to be the only procedure which would be likely to succeed in these small joints.

A clearer understanding of the mechanisms responsible for stiffness in flexion or extension and the availability of refined surgical instruments and techniques have made practicable surgical procedures to functionally mobilize the proximal interphalangeal joint.

Curtis has summarized the anatomical factors other than joint ankylosis that might cause limitation of proximal interphalangeal joint motion.

Stiff in Extension—Limitation of Flexion

1. Scar contracture of dorsal skin.
2. Extensor tendon adherence or contracture.
3. Interosseous muscle or tendon adherence or contracture.
4. Adherence of retinaculum to lateral capsular ligaments.
5. Collateral ligament contracture.
6. Adherence of palmar capsule to head of proximal phalanx.
7. Bone block or exostosis.
8. Adherent flexor tendons within the flexor retinaculum.

Stiff in Flexion—Limitation of Extension

1. Scar contracture on palm skin.
2. Contracture of palmar fascia (i.e., Dupuytren's).
3. Contraction of flexor tendon sheath.
4. Flexor tendon adherence or contracture.
5. Volar plate adherence or contracture.
6. Accessory palmar ligament contracture.
7. Retinacular ligament adhesion to collateral ligaments.
8. Adherence of collateral ligaments to lateral aspects of proximal phalanx.
9. Bone block or exostoses.

Preoperative X-rays of the proximal interphalangeal joint and a detailed examination will help establish the need for surgery and sometimes the probable causes of limitation of motion. True bony ankylosis may be demonstrated. Full range of motion in the other joints of the finger and normal function of tendons bridging the area to move the distal phalanx suggest capsular problems. Tightness of intrinsic muscles is readily demonstrated as well as fixation of the long extensor and flexor tendons.

Surgical approach to the proximal interphalangeal joint may be dorsal or mid-axial bilaterally. A lazy S-curved incision along the dorsum of the finger allows wide exposure of the dorsal and bilateral aspects of the joint for joints stiff in extension. (**A**) A bilateral mid-axial incision may be best for approaching the joint stiff in flexion. (**B**)

A systematic attempt to establish which factors are responsible for fixation of the joint in extension is carried out in a logical sequence. If the preoperative examination suggests capsular collateral ligament tightness, one should section these first and test for passive flexion. The collateral ligaments are exposed by elevating the retinacular ligament and sectioning the collateral ligament close to the proximal phalanx. (**C**)

Bone and Joint Reconstruction

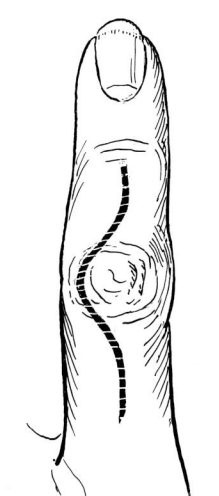

A

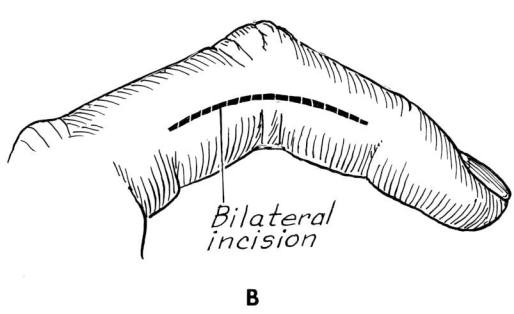

Bilateral incision

B

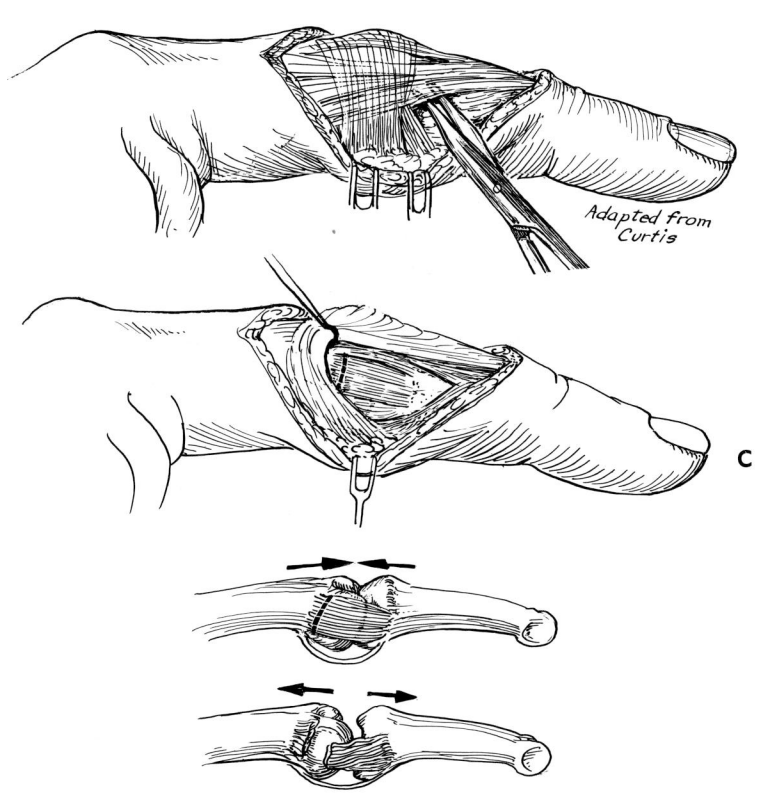

Adapted from Curtis

C

255

60 — Stiff Proximal Interphalangeal Joints

To examine the joint more completely may require the surgeon to section the retinacular ligament. In this way, the joint may be examined for exostosis. (**D**) The ligament is repaired after such elective section.

If interosseous tightness exists, a release of the intrinsic lateral band is carried out. (See Section 86.) Adherence of the extensor mechanism is released by working under the lateral bands by blunt dissection.

Function of the flexors may be checked once the joint can be put through a full range of motion. This is done by picking up the flexor through a small palmar incision and testing its effect on the mobilized proximal interphalangeal joint. If the tendon is adherent, it should be freed to complete the procedure. (**E**) The tendon sheath flap, opened to expose the flexor tendon, may be passed between the flexors and the volar plate and phalanges to avoid readhesion. (**F, G** and **H**) If the joint is still held in extension, release of the volar capsule is done.

Three or four days after the operation, gradually increasing range of motion exercises and dynamic splinting are started. These are continued until the patient's own muscles move the joint through the same range as one achieves passively.

The approach to the proximal interphalangeal joint stiff in flexion is similarly comprehensive and sequential. Preoperative x-rays and meticulous examination may give clues as to the most likely cause of stiffness. When skin scar contracture is an obvious cause of finger flexion contracture, one of the release procedures followed by flap or grafting techniques described in this volume may be used. (See Sections 6, 7 and 21.) Treatment of Dupuytren's contracture and combined palmar fascia and skin release are discussed elsewhere in this book. (See Section 87.) Palmar joint capsule tightness may be released by elevating the capsule from its origins on the proximal phalanx while extension traction is used to put it on tension. (**I**)

Adherence of either the flexor profundus or superficialis or both may require simple tenolysis or actual section of the superficialis.

If both tendons are badly deformed, excision for later replacement with a tendon graft after full range of passive motion is achieved in the proximal interphalangeal joint is good judgment. Postoperative splinting and physical therapy are essential parts of restorative procedures on the proximal interphalangeal joints.

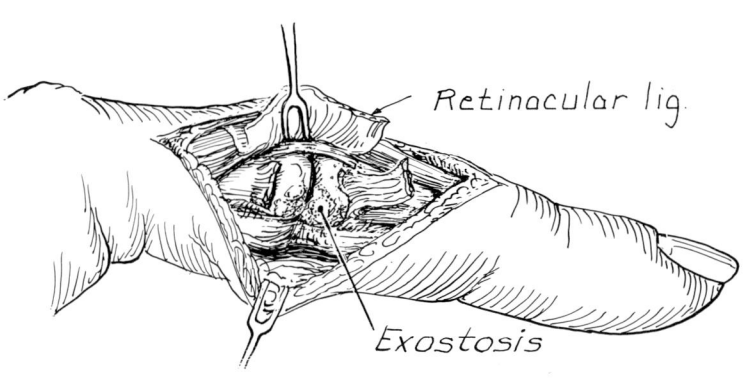

D

Bone and Joint Reconstruction

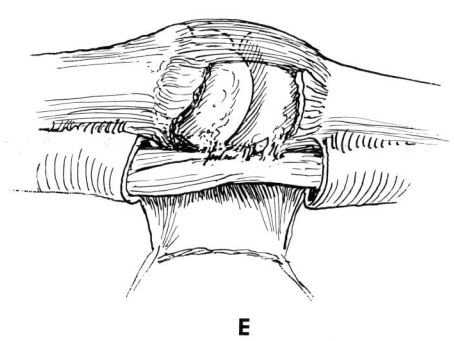

E

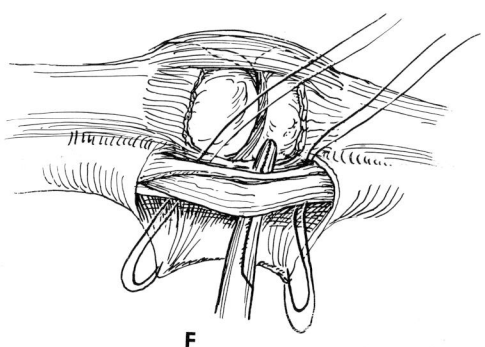

F

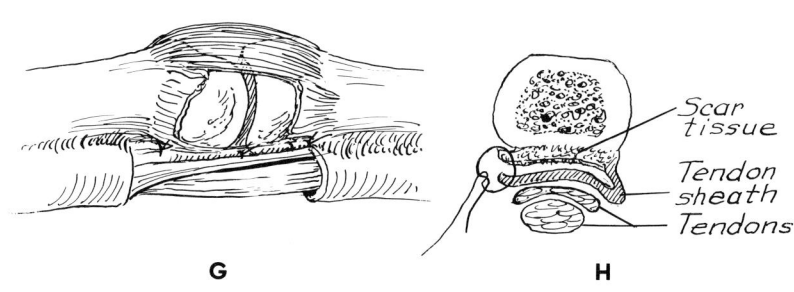

G

H
Scar tissue
Tendon sheath
Tendons

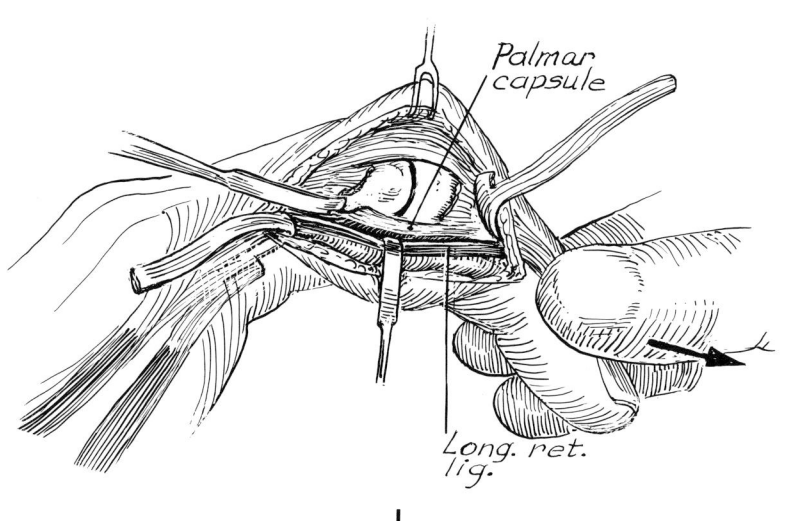

Palmar capsule

Long. ret. lig.

I

61
Bone Grafting

Principles

Bone grafting is essential to overcome deficits in the hand skeleton where bone substance has been lost. In addition, bone grafts are very useful when the surgeon wishes to secure fusion of a joint or healing in a non-united fracture. Autogenous bone grafts are far superior to any of the other types. The choice of donor site depends on whether one wishes to use cortical bone or cancellous bone for the reconstruction.

Cortical Versus Cancellous Bone

For precise fitting and for fixation rendered by the bone graft itself, cortical bone is best. When osteogenesis stimulation is the most important attribute brought by the bone graft, cancellous bone is superior. The two in combination achieve both objectives. In either case, the bone acts largely as a scaffolding for development of new bone which molds itself in response to the stress demands placed upon it.

Donor Sites

The tibia, fibula, ilium, and ribs are common donor sites for new autogenous bone. Bone from the hand itself is very useful if digits or metacarpals are to be amputated. The subcutaneous ulna is a good donor site for small bone pegs.

TIBIA

The best source of thick cortical bone is the subcutaneous surface of the tibia. There is no apparent advantage gained by leaving periosteum on the graft except in a specific circumstance. (See Thumb Reconstruction with Pedicle Flap and Bone Graft, in Section 70.) The advantage of leaving and repairing periosteum at the donor site is that it guarantees prompt bone regeneration. Such donor site periosteum also prevents formation of exuberant irregular callus. The anterior cortex of the tibia alone is usually wide enough to supply small bone grafts such as those used in the hand.

Technique. After incising the skin in curvilinear fashion to offset the skin wound from the tibial donor site, the incision is carried through the periosteum which is elevated with the skin over a sufficient area to expose the tibial donor area. (**A**)

The donor area may be marked out well below the plateau. Drill holes are made through the cortex at the four corners of the graft. (**B**)

An oscillating mechanical bone saw is used to cut the bone between the drill holes. (**C**) One should avoid extending the saw cuts beyond the drill hole areas since such a split may be the weak point which will initiate a fracture early postoperatively. This is particularly important at the distal end of the donor site.

The graft may be pried out with an osteotome. (**D**)

The periosteum is draped back in place with the skin flap. Care must be exercised for several months postoperatively to avoid undue stress on the weakened tibia. Fracture through the donor site may occur with minor trauma. (**E**)

Cortical bone obtained from the tibia is excellent for construction of fitted pegs and small bone substitutes. It may be carved and fitted, using mechanical bone tools, bone cutters, and rongeurs. (**F**) Such bone carpentry is not possible with cancellous bone.

Bone and Joint Reconstruction

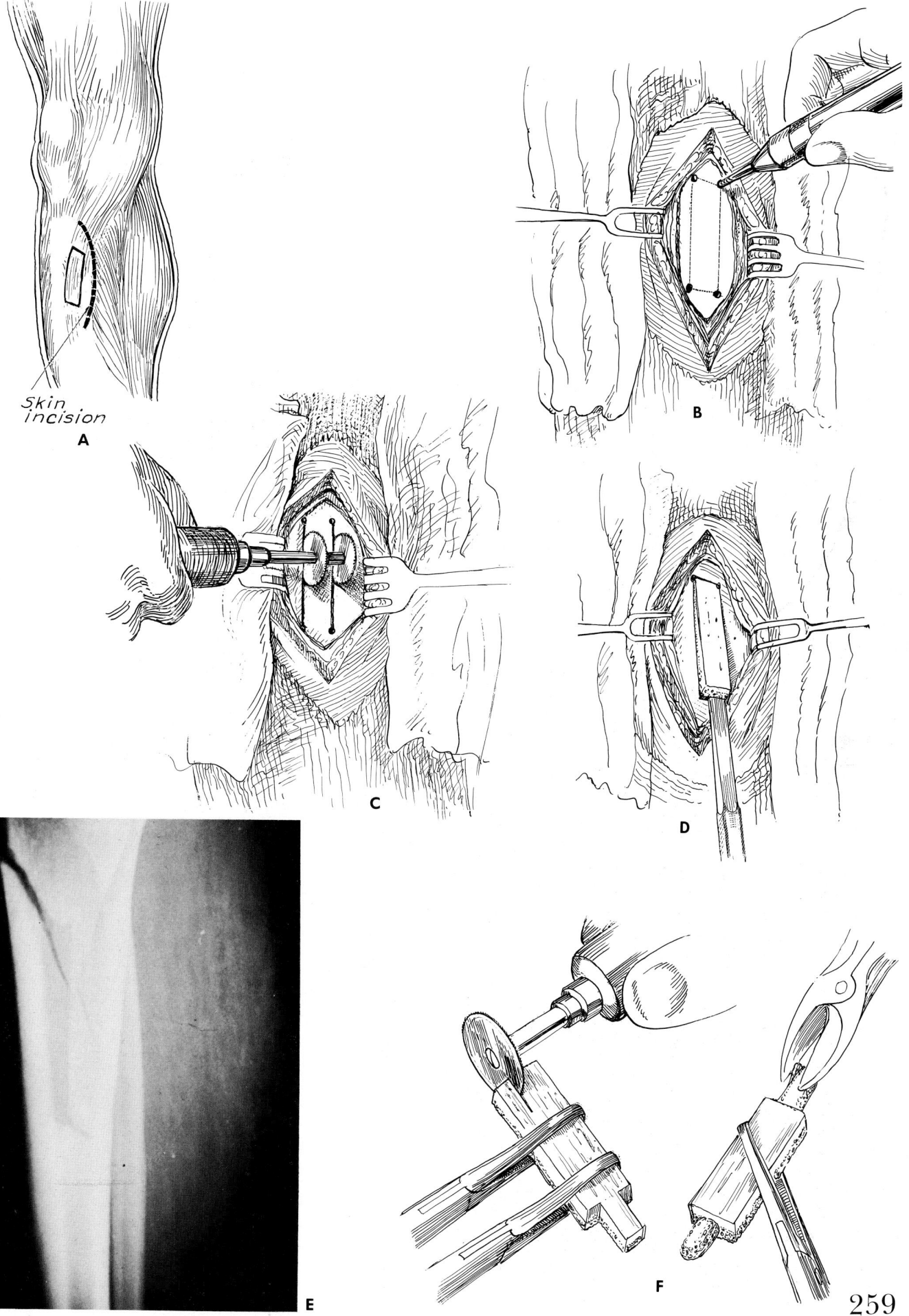

259

61 — Bone Grafting

One may take periosteum with the bone graft by incising it beyond the projected outline of the bone graft. (**G**) The periosteum is elevated toward the graft but is left attached to it. (**H**) Such attached periosteum may be helpful as an anchor for soft tissue placed over the bone graft. (See Thumb Reconstruction with Bone Graft, Pedicle Flap and Island, Section 70.)

The Iliac Bone

The iliac bone is an excellent source of cancellous bone for bone grafts. The variety of shapes and ratio of cancellous to cortical bone in different parts of the ilium make the choice of a site within the ilium important. In the supine position the anterior one-third of the iliac crest is available. If the patient is prone, one may choose to remove bone from the posterior one-third of the crest. (**I**) Vertical grafts through bone cortices may be taken. (**J**) Generally, however, one may obtain a large enough graft for hand operations and still may preserve one cortex and the crest of the ilium.

An incision is made above the palpable iliac crest and it is carried down to the crest itself. The muscle origins along the crest are reflected to gain access to the ilium below the crest itself. (**K**)

The crest may be reflected up from the rest of the ilium by cutting it free with an osteotome. (**L**) One may then subperiosteally dissect the muscles from the outside surface or visceral medial surface so that the donor site may be scored or marked out. By splitting the ilium, one may leave one cortex intact and remove cancellous bone with the other cortex en bloc. The crest of the ilium is replaced and the muscle fascia is repaired with sutures.

Alternatively, one may remove bone directly from the crest of the ilium, with little dissection of structures from the ilium itself. (**M**)

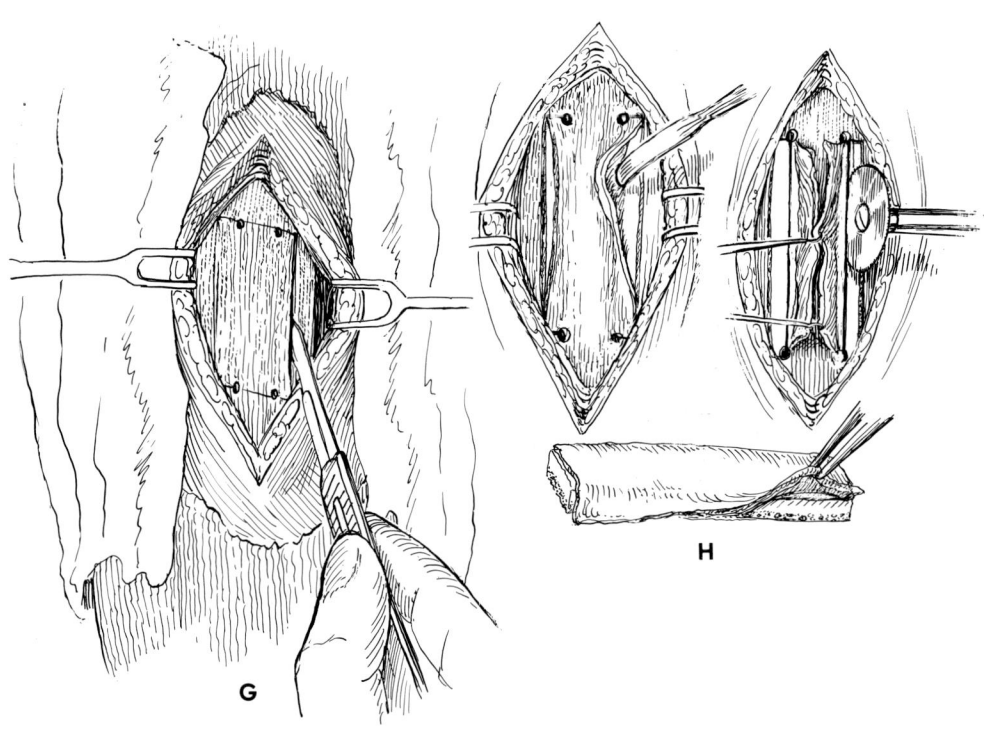

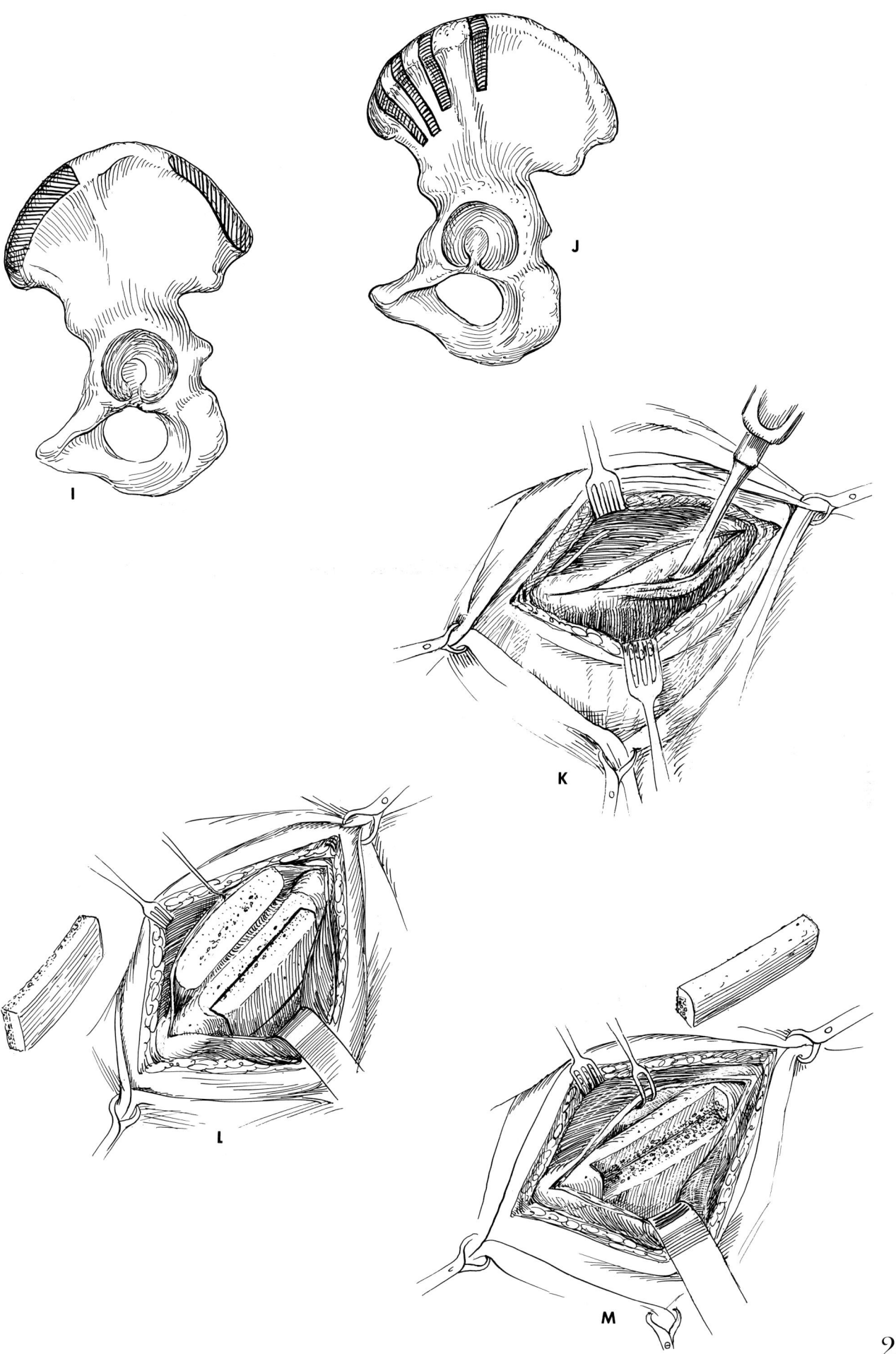

Rib

Rib bone grafts are readily obtainable by simply incising skin overlying the rib below the axilla. The incision is carried down to the rib through its periosteum. (**N**) Subperiosteal rib dissection, using chest periosteal elevators, exposes the rib so that it may be removed without injury to intercostal structures or pleura. (**O** and **P**)

A rib cutter may be used to section the rib anteriorly. (**Q**) After the rib has been cut, it may be elevated out of the wound to facilitate dissection dorsally. A second cut frees the rib graft. The periosteum is repaired and the wound is closed. (**R**) A rib graft is most adaptable, for if it is split longitudinally to expose the marrow cavity, the cortical component of the rib may be shaped to fit the recipient site using saws, drills, osteotomes, and rongeurs. (**S**)

The Ulna

The subcutaneous ulna below the elbow is a very convenient donor site for small cortical grafts. Bone pegs for joint fusion or phalangeal and metacarpal nonunion are commonly obtained from the ulna. A small incision offset from the donor site along the subcutaneous ulna ridge is made and carried to the ulna. (**T**) A small bone graft can be cut, using an osteotome or fine mechanical drills and burrs. (**U** and **V**) The graft should be taken at least two inches below the olecranon to avoid weakness over the elbow joint. Only small grafts should be taken from the ulna since weakness and fractures may result from overzealous removal. (**W**)

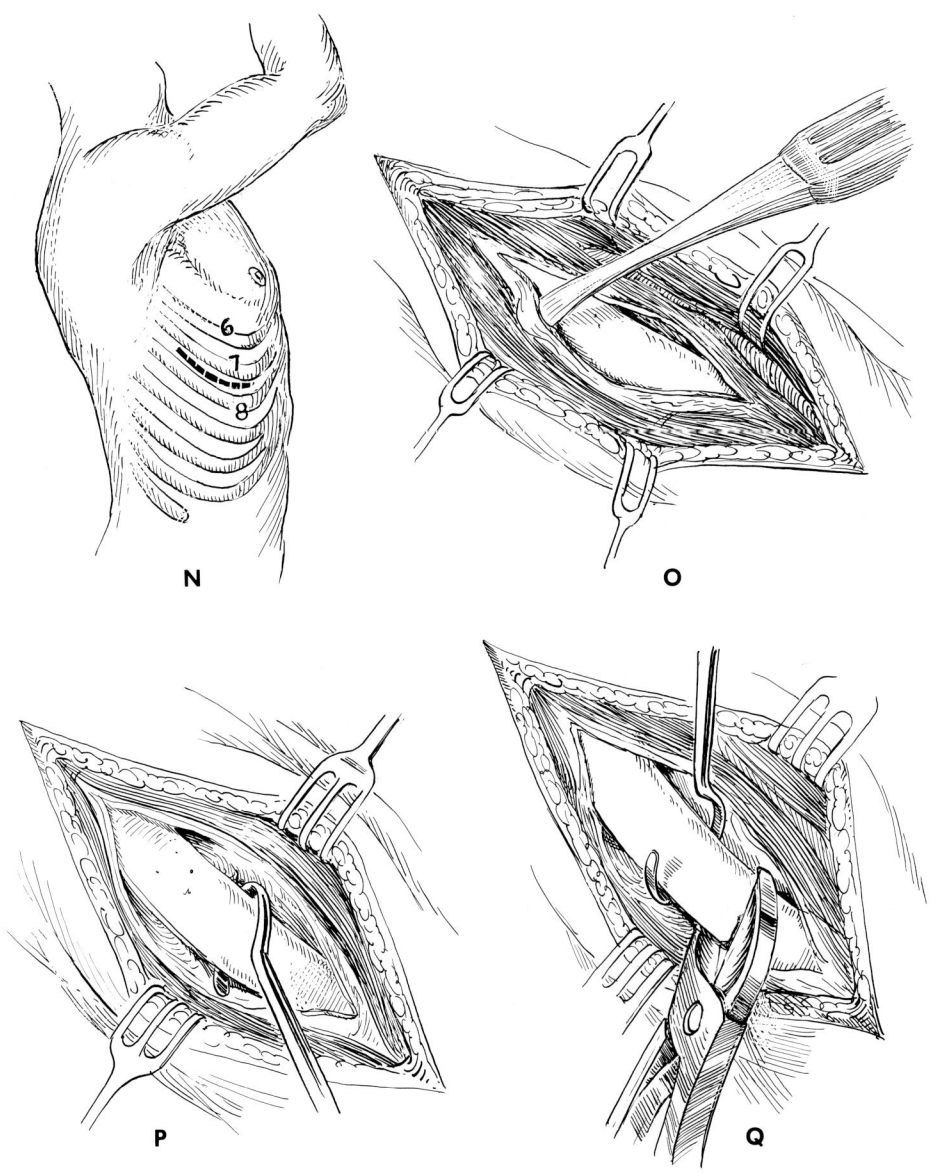

Bone and Joint Reconstruction

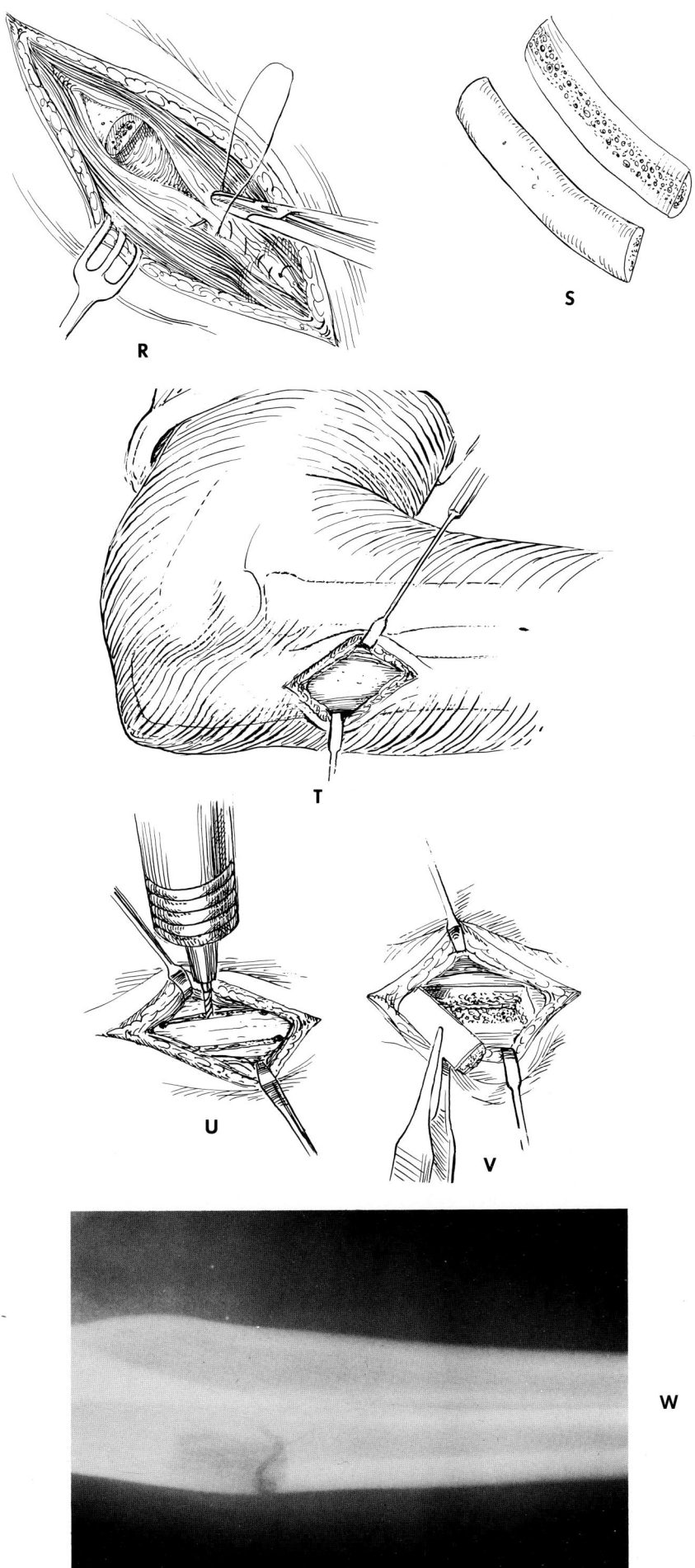

263

61 – Bone Grafting

Bone From the Hand Itself

Amputation of digits or metacarpals makes available excellent bone for grafting in the hand. If traumatically amputated parts of the hand are brought to the hospital with the patient, bits of bone from these parts are useful as free bone grafts. (See Section 39.) In major skeletal reconstruction, parts of the hand may be shifted from one place to another. When this is done there is frequently superfluous bone available for use as bone pegs or for substitutes for lost bone substances. (See Section 69.)

Example

A 21 year old boy sustained a traumatic amputation of the thumb, index finger, long finger and tip of the ring finger in a large mechanical paper cutter. (**X**) The patient brought the amputated parts to the hospital with him.

Reconstruction of the patient's thumb was of highest priority. The proximal phalanx of the amputated thumb was dissected from the prepared amputated part and was trimmed to serve as a bone graft on the first metacarpal. The bone graft was fixed in place with a bone peg made from a portion of the index metacarpal, which was amputated at its proximal one-third. A Kirschner wire was inserted through graft and metacarpal. (**Y**)

The whole hand was carried to the contralateral abdominal wall for application of a double pedicle flap. (**Z**)

Three weeks later the pedicle flap was released from the abdomen and the patient was left with a bone graft–pedicle flap–thumb reconstruction. (**AA**)

To give sensibility, better permanent blood supply, and sudomotor function to the thumb, a secondary island pedicle flap was transplanted from the ulnar side of the ring finger to the reconstructed thumb. (**BB**) The patient did well with his rehabilitated hand. (**CC**)

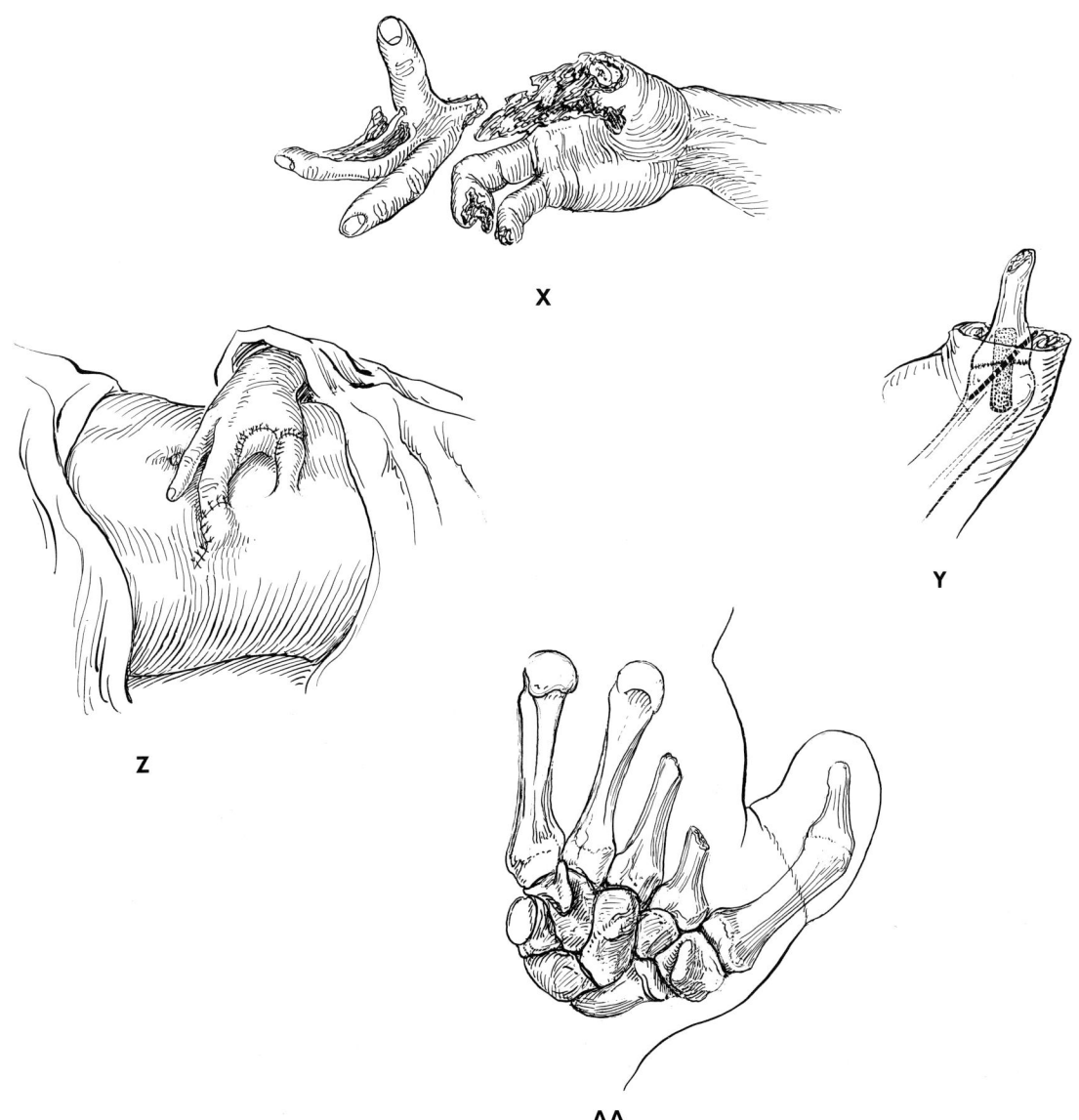

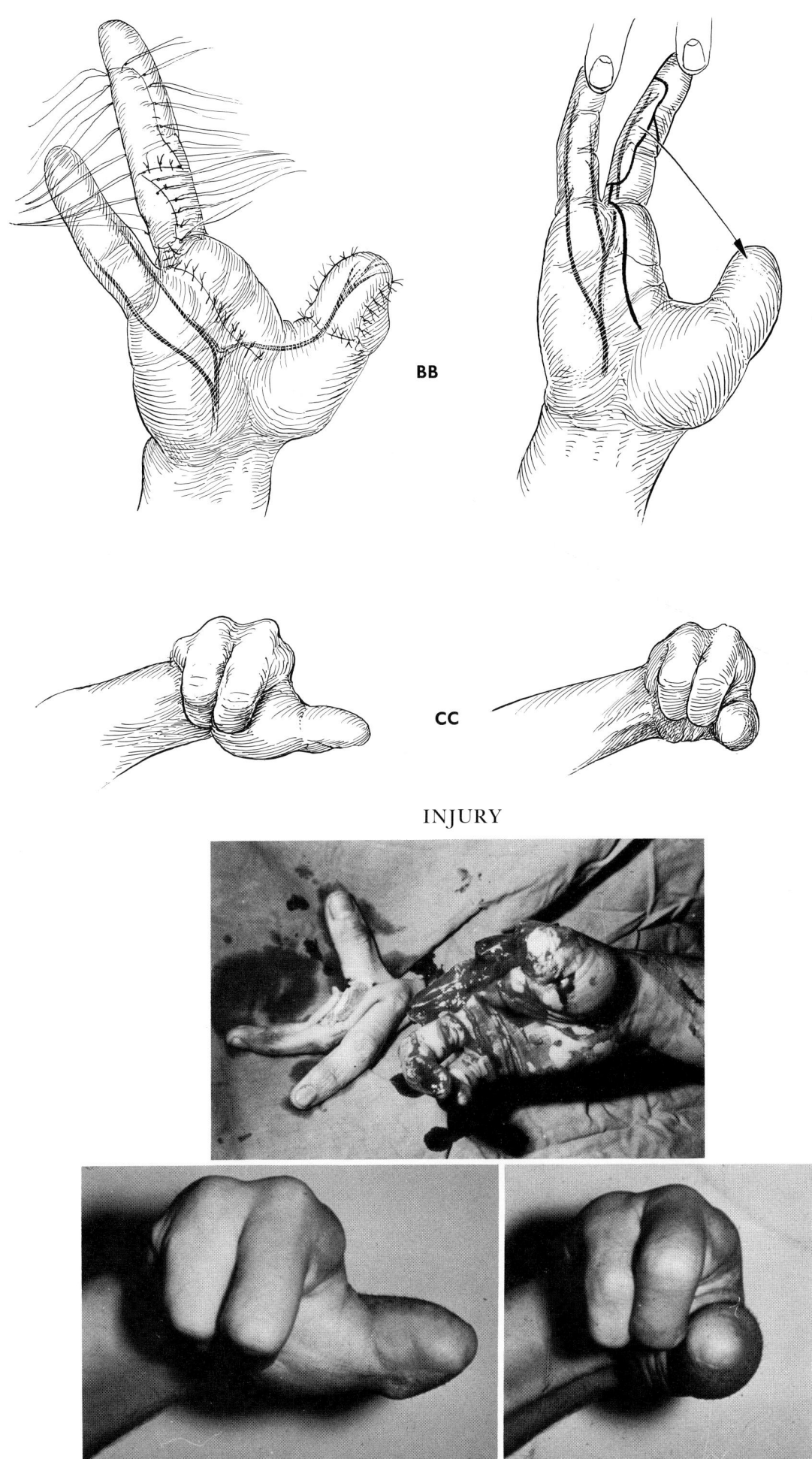

BB

CC

INJURY

RESULT

265

62
Use of Bone Grafts in the Phalanges

Phalangeal Bone Grafts

Bone grafts of a phalanx may be called for when there is traumatic loss of bone substance or at the time of elective bone tumor excision. For example, an osteoid osteoma of the proximal phalanx causes swelling and disabling pain. Its nidus must be removed for cure. This frequently will so weaken the proximal phalanx that a primary autogenous bone graft should be used.

The tumor removal may be carried out with accuracy and precision, using power driven cable instruments. Burrs and drills of small size as used in dentistry may allow removal of the tumor with preservation of one bone cortex.

Should threat of fracture be great or should fracture occur at the weak point, a bone graft from one of the donor sites described may be used to fill the defect.

Additional internal fixation over that provided by careful dowel or mortise bone carpentry may be required. If it is, a temporary Kirschner wire may be placed across the site.

Phalanx bone grafts require immobilization for 8 to 10 weeks for stable union.

Traumatic loss of phalangeal bone substance is a more common indication for a phalangeal bone graft.

Example

The left thumb proximal phalanx of a young boy was lost in a severe infection. The thumb itself was left completely flail and useless. The distal phalanx remained intact. (**A**) A bone graft substitution was decided upon.

The recipient bed was dissected free of scar tissue, and the bone ends were prepared to receive the graft dowels by drilling into the medullary cavities. The defect length was carefully measured and a cortical bone graft about an inch longer than the defect was taken from the tibia. (See Tibial Bone Graft, Section 61.) Dowels were created at both ends of the graft, using a motorized saw; dental burrs could have been used. (**B**)

The proximal dowel was forced into place down to the bone graft shoulders. (**C**) With

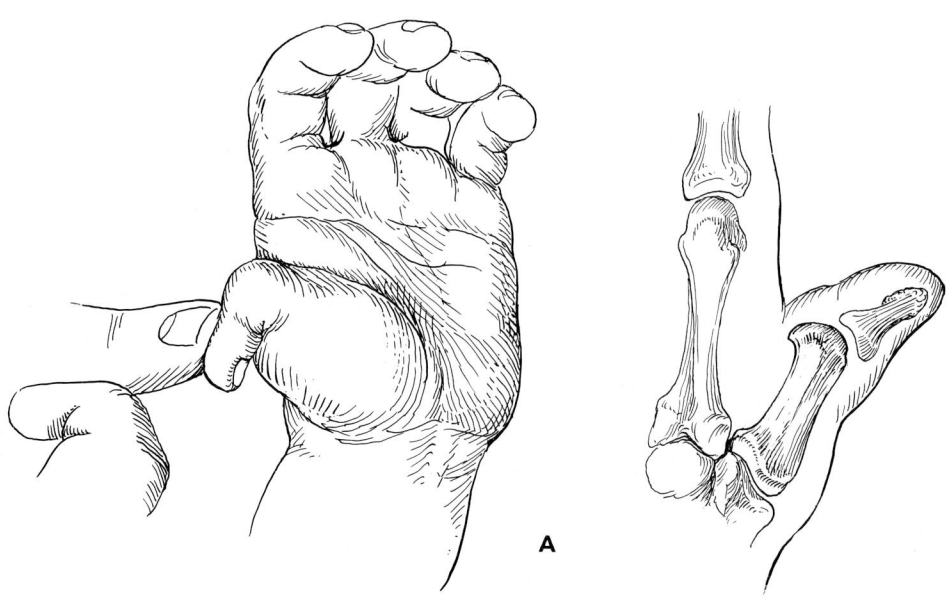

Bone and Joint Reconstruction

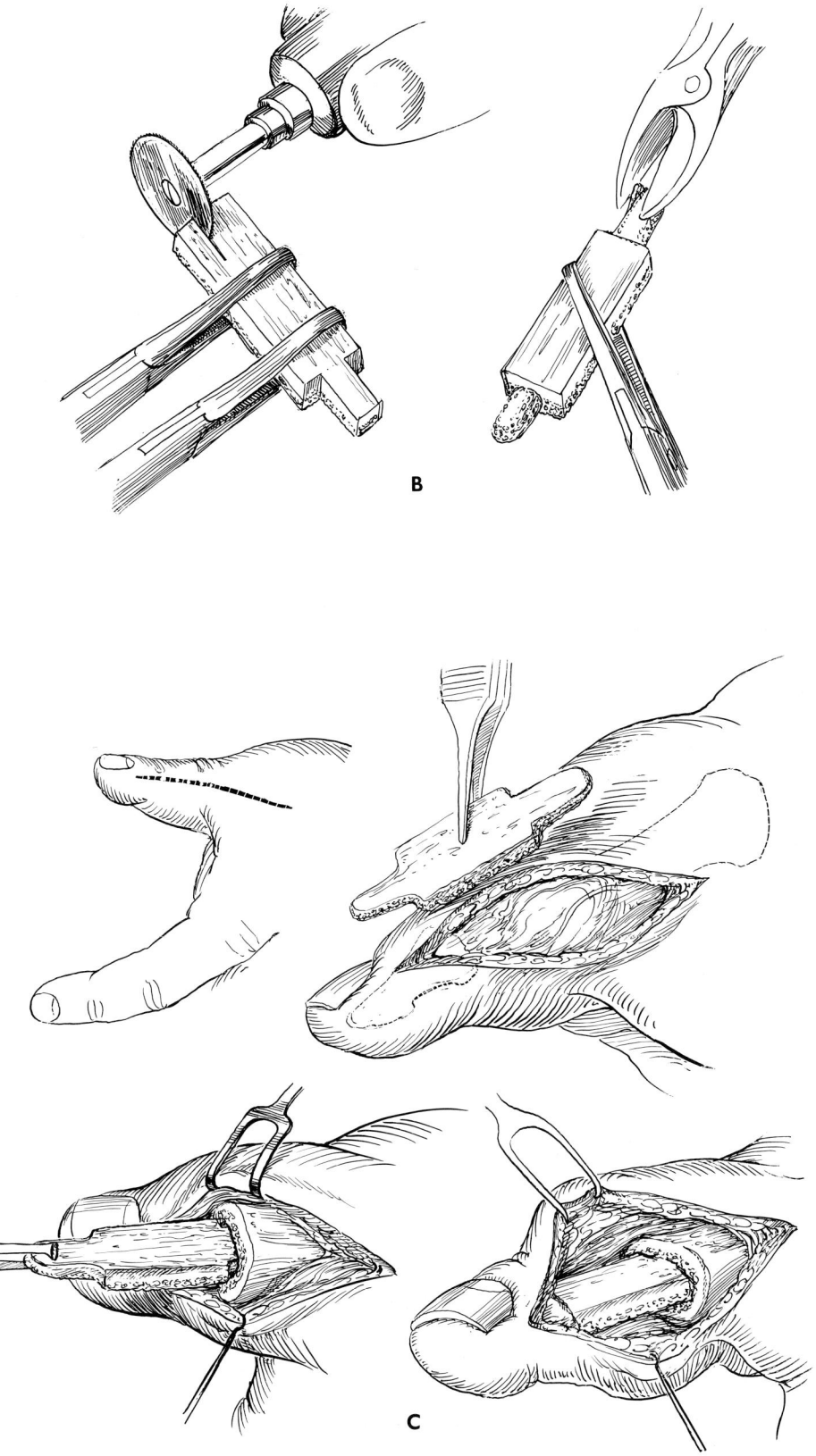

267

62 – Use of Bone Grafts in the Phalanges

maximum traction and manipulation the distal phalanx was seated over the distal bone graft dowel. The bone graft fitted in this manner was stable and required no other internal fixation. (**D**) After careful closure of the soft tissues to maximally eliminate dead space, the whole thumb and the hand proximal to the metacarpophalangeal joints of the fingers was immobilized in a plaster cast.

Immobilization was maintained for eight weeks to secure good union and bone graft take. The bone graft remodeled over many months thereafter as the thumb was progressively used. Excellent function was restored. (**E**)

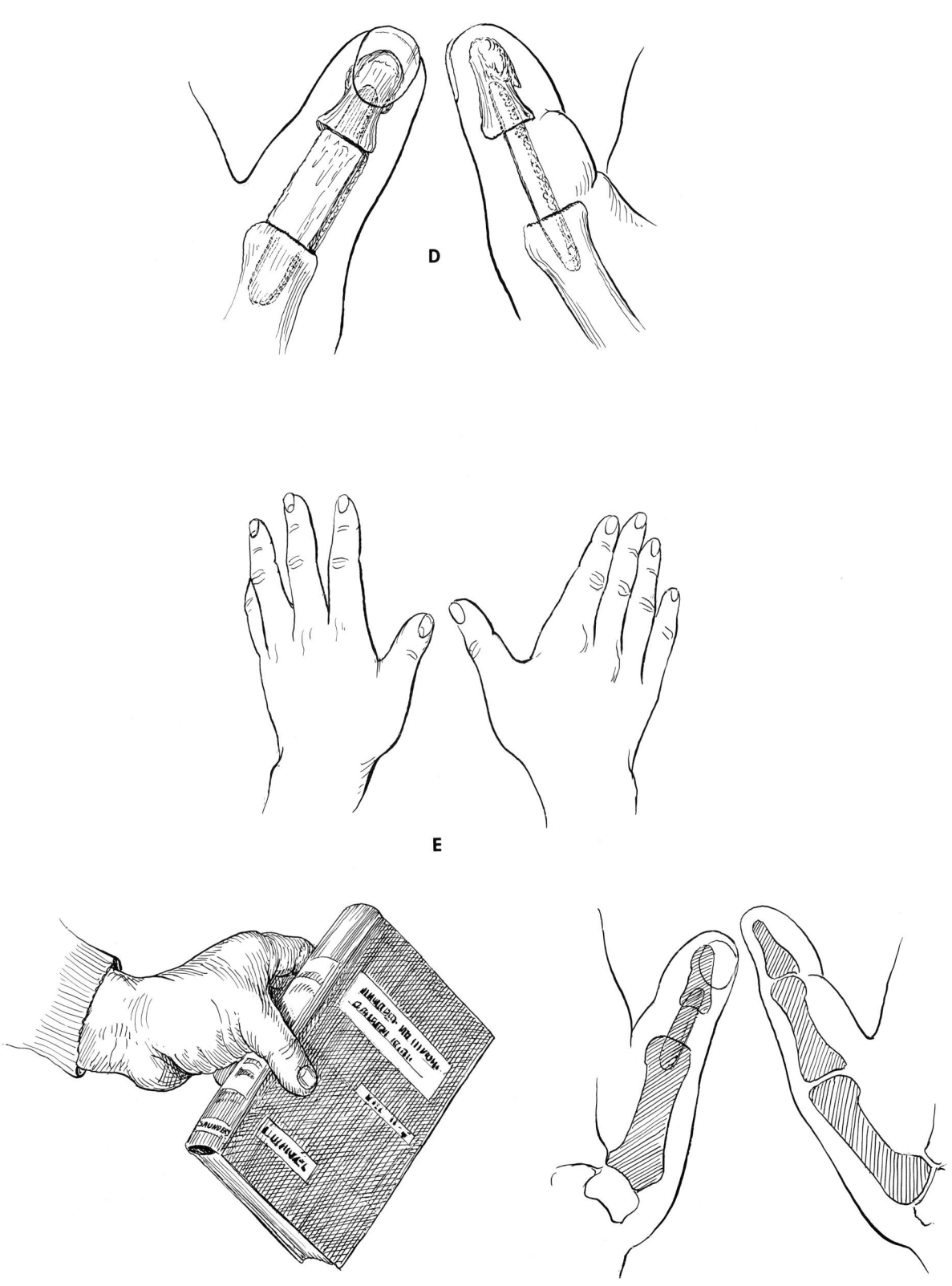

Bone and Joint Reconstruction

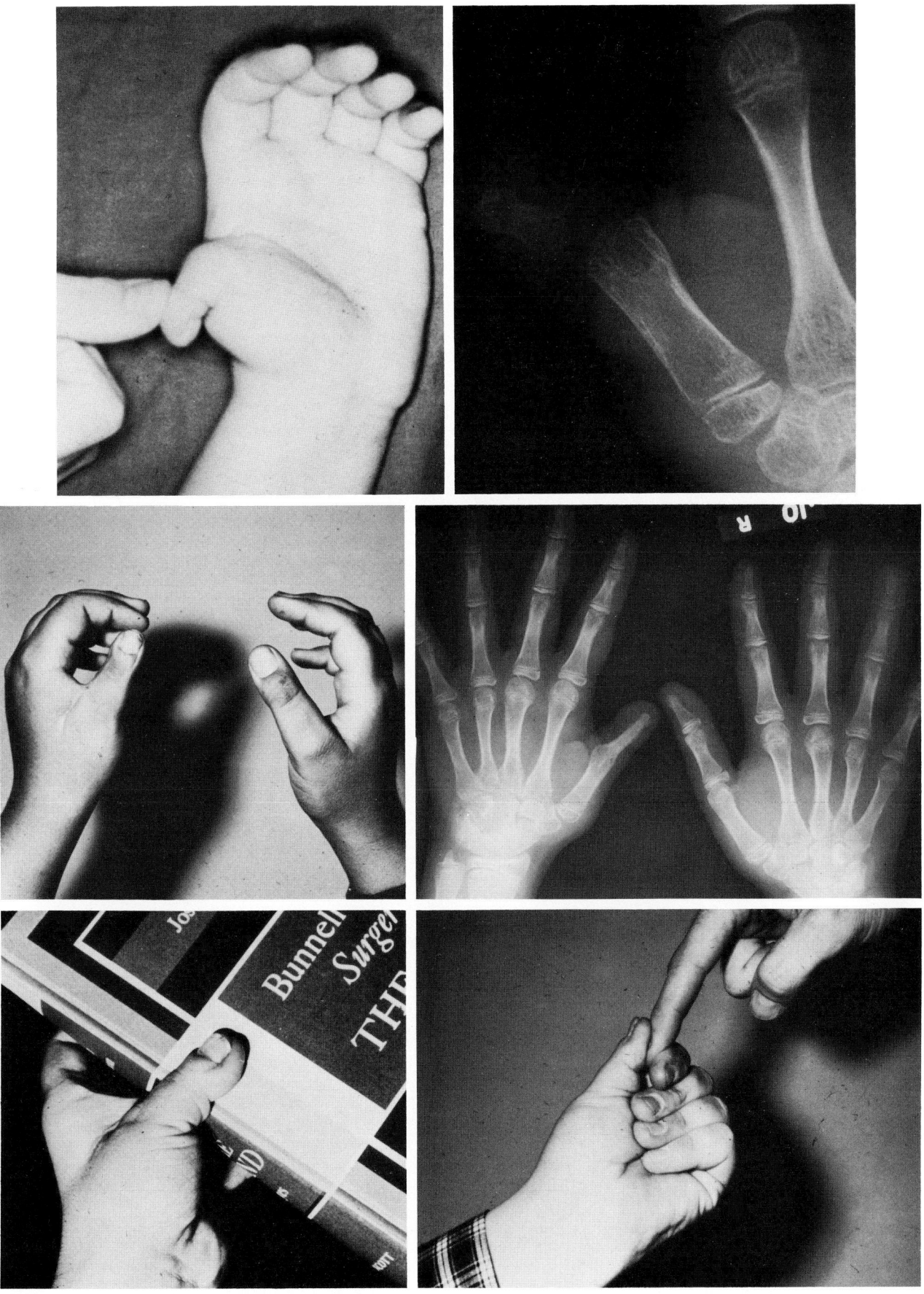

269

63
Metacarpal Bone Grafting

Principle

Missing bone substance in any of the metacarpals in the presence of a digit worthy of salvage can best be substituted for by an autogenous bone graft. Decision for or against salvage will depend on numerous factors, including the presence or absence of other digits, the residual anatomical prerequisites for function such as active muscles with tendons, sensibility, and movable joints, and the occupational or cosmetic need for the finger by the specific patient. Skin and soft tissue cover must be the optimum obtainable over the bone graft recipient site. Full thickness flap coverage is frequently essential to create a proper bed for the bone graft and subsequent tendon restoration which may be necessary.

The best bone for small precision-fitted grafts in the hand is cortical bone. It may be obtained readily from the subcutaneous tibia.

Example

A palmar to dorsal through-and-through gunshot wound resulted in loss of bone substance in the third metacarpal of this 23-year-old soldier. The metacarpophalangeal joint, flexor and extensor tendons, and digital nerves were all intact. Soft tissue cover was adequate to consider a metacarpal bone graft. With the prerequisites met (a worthwhile digit, an M. P. joint, and adequate soft tissue cover) the metacarpal defect was exposed through a dorsal incision that would not leave a wound over the bone graft area itself. (**A**)

The region of bone deficit was cleared of scar and the finger was pulled distally to see if full length could be restored. Length could not be fully restored and some shortening was accepted as appropriate. (**B**)

The metacarpophalangeal joint and the metacarpal head were intact and they were carefully preserved. The metacarpal bone ends were cut square to prepare for proper seating of the bone graft. The distal cut end was drilled out to receive a dowel peg to be fashioned on the end of the bone graft. (**C**)

At the proximal end of the metacarpal, a seat was unroofed to receive the proximal end of the bone graft. Its base was beveled at 45 degrees to hold the bone graft in place.

The tibial cortical bone graft was taken, using a double bladed mechanical bone saw with blades fixed at appropriate width to cut a substitute for the metacarpal. The subcutaneous tibia was exposed through a curved incision around the donor site. The periosteum over the site was elevated with the skin flap, using a periosteal elevator. With the periosteum retracted, drill holes were made at the four corners of the donor site and the bone saw was slowly advanced up and down the site in the middle of the wide superior portion of the tibia until the cuts were through the cortex. The graft was planned with adequate length to construct a bone graft with a protruding dowel or peg. This was determined by precise measurement of the distances from proximal to distal prepared ends of the metacarpal with full traction on the finger. Transverse cuts were made with a small, single saw blade at the ends of the bone graft. The cuts were not carried beyond the corner drill holes lest the cut create a weak point for the start of an unwanted fracture. (See Section 61.)

Using mechanical saws and cable type drilling and shaping tools, the bone graft was shaped precisely to fit the metacarpal defect. A dowel was left on the distal end, and the proximal end was cut at a bevel so that it would be held in its seat in the proximal end of the recipient metacarpal. (**D**)

The bone graft dowel was forced into the distal recipient area to the shoulders of the bone graft. With maximal traction on the finger, the proximal end of the bone graft was snapped into its constructed seat. (**E**) No further internal

Bone and Joint Reconstruction

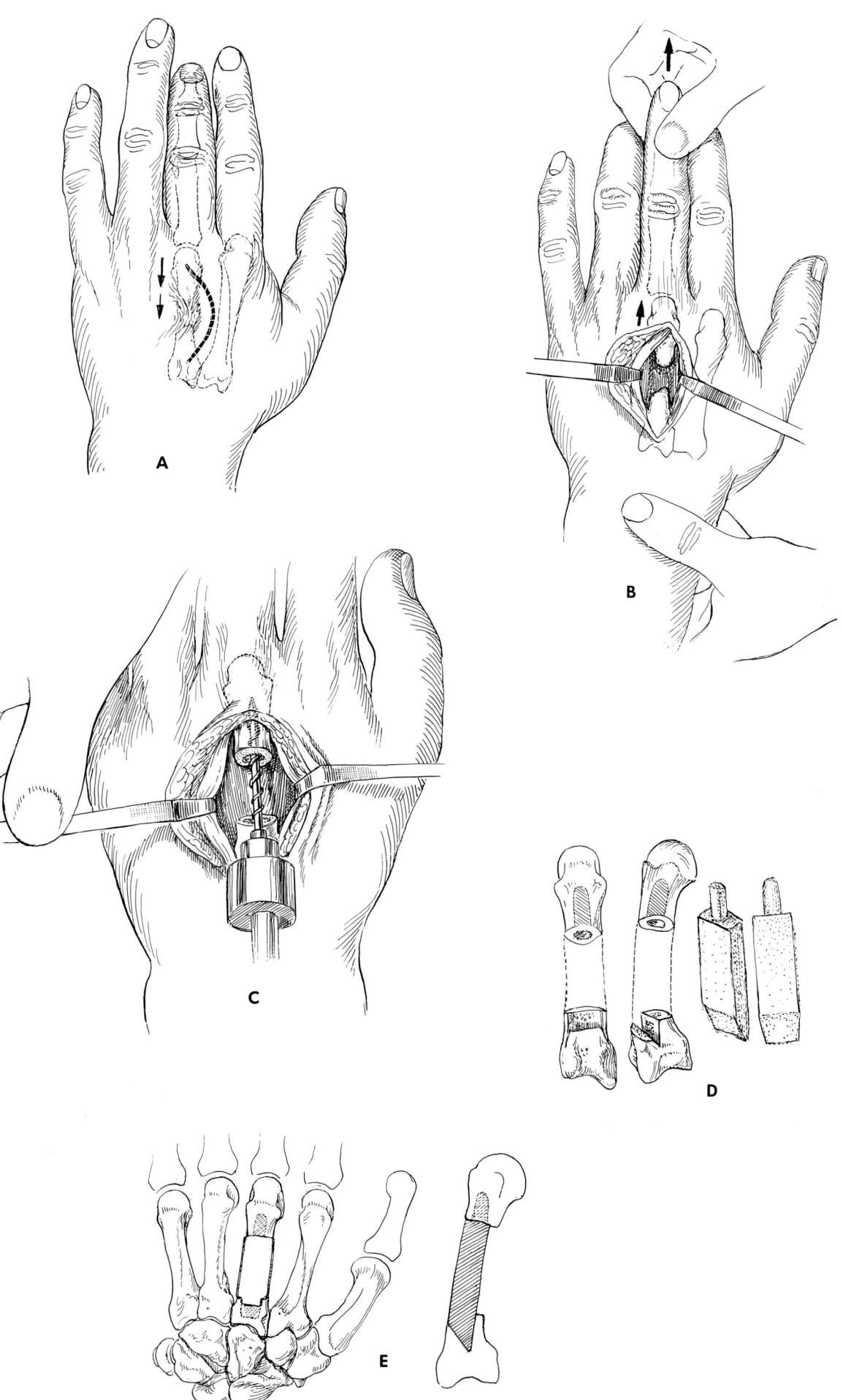

271

63 – Metacarpal Bone Grafting

fixation was necessary. Additional stability could have been acquired by insertion of small Kirschner wires but this was not necessary.

Soft tissues were carefully closed over the graft in a manner which best eliminated any dead space around the graft. The hand was immobilized in a position of function in a fitted split plaster cast. It was immobilized to the level of the proximal interphalangeal joints for ten weeks with one cast change at two weeks to check the wound. After solid union occurred, physical measures to regain motion in the metacarpophalangeal joint were initiated. The patient regained useful but incomplete motion.

PREOPERATIVE

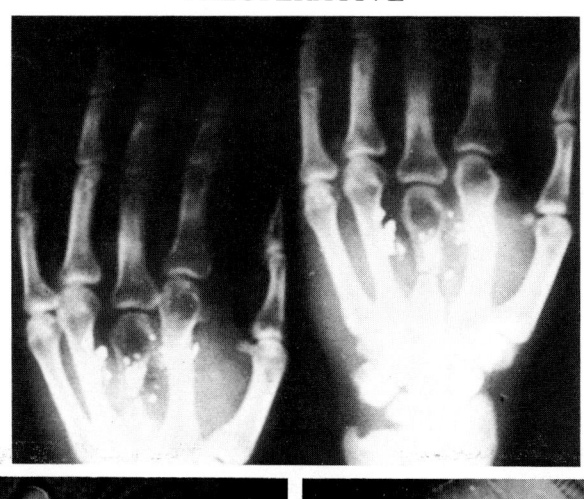

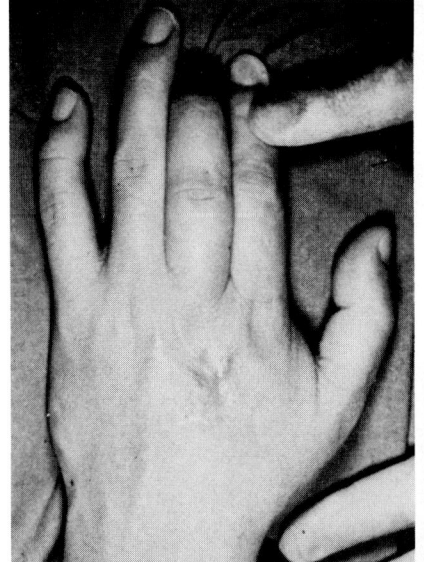
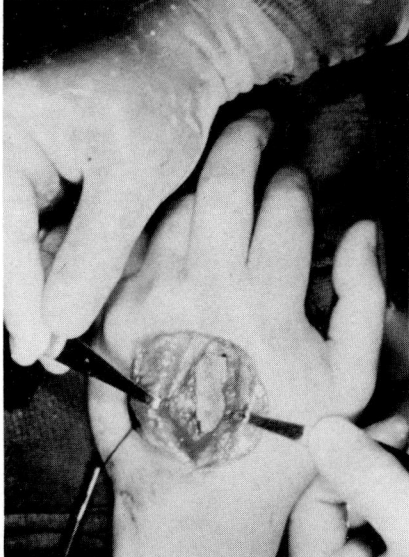

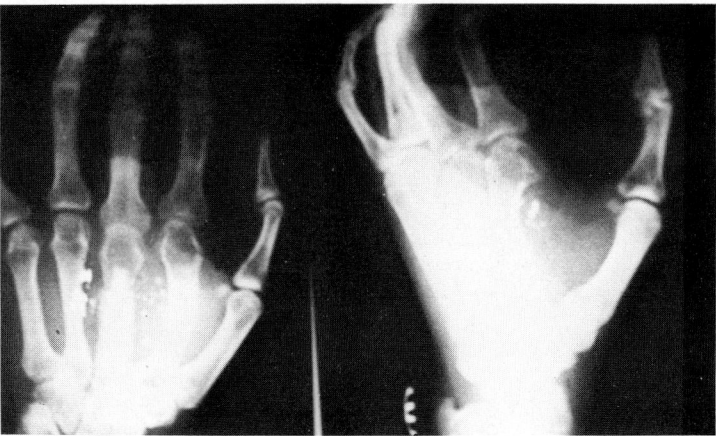

POSTOPERATIVE

Bone and Joint Reconstruction

Technical Variations

A variety of bone carpentry techniques may be used to make a secure bone juncture at each end of the graft. (**F**)

If the metacarpal head is missing and the finger is still worth saving, the bone graft may be carried into the proximal phalanx with palmar angulation of 30 to 45 degrees at the site of the previous metacarpophalangeal joint. (**G**)

If the proximal metacarpal is missing, the bone graft may be seated into the carpal bones. (**H** and **I**)

More than one metacarpal graft may be inserted simultaneously. Dowel construction may be preferred at both ends of the bone graft where circumstances warrant it. (See Section 62.)

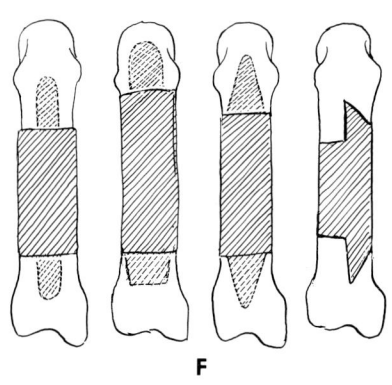

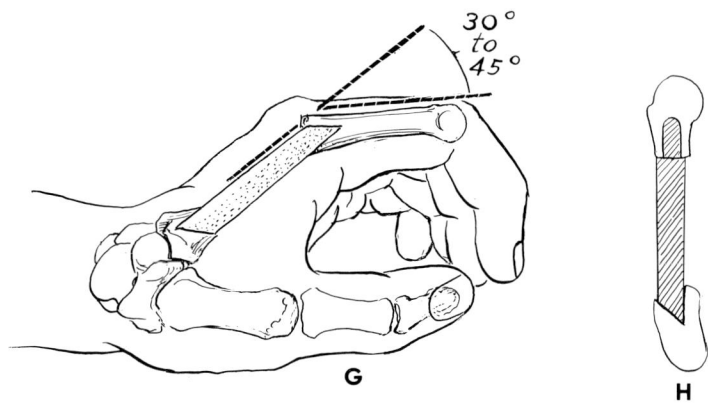

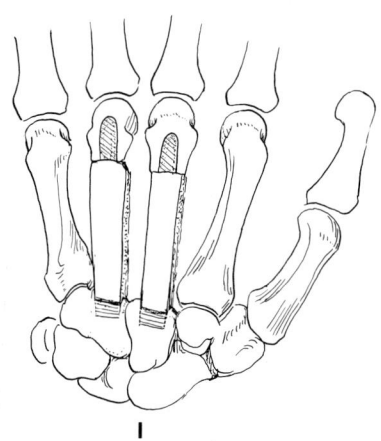

63 — Metacarpal Bone Grafting

THE THUMB METACARPAL

Principle

The absent thumb metacarpal or a thumb metacarpal with missing bone is a compelling indication for bone grafting. The technique is exactly that described for the finger metacarpals. If the metacarpal head is missing, the bone graft is fused to the proximal phalanx with a 30 degree angle of flexion. (**A**)

Example

The thumb metacarpal of a 35-year-old male was blown out by a gunshot wound but the thumb distal to the injury survived. The initial wound healed with marked contraction at the site of bone loss. A large abdominal pedicle flap was used to cover the defect left when scar excision was carried out. The thumb was held in traction to maintain its length during soft tissue reconstruction. A metacarpal bone graft was performed, using the technique described above. Positioning of the bone graft was determined by placing the thumb in full fist posture. (**B**) Stable union in this position resulted in good restoration of function. (**C**)

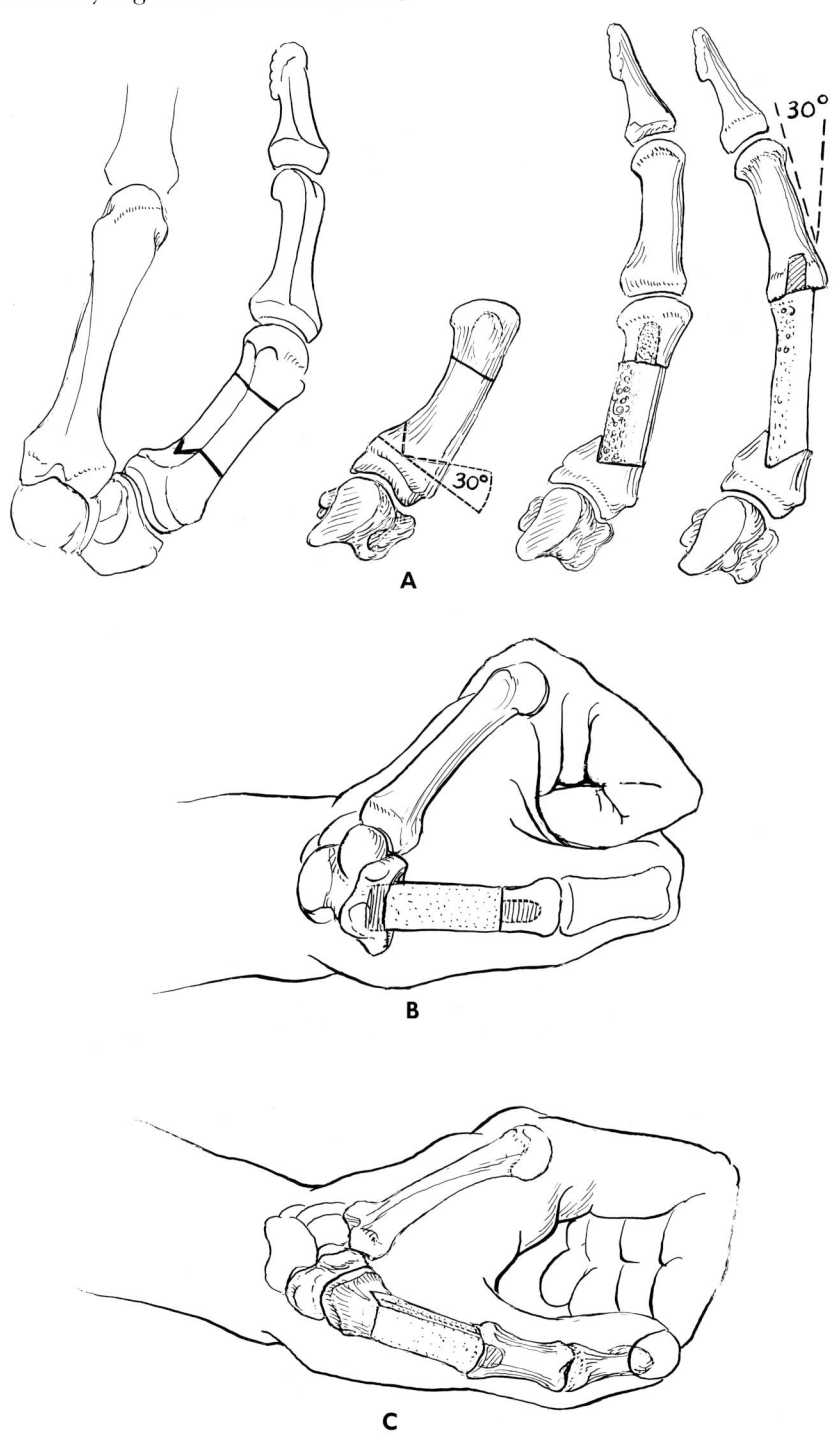

FIRST METACARPAL STABILIZATION

Bone blocks may be used to stabilize and fix the various mobile components of the transverse metacarpal arch.

For example, fixation of the thumb metacarpal for function of the thumb phalanges to flex against the other fingers is sometimes appropriate.

In paralytic states where there are no available muscles to position the thumb metacarpal for useful thumb function, a first web space bone block may be the best method for fixation of the positioned metacarpal to the stable index metacarpal. (**A** and **B**)

A block of cancellous bone may be fitted between the first and second metacarpals, with the first metacarpal in palmar abduction. (**C**) Kirschner wire fixation and external immobilization for eight to ten weeks will result in solid fixation of the previously mobile first metacarpal.

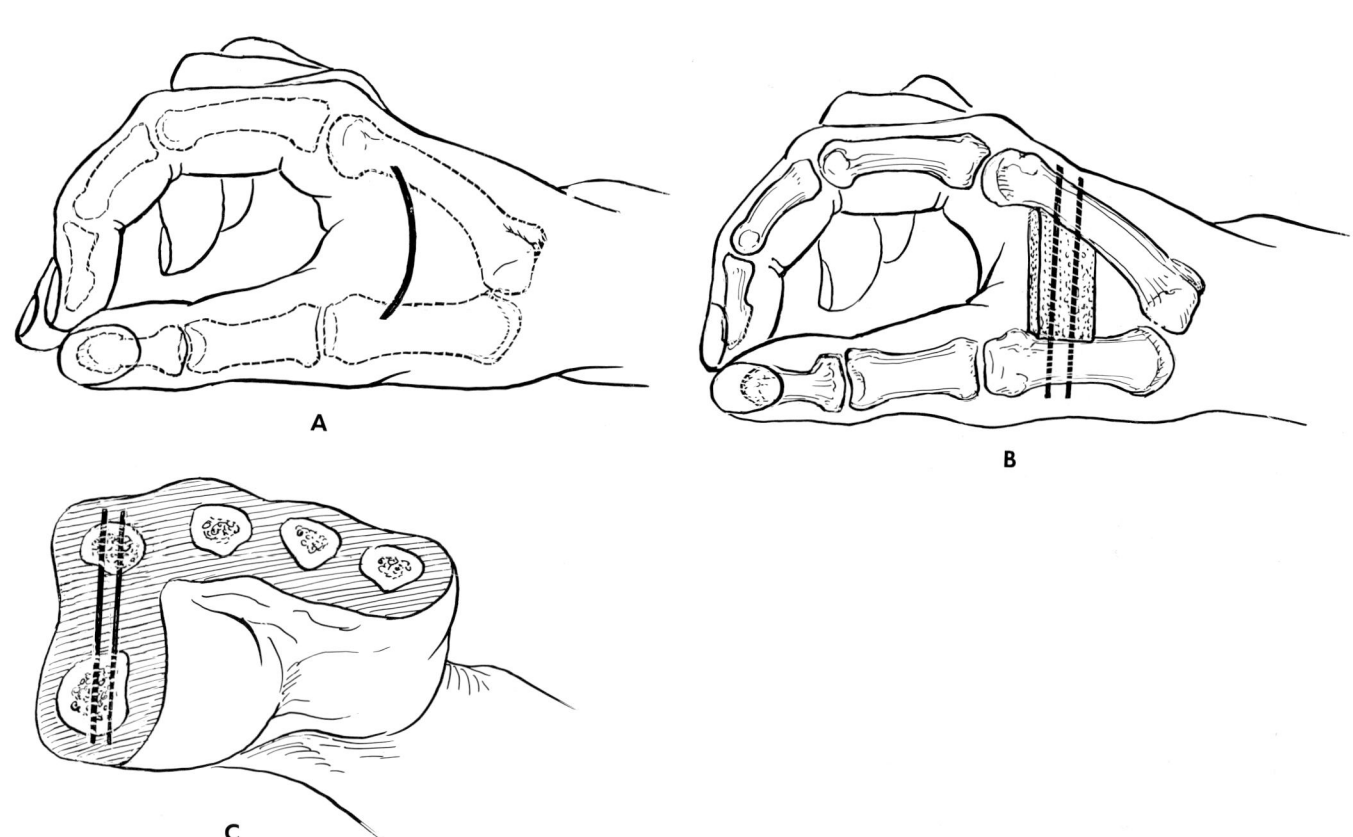

64

Fusion of Thumb Metacarpophalangeal Joint

Principles

Surgical fusion of joints in the hand is less frequently proposed than it was prior to the advent of synovectomy, arthroplasty, silastic spacers, and ingenious tendon transfers. Nonetheless, joint fusion, wisely applied, may improve function both by lending functional stability to the hand and by freeing active muscle tendon units for transfer to improve overall function.

Thumb

Among the joints most commonly chosen for surgical fusion is the thumb metacarpophalangeal joint. Its range of motion varies widely among individuals but when the carpometacarpal and interphalangeal joints are normal, it can be fused without creating a very significant reduction in function. The gain in function achieved by fusion of this joint is great when it is unstable, painful, or malpositioned because muscle pull is unbalanced by selected paralyses. The procedure is done in combination with tendon transfers for intrinsic muscular paralysis to augment thumb positioning function and to avoid recurvatum deformity at the metacarpophalangeal joint.

A dorsal incision longitudinally placed over the joint, or a gently curved incision dorsally and radially will provide good access to the joint. (**A**) The joint is entered radial to the extensor mechanism. (**B**) Enough of the joint capsule is cut to allow elective dislocation of the joint. (**C**)

The joint surfaces are removed using a small sharp osteotome. The surfaces are placed in a plane so that when the cut ends abut one another, the joint assumes the proper position desired for fusion. The thumb metacarpophalangeal joint should be fused at about 20 degrees of flexion and 5 to 10 degrees of pronation, a position assumed with the hand in a full fist position. (**D**) A longitudinal and an oblique Kirschner wire suffice to acquire stable internal fixation. The wires are cut short beneath the skin and the skin wound is closed. External plaster immobilization is maintained for about two months. A bone graft peg may be used for additional security for gaining union. Experience has shown that this joint will fuse quite reliably if one adheres rigorously to detail and insists on immobilization as described.

Additional raw bone to raw bone surface may be gained by a variety of bone carpentry methods, producing fitted angles or a ball and socket. (**E**)

Bone and Joint Reconstruction

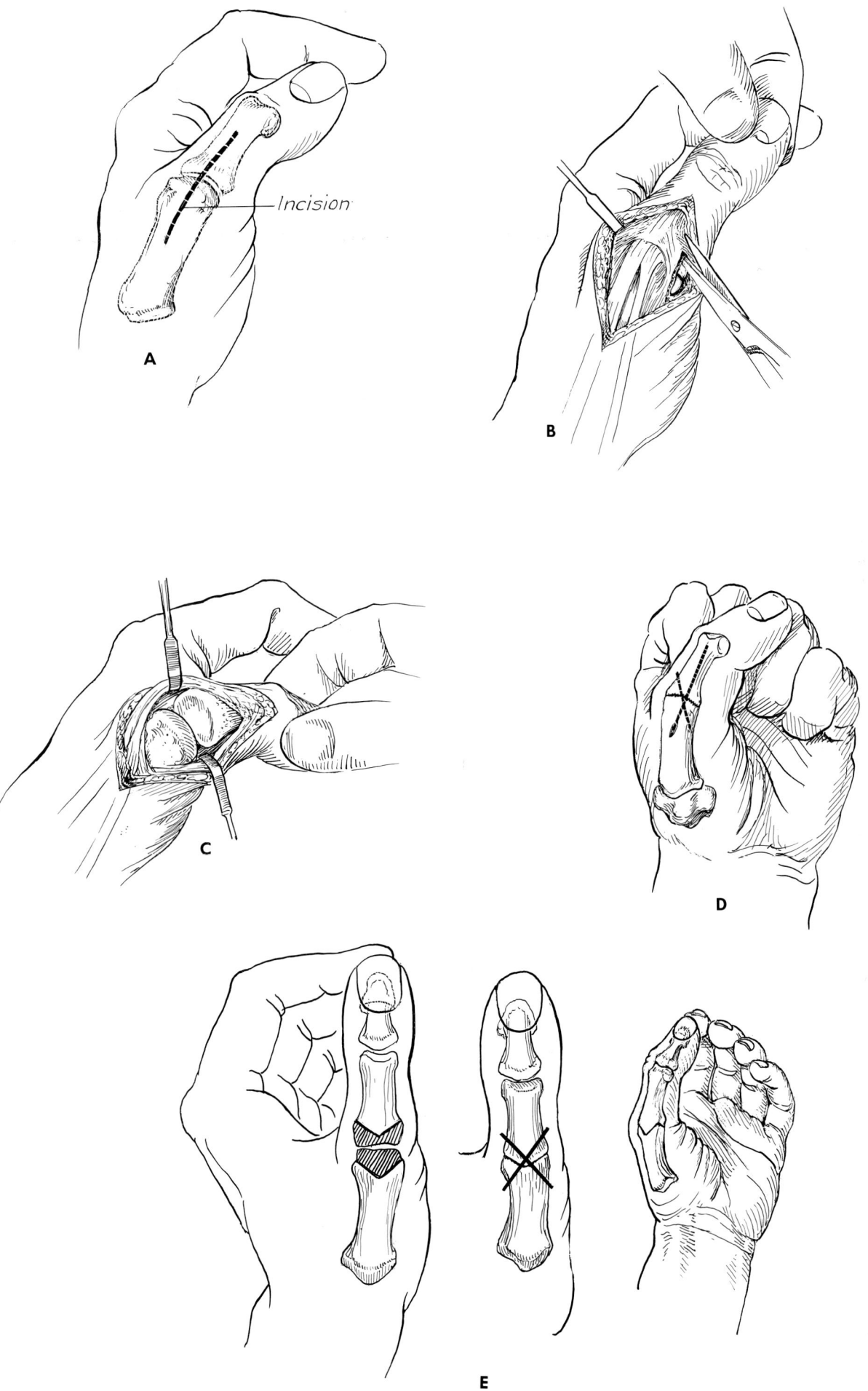

64 – Fusion of Thumb Metacarpophalangeal Joint

Example

A 60-year-old housewife with arthritis lost her capacity to pinch between her thumb and fingers bilaterally because of palmar subluxation and instability of her thumb metacarpophalangeal joints. Palmar subluxation made extension of the joint impossible. The interphalangeal joint was constantly held in hyperextension to attempt to compensate for metacarpophalangeal joint inability to extend. Lateral stability of the metacarpophalangeal joint was destroyed, and when pinching between the thumb and index finger was attempted, the thumb fell away to a radial deviated posture at the joint, making effective pinch impossible. (**F**)

The metacarpophalangeal joint of the left thumb was fused in a nearly straight position, with some pronation rotation. A bone peg fashioned from a bone graft taken from the ulna was placed into the medullary cavities of the metacarpal and proximal phalanx across the fusion site. (**G**) The stability thus gained was augmented by inserting one oblique Kirschner wire across the fusion site after rotation of the thumb into enough pronation for pulp-to-pulp opposition with the fingers.

After ten weeks of healing, the patient rapidly gained a powerful, effective pinch and was free of pain at the metacarpophalangeal joint. (**H**)

The right thumb was less deformed but after fusion of the left thumb, the function of the left thumb was vastly superior to that of the right. (**I**)

Subsequently, the patient elected to have fusion of the right thumb metacarpophalangeal joint.

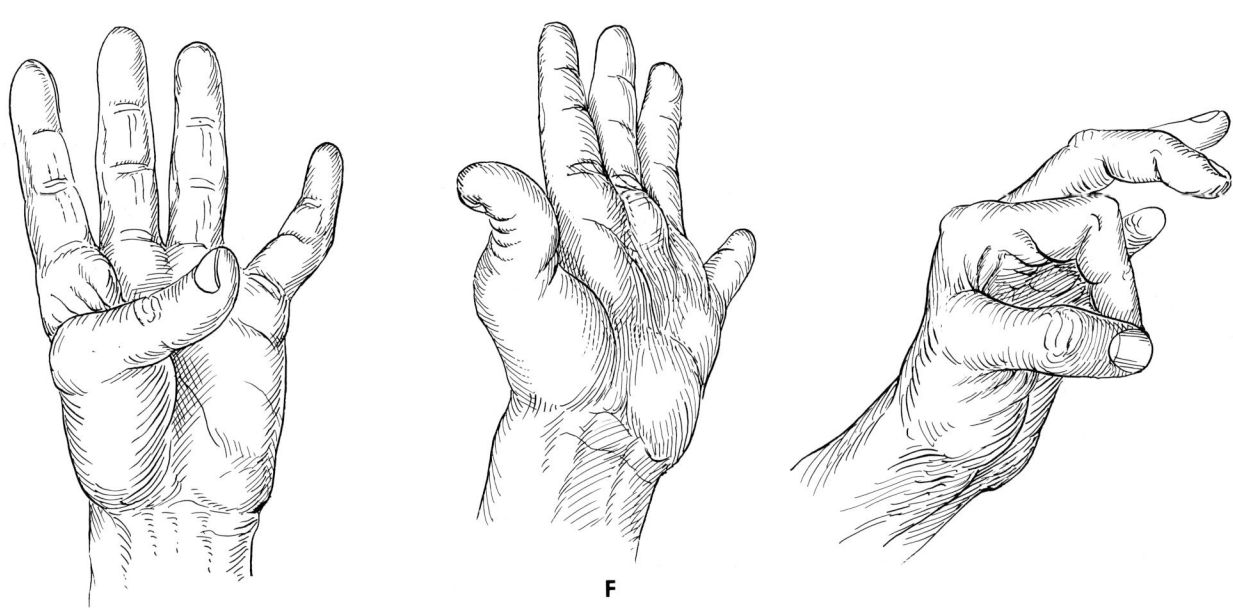

F

Bone and Joint Reconstruction

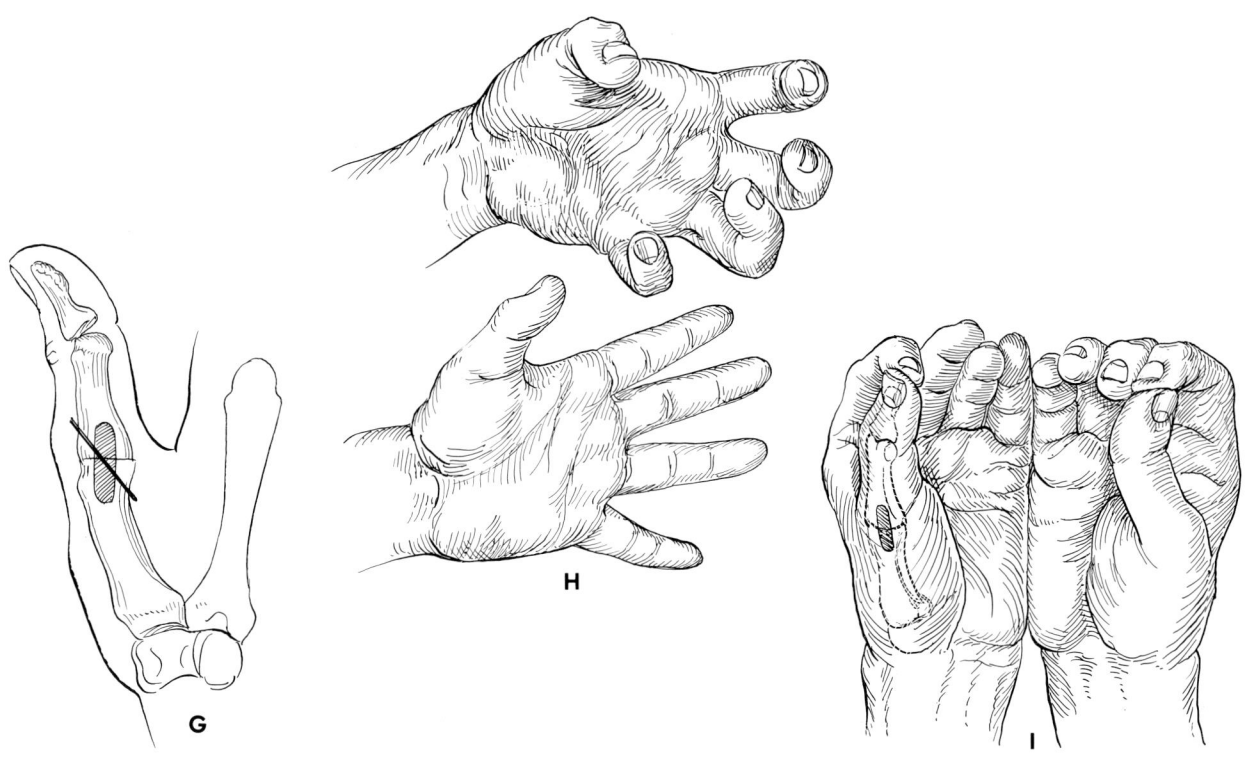

PREOPERATIVE   POSTOPERATIVE

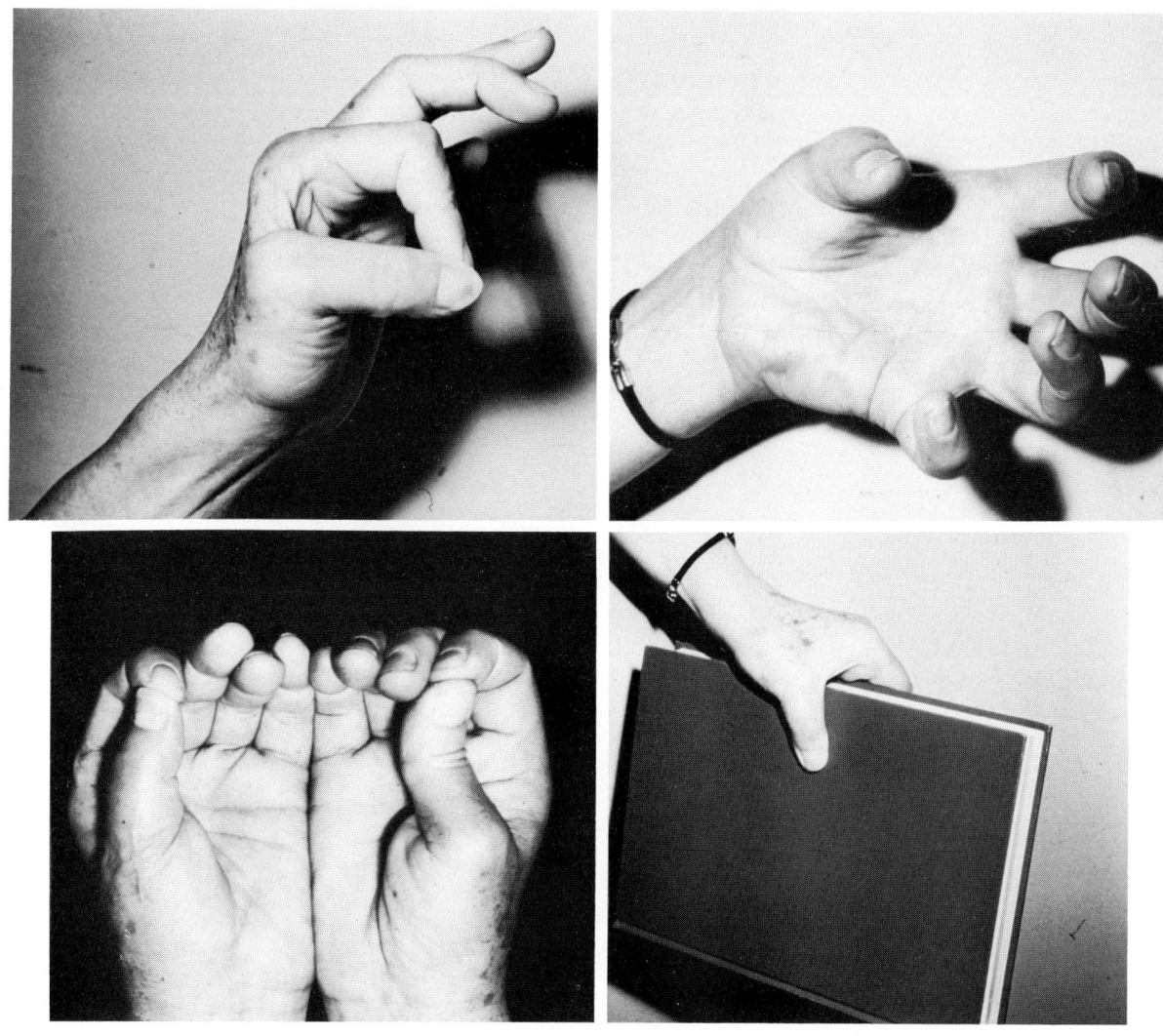

POSTOPERATIVE   PREOPERATIVE   POSTOPERATIVE

279

65

Fusion of Thumb Carpometacarpal Joint

Principle

The joint between the first metacarpal and trapezium is a saddle joint with lax capsular ligaments. It has a wide range of motion and is exposed to constant wear and tear. The joint is commonly disrupted in traumatic incidents and it is frequently in danger of destruction in arthritis. If the joint is very painful, the patient will hold the thumb against the stable hand or even carry the thumb in the clenched fingers. The range of abduction is lost quickly and the thumb becomes secondarily fixed to the side of the hand. Although arthroplasty and silastic implants are now used in the carpometacarpal joint, fusion still offers the greatest stability. It is particularly indicated if the other thumb joints are normal.

The position of fusion is the relationship of the first metacarpal to greater multangular assumed when one makes a tight fist.

The surgical approach to the joint may be made through the anatomical snuff box area, with care not to injure the dorsal branch of the radial nerve superficially and the radial artery deeply.

Example

A 45-year-old physician sustained a fracture dislocation (Bennett's fracture) of the right thumb carpometacarpal joint in a skiing accident. Repeated subsequent subluxation left the patient with a painful, unstable carpometacarpal joint. Fusion was chosen as a logical treatment.

A gently curved incision was planned over the anatomical snuff box and between the extensor pollicis longus and brevis. (**A**)

The dorsal branch of the radial nerve was observed and protected superficially and dissection was carried to the metacarpotrapezial joint, which was opened.

With the hand in ulnar deviation, the carpometacarpal joint was thrown out into the wound.

The joint surfaces were removed with a sharp osteotome, creating flat surfaces which would abut squarely with the first metacarpal in the relationship to the trapezium it assumed in a full fist position. (**B**)

By passively subluxating the joint, it was easily possible to drill a small hole in the trapezium and the proximal metacarpal to receive a small bone peg. (**C**)

A bone peg was readily procured from the proximal subcutaneous ulna, as described under bone graft donor sites. (See Section 61.) The bone peg was inserted into the metacarpal and then, by traction on the thumb, the fusion site was distracted enough for insertion of the protruding bone peg into the hole in the trapezium. (**D**)

Bone and Joint Reconstruction

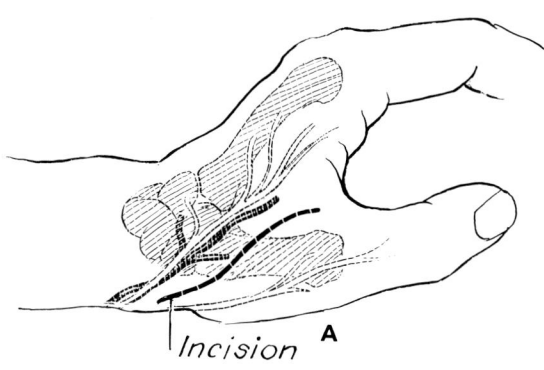

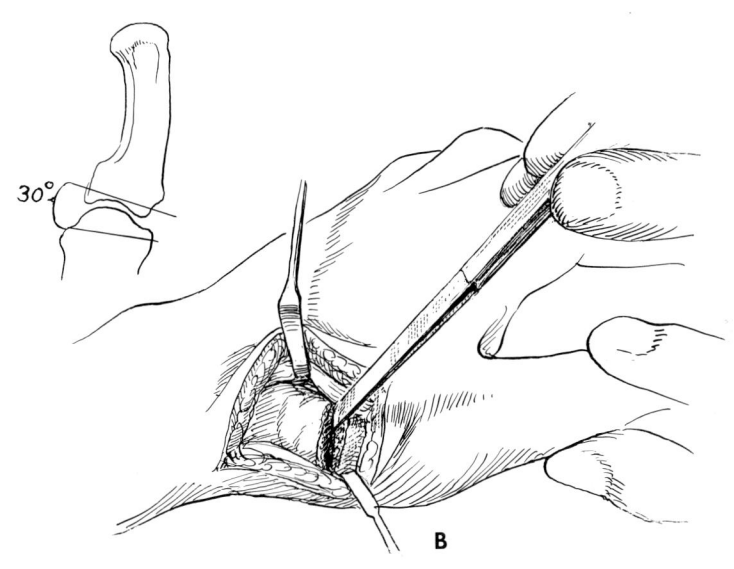

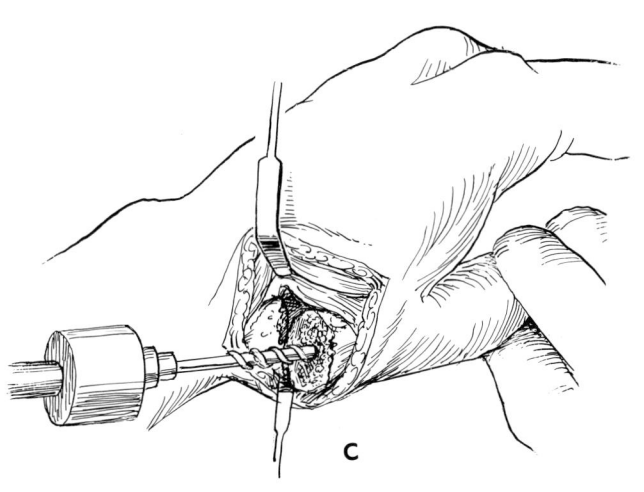

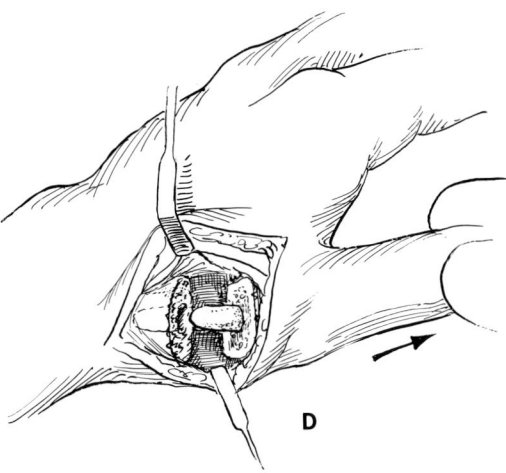

281

65 – Fusion of Thumb Carpometacarpal Joint

After the bone graft was inserted, a Kirschner wire across the fusion site gave further secure immobilization. (**E**)

External immobilization was rigorously maintained for ten weeks. Fusion was solid and the patient gained good strength and function without pain.

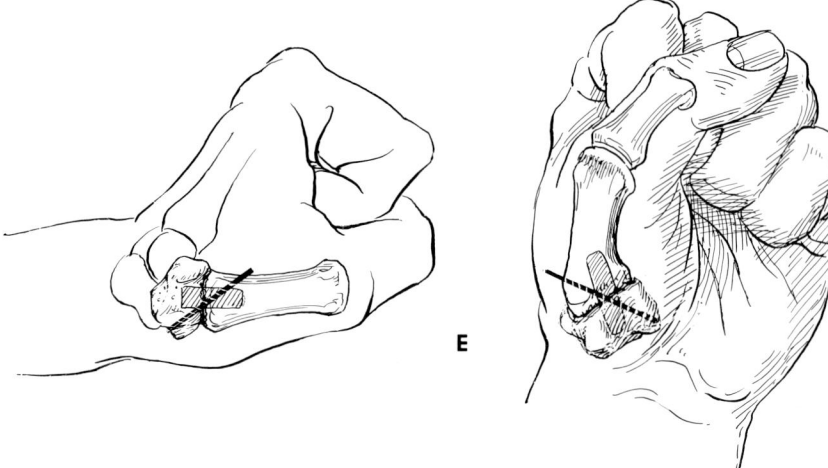

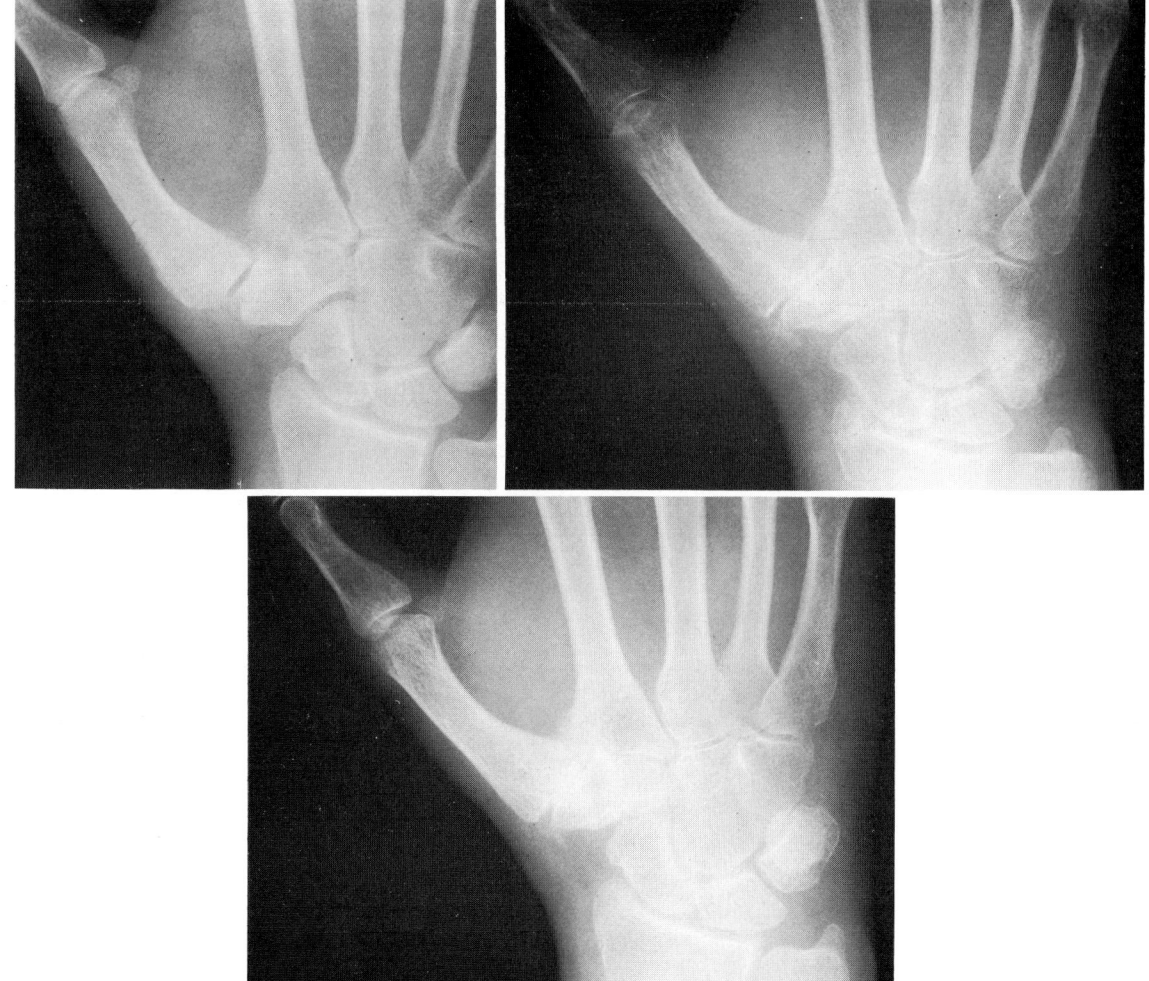

66
Fusion of Digital Joints

METACARPOPHALANGEAL JOINTS

Thumb

See Section 64.

Fingers

Fusion of finger metacarpophalangeal joints is rarely indicated. Arthroplasty and silastic prosthesis replacement have so many advantages for finger metacarpophalangeal joints that one or the other generally should be chosen over fusion. If a fusion must be done, it should be carried out in a manner similar to that described for the thumb. The position for fixation is determined by pulp-to-pulp pinch between the finger and the thumb. (**A**) The surgeon must pay strict attention to the rotation angle at the metacarpophalangeal joint to avoid the crossing of fingers in flexion.

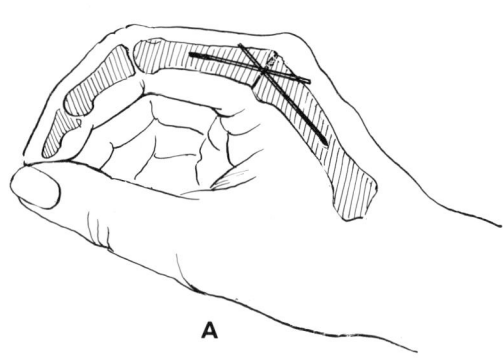

A

INTERPHALANGEAL JOINTS

Thumb

The interphalangeal joint of the thumb requires fusion fixation in rheumatoid disease when the joint support is destroyed and there is abnormal angulation which interferes with function. (**A**) In addition, the interphalangeal joint of the thumb may be fused to shift the primary influence of the flexor pollicis longus to the metacarpophalangeal joint. Occasionally injuries will destroy the extensor flexor tendon influence on the joint beyond repair and, if the joint is malpositioned or painful, it is best fused. To return optimum thumb pulp pinch the joint should be fused in 10 to 15 degrees of flexion. The joint may be approached through a dorsal longitudinal straight or gently curved incision. A mid-axial approach may also be used. (**B**) The joint is entered by sectioning across the extensor mechanism. The joint surfaces are removed at the proper angle with a small osteotome. To assure fusion, particularly in an arthritic, a bone peg should be placed across the fusion site. A square-edged bone peg is helpful in immobilizing the fusion site and in assuring that there is adequate local bone for union. Kirschner wire insertion further insures fixation. Sometimes deformity is such that both the M.P. and I.P. joints are best fused. (**C**)

Fingers

The proximal and distal interphalangeal joints may be fused by the technique described above. Fusion of the distal interphalangeal joints is commonly indicated in rheumatoid arthritis. Fusion of the distal interphalangeal joints is frequently very helpful to the patient in regaining pinch function. Fusion of the proximal interphalangeal joints is far less frequently indicated, particularly with the many procedures now available to mobilize fixed proximal interphalangeal joints and to alter muscle balance at this level.

When fusion of interphalangeal joints is indicated, the flexion angle is determined by positioning the finger in pulp-to-pulp pinch with the thumb. (**D, E** and **F**)

Rotation angle must be carefully controlled to avoid collision with other fingers or crossing of fingers in flexion. (See Section 59.)

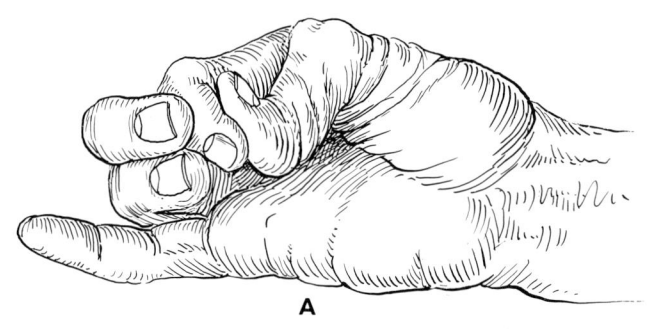

A

Bone and Joint Reconstruction

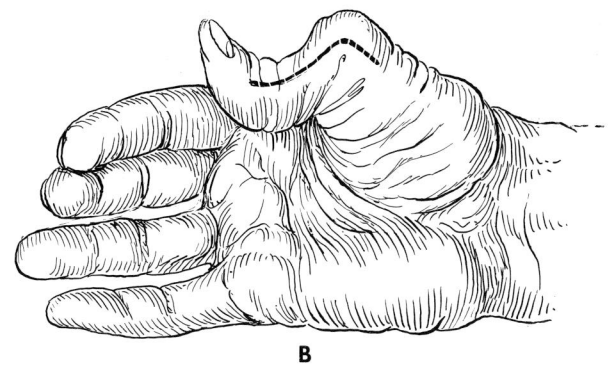

B

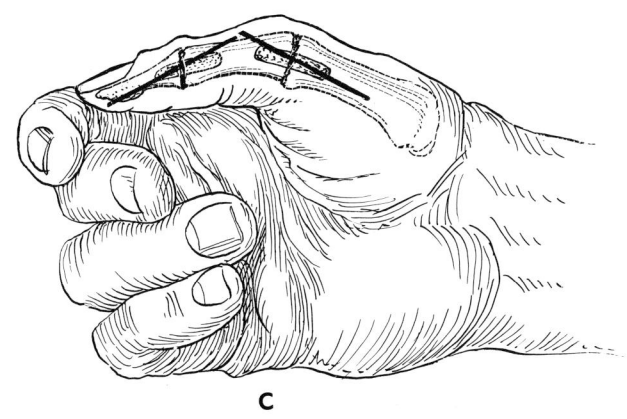

C

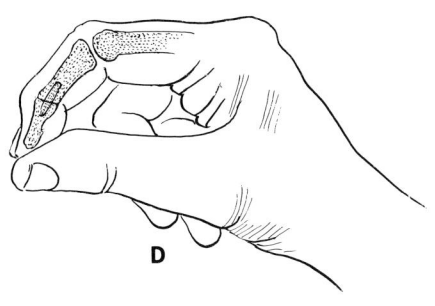

D

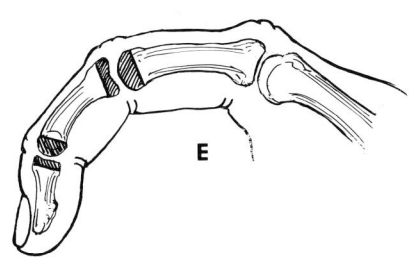

E

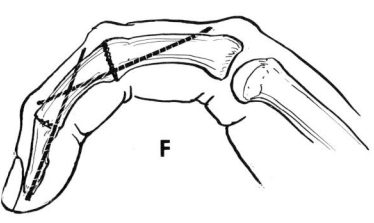

F

66 — Fusion of Digital Joints

Example

A crush injury of the right index finger was sustained by a 35-year-old female patient. It resulted in disruption of the distal interphalangeal joint and loss of skin and soft tissue. Healing with contraction of the wound resulted in ulnar deviation of the distal phalanx and poor skin and soft tissue coverage with an unstable scar. (**G**)

Fusion of the distal joint in a position of function would restore functional pinch. Proper skin and soft tissue cover is an absolute prerequisite for joint fusion; therefore, distal interphalangeal joint fusion coupled with a cross finger pedicle flap was elected as the best treatment.

The scar was excised and the distal interphalangeal joint was exposed. Osteotomies to remove the proximal distal joint surfaces were done using small sharp osteotomes. The osteotomies were made in such a way that with the osteotomies in coaptation the tip of the finger was in normal position for pulp-to-pulp pinch with the thumb. (**H**)

A small bone peg was fashioned from the subcutaneous ulna. (See Section 61.) The peg was placed across the fusion site into the medullary cavity of the middle and distal phalanges.

With the finger properly positioned, a Kirschner wire was passed through the distal phalanx and across the fusion site into the dorsal cortex of the middle phalanx. (**I**)

The soft tissue defect over the fusion on the dorsal ulnar aspect of the index finger was covered by a cross-finger pedicle flap from the adjacent long finger. (**J**) (See technique in Section 13.)

The fingers were immobilized in the connected position for three and a half weeks after which the pedicle from the long finger was sectioned and the flap was fitted into the remaining defect in the index finger. (**K**)

The index finger was kept splinted for eight weeks, after which graded activity was allowed. The patient's ability to manipulate objects and pinch with the thumb and index finger was greatly improved. (**L**)

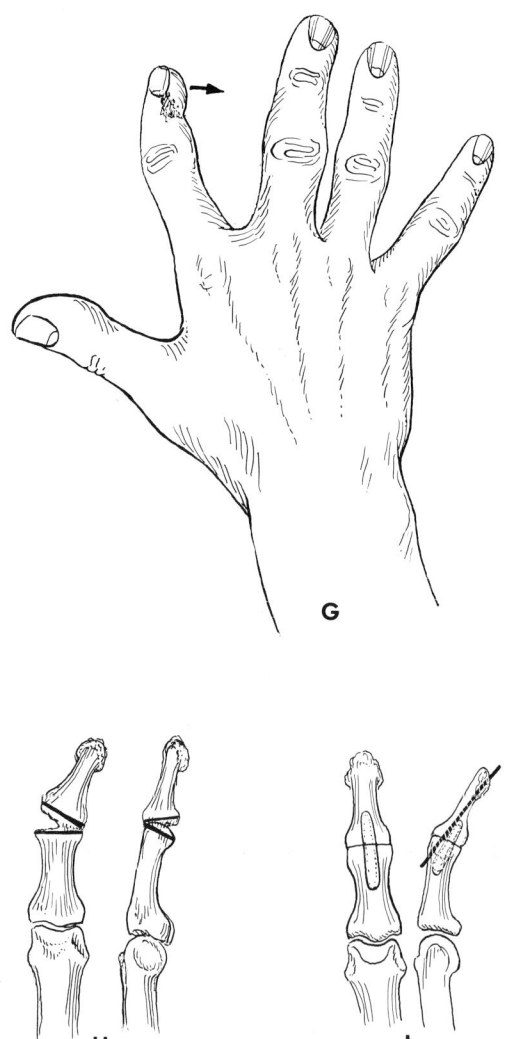

Bone and Joint Reconstruction

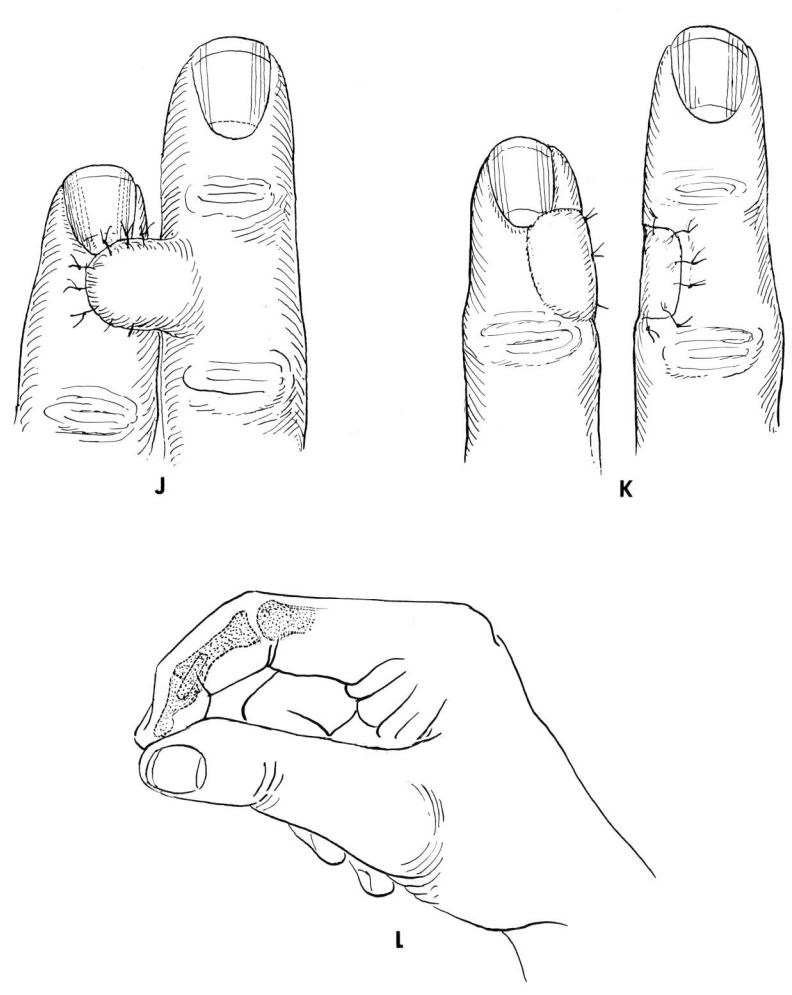

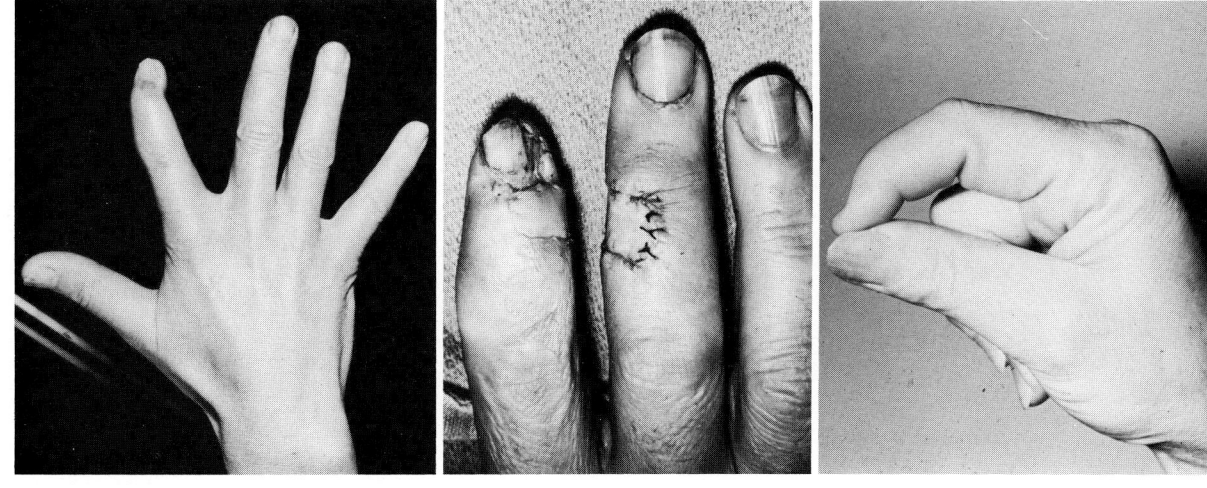

287

67

Fusion of the Wrist Joint

Principle

A wrist which is painful on motion and which is destroyed to the point of uncontrollable subluxation will only be stable enough to withstand major stress if it is fused.

The central fixed unit of the hand beyond the wrist consists of the second and third metacarpals. A fusion of the wrist is complete only if there is solid union across the carpus from the radius to these two metacarpals.

A bone graft across this area produces the most reliable fusion. Iliac bone with a rather thin cortex and associated cancellous bone is best adapted for the purpose.

If both wrists are to be fused, a procedure infrequently indicated in my view, the dominant one should be fused in 15 or 20 degrees of extension and the other in a nearly straight position or even flexed a few degrees. The pattern of fusion should be carefully worked out with each patient, taking into serious account the patient's desires and needs.

Temporary fixation of the wrist with a large pin may be tried prior to fusion so that the patient may better understand the disadvantages as well as the advantages of fusion.

Example

A 52-year-old woman with advanced rheumatoid arthritis developed severe palmar subluxation of both wrists at the radiocarpal joints. (**A**)

Fusion of the left wrist was elected.

A dorsal linear curved incision longitudinally oriented and a bit to the ulnar side of center allowed adequate exposure.

The extensor tendons were dislocated from their tunnels, which were unroofed over the wrist dorsum by excision of the dorsal retinaculum. The wrist dislocation was reduced.

A recipient bed was outlined, which created a seat in the distal radius, crossed the carpus, and extended about 2 cm. into the bases of the second and third metacarpals. (**B**)

The extensor carpi radialis longus and brevis were released from their insertions.

Once the neutral wrist position was decided upon, a trough of bone on the dorsal cortical surface of the distal radius and carpal bones was removed with the wrist held in the chosen position. Enough bone was removed to accommodate a bone graft. The removed cancellous bone was saved to pack into the joints and around the graft. The radiocarpal joint was vigorously curetted to remove joint cartilage surfaces, and bits of cancellous bone were forced into the old joint space. (**C**)

An osteotome inserted distally in the depths of the recipient site was advanced into the bases of the second and third metacarpals. The resulting split was widened enough to receive the thinned end of the bone graft. (**D**)

A bone graft was taken from the iliac crest area. The deep surface cortex was removed as part of the graft while the superficial cortex was left in situ. By careful examination of the iliac crest a portion with about the right curve was found, outlined, and removed with an osteotome and mallet.

The bone graft was shaped precisely to fit the recipient bed and it was thinned to consist almost solely of cortex at the distal end. It was tapped into place in the split in the base of the metacarpals with the wrist flexed. (**E**)

Bone and Joint Reconstruction

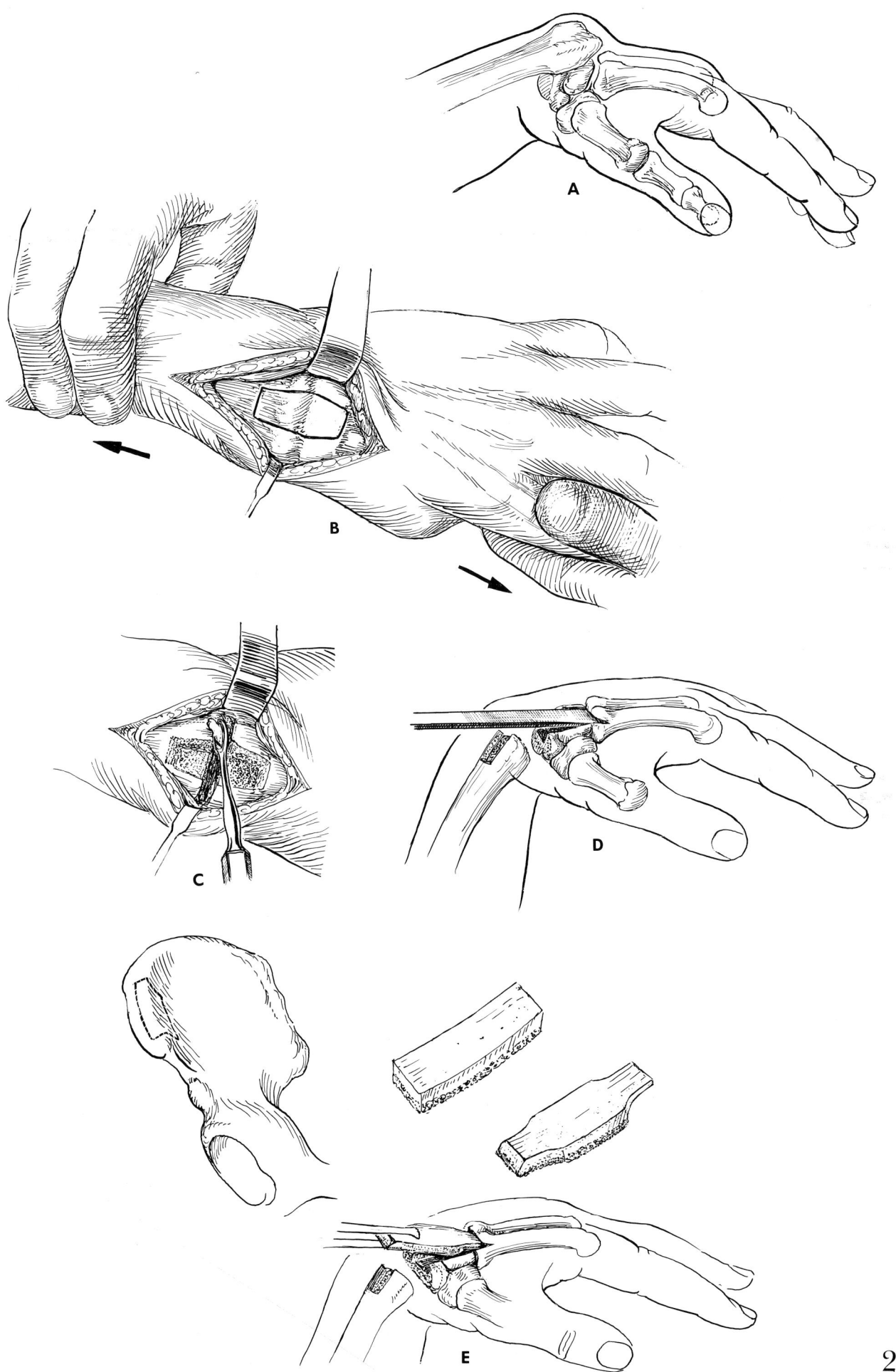

67 — Fusion of the Wrist Joint

The bone graft was inserted in place across the created carpus trench and into the seat in the distal radius as the wrist was brought into neutral position. (**F**)

A large pin placed through the second metacarpal and into the distal radius was used to stabilize the wrist in proper position. The bone graft did not require further internal fixation.

Residual soft tissue was closed over the bone graft, and the tendons were allowed to fall into their natural position. (**G**)

A dressing and immobilizing plaster splint was applied and left for about ten days. After this, the wound was inspected and the splint was replaced by a snug plaster cast from the metacarpophalangeal joints to just below the elbow. Eight to ten weeks of strict immobilization followed. Solid fusion resulted. (**H**)

With fusion across the wrist of radius carpals and second and third metacarpals the anatomical back bone of the hand is solidly fixed. Motion is preserved in the first metacarpal, with its wide range of motion, and in the fourth and fifth metacarpals, with their more limited mobility. (**I**)

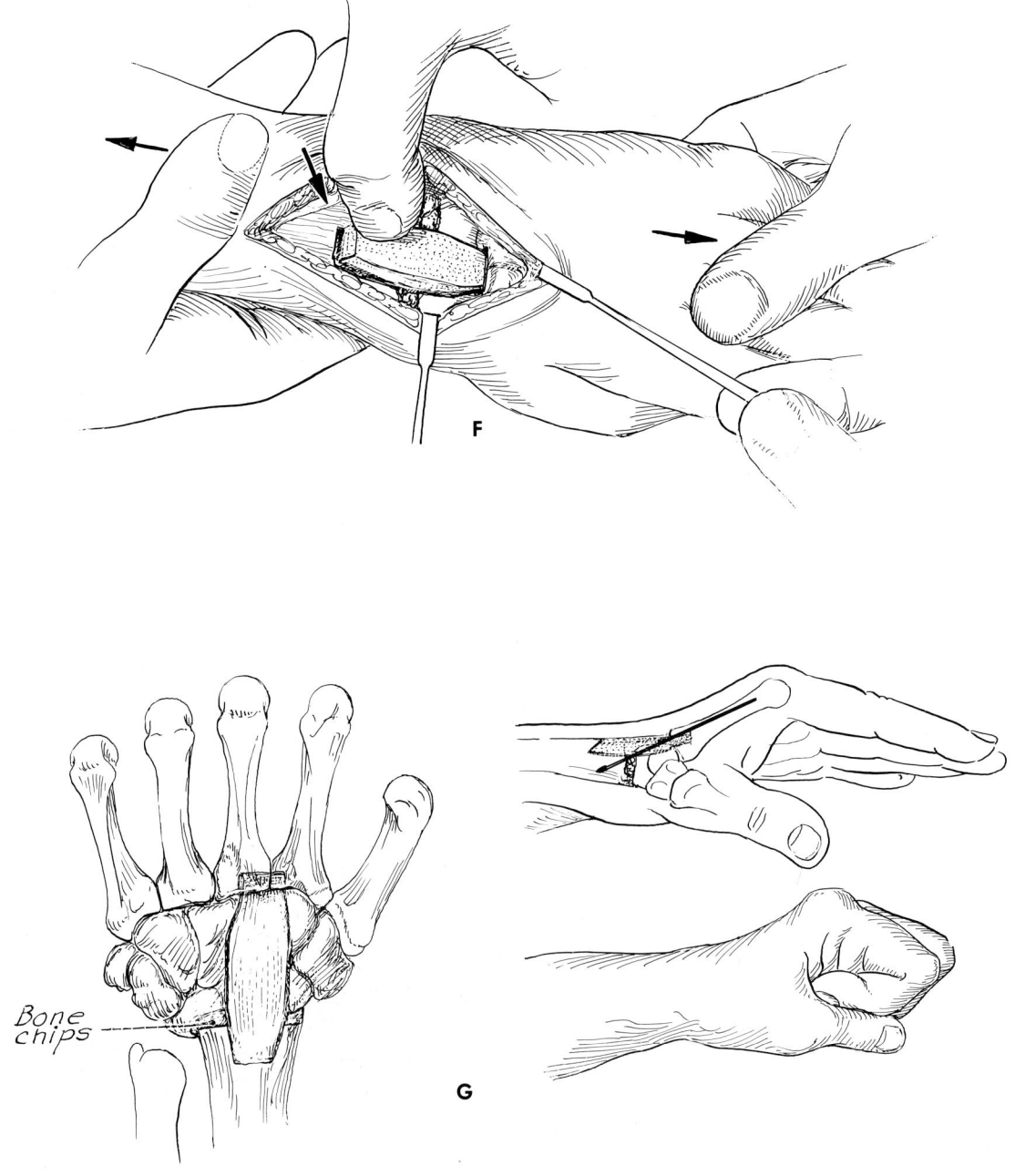

290

1

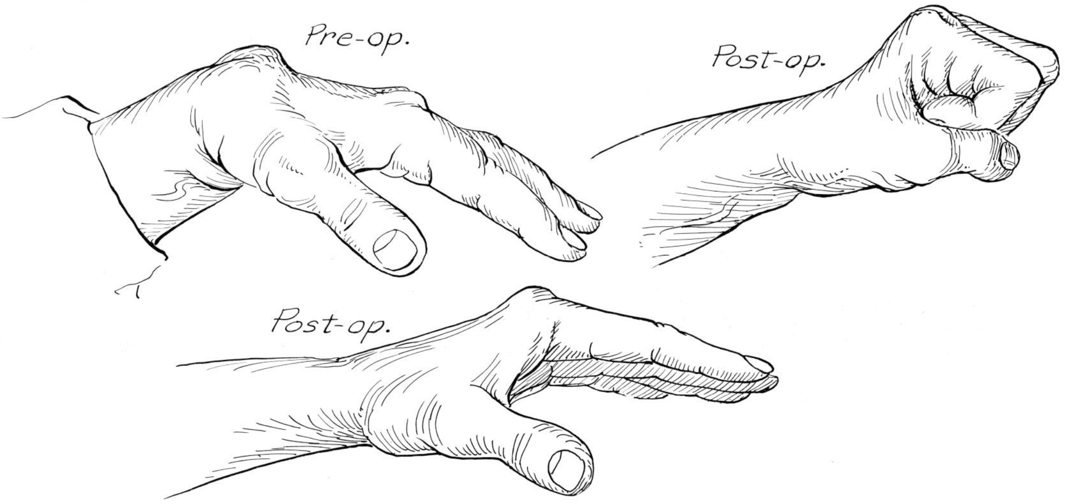

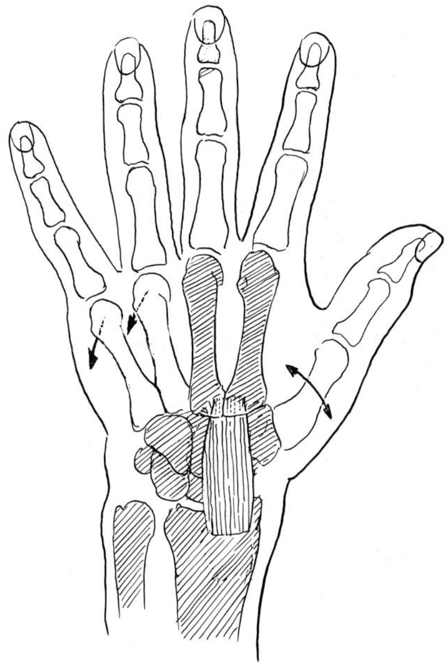

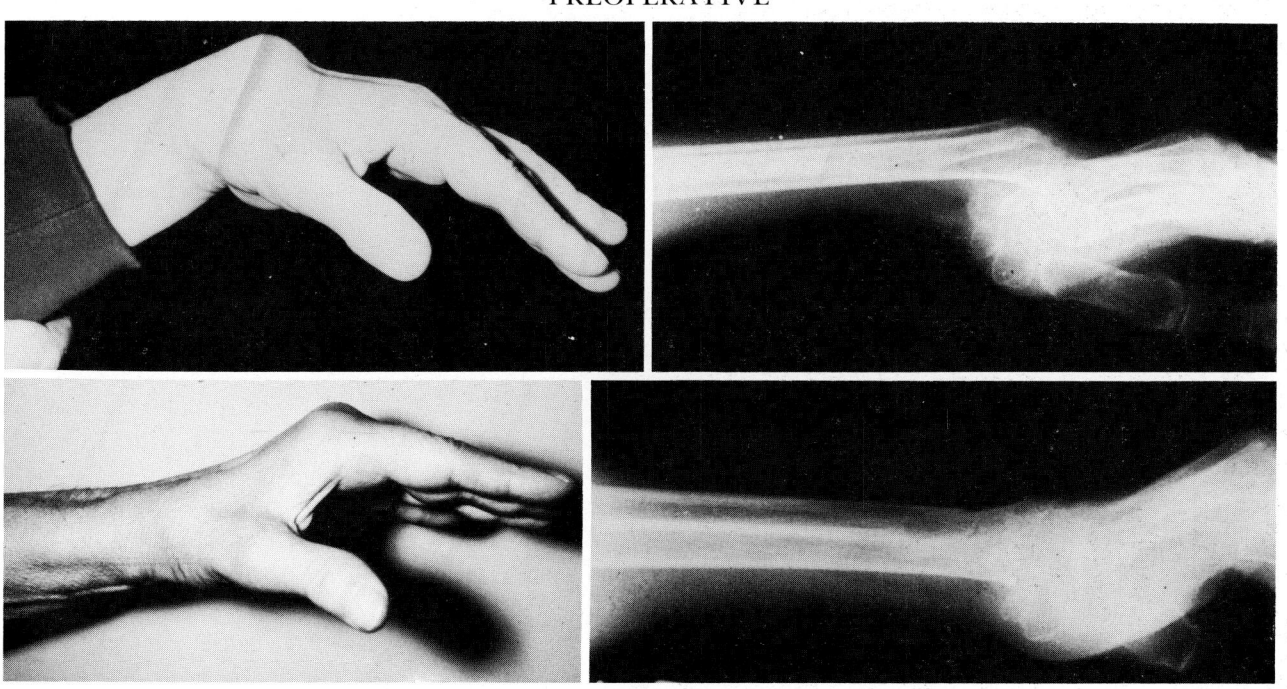

PREOPERATIVE

POSTOPERATIVE

Reconstruction of the Thumb

68

Reconstruction of the Thumb

The compleat hand surgeon must be well aware of the many procedures which will improve function in the thumb after it has been disabled or amputated. The ideal thumb is mobile over a wide range, with stability in any position lent to it by the dynamic tension of opposing muscle groups. It must be of adequate length to act against the fingers and palm, and it must have oppositional capability. Critical sensibility in the thumb is a key to man's ability to assess objects touched and to afford protection of the thumb from injury. Ideally, the thumb should look normal and should possess a nail. Injury or amputation reduces the thumb in varying degrees from this ideal.

The surgeon's time is generally well invested if he can help the patient overcome some of the elements responsible for thumb disability. Thumb mobility is dependent upon intact functional joints, adequate soft tissues and skin (especially in the first web space) and free-moving tendons. Stability and dynamic positioning of the thumb depend upon joint capsules and ligaments as well as intact innervated extrinsic and intrinsic muscles with their tendons. When muscle tendon function is lost or ligaments are disrupted, selected tendon transfers or joint fusions must be done to restore stability and positioning capability. These problems have been addressed elsewhere in this atlas.

Subtotal Amputation of the Thumb

A shortened thumb may function quite adequately to meet the needs of many individuals. If any part of the proximal phalanx remains, the thumb nub with intact sensibility may be opposed by intact index and long fingers. (**A**) Manipulation of buttons and small objects is possi-

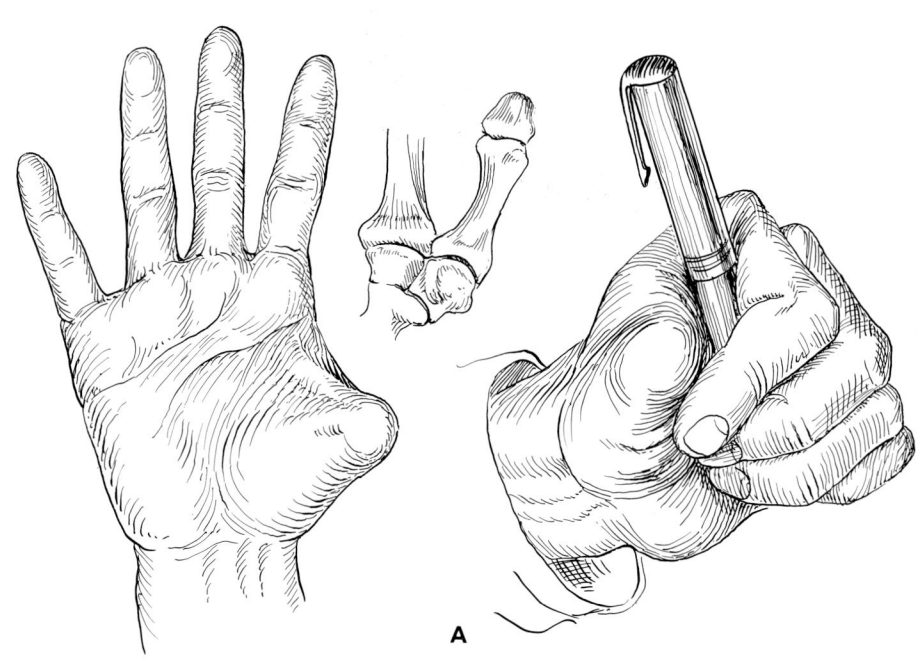

68 — Reconstruction of the Thumb

ble but the performance of such activities is rather clumsy. (**B**) The thin hand with long fingers functions better after thumb loss at this level than does the stubby fat hand.

If function is not satisfactory to the patient, one may choose surgically to deepen the web space or to add length to the thumb by ingenious local surgery.

Local Soft Tissue Advancement and Bone Graft

A limited addition to thumb length may be achieved by advancing a cap of local skin and subcutaneous tissue on a pedicle. The incision is placed well proximal over the mid-metacarpal area. It is a curved, transverse incision circumscribing the dorsal two-thirds of the metacarpal. This leaves a palmar pedicle for blood supply. The whole caplike flap is advanced distally to expose the bone amputation site. The bone end is freshened and extended by inserting a bone graft. The length of the graft is limited by the extent of soft tissue advancement acquired by the pedicle advance. The bone graft preferably is cancellous but may be cortical and is fixed with a Kirschner wire.

The pedicle cap is seated snugly over the graft to avoid any dead space and is sutured down to dorsal fascia leaving a dorsal elliptical defect. A free full thickness or thick split thickness skin graft is applied to the flap donor area. A tie-over stent dressing may be used over the graft if it is carefully applied in a manner which will not impede blood flow in the pedicle. After six or eight weeks of healing, the patient is allowed progressively to use the thumb.

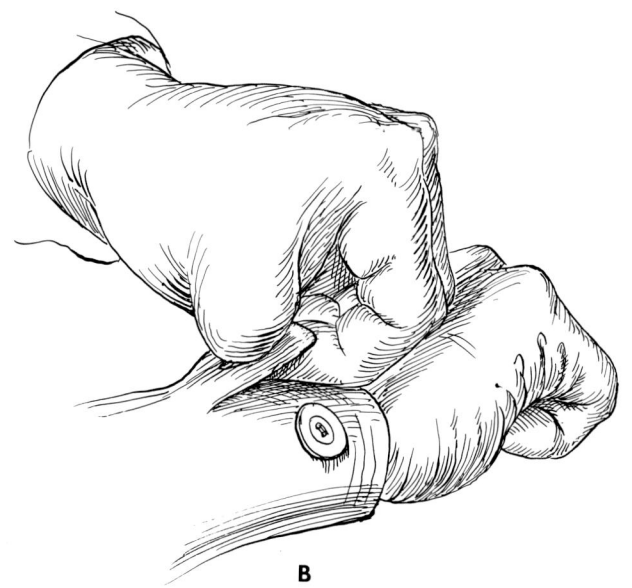

B

Reconstruction of the Thumb

Deepening the First Web Space

Subtotal amputation of the thumb which leaves the entire first metacarpal intact may be improved functionally by deepening the first web space. In effect, this phalangizes the distal metacarpal to create a space to receive objects to be held or picked up between the short thumb and the adjacent metacarpal. It also removes some of the tethering effect of the web space soft tissues and thus liberates the first metacarpal, to allow some additional range of motion.

Deepening of the first web space is a very contributory element in the rehabilitation of individuals who have suffered loss of the thumb and all fingers. The effect of deepening the first web space under these circumstances is augmented by amputation of the second metacarpal to widen as well as deepen the space between the thumb metacarpal and the rest of the hand. There is a compelling indication when all fingers and thumbs are lost on both hands.

Example

A fifty-year-old female patient, victim of a severe frostbite injury, sustained amputation of both thumbs through the proximal phalanx and all fingers at the level of the metacarpophalangeal joints. (**C**) The patient's function was sharply reduced and her best effective prehension was performed by using one hand against the other.

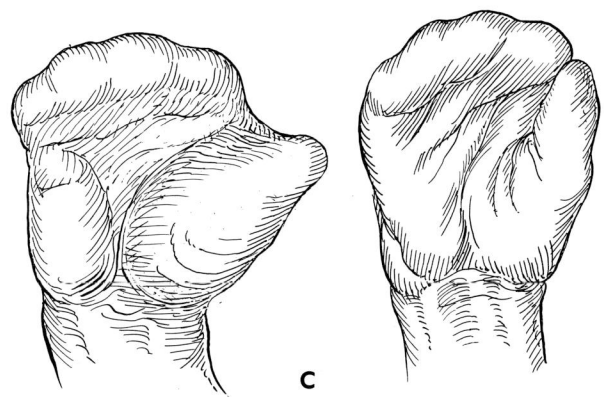

68 – Reconstruction of the Thumb

Two years after injury, the patient elected to undergo surgical phalangization of the first metacarpal and creation of a substantial cleft between it and the rest of her right hand by amputation of the second metacarpal. Skin and soft tissue coverage in the hand was adequate, and the patient was capable of moving the first metacarpal through a full range of motion.

Incisions were planned to construct a web flap for the base of the projected web space to avoid a scar which would restrain spreading of the cleft to encompass large objects. The flap was designed with its proximal base on the dorsum of the hand and its tip at the leading edge of the existing web. On the palmar aspect, a linear incision was planned from the midpoint of the leading edge of the web to the palm, at a point projected as just proximal to the midpoint of the planned new deepened web space. (**D**) Since the second metacarpal was to be amputated, this point was placed over the proximal position of this bone. The laterally based flaps created by this linear incision were planned so that they could be used to resurface the opposing sides of the new cleft.

The dorsal incisions were made, and the soft tissue over the second metacarpal was elevated to expose the second metacarpal. The periosteum over the second metacarpal was incised, and the metacarpal was amputated in the manner described under index ray amputation (see Section 33). The first dorsal interosseous muscle, which was somewhat atrophic, was allowed to fall back into the wound where it added soft tissue padding over the third metacarpal. (**E**) Had the first dorsal interosseous created any impingement in the planned cleft it would have been partially resected. The adductor pollicis attachment to the first metacarpal was recessed from the distal metacarpal for one and one-half centimeters and the muscle was pressed against the first metacarpal over sufficient length to phalangize three or four centimeters of the metacarpal.

The palmar linear incision was made and then progressively lengthened as dissection continued, and the dorsal flap was pulled through the cleft to measure how far proximal it would reach. Once that was determined, a transverse incision was made to receive the squared end of the dorsal flap. The palmar flaps were then undermined to allow closure of the skin over the opposing surfaces of the new cleft. The dorsal flap was sutured in place, (**F**) and the lateral flaps were adjusted and closed. (**G**)

Healing occurred promptly and the patient gained new capabilities in prehensile function. She elected to have a similar procedure done for the left hand six months later.

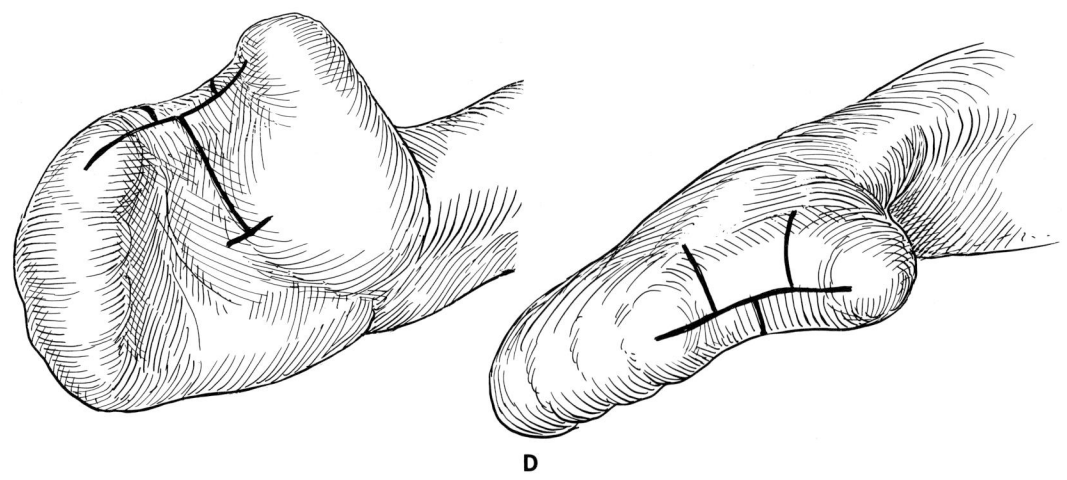

D

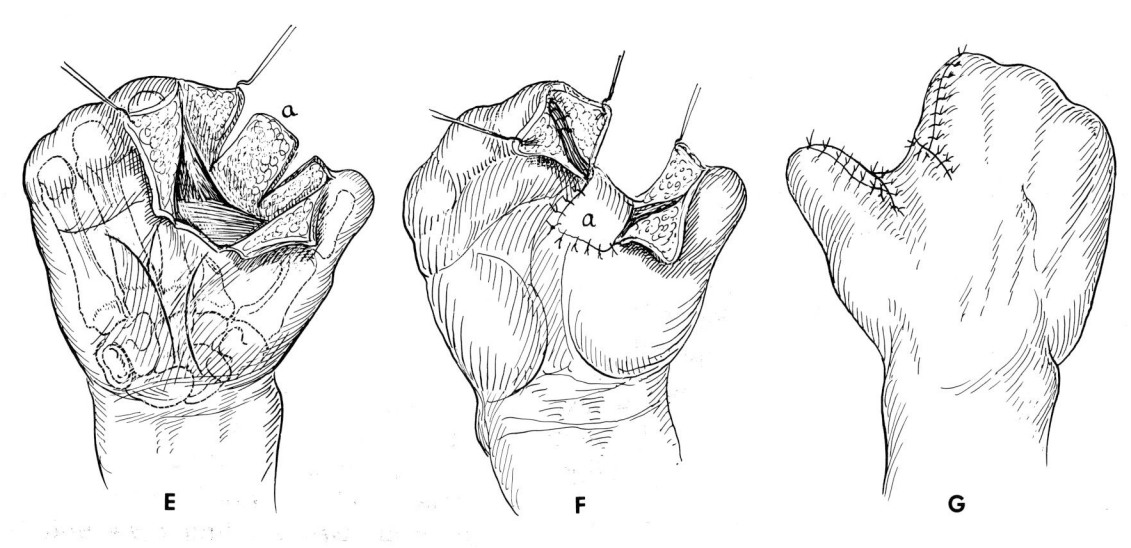

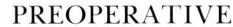

PREOPERATIVE POSTOPERATIVE

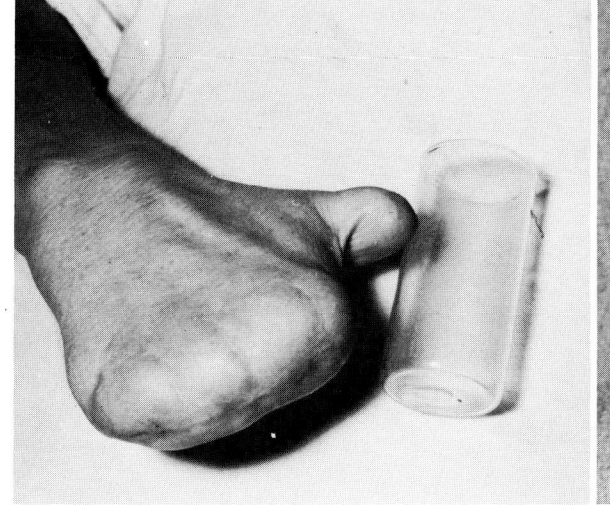
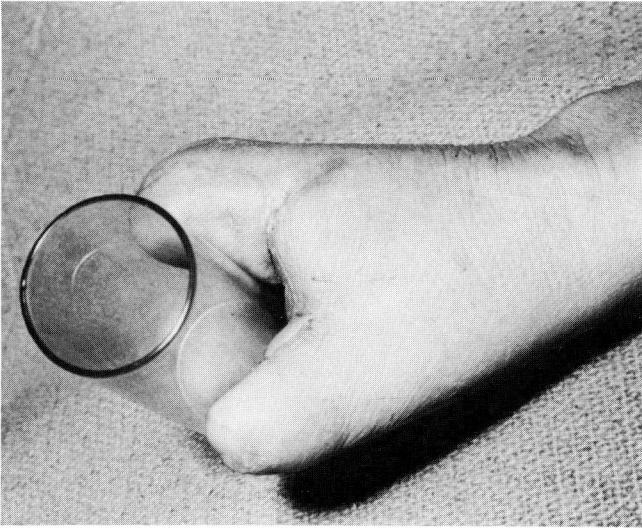

69
Thumb Reconstruction by Pollicization

Principle

A finger may be transferred to the thumb position to substitute for absence of the thumb. Each of the four fingers in the hand has been used at one time or another as a thumb substitute. Of the four fingers the index is most preferable in my view. Since Littler refined the pollicization procedure, it has become the standard technique for thumb reconstruction for total thumb loss and for most losses proximal to the metacarpophalangeal joint. It is the only reasonable procedure for reconstruction after total amputation loss of the thumb or in cases of congenital absence of the thumb ray.

When the loss is subtotal with an intact carpometacarpal articulation and functioning thenar muscles, considerable thought must be given to the decision for pollicization versus tubed flap bone graft island pedicle reconstruction or other less spectacular procedures. When the contralateral thumb is sound, the patient's functional needs may not require any surgical reconstruction.

POLLICIZATION FOR SUBTOTAL THUMB LOSS

Patients who have sustained amputation of the thumb at the metacarpophalangeal joint or across the metacarpal must be carefully evaluated to determine the indication for surgical thumb reconstruction. The patient's need for a mobile, sensitive, functional oppositional unit may be the indication for pollicization. Any finger in the hand may be transferred to the thumb position, but the numerous virtues of the index finger for this purpose make it reasonable to describe the technique for index finger pollicization in this volume.

Careful measurement and design of skin flaps and osteotomy sites will pay great dividends as one assesses the final result. Incisions are planned in such a way that the projecting index finger after transfer will extend peripherally to the proximal interphalangeal joint level of the long finger. Measurement may be made by placing the hands together and measuring the length necessary to match the normal thumb length.

When the index finger itself is damaged and has reduced function, the indication for its use may be even clearer, since sacrifice of a finger with reduced function is less significant than loss of a normal finger.

Scars which cross the web space from the reconstructed thumb to the long finger should be broken up to avoid scar contracture which will limit the range of motion of the reconstructed thumb.

The index finger is transferred, preserving its proper digital vessels and nerves, the dorsal branches of the radial nerve, the flexor and extensor tendons and a dorsal vein. The proper digital vessels to the radial side of the long finger must be ligated and cut to allow mobilization of the index finger. The proper digital nerve is carefully preserved but is split away from the proper digital nerve to the long finger proximal enough into the common digital nerve to allow free mobility of the index finger for shift to the thumb position. The first dorsal interosseous muscle is retracted at its insertion into the index finger and, after the finger is shifted, the muscle insertion is transferred to the long finger lateral band.

Example

A fifteen-year-old boy had sustained an amputation of his right thumb in a traumatic incident four months before consultation. Amputation occurred at the metacarpophalangeal joint, and no significant residual soft tissue defect existed. (**A**) The patient elected reconstruction of the thumb by pollicization of the index finger of his dominant hand.

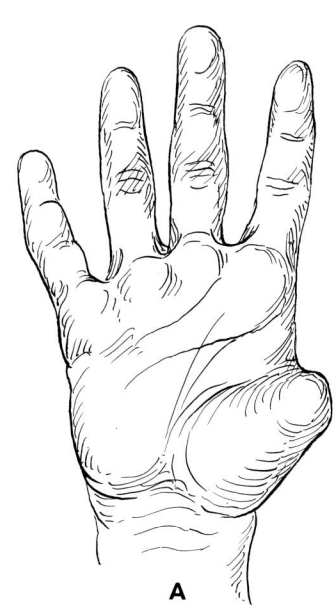

X-rays of both hands were taken for use in planning the osteotomy sites across the proximal phalanx of the index finger and first metacarpal to reconstruct a thumb of proper length, leaving sufficient bone for a proper mortise to add stabilization during healing. (**B**)

An incision to resect the amputation scar was marked out. An incision circumscribing the index finger over the proximal portion of the proximal phalanx measured back from the tip to give the thumb proper length was also marked out. An incision to join the two was planned as W-shaped and curvilinear to avoid a scar straight across the leading edge of the first web space. (**C**) First web space structures were exposed by dissecting in the areolar subcutaneous plane. A dorsal vein and branches of the dorsal branch of the radial nerve to the index finger were preserved.

Dissection around to the palmar aspect of the first dorsal interosseous exposed the lumbrical and the lateral band on the radial side of the finger. Continued dissection palmar to the lumbrical exposed the proper digital vessels and nerve to the radial side of the index finger. This neurovascular bundle was very carefully preserved. The insertion of the first dorsal interosseous muscle was sectioned from the finger, and the muscle was dissected away from the second metacarpal, preserving its aponeurotic insertion for later transfer to the long finger. (**D**) The extensor tendons were retracted ulnarward. The second metacarpal was subperiosteally freed all around from interosseous origins. It was sectioned across its proximal quarter.

The extensors were then retracted radially and the intertendinous bridges to the long finger extensor digitorum were cut. The metacarpal thus mobilized could be reflected from its bed to expose the first palmar interosseous muscle and the intermetacarpal ligament between the volar plates of the index and long finger metacarpophalangeal joints. Section of the intermetacarpal ligament was carried out, being careful not to injure the neurovascular structures just palmar to it. The whole ray was now mobile and, by rolling it toward the radial side of the hand, the neurovascular bundle on the ulnar side of the index finger was readily exposed. The bundle was freed and traced back to the branching of the common digital artery into the proper digital artery to the adjacent sides of the index and long fingers. Once satisfied that the common to proper artery on the ulnar side of the index digit was intact, the proper branch to the long finger was doubly ligated and cut.

As more mobility was gained, the common digital nerve was seen splitting into proper digital nerves to the adjacent sides of the index and long fingers. (**E**) The proper digital nerves were split proximally by carefully incising the nerve sheath between the two major funiculi. With a watchful eye toward preservation of the neurovascular bundle, the metacarpophalangeal joint and volar plate were freed from the palm soft tissues. The metacarpal was removed by disarticulating the metacarpophalangeal joint but it was preserved as a source of bone for use as an intramedullary bone peg between the index proximal phalanx and the thumb metacarpal. (**F**)

The proximal phalanx end and its meta-

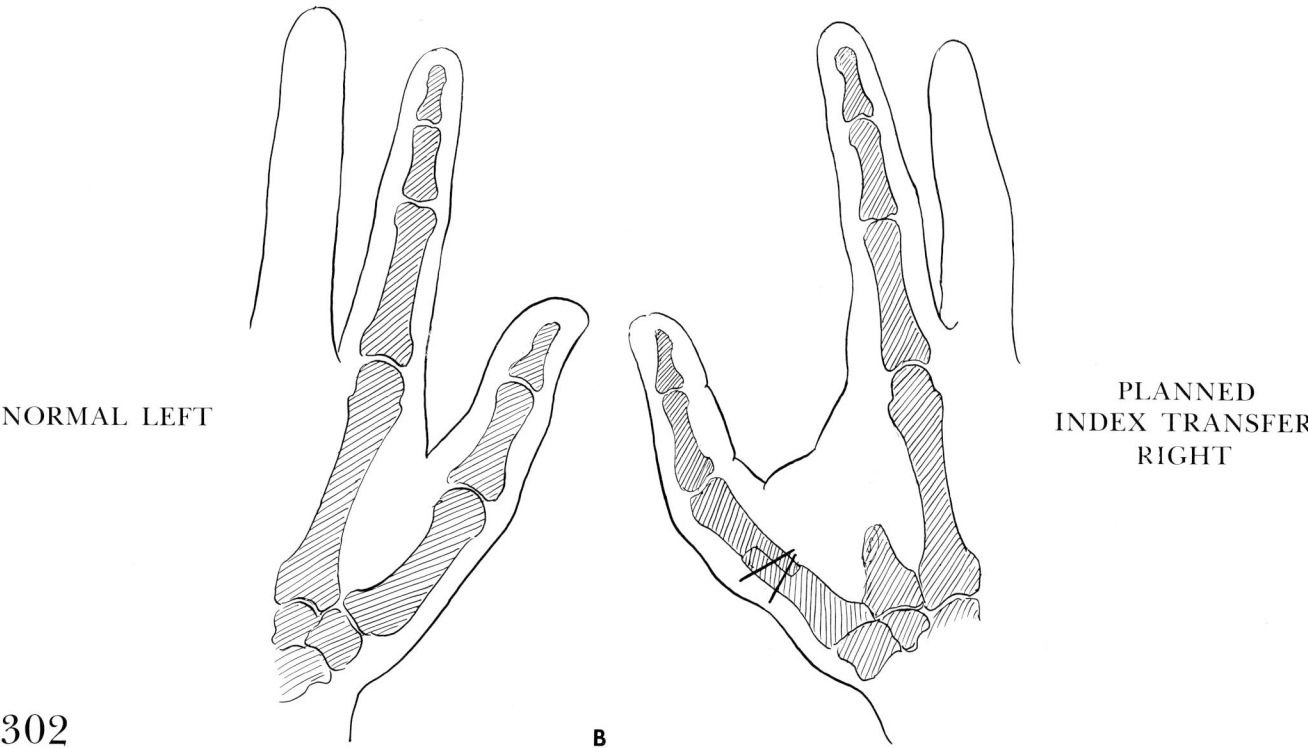

NORMAL LEFT

PLANNED INDEX TRANSFER RIGHT

B

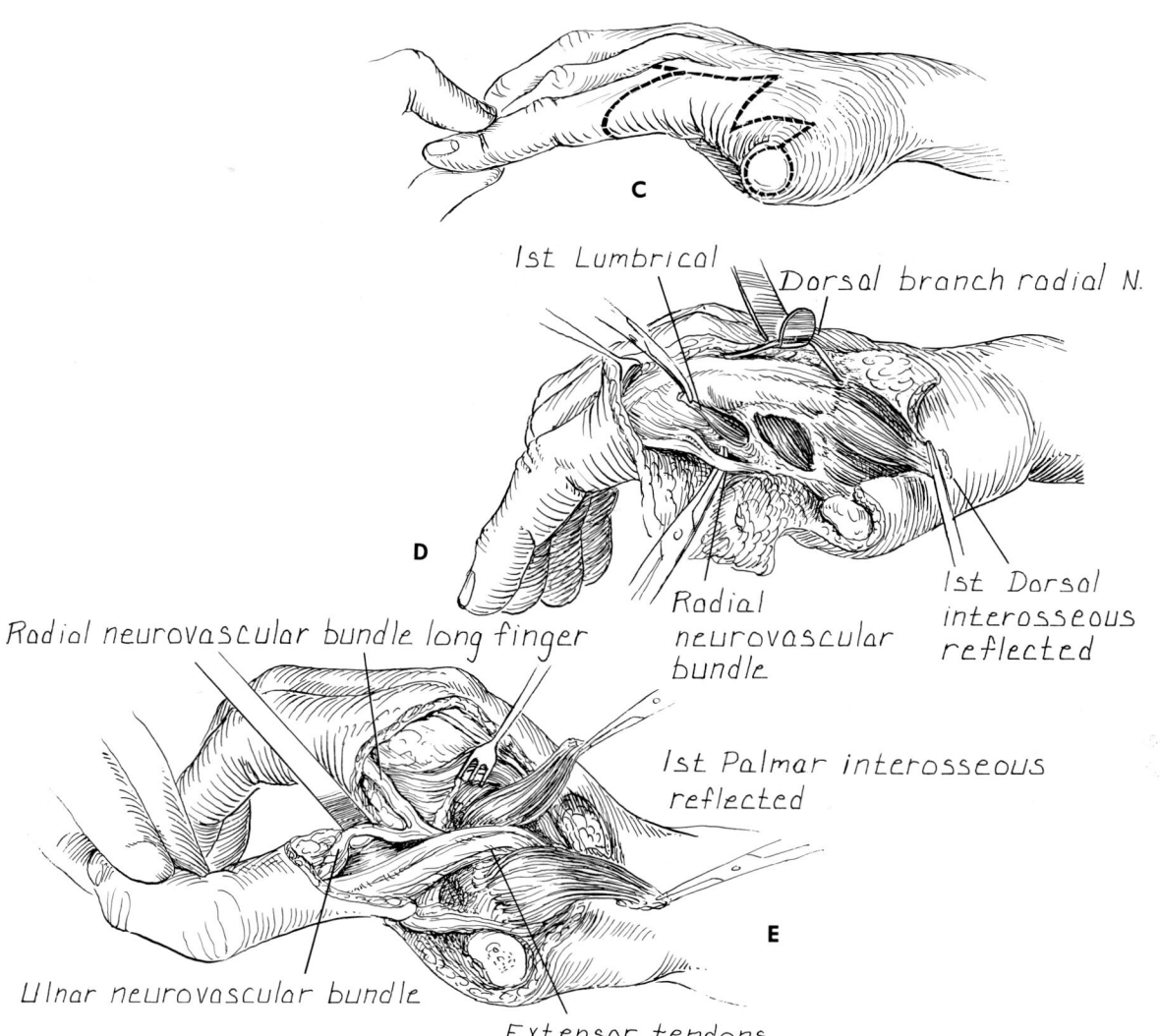
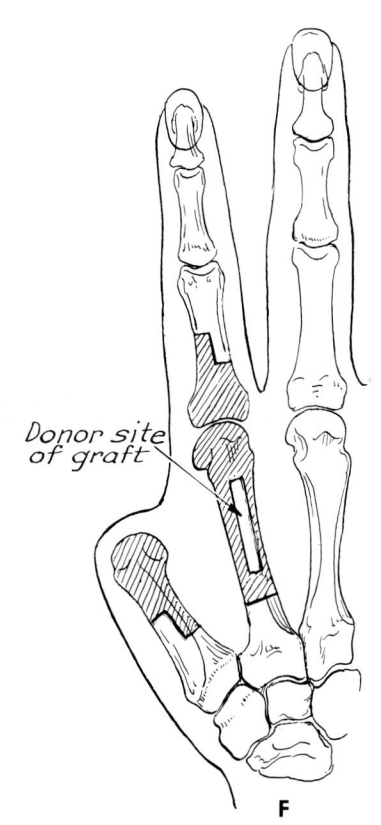

69 – Thumb Reconstruction by Pollicization

carpophalangeal joint surface were dissected free of surrounding soft tissues. The first metacarpal was exposed by dissecting down on its subcutaneous dorsum and the amputated end was cut squarely with a small blade of an oscillating bone saw at the level planned on the x-rays. A mortised recipient end was prepared by appropriate saw cuts. Precise measurements were then made from the first metacarpal bone to the cut end and matched to the measurement from the tip of the index finger to its proximal phalanx, to sum up to the proper length for the reconstructed thumb.

The proximal phalanx of the index finger was mortised to fit the first metacarpal with proper rotation. (**G**) A bone peg was fashioned from the amputated metacarpal for insertion into the medullary canals across the mortised juncture. With all index finger tendons mobilized proximally to swing freely toward the thumb, the finger was transposed and lifted into position with the intramedullary bone peg in position. Two Kirschner wires inserted obliquely across the mortised joint were sufficient to achieve solid internal fixation. The extensor indicis tendon was shortened to take up the slack created by recessing the index finger in transfer. A simple end-to-end tendon juncture was performed. (See tendon repair, Section 77.)

The first dorsal interosseous muscle was allowed to fall ulnarward against the second dorsal and first palmar interossei and its insertion was sutured to the lateral band of the long finger to create a smooth, soft tissue pad in the new first web space. (**H**)

The skin flaps were fashioned to fit and were closed. (**I**) A bulky fluffy dressing was applied with a plaster shell over it in such a way that the transferred index finger tip could regularly be examined.

Immobilization for eight to ten weeks was adequate to assure clinical union of the osteotomy sites. Graded active motion was allowed and within six additional weeks the patient was actively using his reconstructed thumb. In eight months the patient had remarkable dexterity and seemed to be well rehabilitated.

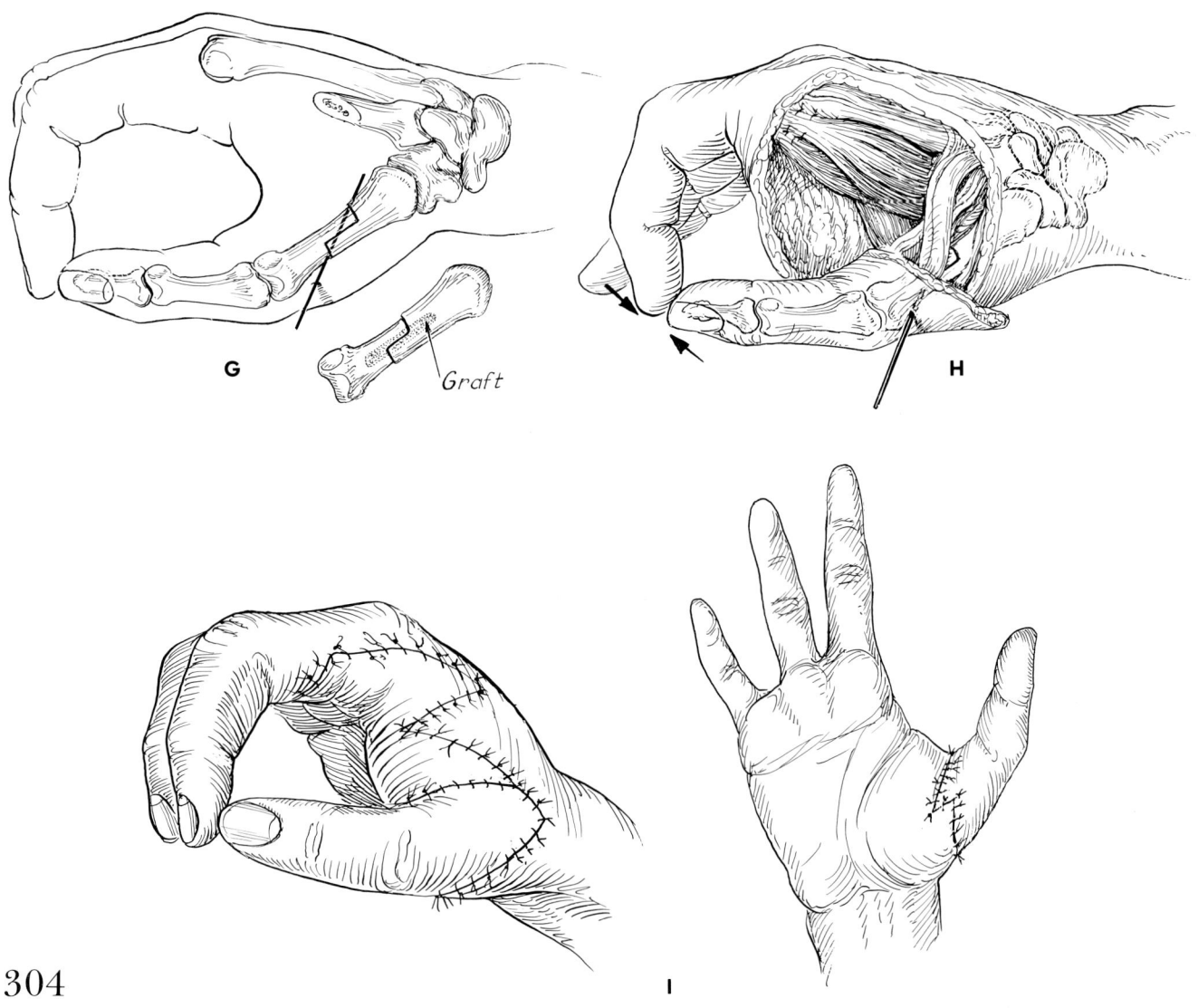

Reconstruction of the Thumb

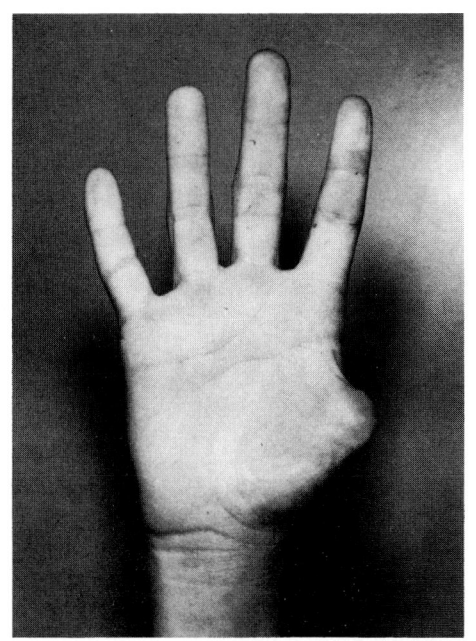
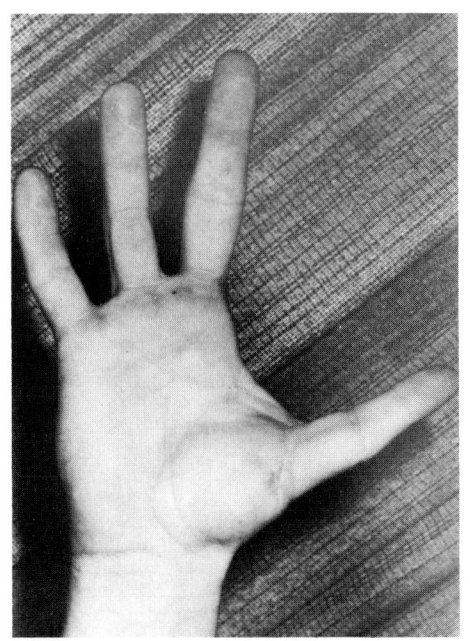
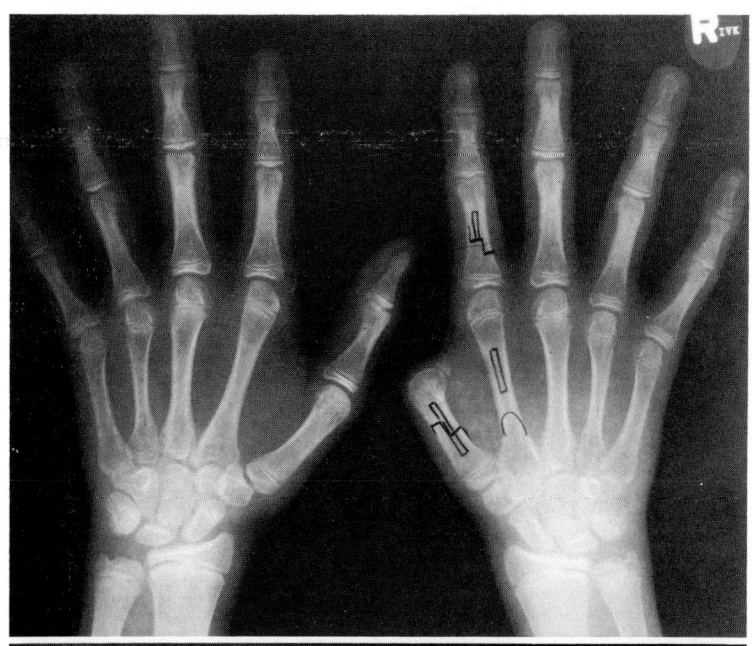
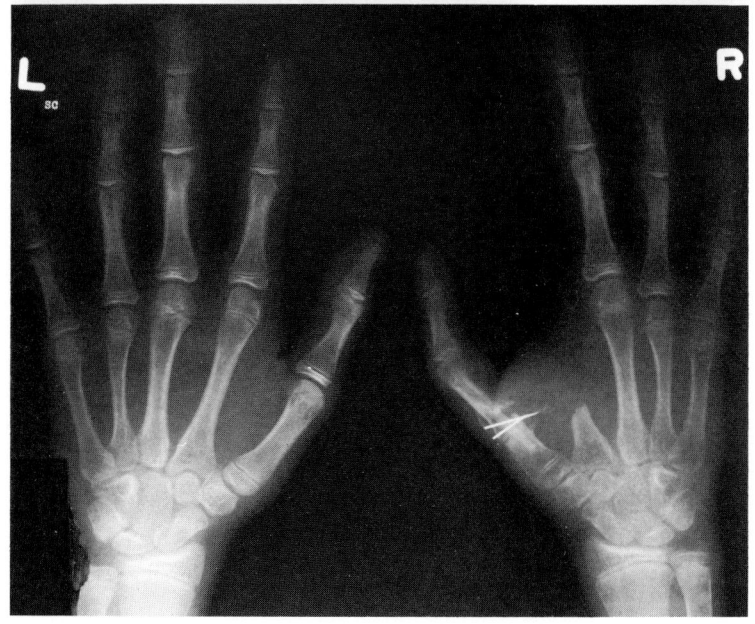

POLLICIZATION FOR CONGENITAL ABSENCE OF THE THUMB

Principle

Congenital absence of the thumb usually means absence of the entire thumb ray and the thenar muscles. Pollicization of the index finger is appropriate in this set of circumstances. Some variation in the technique of pollicization may help to overcome the lack of intrinsic thenar muscles and lack of a carpometacarpal articulation.

The metacarpophalangeal joint is recessed enough to serve as a substitute for the first carpometacarpal joint. The first dorsal interosseous muscle is preserved and redirected to serve as a thenar muscle substitute. The projection of the thumb is directed in such a manner that pulp-to-pulp opposition may be achieved without strong functioning thumb positioning intrinsic muscles.

Although early surgery has been advocated by excellent hand surgeons I prefer to carry out pollicization at the age of four or five years.

Example

A four-year-old male patient with congenital absence of both thumb rays unassociated with other anomalies was brought for consultation by his parents. (**A**)

After detailed discussion over several months, pollicization of the index finger on the dominant left hand was decided upon. The thumb and its metacarpal and thenar muscles were absent.

An **S**-shaped incision was planned, starting at the mid-dorsal base of the index finger and ending at a point from which the reconstructed digit should project from the hand. (**B**) The incision outline was continued around the base of the index finger to completely circumscribe it. The point of skin at the mid-dorsum was to be transferred to the proximal extreme end of the curved incision.

Dissection in the areola plane quickly exposed the first dorsal interosseous muscle. Its aponeurotic attachment to the index finger was sectioned and the muscle was reflected up from its origin on the second metacarpal. (**C**) The extensor tendons to the index finger were exposed and the extensor digitorum was sectioned at the proximal metacarpal level. (**D**) The extensor indicis lying on the ulnar side of the extensor digitorum was left intact.

The index metacarpal was then freed from the intrinsic muscles on the ulnar side in preparation for osteotomies. The proximal osteotomy was planned close to the base of the metacarpal with the cut at right angles to the planned projection of the reconstructed thumb. The distal osteotomy was planned across the metacarpal at the epiphysis, just proximal to the metacarpal head. A bone peg was to be fashioned from the superfluous metacarpal. (**E**)

With the osteotomies completed and the bulk of the metacarpal removed, the proximal metacarpal was reamed out, using an osteotome held in the projected position for the reconstructed thumb. (**F**) The hole thus created was deepened into the carpus for 0.5 centimeter.

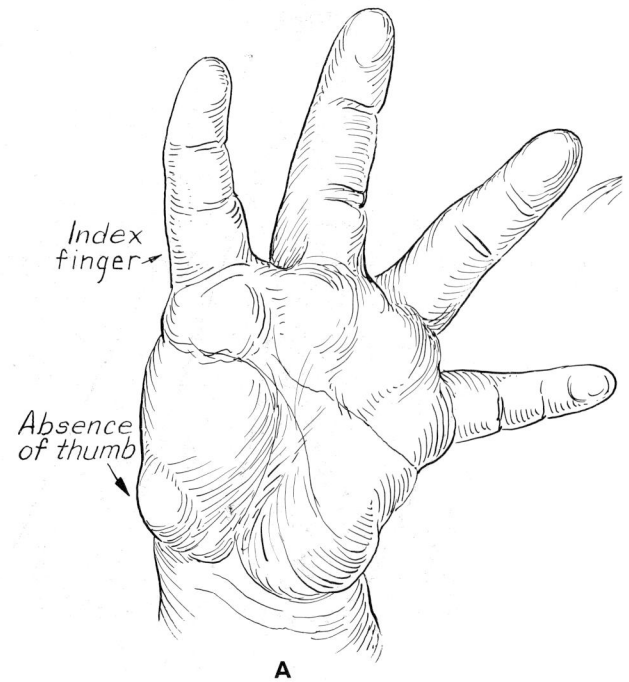

A

Reconstruction of the Thumb

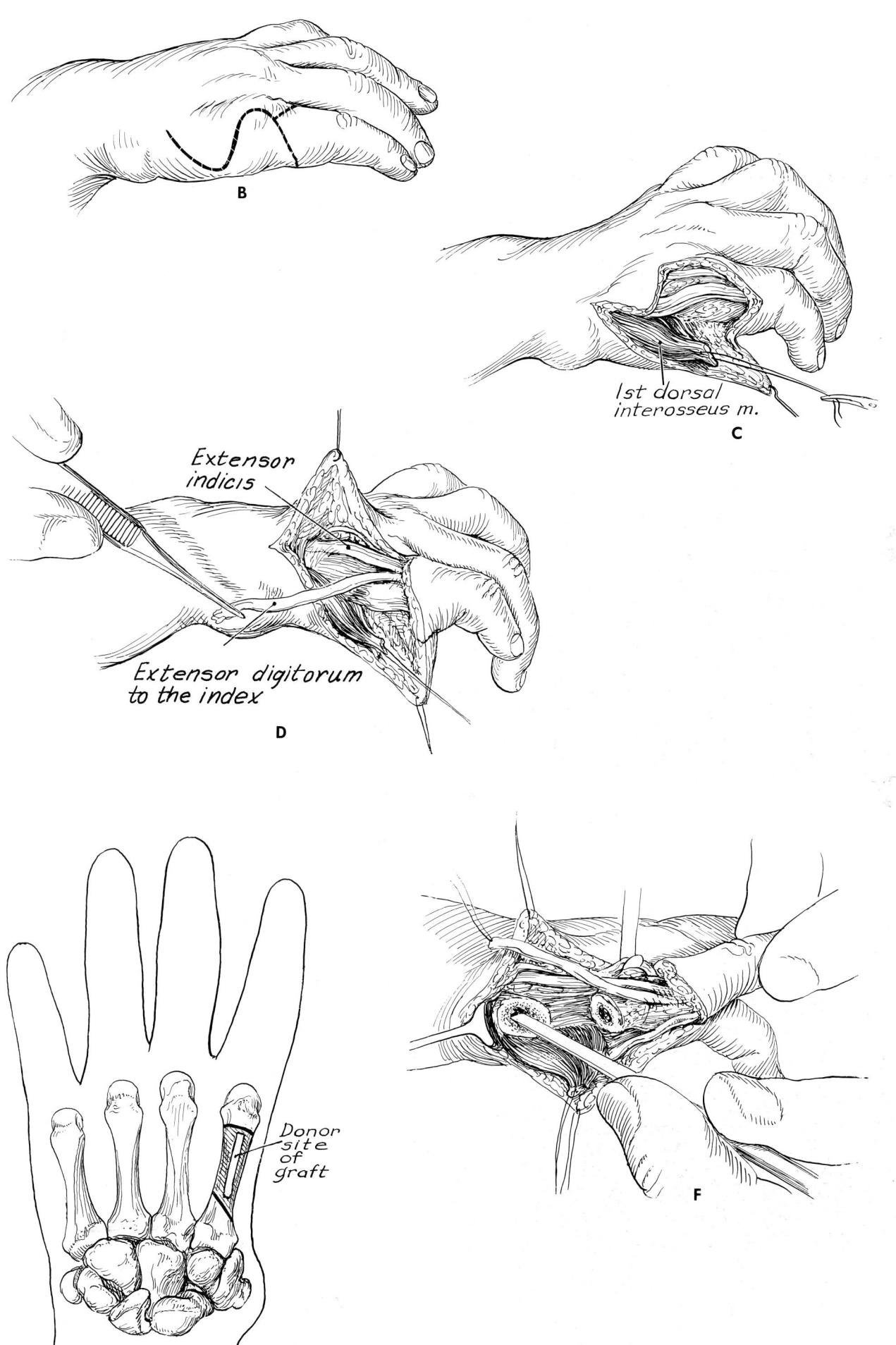

307

69 – Thumb Reconstruction by Pollicization

The management of the neurovascular bundles and flexor tendons, the dorsal nerves and veins, and extensor indicis tendon was described in the management of pollicization on page 302. A bone peg was fashioned from the amputated metacarpal and inserted into the reamed-out recipient site in the proximal part of the metacarpal and carpus. The distal metacarpal and finger were transferred to the thumb position, and the metacarpal head was seated over the projecting bone graft. A Kirschner wire was placed across the osteotomy site with the finger properly positioned. A second Kirschner wire was placed through the proximal metacarpal and carpus, impaling the bone graft. (**G**)

With the transferred finger in satisfactory position, the first dorsal interosseous muscle was positioned to substitute for the absent abductor pollicis brevis. The split between the extensor digitorum and extensor indicis was carried far enough distal to allow the extensor digitorum to fall palmar to the proximal interphalangeal joint. (**H**) The extensor digitorum was then threaded through the aponeurotic end of the muscle and fixed with enough tension to extend the distal interphalangeal joint and flex the proximal interphalangeal joint. (**I**)

The extensor indicis was shortened by the technique described for pollicization for traumatic thumb loss on page 304. The skin flaps were closed and a bulky dressing and plaster shell were applied. (**J**)

The plaster shell was carried above the elbow, which was placed in comfortable flexion. This avoided the problem of cast slippage so common in active children. The dressings were changed in two weeks, sutures were removed, and a snug fitted plaster cast from mid-upper arm to the tip of the reconstructed thumb leaving the fingers free was applied. All external immobilization was removed eight weeks after surgery. The distal Kirschner wire worked out spontaneously a month later.

The patient gained excellent prehensile function and the ability to pinch and manipulate objects between his reconstructed thumb pulp and remaining fingers. Abduction ability using the transferred first dorsal interosseous was readily demonstrable. The same procedure was carried out on the right hand.

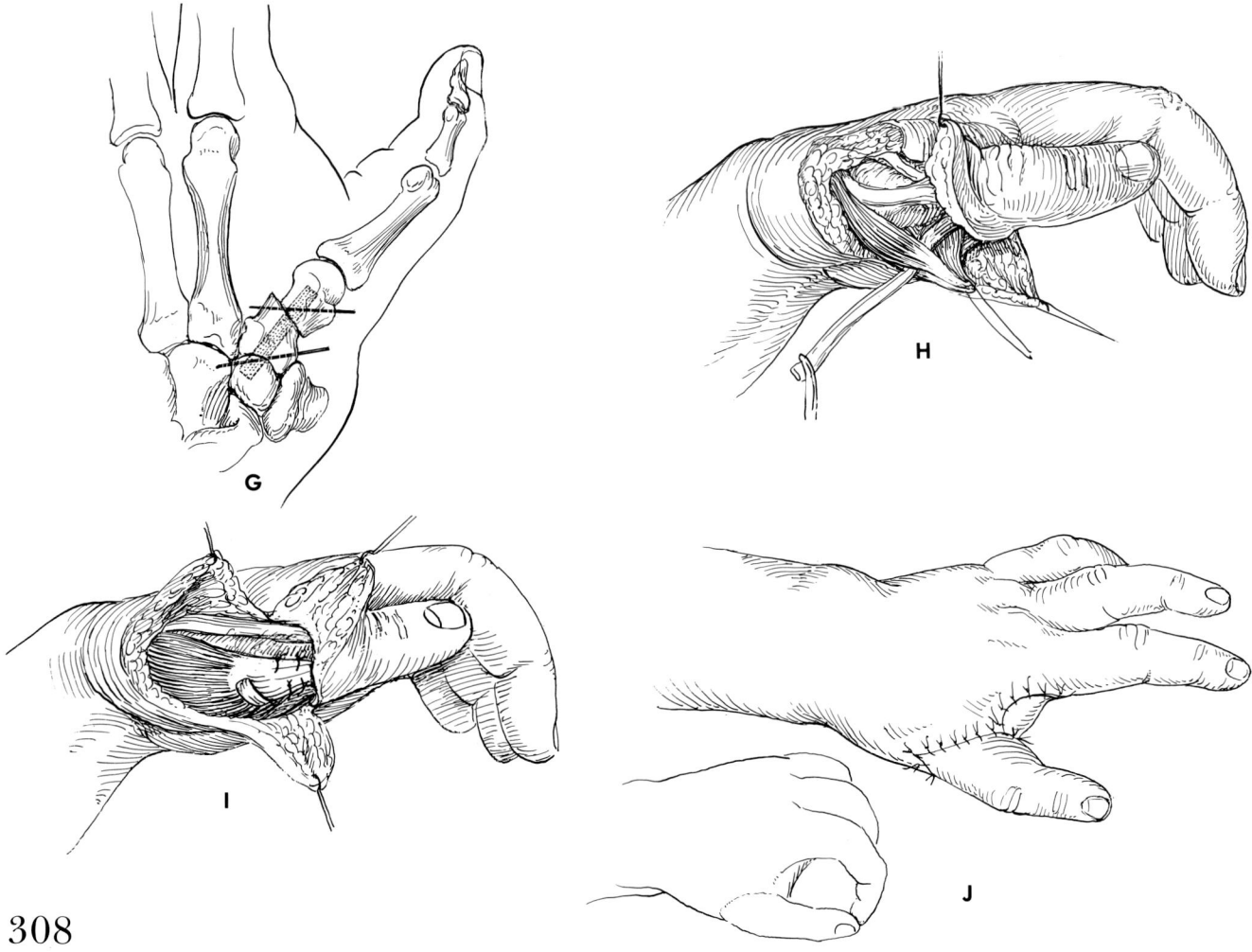

Reconstruction of the Thumb

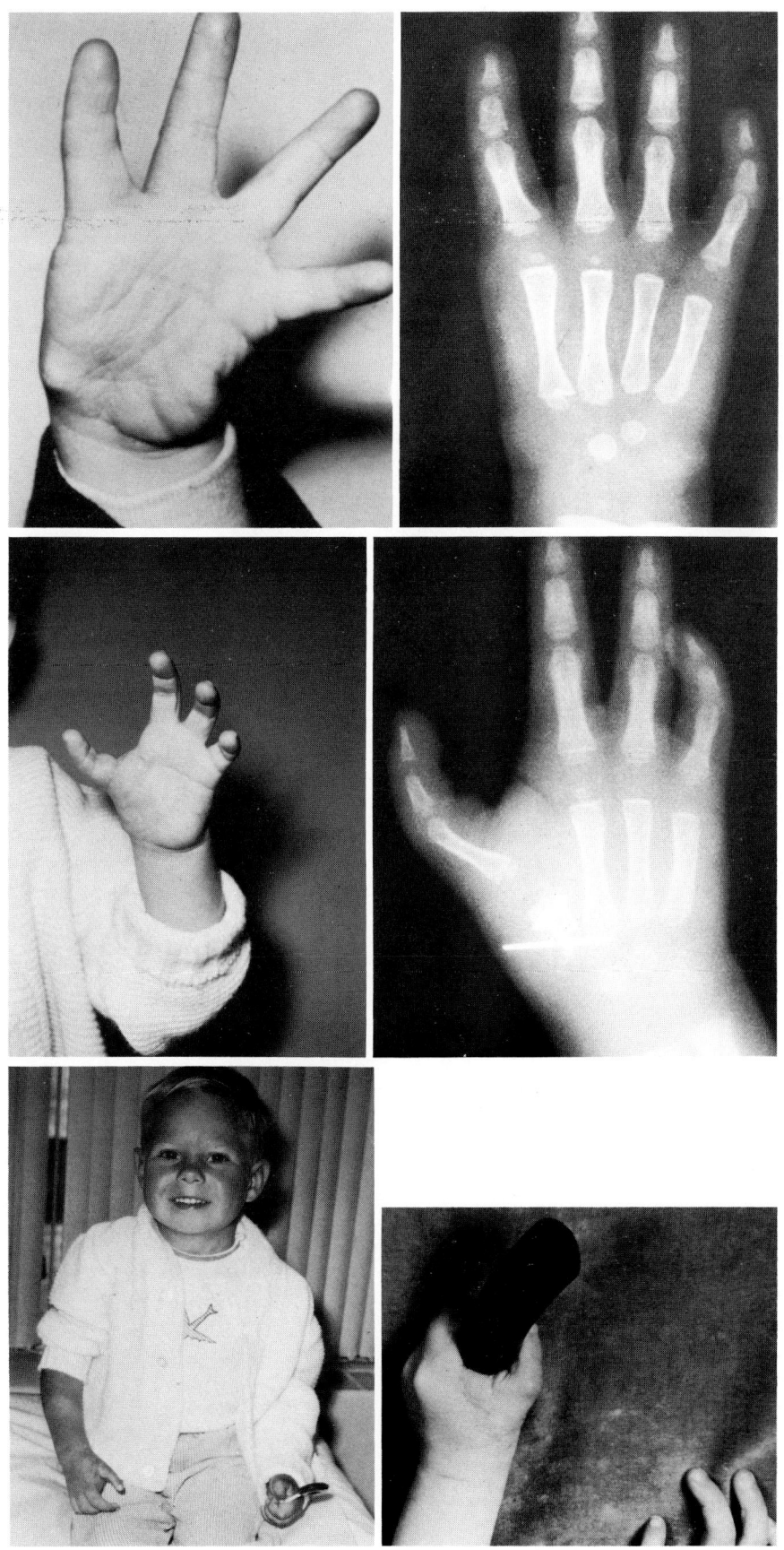

309

70
Pedicle Flap, Bone Graft, Island Flap Reconstruction of the Thumb

Principle

The technique for thumb reconstruction suggested by Nicoladoni near the turn of the century and used by a number a surgeons in the first quarter of this century consisted of a distant pedicle flap for soft tissue reconstruction with a free bone graft for skeletal support. The procedure fell into disuse, being replaced by digit transposition which was popular during both World Wars. Littler's refined pollicization procedure all but eliminated the more tedious and less satisfactory tubed pedicle flap, bone graft method. The great advantages of motion, reliable blood supply, and, particularly, sensibility in the pollicized finger were evident.

Moberg and Littler further refined the transfer of tissues in the hand solely on neurovascular pedicles so that skin and subcutaneous tissue could be moved about to achieve both adequate vascularized soft tissue coverage and critical sensibility without major sacrifice of function in the donor finger. This innovation revived interest in the tubed pedicle flap, bone graft method as an acceptable alternate to finger pollicization, but only when the loss was *sub*total, with metacarpal and thenar muscles preserved. The neurovascular island pedicle technique now meant that the reconstructed pedicle flap, bone graft thumb could be resurfaced using soft tissue with reliable blood supply and protective and perceptive sensibility. The technique has the following advantages:

1. No finger is sacrificed.
2. The reconstructed thumb has sensibility and sudomotor function.
3. Hand skin, with its unique characteristics, is used on the working surface of the thumb.
4. Blood supply to the thumb and bone graft is enhanced.
5. The thumb may be contoured to look like the normal thumb on the other hand.

The disadvantages of the technique are:

1. It requires more than one operative procedure.
2. No phalangeal joints exist in the reconstructed thumb.

Where phalangeal joint function is important in thumb reconstruction there is no substitute for finger pollicization.

Example

A 20-year-old male patient sustained an amputation of his right thumb just distal to the metacarpophalangeal joint while repairing an automobile engine. (**A**) After a year the patient sought advice and, after considerable discussion and explanation of the variety of possible reconstruction techniques, the patient elected to undergo reconstruction by distant pedicle flap, bone graft, and island pedicle flap technique. The amputation site scar was resected in preparation for attachment of a one-stage tubed pedicle flap.

The tubed flap, elevated in the infraclavicular area of the opposite chest wall, was designed so that the hand would be immobilized in a comfortable, elevated position with the fingers curled into the axilla around the pectoral fold. The longitudinal tubing scar was placed in the midpalmar aspect of the thumb, since it would ultimately be replaced by a vascularized sensory island pedicle flap. The chest pedicle flap was carefully thinned by removal of excess fat so that it could be tubed without tension and so its size would be that of normal thumb. The donor area was closed by suture. The free edge of the tubed pedicle was sutured to the prepared thumb stump. The arm and hand were immobilized to the chest with adhesive tape. (**B**)

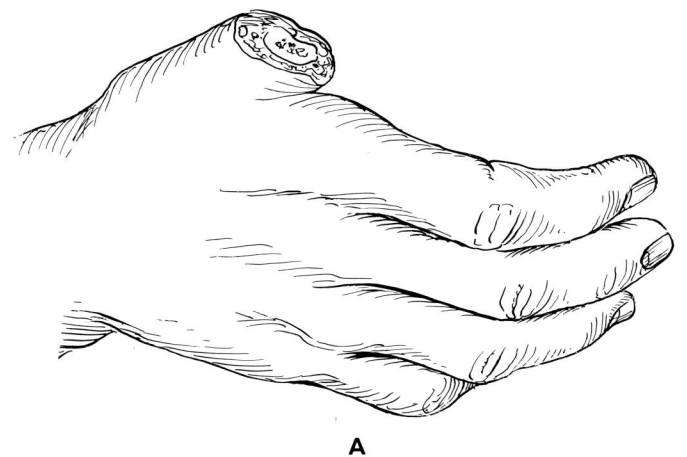

A

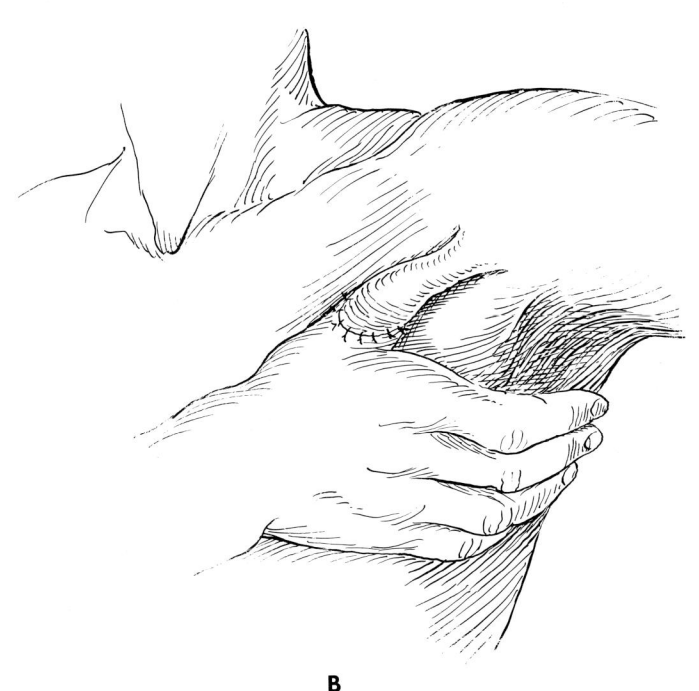

B

70 — Pedicle Flap, Bone Graft, Island Flap Reconstruction of the Thumb

The tubed pedicle attached to the thumb stump was allowed four weeks to heal completely. It was then released from the chest wall, leaving it long enough to construct a thumb of normal length. (**C**) Possibly, the release procedure could have been combined with the bone graft insertion and island pedicle application.

The bone graft-island pedicle stage was done at a time of election two months after the pedicle flap had healed and softened.

The tubed pedicle flap thumb was opened by excising the palmar midline scar. (**D**) The incisions on the medial and lateral surfaces of the pedicle flap thumb were planned to receive the full width of the island flap while retaining a nearly normal total thumb circumference. Additional fat was removed from the reopened tube of soft tissue to provide sufficient space to accommodate the bone graft. (**E** and **F**).

A cortical bone graft of appropriate length to construct a nearly normal length thumb plus an extra 2 centimeters for bone dowel construction was taken from the tibia. (See Section 61 for technique.) In this instance since the bone graft was to serve as the architectural support for the thumb, the periosteum was left on the bone graft. A skirt of periosteum 0.5 centimeter wide was left to use as a substitute for dermal stabilizing ligaments. (Cleland's ligaments.)

A bone dowel with square edges was fashioned to be inserted into the nub of the proximal phalanx. The bone at the thumb amputation site was prepared by cutting it sharply at right angles. A drill hole was made to receive the bone graft dowel. The bone graft was forced into position with the periosteal surface toward the palm. (**G**)

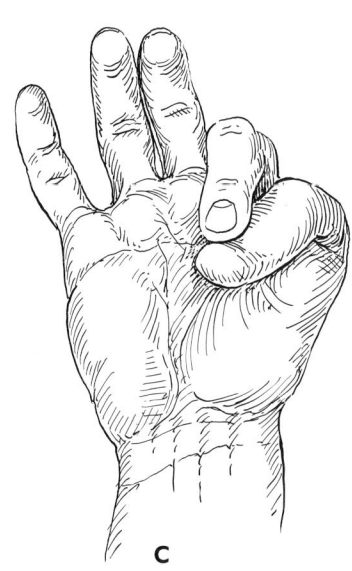

C

Reconstruction of the Thumb

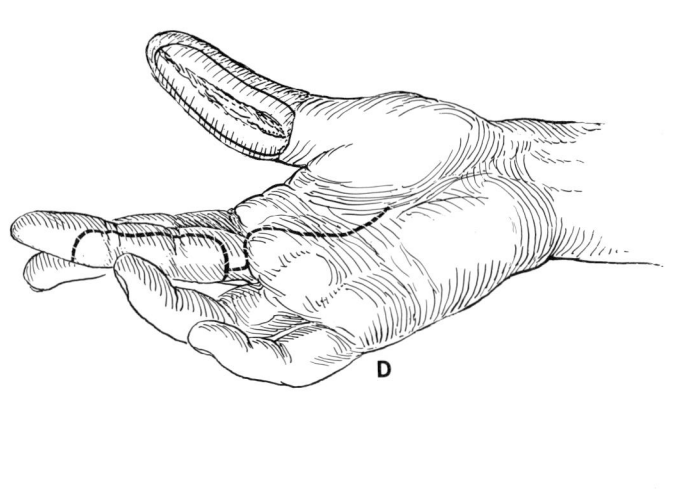

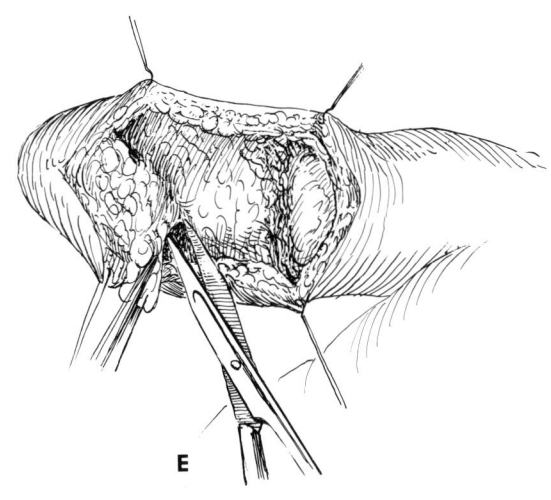

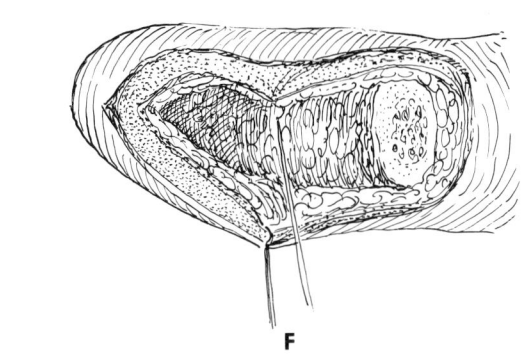

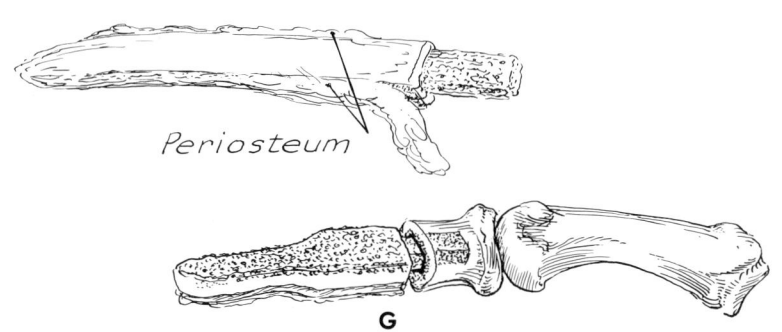

Periosteum

313

70 – Pedicle Flap, Bone Graft, Island Flap Reconstruction of the Thumb

The island pedicle flap was planned in the ulnar side of the long finger to take sufficient soft tissue to resurface the whole palmar aspect of the reconstructed thumb and its tip. (**D**) The finger flap would better have been taken well out on the distal phalanx pulp, incising around the nail and bed dorsally. Few nerve fibers are cut across by this maneuver since the area of supplied sensibility distally is moved as part of the flap. The tip shape is useful in lending normal contour to the reconstructed thumb tip.

The island pedicle flap in this case was elevated from the long finger by the technique outlined in Section 15. It was passed through a tunnel to the thumb, which was bluntly dissected beneath the palmar fascia in the proximal palm. At this part in the procedure all of the elements to construct the thumb were present at the thumb site.

The pedicle flap thumb was draped over the bone graft for final shaping of the bone with fine rongeurs. With the chest pedicle flap skin draped over the dorsum of the bone graft, the skin edges were trimmed back so that they would comfortably reach the junction of the periosteum with the bone graft on both sides. With the skin held in that position the island pedicle flap was draped over the palmar surface of the bone graft, and a line was drawn around it on the dorsal pedicle flap skin. An incision was made along the line, down to but not through the dermis. The epidermis and superficial dermis were removed from the free edges of the dorsal pedicle skin.

The dermal leading edges of the pedicle flap were sutured to the periosteum to stabilize the thumb soft tissues to the base architecture. (**H**) The island pedicle flap was fitted over the palmar surface, where it was sutured in place as cover for the thumb's working surface. (**I**)

The newly constructed thumb was held rigorously immobilized for eight weeks, after which x-rays were taken. Eight to 12 weeks were sufficient to achieve clinical union. After clinical union, progressive activity was allowed. The bone graft slowly remodeled into a large phalanx-shaped bone of length equal to the combined phalanges of the left thumb. (**J**)

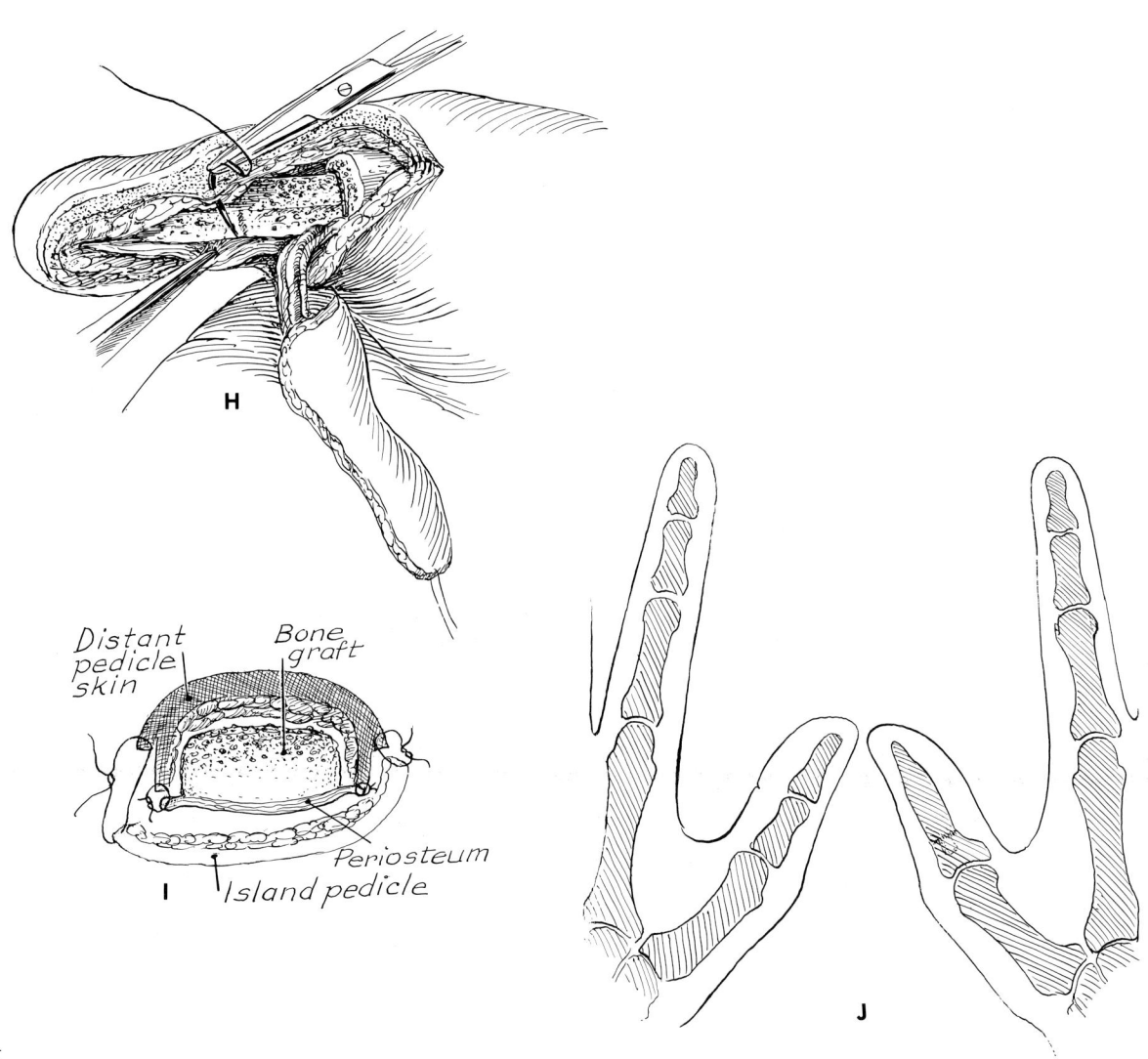

The patient regained remarkably good function, and after several months he noted a little motion at the metacarpophalangeal joint. He became a carpenter's apprentice and was able to achieve working foreman status, which required extensive use of the reconstructed thumb. He was able to pinch against each of his four fingers. (**K**) Missing was his ability to flex the thumb into the palm, since he had very limited metacarpophalangeal joint motion and no interphalangeal joint at all. (**L**)

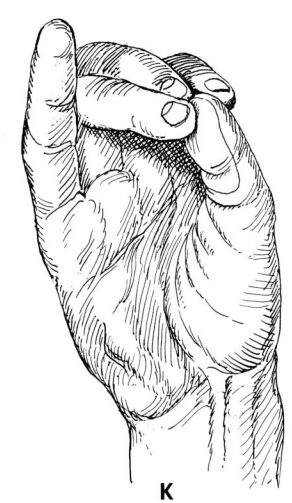

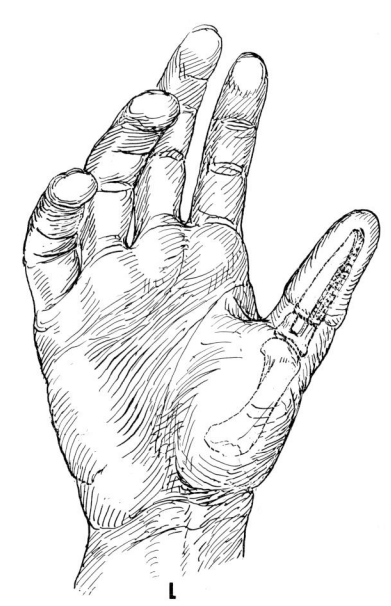

STAGE ONE

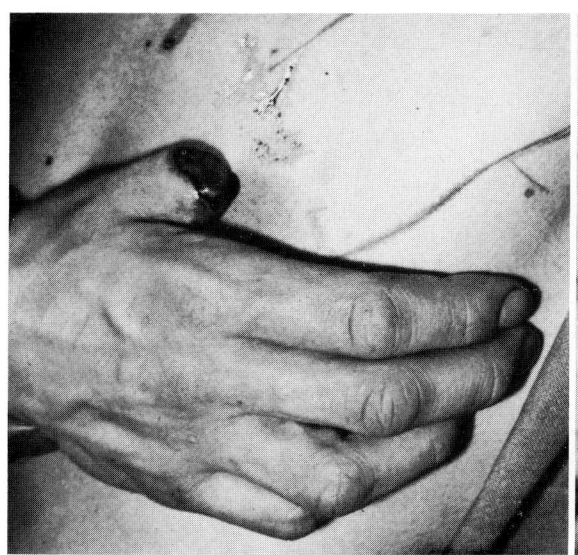

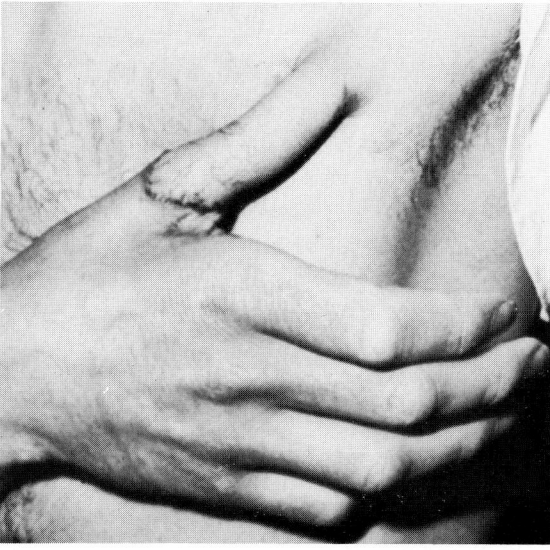

70 – Pedicle Flap, Bone Graft, Island Flap Reconstruction of the Thumb

STAGE TWO

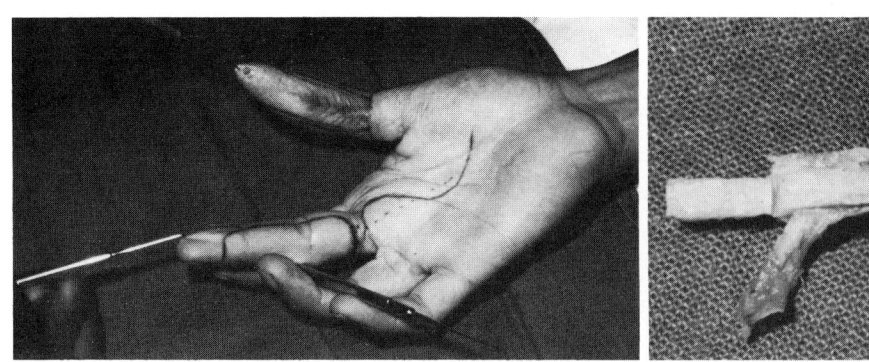
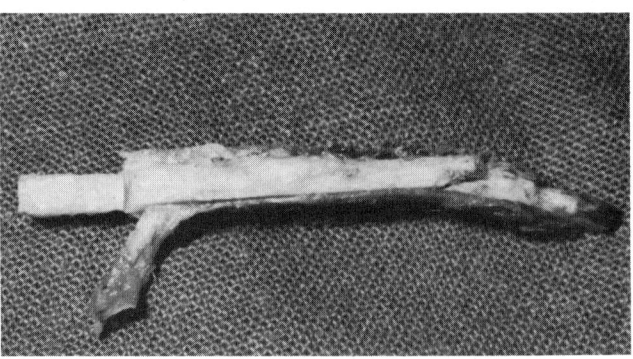

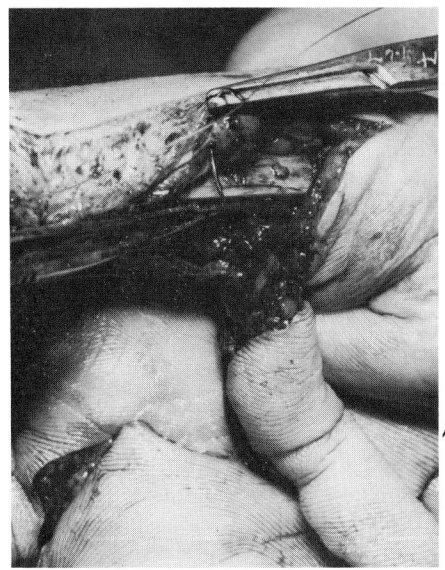
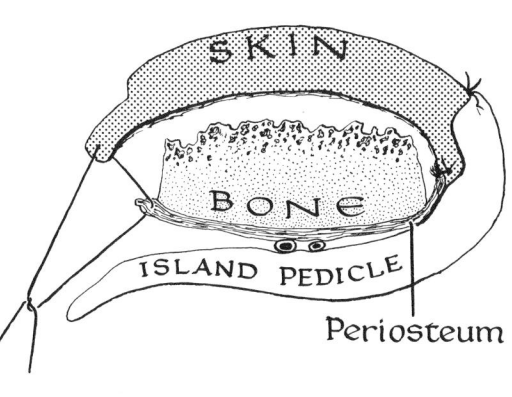

PREOPERATIVE   POSTOPERATIVE

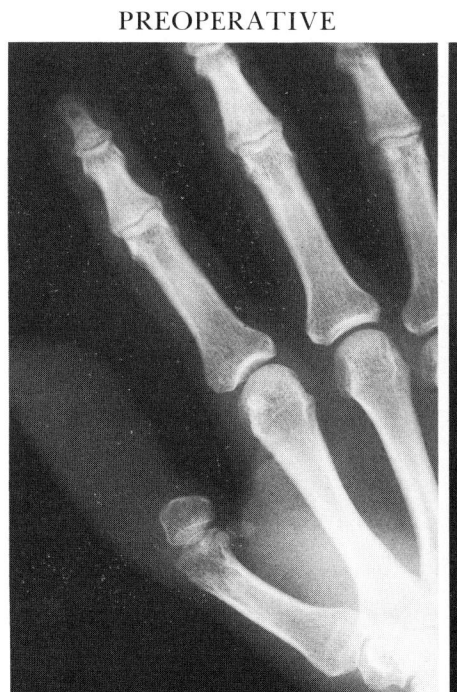
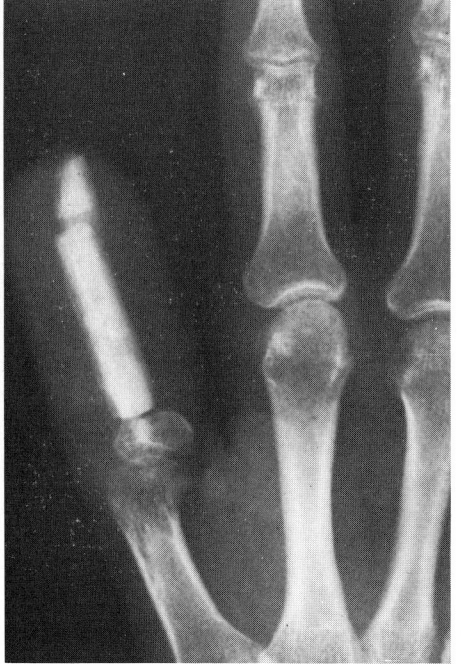

POSTOPERATIVE RESULT

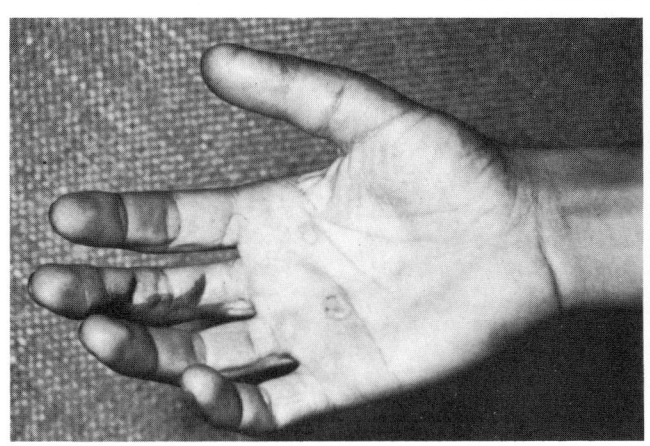
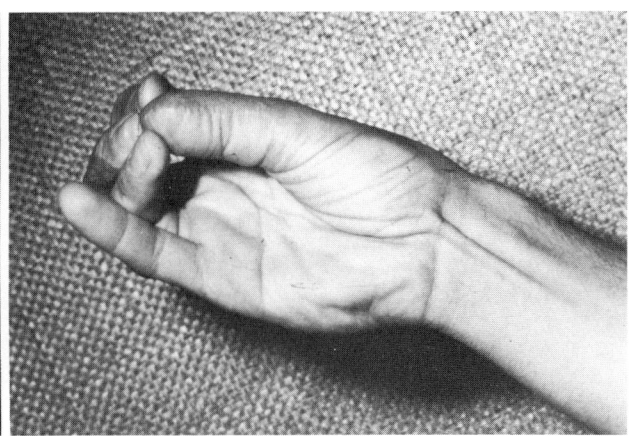

POSTOPERATIVE X-RAYS
LEFT RIGHT.

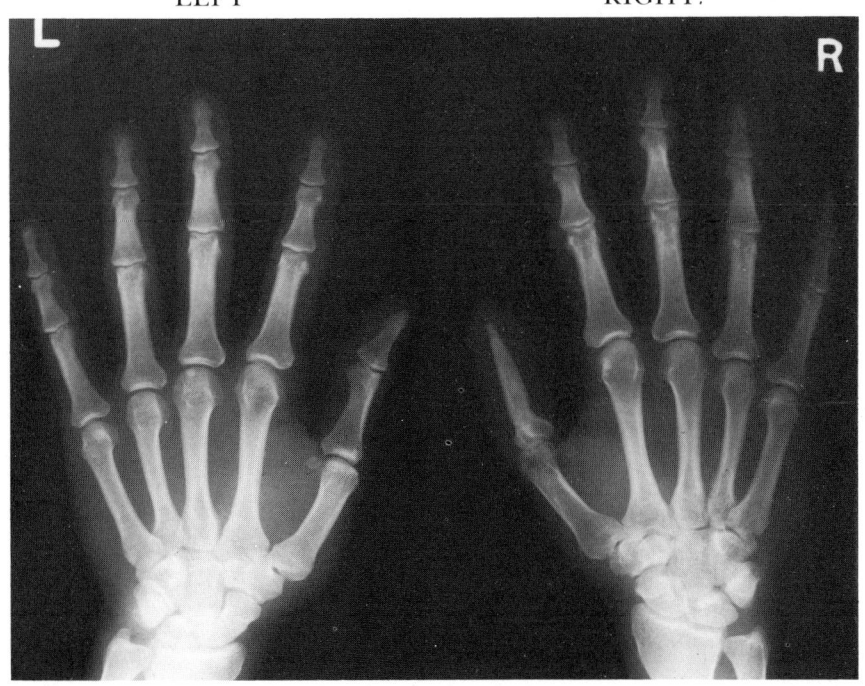

Surgery of Rheumatoid Arthritis

71

Wrist Arthroplasty

Principle

The most common deformity requiring wrist arthroplasty is that created by arthritis. The usual sequence of events is destructive synovitis in the wrist progressing to destruction of the palmar lip of the distal radial articular area and subluxation of the carpus palmar to the radius at the radiocarpal joint. The resulting deformity is disabling and sets the stage for disruption of the extensor tendons. The wrist subluxation destroys the normal balance of the long extensor and flexor tendons as they influence the phalanges. A position of nonfunction results. It consists of hyperextension of the metacarpophalangeal joints and flexion of the interphalangeal joints. If there is destruction of the metacarpophalangeal joint mechanism, these joints may also subluxate into the palm with guttering of the extensor tendons and classical ulnar deviation of the fingers.

The recessed position of the subluxated wrist shortens the distance between the origin and insertion of the flexor tendons. It robs them of power, leaving digital flexion both incomplete and weak. Fusion after relocation of the wrist produces a good, rugged restoration but it precludes wrist motion. If one wrist is fused and the other is badly deformed, arthroplasty may be indicated for the second wrist.

The technique for wrist fusion is described in Section 67.

Arthroplasty of the wrist may be accomplished by a variety of methods. One useful technique consists of excision of the distal ulna and shortening of the distal radius, leaving a palmar shelf of cortex to prevent palmar subluxation of the carpus.

Example

A 52-year-old woman with advanced rheumatoid arthritis developed severe palmar subluxation of both wrists at the radiocarpal joints. The left wrist was treated by fusion (see Section 67.) Arthroplasty of the right wrist was elected as appropriate treatment. Typically, the palmar lip of the distal radius was eroded and the carpus was subluxated palmar to the radius. A *large* palmar spur was evident on the distal radius. Flexion of the fingers and thumb was weak and incomplete, and the wrist was painful and unstable. (**A**)

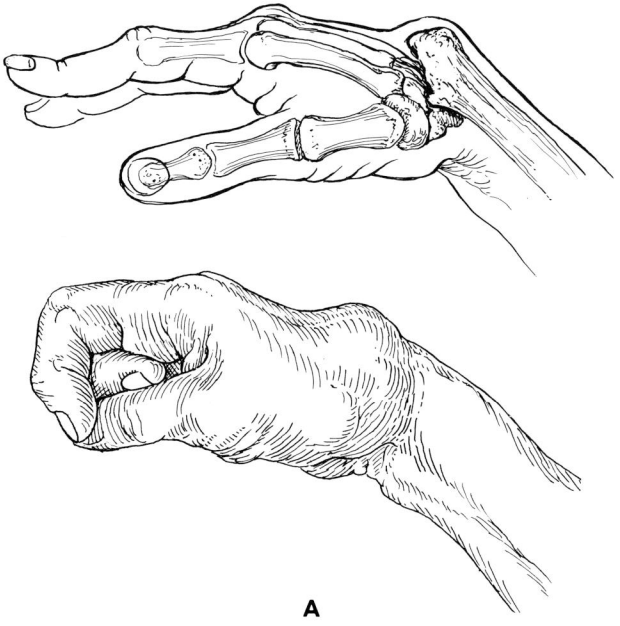

71 — Wrist Arthroplasty

Through an **S**-shaped incision on the dorsum of the wrist extensor tendon synovectomy was performed and the extensors were reflected ulnarward and radially to expose the distal radius and ulna. (**B**)

The palmar spur was removed with rongeurs, (**C**) and the distal ulna was removed by osteotomy. (**D**) The distal radius was fully exposed by dissection of tendons and other soft tissues from it for a distance of two centimeters. The distal radius was shortened dorsally until the palmar cortex protruded distal to it by about a half centimeter as a palmar cortical shelf.

Shortening of the distal radius was continued, maintaining the relationship between the dorsal and palmar cortex until the wrist joint could be reduced without undue tension. (**E** and **F**) This was tested by reducing the dislocation and then passively extending and flexing the wrist for range of motion. Tension on the extensors and flexors which sharply limits such motion suggests the need for further shortening. Too much laxity in the wrist extensors would suggest the need to shorten these tendons.

The articular surface of the carpal bones was protected from injury to help prevent unwanted fusion of the radiocarpal joint. With the wrist in reduced position two Steinmann pins were threaded through the distal radius across the arthroplasty into the carpals. (**G**)

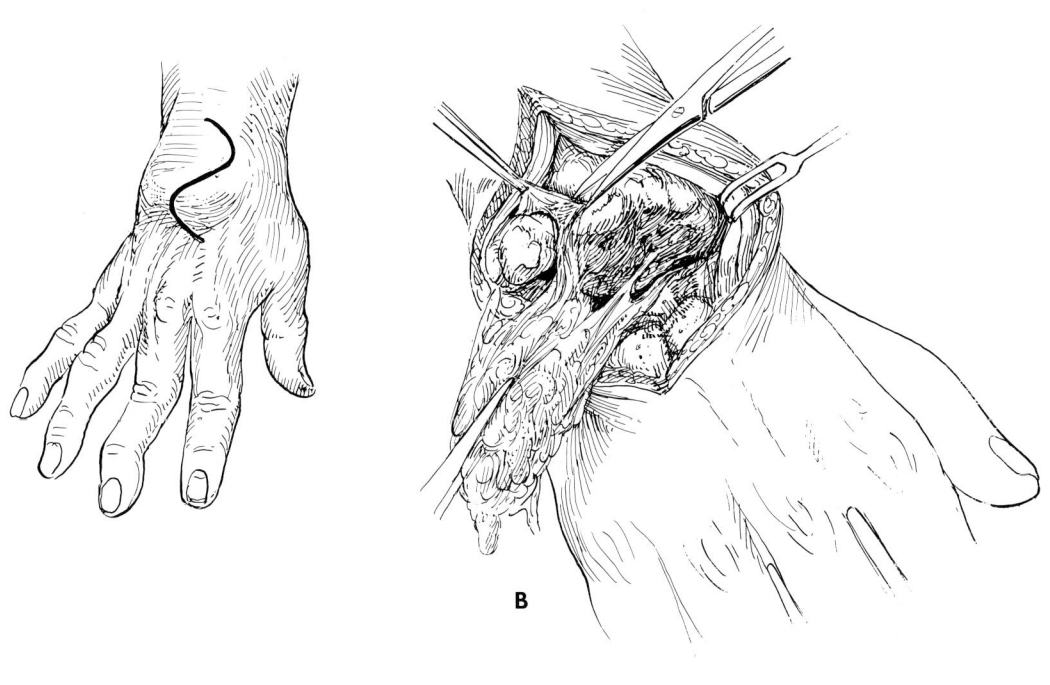

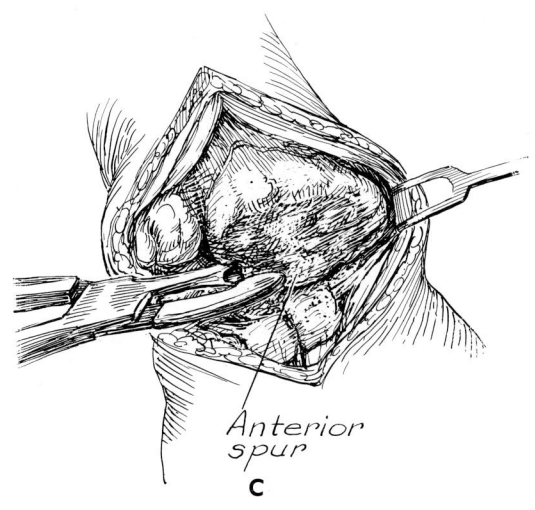

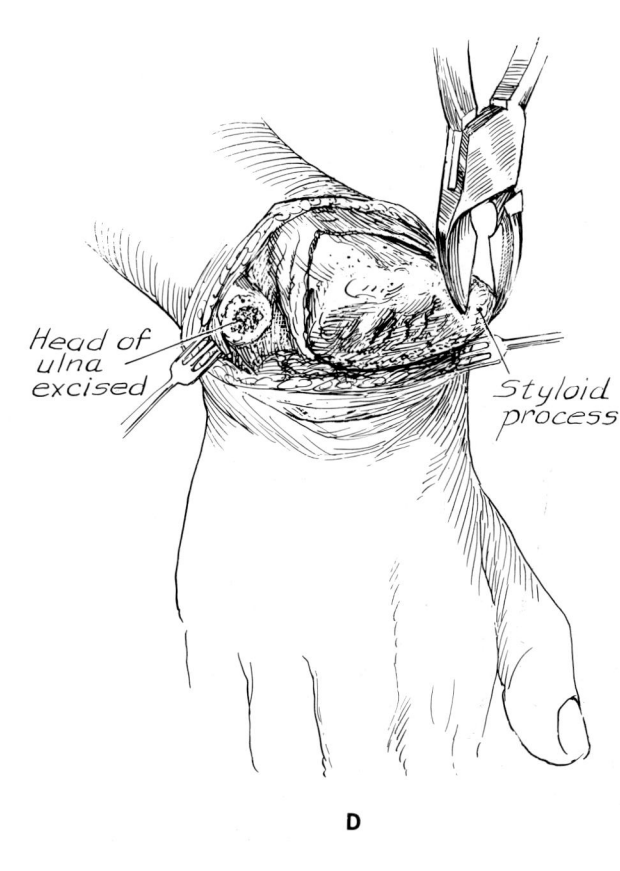
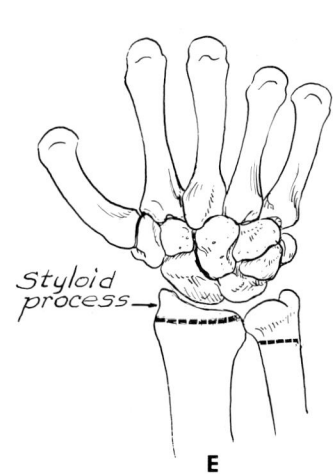
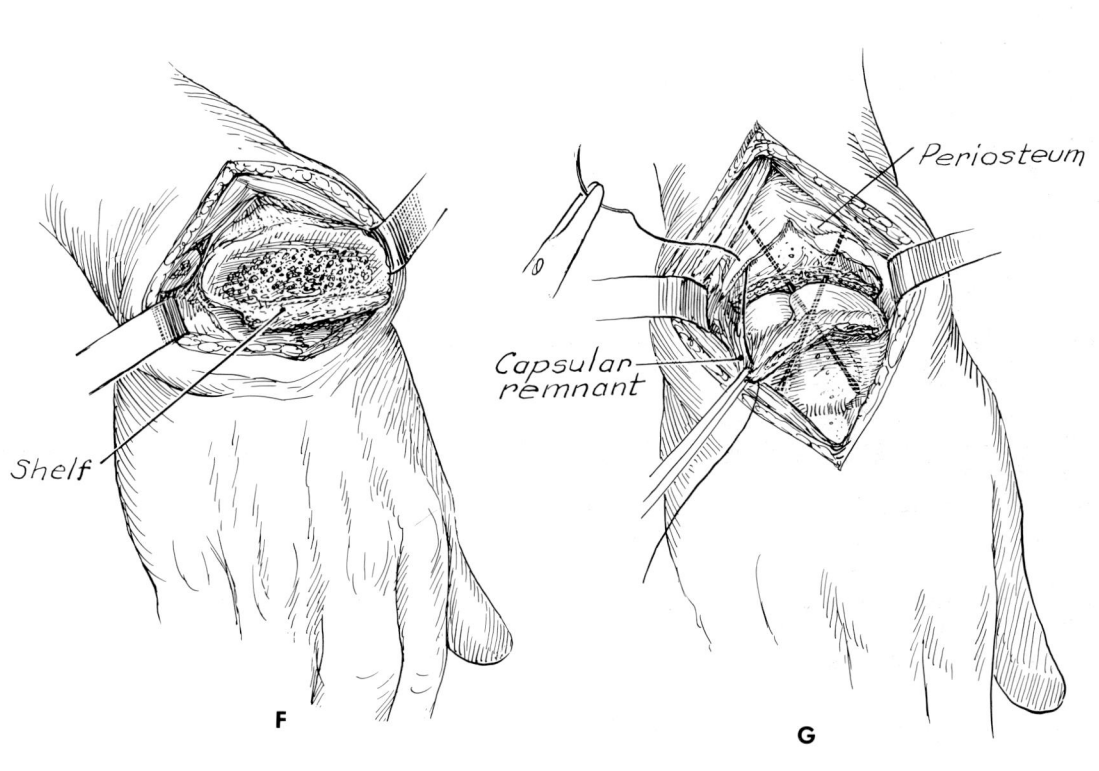

71 – Wrist Arthroplasty

The capsular structures were loosely sutured and the extensor tendons were allowed to fall back in place. The extensor carpi radialis longus and brevis and the extensor pollicis longus were shortened for balance. The subcutaneous tissue and skin were closed.

The pins were removed after six weeks of immobilization and graded motion was started. One should not urge the patient to try to regain a wide range of motion since it will jeopardize stability of the arthroplasty.

The palmar shelf of bone persisted and helped to prevent recurrent palmar subluxation that had existed preoperatively. (**H** and **I**)

The patient had some ulnar deviation posture at the wrist with 45 degrees of deviation motion. She regained 15 degrees of flexion and 25 degrees of extension, a gain of about 40 degrees of motion. (**J**)

Finger extension and flexion were improved in strength and range. (**K**)

PREOPERATIVE

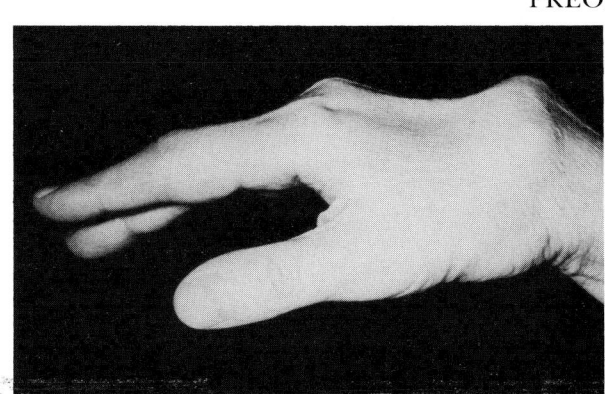
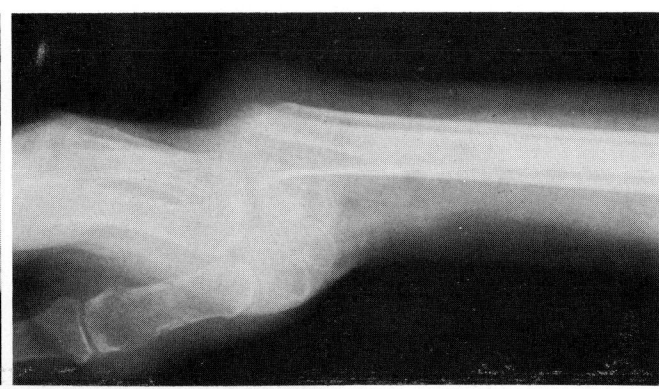

POSTOPERATIVE

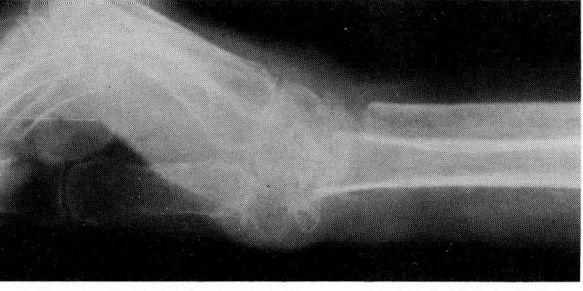

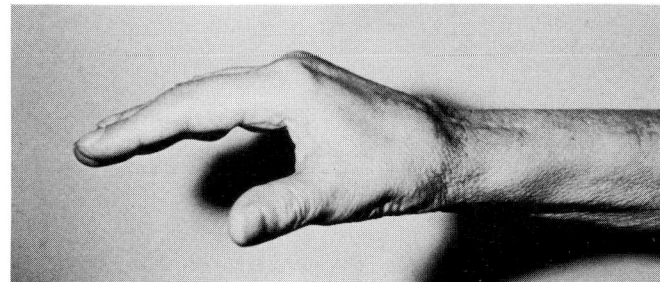
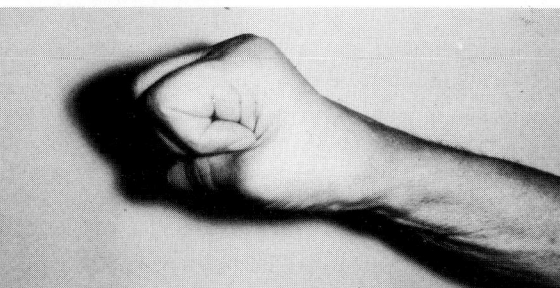

RESULT

K

72

Metacarpophalangeal Joint Synovectomy

Principle

Synovectomy has proved successful in impeding the progressive destruction which occurs too commonly in rheumatoid arthritis. The procedure is recommended before deformity becomes severe. It may be appropriate to discuss synovectomy with patients who are suffering from disabling pain in joints and, particularly, with patients in whom synovial bulging is evident. The suggestion of early destruction of supporting stabilizing structures and beginning deformity makes synovectomy more justified. (**A, B,** and **C**)

If synovectomy is done early in the course of the disease, one must caution the patient that the procedure will not increase the range of motion in the joints; in fact, it may further limit the existing range. Such an "arrestive" synovectomy must be carefully considered for proper indications.

Synovectomy in a hand already undergoing deforming changes is more readily justified. The procedure is combined with corrective measures for the developing ulnar drift. The forces pulling fingers into ulnar deviation are well known, and in certain strain positions such as finger flexion, stress is placed on the structures which counter those forces. The very structures which balance the palmar and ulnar pull are those stretched and weakened in rheumatoid arthritis. Most significant is destruction of the radial collateral ligaments and the thin dorsal aponeurosis on the radial side of the extensor tendons which holds them centered over the metacarpophalangeal joint in flexion. As these supports give way, a cascade of events occurs which tends to increase the deformity to a point where it becomes fixed.

When synovectomy is performed, centralization of the extensor tendon, release of ulnar intrinsics to the proximal phalanges, and, sometimes, transfer of these to the radial side of the next ulnar finger tend to overcome the tendency toward ulnar drift.

Centralization of the extensor may be achieved by reefing the dorsal aponeurosis on the radial side of the extensor, usually with a longitudinal incisional release on the ulnar side. The transverse lamina or hood may be fixed to the dorsum of the proximal phalanx, or the tendon itself may be fixed at this point. Interphalangeal extension is then more dependent upon the intrinsic muscles than usual.

Example

A fifty-year-old housewife with a 15-year history of rheumatoid arthritis developed progressive ulnar drift of her fingers at the metacarpophalangeal joints. She noted progressive palmar drop of the proximal phalanges and inability to fully extend her metacarpophalangeal joints of both hands. Early boutonniere deformity was evident in the long, ring, and little fingers on the left. (**D**) She was suffering from

Surgery of Rheumatoid Arthritis

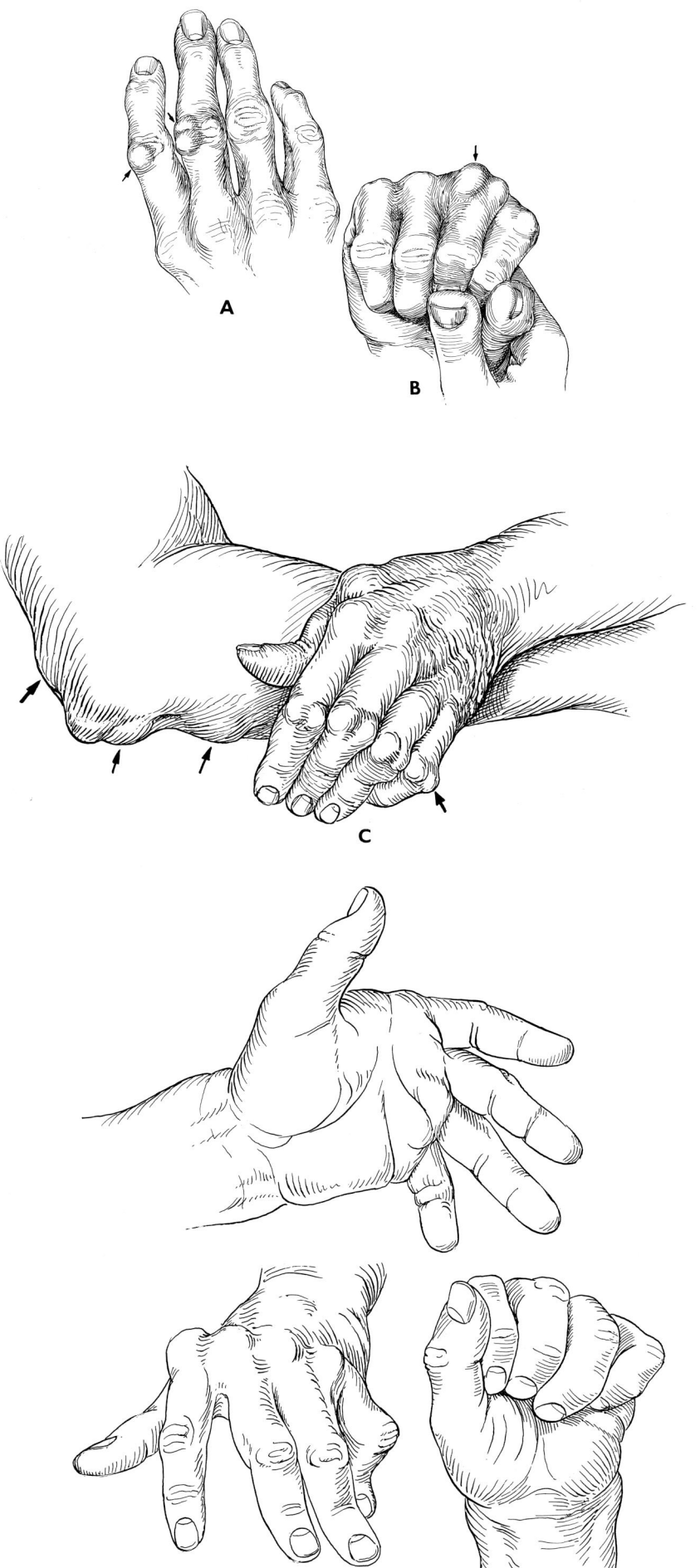

327

72 – Metacarpophalangeal Joint Synovectomy

considerable pain in her metacarpophalangeal joints and the extensor tendons were displaced ulnarward. (**E**)

Metacarpophalangeal joint synovectomy was elected after thorough discussion with the patient.

The procedure was performed through a transverse incision on the dorsum of the hand, a centimeter proximal to the knuckles. (**F**)

The dorsal blood vessels and sensory nerves were carefully preserved during dissection.

The extensor tendons were dislocated to the ulnar side of the metacarpophalangeal joints in all four fingers.

The proximal end of the dorsal expansion of the extensor mechanism was identified and separated from the underlying joint capsule on the radial side of the extensor tendons. (**G**)

Longitudinal incisions through the dorsal expansions were planned to preserve the expansion for repair by imbrication. (**H**)

With the dorsal fascia reflected, the joint capsule was opened and preserved and a dissection plane between it and the diseased hypertrophic synovium was developed. (**I**)

The diseased synovium was dissected up to the articular cartilage where it separated from the metacarpal head. Traction on the synovium being removed allowed thorough dorsal removal. Less adequate removal was possible around the collateral ligament areas and palmar aspect of the joint. The radial collateral ligament was preserved since it had not been destroyed by the disease and stress.

It was possible to repair the joint capsule after reduction of a partial subluxation of the metacarpophalangeal joint. The dorsal expansion incision was closed by imbrication of its edges to recentralize the extensor tendons. Relaxing incisions in the expansion on the ulnar side were necessary to centralize the extensor tendons of the long, ring, and little fingers.(**J**) The abductor digiti minimi insertion into the little finger was sectioned to allow relaxed corretion of the ulnar deviation and subluxation of the metacarpophalangeal joint.

After closure of the wound the hand was wrapped with a bulky dressing and a palmar splint was applied with the fingers in slight radial deviation and extension at the metacarpophalangeal joints. After five weeks of splinting, the patient was allowed progressive active motion during the day. A night splint was prescribed for an additional two months.

The patient's ability to extend the metacarpophalangeal joints improved and she had no pain in the metacarpophalangeal joints. This was reflected in an increase in grip strength but insignificant improvement in range of flexion of the metacarpophalangeal joint.

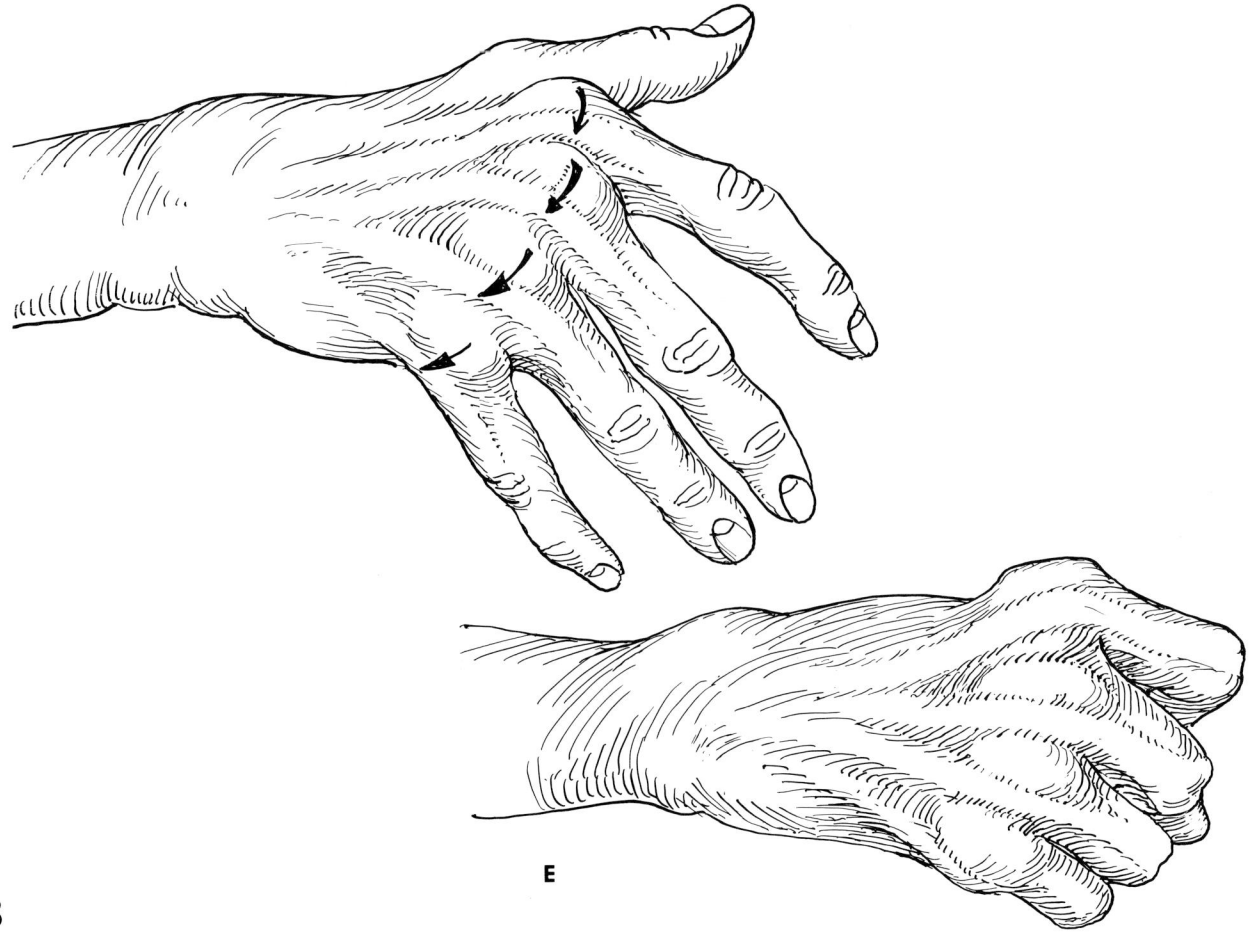

E

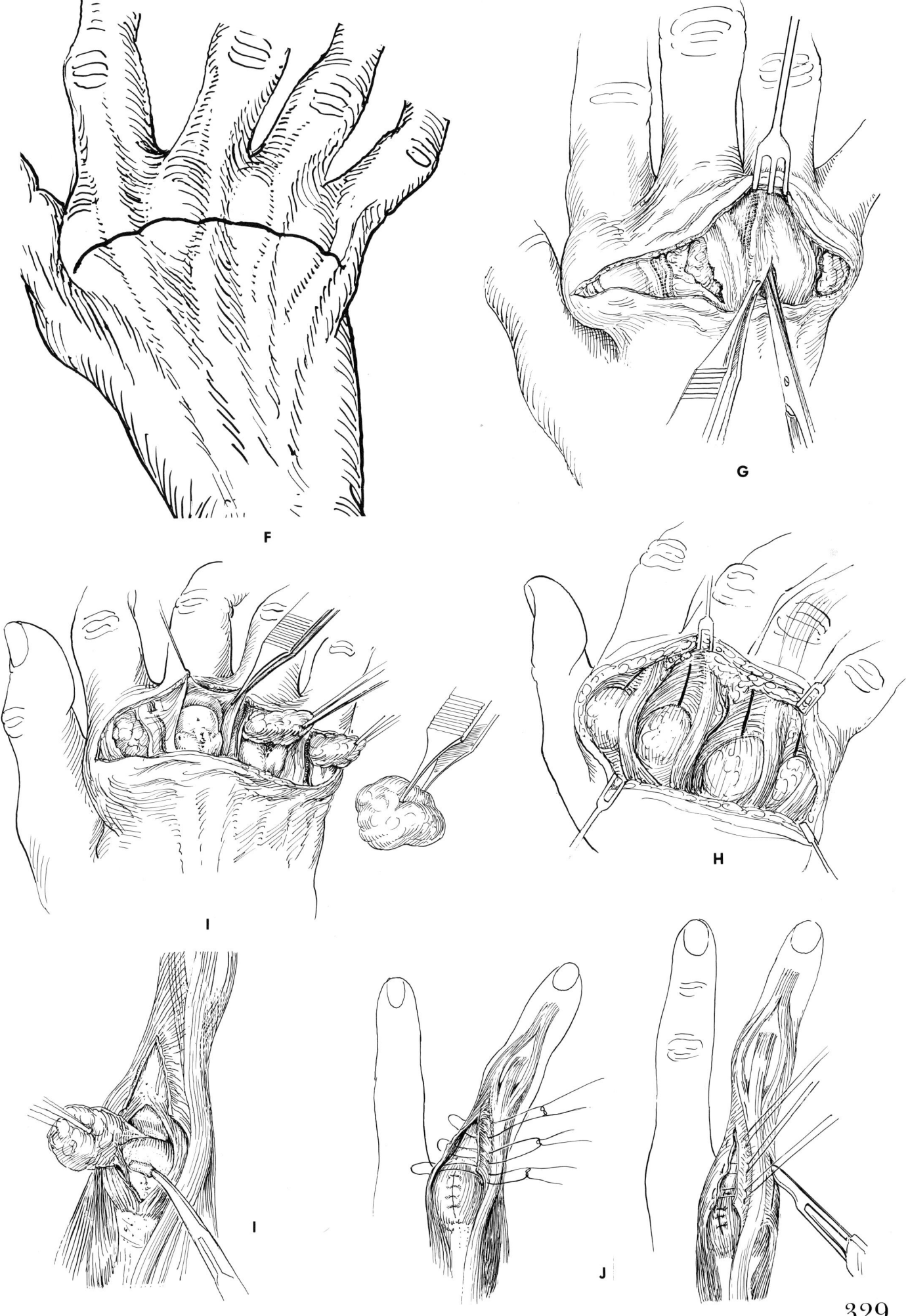

329

The purpose served by the procedure was to reduce the palmar subluxation of the metacarpophalangeal joints, to correct ulnar deviation and to eliminate the severe pain felt in the metacarpophalangeal joints. Reduction of pain and improvement of efficiency of the long flexors by metacarpophalangeal joint correction resulted in improved strength in flexion.

Extension ability at the metacarpophalangeal joints was improved by recentralization of the long extensor tendons. Pinch was augmented by correction of the ulnar drift of the fingers away from the thumb and elimination of pain at the metacarpophalangeal joints. Small gains in functional ability were much appreciated by the patient, as is true with most patients with arthritis. In addition, even though functional gains were minimal, the cosmetic correction was gratifying to this patient.

Preoperatively the patient's hand functioned in extension and flexion as shown. (**K**) Note the deforming palmar subluxation of the metacarpophalangeal joints in extension. Failure to fully extend was a result of this subluxation and the inability of the extensors to effect extension. The extensors lost their fulcrum for extension action as the tendons slipped from the top of the metacarpal head to the gutter on the ulnar side. The extensors then added to the forces causing ulnar deviation of the fingers at the metacarpophalangeal joint. Efficiency in metacarpophalangeal joint flexion by intrinsic and long flexors was sharply curtailed by subluxation of the metacarpophalangeal joints and resulting recession or shortening. Diminished efficiency of the long flexors and metacarpophalangeal joint pain weakened flexion power at the interphalangeal joints.

After surgical correction the appearance and function of the hand improved. (**L**) Once healing was complete the metacarpophalangeal joints were nearly pain free on active and passive motion. Centralization of the extensor tendons improved efficiency of metacarpophalangeal joint extension, and the subluxation tendency was diminished. Although the range of motion in flexion of the metacarpophalangeal joints was not increased, grip strength and efficiency of flexion of the interphalangeal joints was improved.

The patient asked for corrective surgery on the left hand and this has been performed.

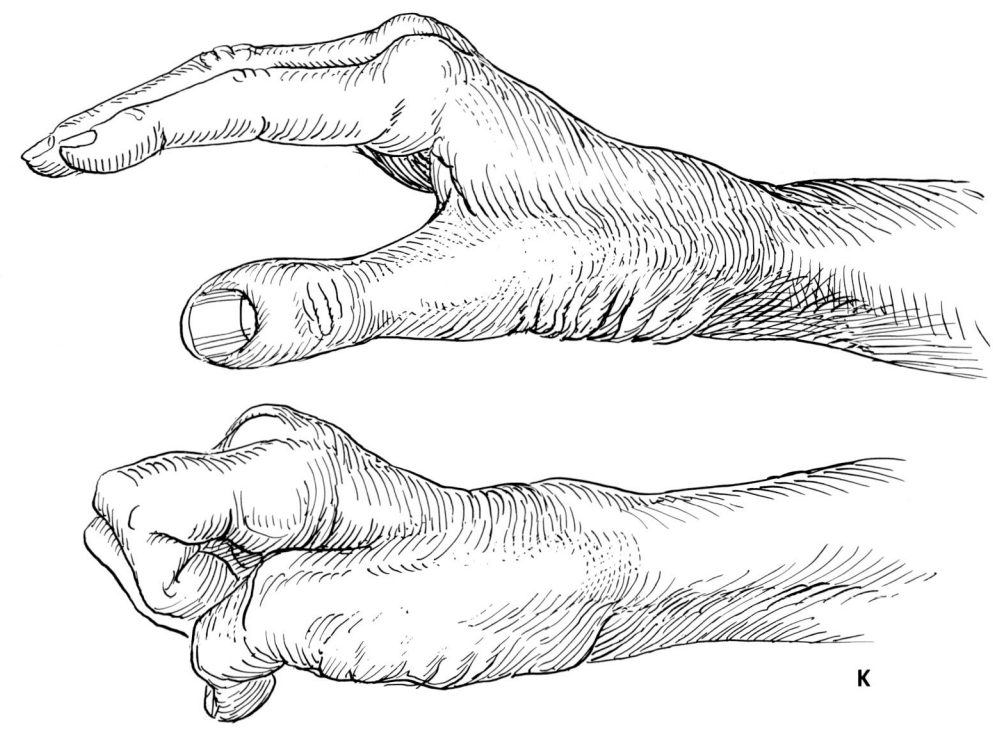

PREOPERATIVE

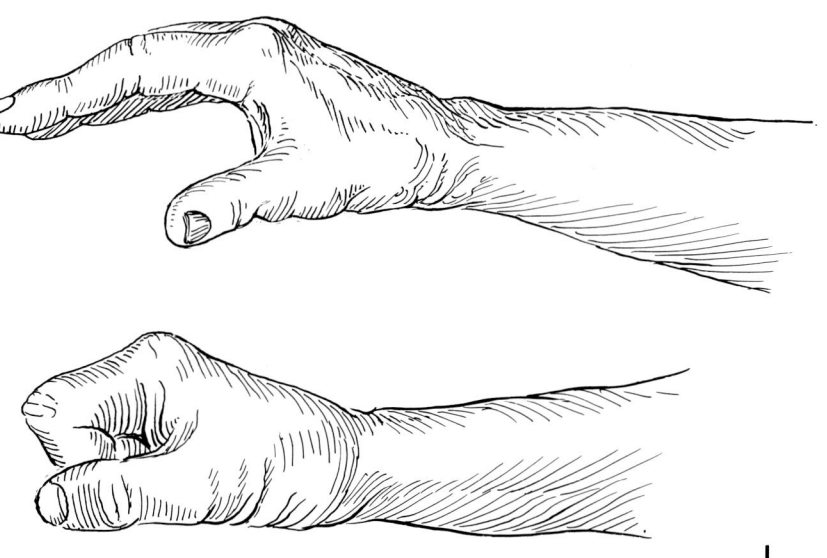

POSTOPERATIVE

73 Finger Arthroplasty

With x-ray and clinical evidence of deforming destruction of the head of the metacarpal in arthritis, arthroplasty may be the operation of choice for metacarpophalangeal joint reconstruction. Whenever metacarpophalangeal synovectomy is done for this disease, one should be prepared to perform an arthroplasty if the indication is evident on joint exploration. Palmar subluxation of the proximal phalanx is the rule as ligamentous support gives way. (**A** and **B**)

Many ingenious methods have been designed to keep the joint from resubluxating following arthroplasty. The simplest arthroplasty for the metacarpophalangeal joints consists of opening the joint, resecting the head of the metacarpal, and shaping it for articulation with the proximal phalanx. Some variations on this theme are worthy of mention.

Access to the metacarpophalangeal joints is acquired through the dorsal aponeurosis. The approach is the same as that described for implant arthroplasty. (See p. 334.) After a long period of palmar subluxation, it is not possible to relocate the proximal phalanx over the distal end of the metacarpal head. Ligamentous and intrinsic muscle shortening reins the proximal phalanx into the flexed subluxed position. Shortening the metacarpal by resecting the distal end will allow easy relocation of the finger on the metacarpal.

The metacarpal head may be shaped like the roof of a house, with the ridge placed horizontally and at an angle to allow the flat end of the proximal phalanx to teeter into flexion and extension but not deviate in an ulnar or radial direction. (**C**)

Resubluxation may be prevented by fixing the extensor tendon to the dorsum of the proximal portion of the proximal phalanx. (**D**)

Alternatively, the extensor may be shortened and its superfluous portion used as a spacer in the new joint by using the Vainio modification. The extensor tendon is cut across proximal to the metacarpophalangeal joint by about 1.5 cm. (**E**) The long distal end of the tendon is dropped into the joint space and sutured to the palmar capsule. (**F**) The proximal tendon end is sutured to the extensor at the dorsum of the proximal end of the proximal phalanx. Vainio recommends repair of the collateral ligaments by reinserting them onto the dorsolateral aspect of the metacarpal just proximal to the site of resection of the metacarpal head. (**G**)

After fibrous or even bony ankylosis the metacarpophalangeal joint may be remobilized by arthroplasty. (**H**)

NORMAL

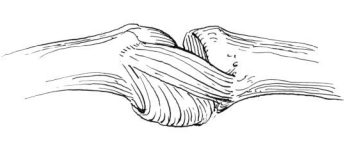

A

METACARPOPHALANGEAL SUBLUXATION

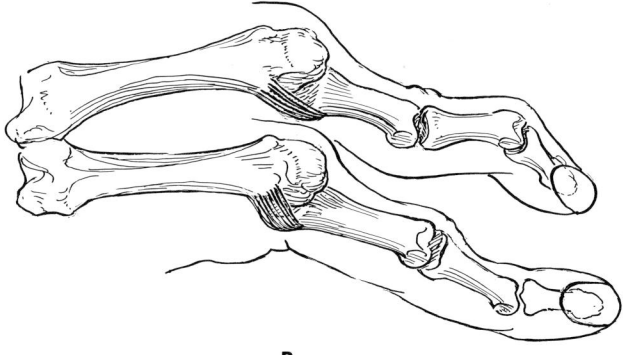

B

Surgery of Rheumatoid Arthritis

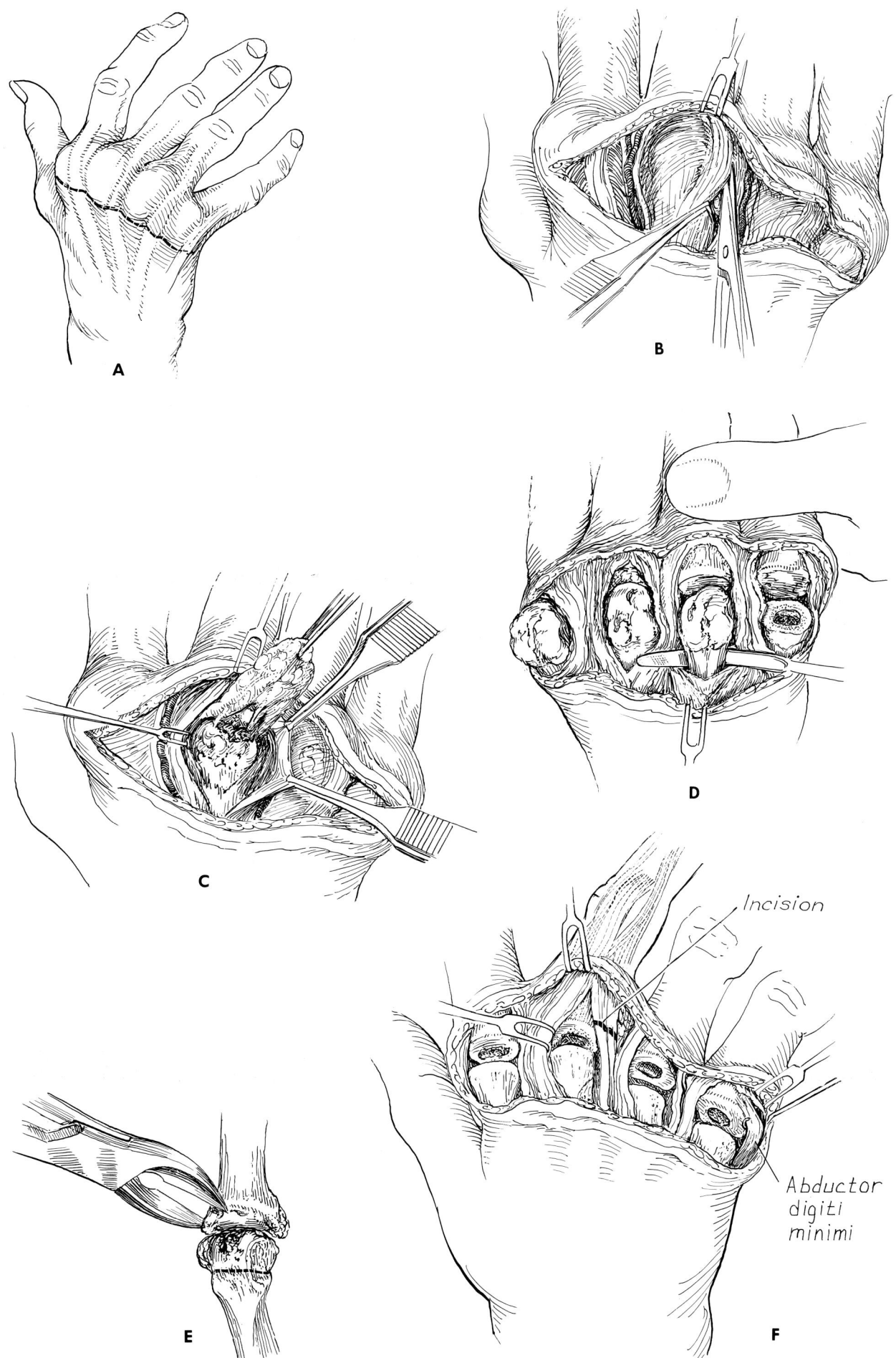

335

The bone ends are prepared to receive the silicone prostheses by reaming out the medullary cavity with a broach or special drill. Test implants are used to determine proper size. The largest possible implant should be used. (**G**)

The proximal stem of the chosen implant is inserted into the prepared metacarpal recipient area with the proximal phalanx palmar subluxated. The implant is handled with blunt instruments and "no touch" technique to avoid damage and weakening of the formed silicone. Once it is well seated in the metacarpal end, the proximal phalanx can be manipulated over the distal stem by traction and bending of the prostheses. (**H**) Once the prosthesis is fully seated, passive flexion and extension will reveal a need for further bone trimming or shaping.

The extensor mechanism is closed by reefing the dorsal aponeurosis on the radial side, to center or slightly overcorrect the ulnar shift of the extensor tendon by pulling it radial to the mid-dorsal line of the joint. (**I**)

After skin closure, a soft bulky dressing and plaster splint are applied with the metacarpophalangeal joints in extension. After routine wound checks in the first few days, the hand is put at rest for five days to a week. After this, controlled motion in flexion and extension—without ulnar or radial deviation—is started. Special dynamic splints are used to continue to control the axis of motion. A carefully controlled program of progressive motion is insisted upon over several months after implant arthroplasty.

Proximal Interphalangeal Joint

The normal proximal interphalangeal joints are hinge joints with little lateral mobility. Frequently the choice is made to surgically fuse the joint when it is painful, malpositioned, or destroyed. If the function of the metacarpophalangeal joint of the finger is reduced, the need to preserve mobility in the proximal interphalangeal joint is more compelling. Small spacer implants for the proximal interphalangeal joints may be implanted safely when the prime tendons affecting the joint are intact. The implant arthroplasty is useless unless one can preserve extensor motor function by saving or reconstructing the central extensor slip.

Through a dorsal longitudinal curved incision over the joint, the extensor mechanism is exposed. The joint may be entered lateral to the central slip or by splitting it longitudinally proximal from its insertion into the proximal phalanx. (**J**)

Preparation of the implant

1. Boil implants with distilled water and non-oily mild soap for 20 minutes.
2. Rinse thoroughly in distilled water.
3. Wrap in lint-free cloth or place on clean open tray and autoclave by one of the following methods:
   a. High speed instrument sterilizer   3 minutes at 270° F
   b. Standard gravity sterilizer   30 minutes at 250° F
   c. Prevacuum high-temperature sterilizer   Normal cycle at 250° F
4 Use no-touch technique with blunt instruments.

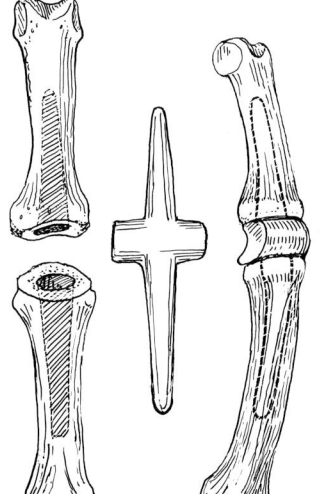

G

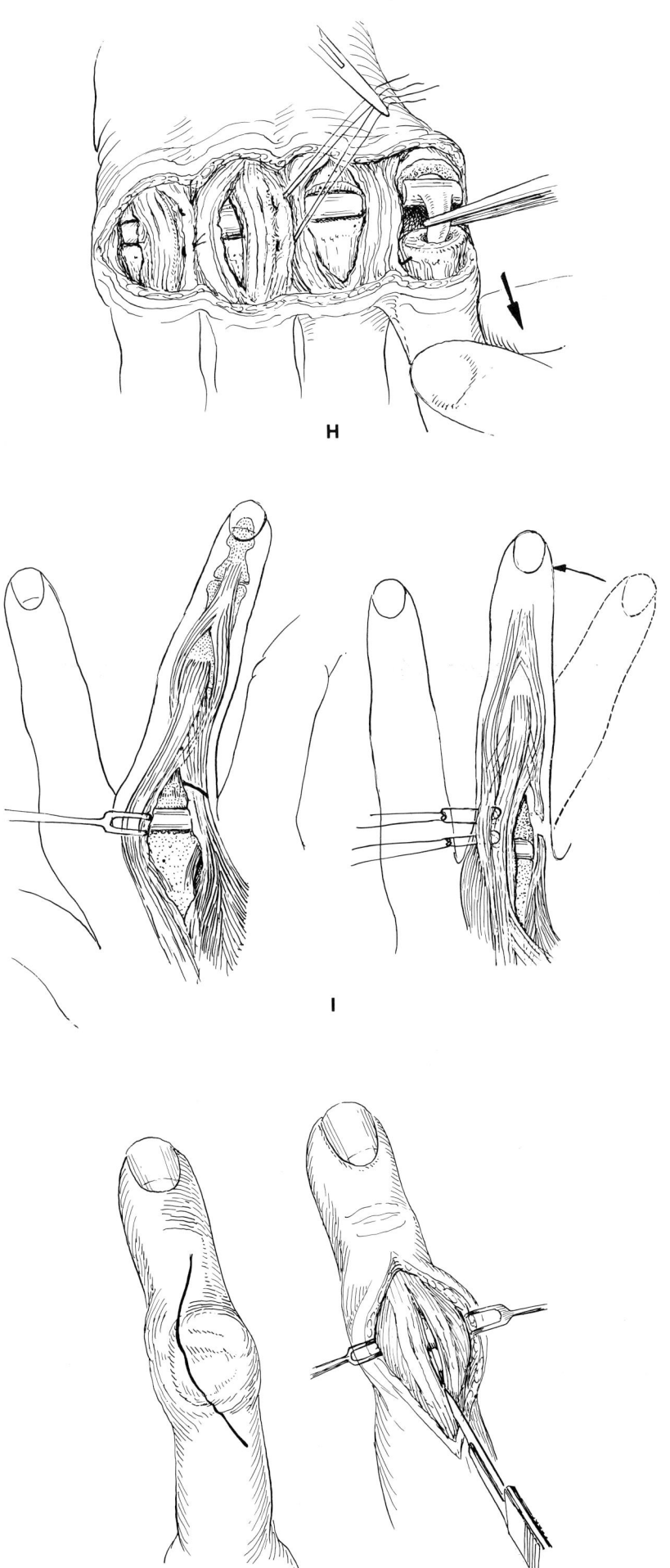

73 — Finger Arthroplasty

With the joint subluxated, the bone ends are treated in the same manner as outlined under metacarpophalangeal joint implant arthroplasty. (**K**) The spacer prosthesis is inserted and the extensor mechanism is repaired. (**L and M**) Motion is started after the first postoperative week but strictly in the flexor-extension plane.

Joint Prosthesis — Niebauer vs. Swanson

The Niebauer prosthesis is a hinged prosthesis with Dacron mesh through its center and covering the stems. The Swanson prosthesis is fashioned solely of silicone. (**N**)

With the Niebauer prosthesis adhesion to bone occurs at the stems, and no piston movement or slippage occurs. This may lend lateral stability beyond that acquired from the natural scar substitute for collateral ligaments. (**O**) Piston motion of the stems is considered an advantage of the Swanson prosthesis by its advocates. There may be less stress wear and more range of motion with the slippage.

The prostheses are manufactured in five sizes, with reamers or broaches to match.

When either prosthesis is used, enough bone must be removed to allow easy relocation of the proximal phalanx on the metacarpal. If significant tension exists at the time of operation, more bone should be removed. This avoids the problem of buckling of the prosthesis. Niebauer suggests cutting across the metacarpal so the end angles about 10 degrees toward the radial side of the hand. (**P**)

Further protection against recurrence of ulnar drift by deviation at the metacarpophalangeal joint may be provided by sectioning the interosseous tendons on the ulnar side of each finger. Added defense against drift is provided by transferring the sectioned interosseous tendons to the radial side of the adjacent finger. If interosseous transfer is done, Flatt's recommendation that insertion be to bone or collateral ligament should be followed.

Thumb Carpometacarpal Joint

Disability from a painful, crepitating, subluxating first carpometacarpal joint is a common indication for surgery in rheumatoid arthritis, osteoarthritis, and unstable post-injury subluxation. If retention of motion at this joint is crucial, either synovectomy and ligament reconstruction or implant arthroplasty must be the treatment of choice. Inadequate function and range of motion in the other joints in the thumb makes retention of motion important. Trapezium implants with a stem for insertion of the proximal end of the first metacarpal are made for this purpose. A curved incision to expose the "anatomical snuff box" area between the extensor pollicis longus and brevis is appropriate for an approach to the first carpometacarpal joint. Care must be exercised to avoid injury to the dorsal branch of the radial nerve superficially and the radial artery deeply. The trapezium (greater multangular) is removed, preserving the articular capsule. The proximal end of the metacarpal is prepared to receive the stem of the prosthesis by drilling and reaming the medullary cavity. The stem of the prosthesis is inserted well in place and the round head of the prosthesis is seated in the space previously occupied by the trapezium. Soft tissue and skin closure complete the procedure. (See Section 65, Fusion of Thumb Carpometacarpal Joint.)

Niebauer versus Swanson

Niebauer:
1. *Strength of implant augmented by Dacron.*
2. *Lateral stability with fixation.*
3. *Avoids synovium re-formation around implant in bone which may be subject to continuing rheumatoid destruction (unconfirmed).*

Swanson:
1. *Piston motion of stem in metacarpal and phalanx adds some greater range of motion and generates less stress on prosthesis.*
2. *Shorter period of postoperative immobilization necessary.*
3. *Easily removable when necessary.*

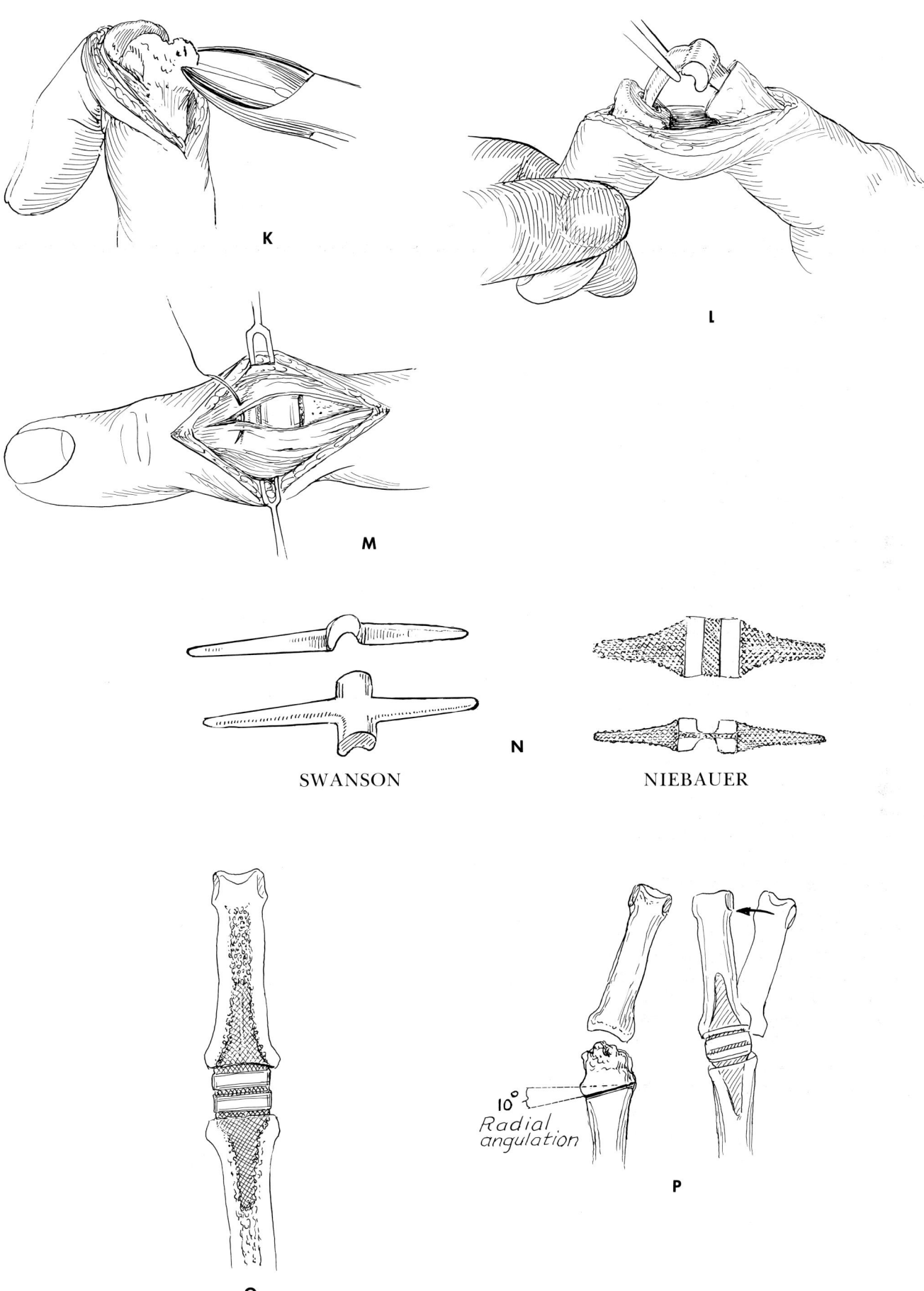

74

Synovectomy of Extensor Tendons at the Wrist

Principle

The synovial membranes surrounding the extensor tendons at the wrist when involved in rheumatoid arthritis pose a threat to the continuing integrity of the extensors. The extensors pass through tunnels beneath the extensor retinaculum at the wrist, and at this point tendon direction changes, creating a need for this pulley-like mechanism. Tendon gliding within the tunnels is assured by the existence of synovium. The inflammation of this synovium in rheumatoid disease causes swelling, thickening, and invasion of the tendons by inflammatory cells.

Clinically, the synovial swelling is evident as it protrudes both proximal and distal to the extensor retinaculum. Drug therapy and immobilization may be adequate to control this dorsal tenosynovitis but if it is progressive despite nonsurgical efforts, one should urge synovectomy.

Example

A 38-year-old woman with a five-year history of rheumatoid arthritis had pain over the extensor surface of her wrist and marked swelling limited to the extensor tendon area for an area three centimeters distal to the extensor retinaculum at the wrist. The mass was boggy and cystic to palpation, and on pressure one could detect transmission to the area beneath the retinaculum and proximal to it in the forearm.

Because of her pain, and the probable threat to the integrity of her extensor tendons, extensor synovectomy was decided upon.

The procedure was done through a lazy-S-shaped incision on the dorsum of the hand and wrist, extending proximal and distal to the extensor retinaculum. (**A**)

The extrasynovial extensor retinaculum was incised at the ulnar border and the retinaculum was reflected radially. By cutting the partitions between the tunnels close to bone, the retinaculum was lifted like a blanket across the wrist. (**B**)

As much of the hypertrophic synovium as possible was excised, being careful not to injure the already weakened extensor tendons. (**C**)

The flap of extensor retinaculum was replaced beneath the tendons and the wound was closed. (**D**)

There was considerable bow-stringing of the extensors after this procedure, but this was little sacrifice to make to save the extensor tendons from progressive destruction, stretching, and rupture. The procedure is commonly combined with resection of the ulna head where this is indicated (see Section 76), and not infrequently it is combined with wrist joint synovectomy.

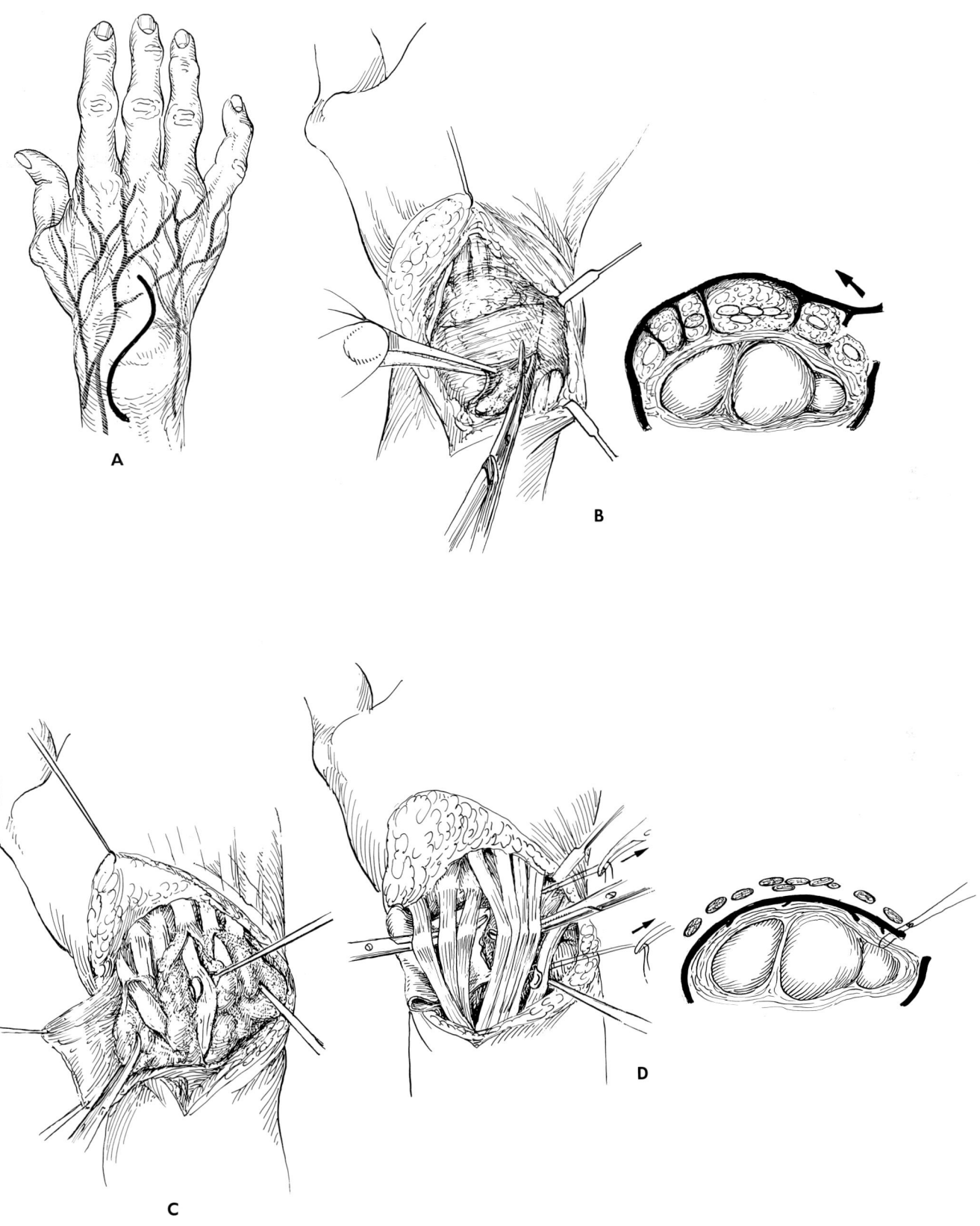

75

Rupture of Extensor Tendons

Principle

Rheumatoid synovitis involving the synovium around the extensor tendons at the wrist, if left unchecked, may ultimately result in destruction of the extensor tendons. Rupture or attenuation and stretching of the extensor tendons leaves the patient unable to extend the metacarpophalangeal joints and robs him of extension strength at the interphalangeal joint levels. Diseased and attenuated extensors are not repairable by suture repair without reinforcement. The best method to restore extension capability is by tendon transfer. Occasionally, one may use a tendon graft to bridge the area of weakness in the extensor. However, it is generally more satisfactory to hook the distal end of the ruptured tendon into a functioning, intact extensor by transfer.

Example

A 50-year-old man with rheumatoid arthritis involving multiple joints developed progressive weakness in extension of the long, ring, and little fingers of his right hand. He developed a finger drop deformity to a disabling degree in these fingers and sought professional help. (**A**)

The patient had excellent strength in the extensor indicis, and a transfer of the extensors of the ulnar three fingers to the indicis was selected for treatment.

Surgical exploration of the dorsum of the hand revealed an undiseased, intact extensor digitorum tendon to the index finger as well as a normal extensor indicis. A side-to-side juncture of the distal ends of the extensor digitorum tendons of the long and ring fingers, as well as the tendon of the extensor digiti minimi, to the extensor digitorum to the index finger was performed while the three dropped digits were held in extension. (**B** and **C**)

The hand was splinted with the fingers in extension at the metacarpophalangeal joints and comfortable neutral position of the interphalangeal joints. Extension splinting was maintained for six weeks, after which graded active motion was permitted. Although complete extension was not restored to the long, ring, and little fingers, the function was much improved. Independent extension of the index finger was undisturbed.

Surgery of Rheumatoid Arthritis

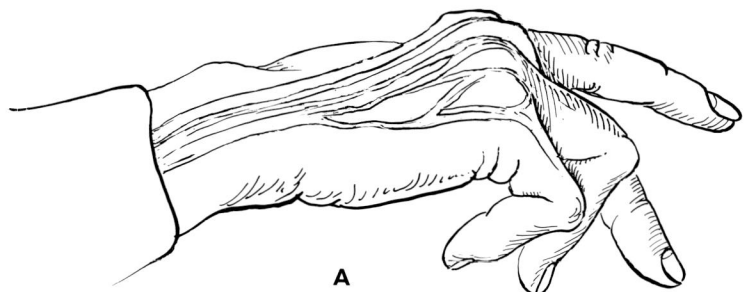
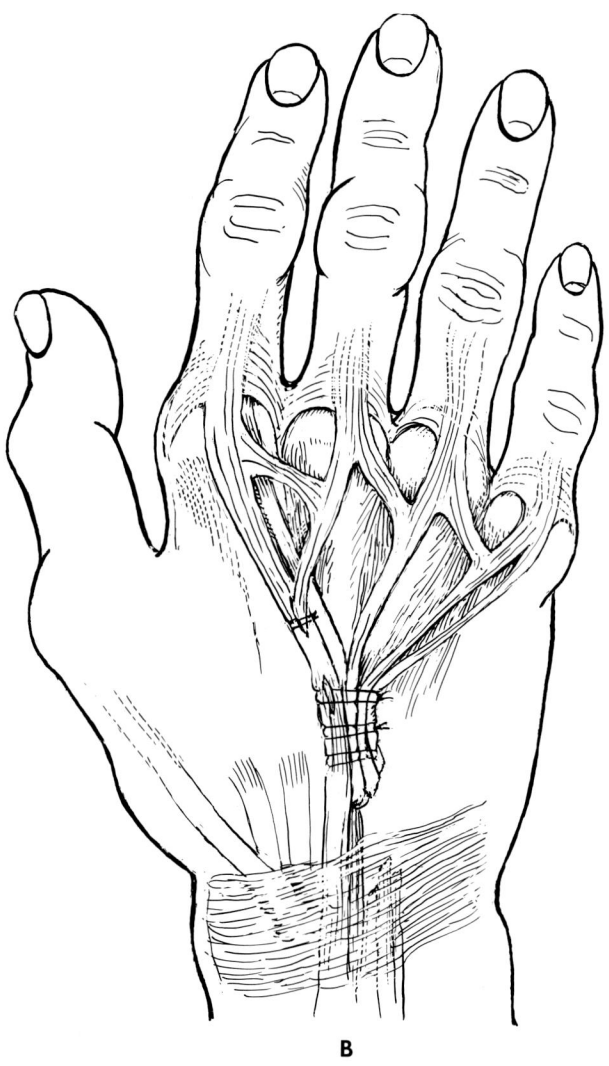
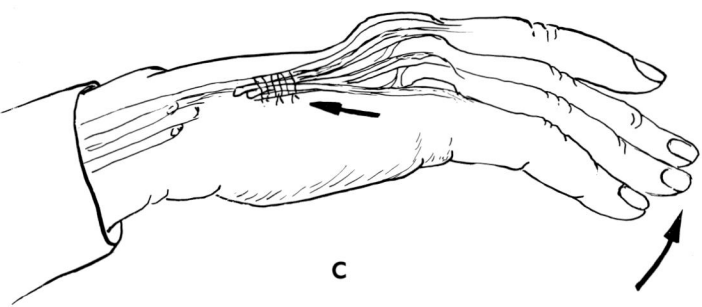

76

Resection of the Ulnar Head

Principle

In rheumatoid arthritis the distal radial-ulnar articulation is frequently involved. The marked synovial swelling around the head of the ulna is readily detectable clinically. Destruction of the ligaments which normally restrain the head of the ulna results in abnormal motion, particularly on supination and pronation. The head of the ulna generally dislocates dorsally. Pushing it back into place elicits considerable pain. Pain and limitation of motion are indications for surgery. The simplest procedure is resection of the ulnar head and the distal 2 centimeters of the ulna. This procedure is *not* done in a growing child. It is a procedure simply done through a longitudinal incision over the ulnar dorsal aspect of the head of the ulna. The dorsal branch of the ulnar nerve is scrupulously preserved.

Example

A sixty-year-old woman with advanced deformities from rheumatoid arthritis came for consultation complaining about pain in the left wrist and a bumping dislocation of the ulnar head on supination. There was marked limitation in her range of supination and pronation which was exaggerated by her pain. She had visible dorsal dislocation of the ulnar head on supination. (**A**)

Resection of the ulna head was done in combination with other reconstructive procedures on the hand. The procedure was performed through a short dorsal longitudinal incision over the ulna head.

The dorsal branch of the ulnar nerve was retracted with the skin and subcutaneous tissue on the ulnar side of the wound.

A limited subperiosteal dissection around the ulna 2 to 3 centimeters from the articular surface was done (**B**) in preparation for a square cut osteotomy, which was done simply with a small-blade oscillating bone saw. (**C**)

The distal ulna and head were dissected out from proximal to distal by reflecting the distal bone fragment up out of the wound. (**D**)

Soft tissue closure in layers filled the residual dead space. Immobilization for two weeks to achieve soft tissue healing was followed by progressive unrestricted free activity.

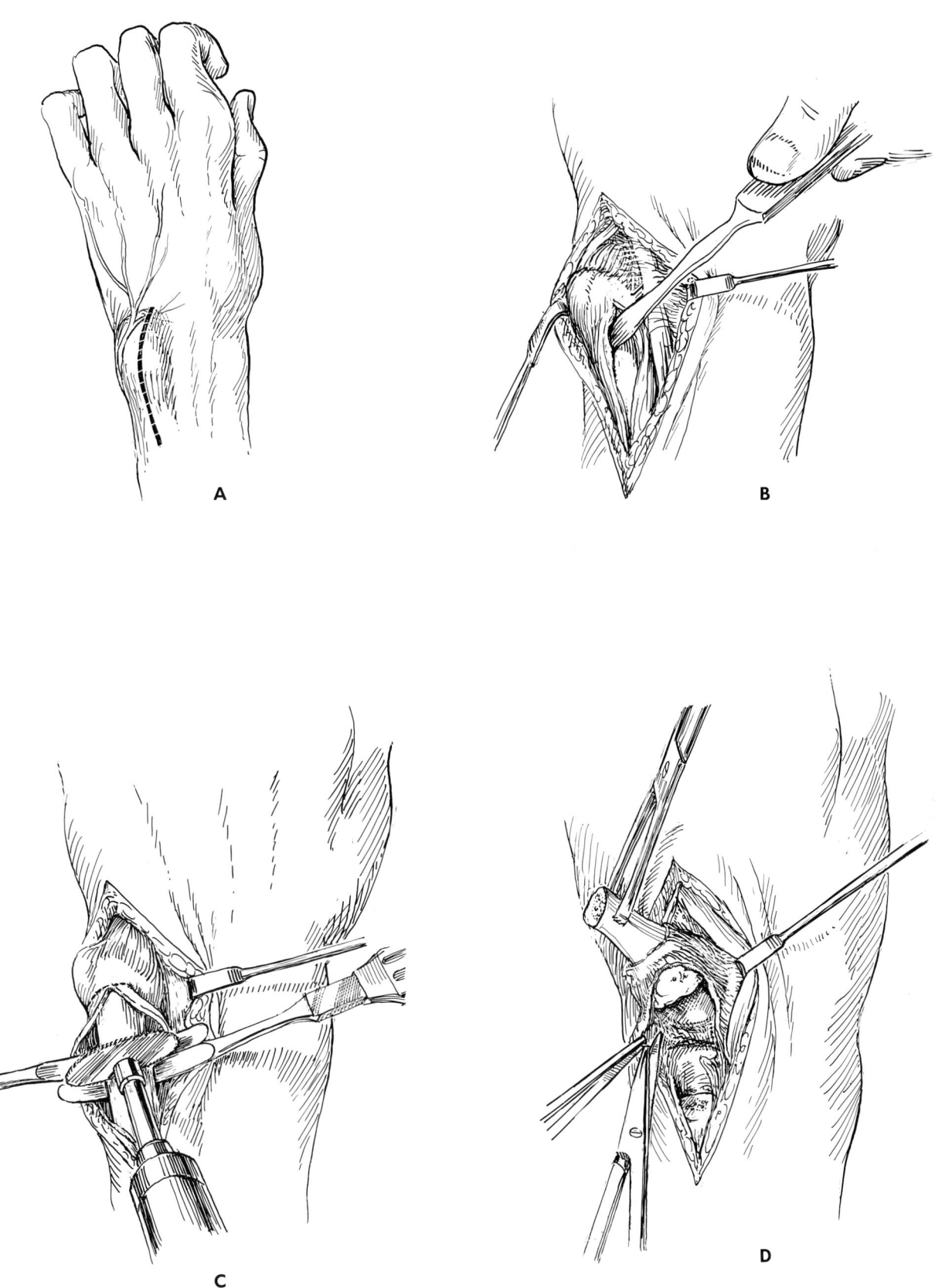

Tendons, Fascia and Muscles

77

Tendon Injuries

Principles

Disruption of tendon continuity may be a result of laceration, avulsion, or destruction by disease. When avulsion injuries occur, the tendon ruptures at its weakest area. This is usually at the musculotendinous juncture, but it may also occur at the site of tendon insertion into bone. Avulsion amputation of digits may result in rupture of the extrinsic musculotendinous units at the musculotendinous junction and removal of the entire tendon from the forearm. Tendon disruption by destruction, which is most frequent in rheumatoid arthritis, is dealt with elsewhere (see Section 75). Traumatic laceration of a tendon is managed in a variety of ways depending on which tendon is lacerated and at what level.

Tendon Repair

End-to-end repair of a transected tendon is best performed with a single non-absorbable, precisely placed suture.

The technique is best initiated by controlling the tendon by securely grasping the cut ends with hemostats. A non-absorbable suture, armed at each end with a swaged-on straight needle, allows placement of the suture. The first pass of the suture is straight across the tendon 1.0 to 1.5 centimeters from the cut end of the tendon. (**A**) The suture is adjusted to equalize the length of suture emerging from each side of the tendon and the first needle is inserted just distal to the first pass, obliquely toward a point about one-third of the way to the cut tendon end.

Before the needle is pulled through, the second needle is passed across the first and then both needles may be pulled through the tendon. (**B**) This avoids spearing the suture with the needle crossing it within the tendon.

The first pass out of the first tendon end is made after the tendon is cut nearly through. (**C** and **D**)

The other cut end of the tendon partially transected close to the controlling clamp. (**E**)

The same needles and sutures are now passed into the freshened tendon end and out the side of the tendon. (**F**) The crisscross technique is continued, being careful that the needles are inserted across one another each time before the suture is passed. This is particularly crucial at this stage since tightening and adjustment of the suture requires unrestricted slippage within the tendon.

The tendon ends are pulled together by tightening the suture ends *one at a time* while the tendon is held atraumatically just proximal to the site of emergence of the suture ends. The tendon should be bunched up slightly to assure good tendon end coaptation. The suture ends are tied when tension is judged to be appropriate. The technique leaves the externalized suture knot away from the site of tendon repair. (**G**)

If a pull-out wire technique is being used, the pull-out wire is placed around the tendon suture before the first pass is made through the tendon.

A

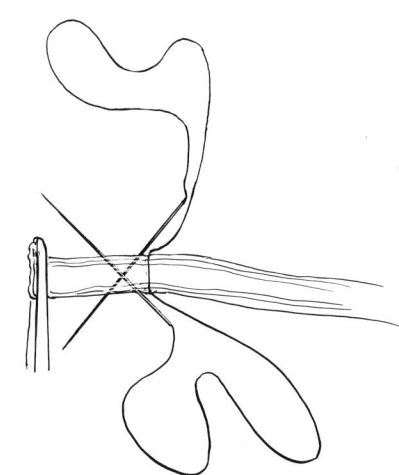

B

Tendons, Fascia and Muscles

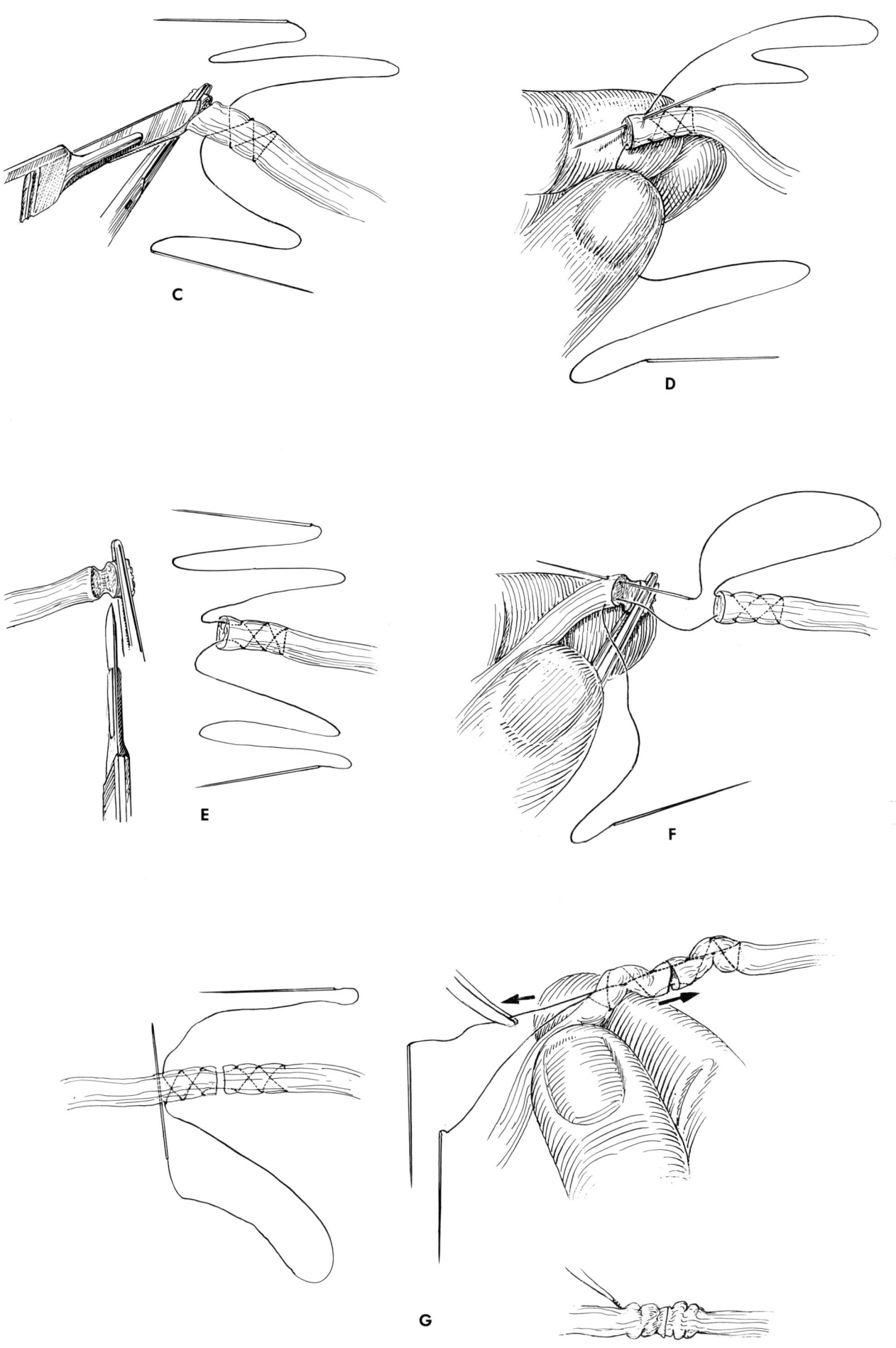

347

78

Flexor Tendon Lacerations

Principles

A knowledge of certain anatomical relationships of the long flexor tendons of the fingers is crucial to the surgeon who intends to treat tendon injuries.

1. Nature has provided fibrous restraining sheaths to prevent bowstringing of the flexor tendons in areas where flexion creates mobile concavity. In the digit the fibrous sheath for the tendons extends from the distal joint to just proximal to the metacarpophalangeal joint. (**A**) The longitudinal arch over the length of the metacarpal is fixed, and at this level there is no fibrous tendon sheath. The flexor surface of the wrist, however, moves from convexity to sharp concavity. The flexor tendons are prevented from bowstringing by the flexor retinaculum at the carpal level. This transverse carpal ligament forms the roof of the carpal tunnel.

Tendon injuries which occur at levels where the range of excursion puts the injury within the rigid tunnels formed by the fibrous structures in the finger and at the wrist require special consideration. This is particularly true in the finger itself, where the profundus and superficialis are in intimate relationship to one another in a tough, immobile fibrous sheath which forms a fitted tunnel for the flexors. (**B**)

Adhesions between this fibrous sheath and the flexor tendons effectively destroy their unique function of flexing the interphalangeal joints.

2. The skin injury associated with injury of the underlying tendons is not a reliable indication of the level of the underlying tendon injury. For example, if laceration in the distal palm occurs with the finger fully flexed, the skin incision may be at the level of the proximal end of the digital fibrous flexor sheath but, as the finger is extended, the cut tendon end is in the fibrous sheath. (**C**) The excursion of the tendon at the site of laceration is almost entirely within the fibrous sheath. (**D**)

If, however, the laceration at the same skin level occurs with the finger extended, (**E**) the tendon excursion at the injury site will be entirely within the palm proximal to the fibrous flexor sheath. (**F**) The distal tendon ends are then readily located in the distal palm by simply passively flexing the finger.

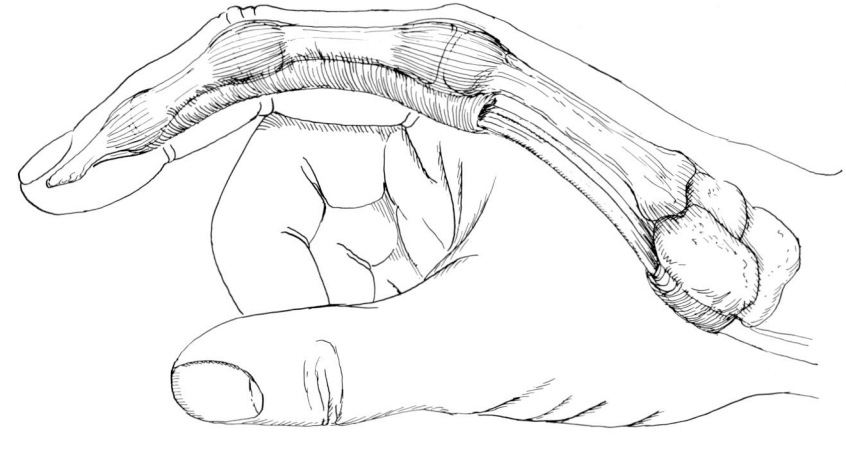

A

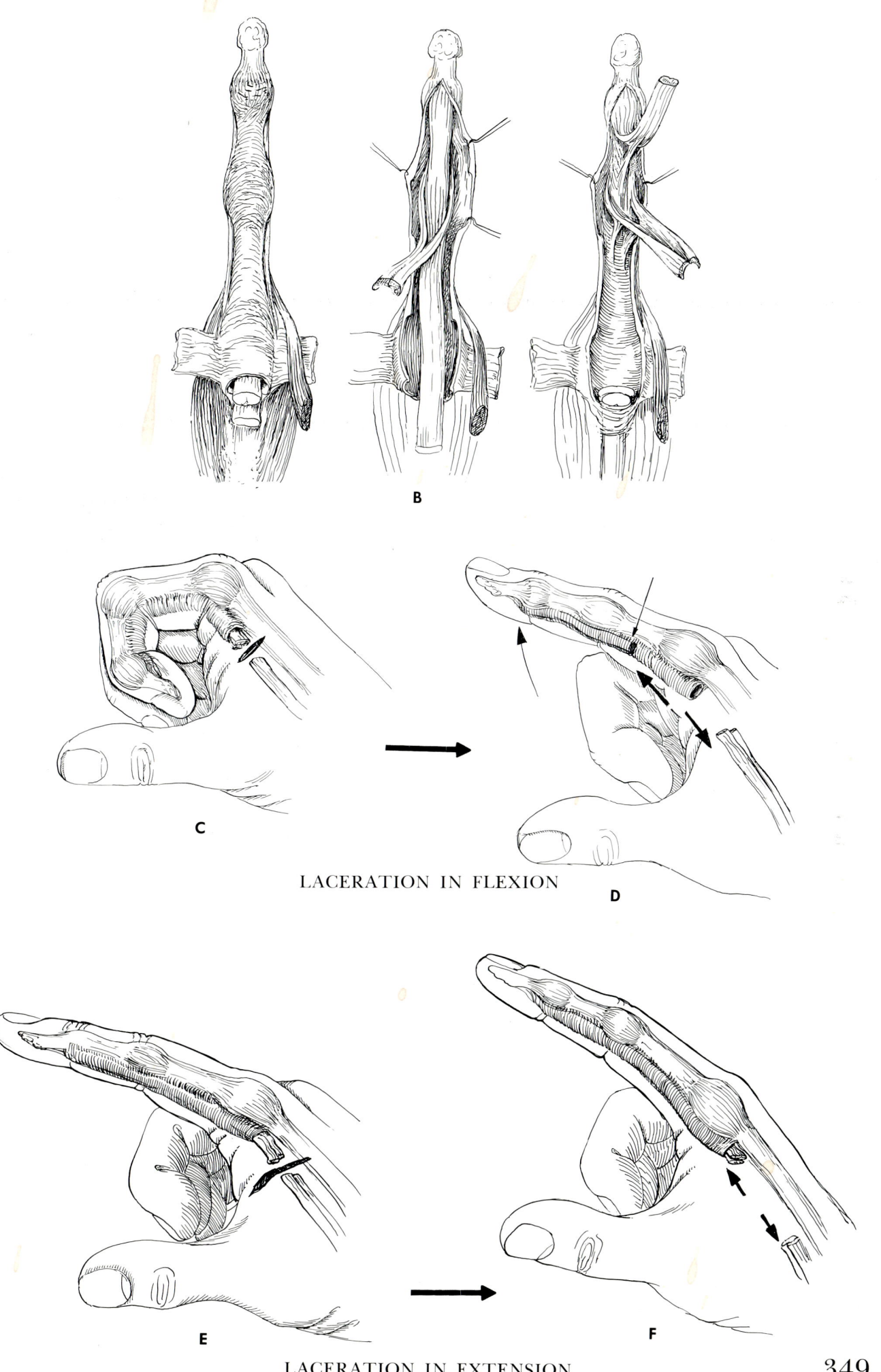

B

LACERATION IN FLEXION

LACERATION IN EXTENSION

3. It is unwise to repair both the profundus and superficialis tendons when they are cut adjacent to one another since the two repairs are likely to adhere to one another. This robs each of its normal range of motion.

4. Function of the flexor digitorum superficialis and the flexor digitorum profundus may be tested clinically in a conscious, cooperative patient. Since the profundus is the only flexor which inserts on the distal phalanx, the ability to actively flex the distal interphalangeal joint confirms the presence of an intact profundus. Transection, rupture, or paralysis of the profundus tendon should be suspected when the distal interphalangeal joint fails to flex when the patient makes a fist.

The diagnosis is further confirmed by specifically testing the patient's ability to flex the distal interphalangeal joint while the other joints of the finger are held in extension. (**G**)

The superficialis tendon splits at the level of the proximal phalanx to allow passage of the profundus through it to the distal phalanx. The two tails of the superficialis insert on the middle phalanx after they coalesce and decussate deep to the profundus tendon. (**H**) Thus the superficialis will not affect the distal interphalangeal joint but is a prime flexor of the proximal interphalangeal joint.

Since a muscle-tendon unit affects every joint between its origin and insertion, the flexor digitorum profundus also may flex the proximal interphalangeal joint. This makes the diagnosis of nonfunction of the superficialis more difficult. Each superficialis flexor has its own muscle belly and each acts independently of the others. The profundus flexors are not as independent since there is a common muscle for the long, ring, and little finger profundus tendons and a variable degree of interconnection between these and the index finger profundus. The diagnosis of disruption of flexor digitorum superficialis function is confirmed by check-reining the profundus by holding the other fingers in extension while the patient actively attempts to flex the finger whose superficialis is being tested. (**I**) Flexon of the finger at the proximal interphalangeal joint while the distal interphalangeal joint remains loosely extended confirms the functional integrity of the flexor digitorum superficialis.

Surgical approach to flexor tendons in the finger is best through a mid-axial incision in the finger. (See Section 6, Incisions.) Once the skin incision is made the surgeon comes upon the skin ligaments of Clelland from the sides of the phalanges to the lateral palmar skin. (**J**) Identification and precise section of these ligaments allows the palmar skin to fall away from the finger to expose the neurovascular structures and the flexor tendon sheath. (**K**)

Such a mid-axial digital incision may be extended onto the palm by designing it in a curvilinear mode to avoid an unbroken longitudinal palmar scar. (**L**) This extension will expose the entire hand and digit long flexor anatomy. The neurovascular structures must be carefully protected at the base of the finger where the skin incision crosses the route of the proper digital nerves and blood vessels.

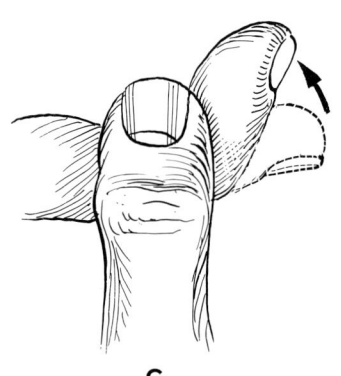

G

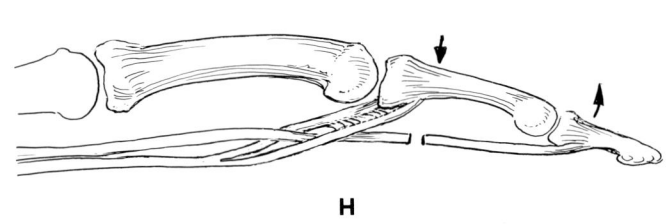

H

Tendons, Fascia and Muscles

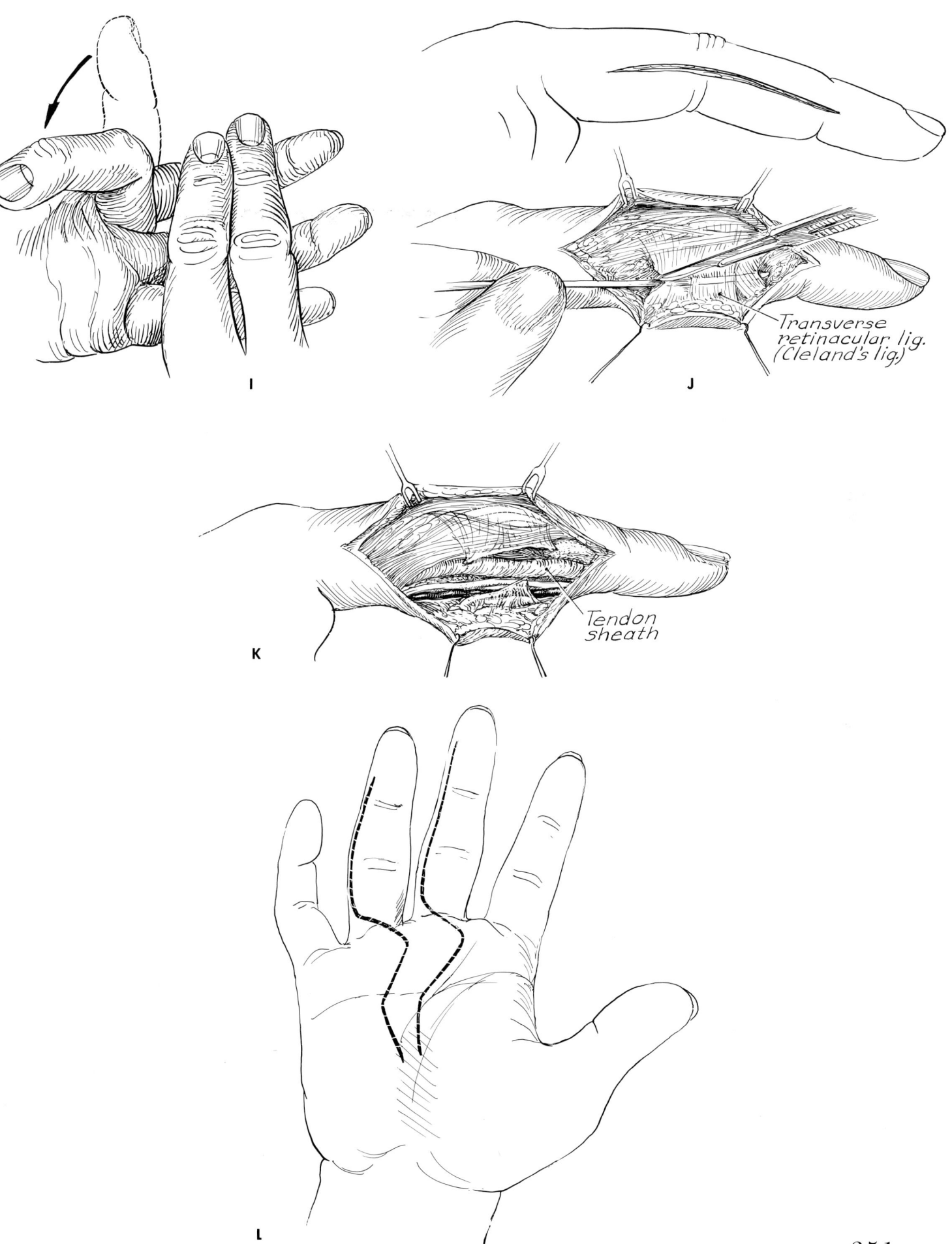

351

Primary Management

When flexor tendons are traumatically divided in the wrist and hand, serious permanent disability may result if inappropriate primary surgery is performed. Experienced surgeons have agreed on what surgery is appropriate when tendons are divided at some levels. They continue to debate the case for or against primary repair of tendons divided within the digital theca over the proximal phalanx and proximal half of the middle phalanx of the finger in adults. There is general agreement that primary repair of a divided profundus tendon is appropriate when division occurs: (1) within 1.5 centimeters of its insertion into the distal phalanx; (2) proximal to the digital theca in the hand and wrist; (3) at any level in a child under 8 years of age.

There is fair agreement that if the profundus and superficialis tendons are divided adjacent to one another in an adult that repair of the profundus should be performed and that the superficialis is best left unrepaired. There is general agreement that the flexor pollicis longus should be repaired primarily when it is sectioned in a clean wound.

No tendon should be repaired in heavily contaminated wounds or in injuries where vascularized skin and soft tissue cover is missing. Following are examples of clean lacerations in adult patients:

Example 1

A laceration of the flexor digitorum profundus occurred 1 centimeter from its insertion on the distal phalanx. (**A**) The wound was clean and appropriate for primary reconstructive surgery.

The proximal cut end of the profundus tendon was reinserted into the distal phalanx using the Bunnell pull-out wire method. This technique attaches the cut end of the profundus tendon into its normal insertion site on the distal phalanx.

The site of insertion was prepared by reflecting the short distal segment of the profundus and dissecting beneath it to create a raw, rough area on the distal phalanx. (**B**) Care was exercised not to injure the palmar capsule of the distal interphalangeal joint.

A pull-out wire was prepared by folding one wire over another, which was armed at each end with fine straight needles. (**C**) The double-armed wire was passed through the tendon in a manner which crisscrossed the wire several times before the ends emerged from the tendon end. The pull-out wire was thus seated at the proximal end of the tendon-holding wire. (**D**)

A straight Keith needle was placed in a drill chuck and inserted into the prepared recipient area of profundus tendon insertion. It was passed through the distal phalanx in such a manner as to emerge from the middle of the fingernail. (**E**) (CAUTION: If the first pass of the needle misses its mark, it should NOT be pulled back through the distal phalanx but thrust on through. To pull the needle back may pull nail and nail bed cells back into the phalanx. This may result in the development of a troublesome cyst in the distal phalanx.) With the chuck removed, the holding wire ends were threaded into the needle and pulled through the distal phalanx and nail.

The tendon end was pulled snugly into the recipient bed and fixed by tying the wires over a button on the fingernail. (**F**) The pull-out wire was inserted retrogradely through the skin in a line so that it would pull the holding wire straight back out of the tendon at the time of removal.

The finger and wrist were immobilized on a moulded palmar splint. The finger was immobilized in moderate flexion with the wrist held in neutral position. (**G**)

After a three-week healing period, the immobilization was terminated and progressive active motion was initiated with the pull-out wire still in place. At four weeks after repair, the button was removed from the nail by cutting the wires at nail level. Gentle, steady pull on the pull-out wire removed the whole wire mechanism. After two months the patient had full restoration of profundus tendon function with a full range of motion.

Tendons, Fascia and Muscles

EXAMPLE 1

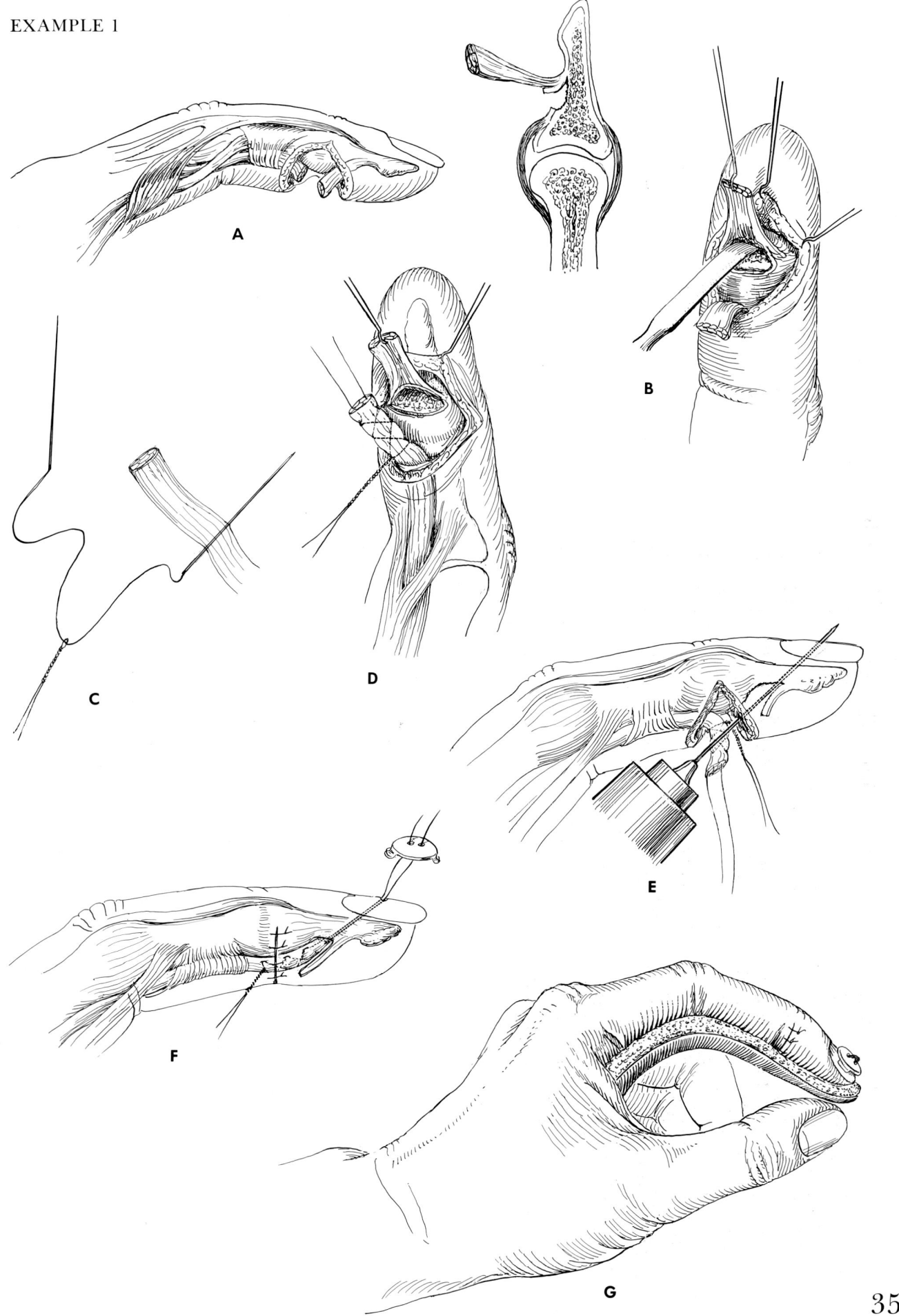

353

78 – Flexor Tendon Lacerations

Example 2

A clean laceration resulted in transection of the flexor digitorum profundus at the level of the proximal phalanx. The flexor digitorum superficialis was intact and functioning. (**H**) Since the wound was clean and sharp, primary reconstruction was appropriate. Consideration was given to primary tendon graft, but simple skin closure without tendon surgery was elected. If the profundus tendon is left unrepaired, the residual disability, the inability to flex the distal joint, ordinarily is not great.

After a variable period, however, the distal joint without flexor tendon support may hyperextend into a position of recurvatum. (**I**) If a decision is made against the need for profundus reconstruction by tendon grafting, either primary or delayed, the distal joint may be fixed in a manner which will prevent hyperextension and support the finger's ability to pinch with its pulp. This may be achieved by joint fusion in a functional position, or better, in my view, by tenodesis of the distal joint. This was achieved in this case by fixation of the distal cut end of the profundus tendon to the middle phalanx. (**J**)

Example 3

A laceration which transected only the flexor digitorum superficialis occurred at the level of the proximal phalanx and left the finger of an adult patient with little immediate disability (**K**) The finger lost some of its ability to flex independently of other fingers and it had lost some strength. The diagnosis of flexor tendon injury limited to the superficialis could easily have been missed unless the ability of the finger to flex while the others were held in extension was tested. Except under very unusual circumstances, the most logical treatment would be to ignore the tendon laceration and to repair the skin and digital nerves if they are injured. The proximal end of the superficialis had retracted well proximally and the distal cut end was well within the tendon sheath. (**L**) Thus there was no need to surgically attend to the cut tendon ends. The patient had little detectable residual disability following recovery. Late recurvatum or swan neck deformity should be watched for in the years ahead.

Example 4

4. Clean transection of both the superficialis and profundus tendons proximal to the fibrous flexor sheath resulted in total loss of ability to actively flex the interphalangeal joints in a young adult male. (**M**) The constraints on therapy necessary when the flexors are transected within the tightly fitted fibrous sheath with its rigid fixation to the digital skeleton do not exist when tendons are divided in the midpalm. Treatment of this injury consisted of precise end-to-end repair of the profundus tendon. (**N**) (See tendon repair technique, Section 77.) The superficialis was left unrepaired, but existing nerve injuries were treated by repair.

Example 5

Laceration of both the flexor digitorum superficialis and flexor digitorum profundus tendons over the proximal phalanx of the left long finger occurred from a sharp knife wound in a young adult male patient. Both digital nerves were intact.

This common and severely disabling injury is a problem for which there is no single proper treatment. If such an injury occurs in an individual over 8 to 10 years of age, many hand surgeons agree that no primary tendon reconstruction should be done and that a later profundus tendon graft produces more reliable results.

Other equally competent experts recommend primary repair of the profundus tendon only and removal of the fibrous flexor sheath over the excursion limits of the repair site. In a very clean cut, seen immediately after injury, a few hand surgeons recommend an immediate primary profundus tendon graft. When the profundus tendon is reconstructed primarily either by repair or graft, the distal cut end of the superficialis should be sutured to the fibrous flexor sheath or proximal phalanx to avoid recurvatum deformity at the proximal interphalangeal joint. In this case primary closure of the skin wound was carried out in preparation for a flexor tendon graft under elective surgical conditions. Three weeks later with the skin wound well healed a full length flexor tendon graft was done. (See Section 79.)

Tendons, Fascia and Muscles

EXAMPLE 2

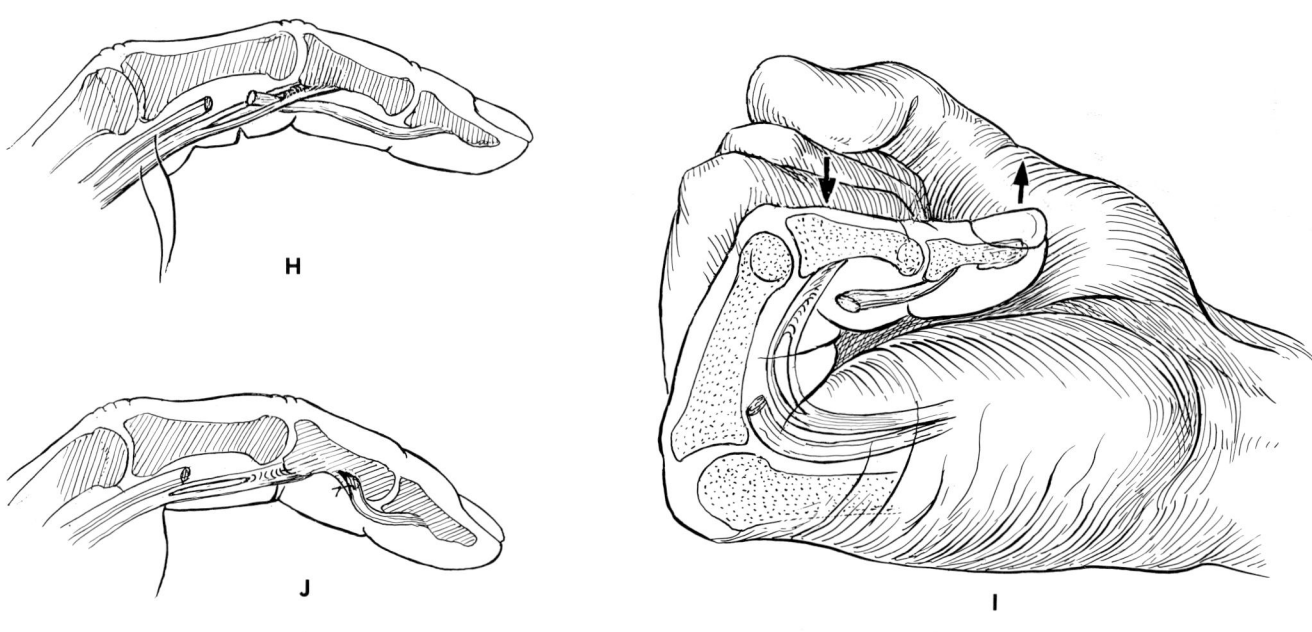

H

J

I

EXAMPLE 3

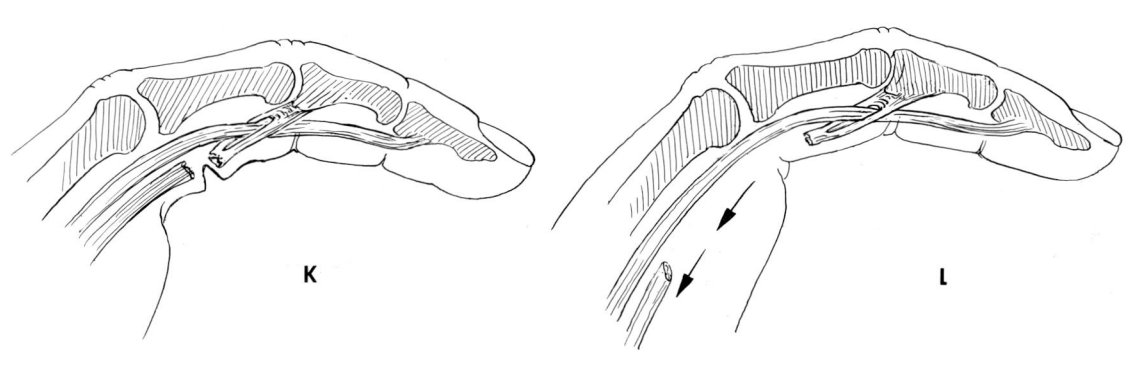

K

L

EXAMPLE 4

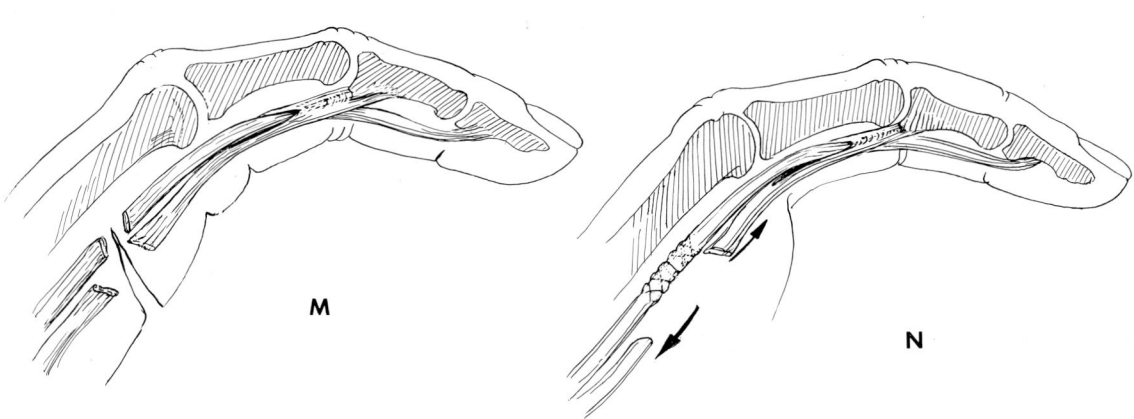

M

N

355

79

Flexor Tendon Grafting

Example

The ideal situation for a profundus flexor tendon graft from palm to distal phalanx existed in the patient who had sustained a laceration of profundus and superficialis tendons without nerve injury in whom no exploration or initial repair had been done. (See Example 5 in Section 78.)

The digital theca was intact; the finger had normal sensibility; scarring was insignificant; and joints had a full range of motion passively. A tendon graft is less likely to succeed in a finger which has been the subject of several surgical procedures, has any skin loss, lacks full sensibility, has any limitation of passive joint motion or has lost its digital theca.

Incisions were planned so that as a minimum one might expose the flexor tendons of the involved finger in the palm and at the site of insertion into the distal phalanx. The area traumatized at the time of original injury generally requires exposure since the fibrous sheath at this level is likely to be contracted. The mid-axial lateral digital incision is excellent. Variation of the incision is appropriate as long as one adheres to the principles for scar placement outlined earlier (see section 6, incisions). The initial incision in the finger was made to expose the distal cut end of the flexor profundus. The thin, translucent part of the fibrous flexor sheath over the distal one-third of the middle phalanx was entered and the distal flexor profundus was reflected out of the wound. (Commonly, there will be no adhesions to the cut tendon end, which rounds off and heals over when it lies free in the digital synovial sheath. If it is adherent, just enough dissection to release it should be done.) A separate incision was made in the palm in such a way that it might join the digital incision should this be necessary. The palm incision was carried through the palmar fascia to expose the flexor profundus and superficialis tendons of the finger. By traction first on the superficialis, then on the profundus, the tendons were reflected out of the finger without further dissection. (If the tendons are adherent in the digital sheath, additional dissection may be required to obtain full release). (**A**)

A probe passed from the palm into the finger within the sheath will pass with ease to the point of the original injury. (**B**) Similarly, one may pass a probe from the distal wound proximally to the point of constriction or obliteration of the digital tunnel.

The scar at the site may be resected allowing free passage from palm to tip. (**C** and **D**)

A doubled wire with its loop fold proximal was passed through the tunnel and left *in situ*. The distal recipient site was prepared as described in the Bunnell pull-out technique in Section 78 (see pages 352 and 353). The palmaris longus tendon was identified by palpation and was removed through several small transverse incisions. (If the palmaris longus is absent as it is in 15 to 20 per cent of people, the plantaris tendon may be used. If both tendons are absent, the second or third toe extensor may be used. (See Section 80.) The tendon graft was immediately threaded through the digit, using the wire pull through. (**E**) The profundus tendon proximally was tested for proximal freedom of motion. The superficialis was pulled distally and cut short after which the cut end retracted above the wrist.

The tendon graft was sutured to the profundus just distal to the origin of its lumbrical. (**F**) A simple end-to-end juncture as described on page 346 was performed. (As an alternate one may use the weaving technique of Brand, described on pages 412 and 413.)

Tendons, Fascia and Muscles

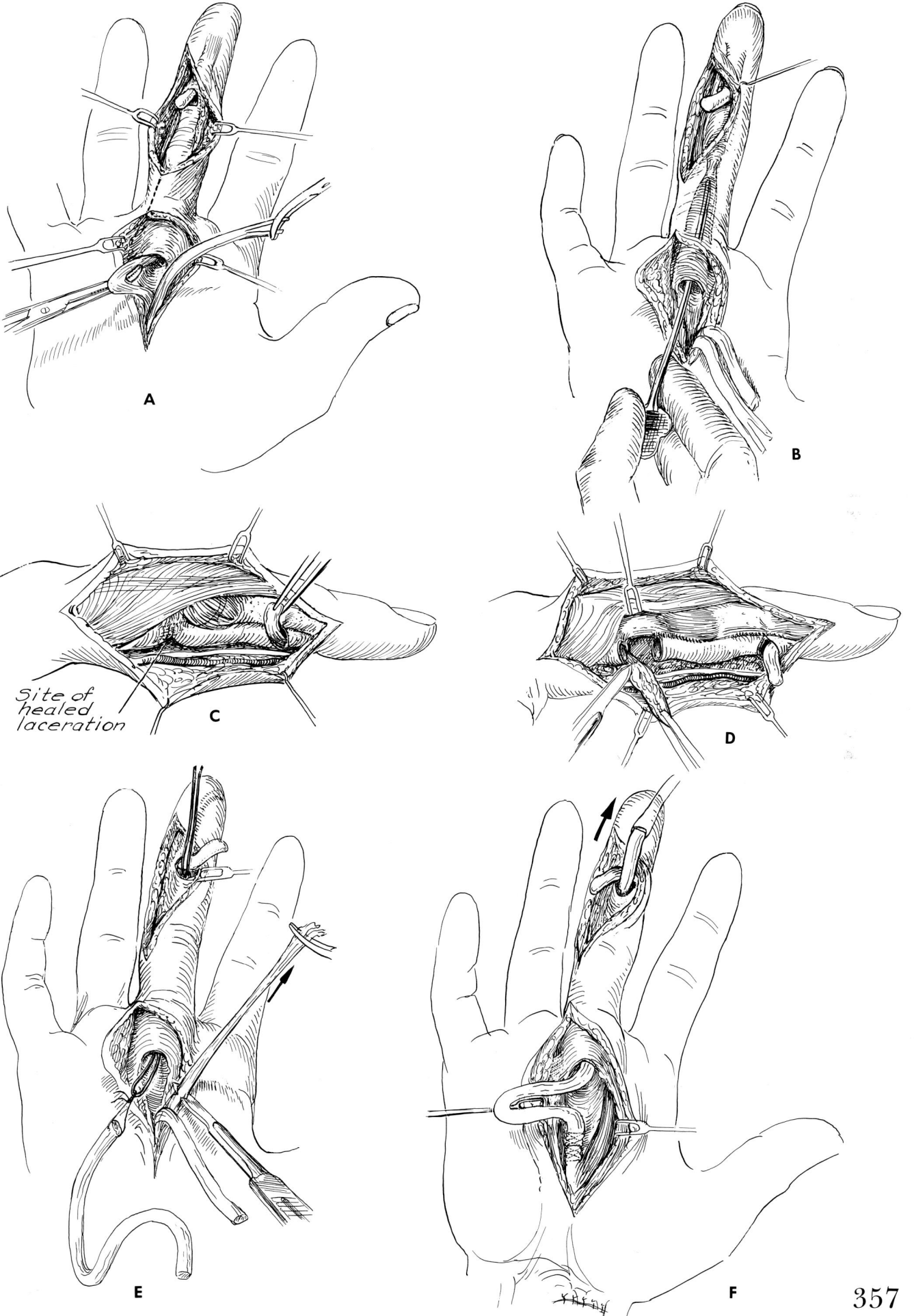

Site of healed laceration

A B C D E F

357

79 — Flexor Tendon Grafting

With the proximal juncture complete, the wounds in the forearm and palm of the hand were sutured closed. **(G)** This avoided the problem of suturing the wounds with the wrist and finger in flexion, essential after both tendon junctures were completed.

The site for distal juncture chosen on the tendon graft requires careful measurement and good judgment. One may apply traction on the tendon with the wrist fully flexed and the digital joints extended. **(H)** The point at which the tendon reaches the recipient site prepared in the distal phalanx may be marked on the tendon.

This may be checked by allowing the hand to sit in a relaxed position, palm up, and noting what length in the tendon graft will hold the finger in proper relationship with the others. If the point double checks, a pull-out wire suture is placed proximal to the site in preparation for distal insertion. The technique for insertion has been described (see pages 352 and 353).

With both junctures complete, passive extension of the wrist resulted in passive flexion of the finger just a few degrees more than normal. Full flexion of the wrist allowed near full extension of the finger by passive traction. Bulky dressings and a plaster splint were applied and left undisturbed for three weeks.

After three weeks of healing, the dressings and splint were removed. Skin sutures were removed and gentle active exercise was started with the pull-out wire still in place, protected by a local dressing. The finger was in neutral position between flexion and extension and little motion was detectable. After one additional week, the pull-out wire was removed and graded increase in active motion over the next month was encouraged.

Blocking flexion of the metacarpophalangeal joint by its intact intrinsic flexors while encouraging flexion of the interphalangeal joints which depended upon the tendon graft was urged.

An exercise block of smooth wood was useful in securing interphalangeal joint motion. The block was made sufficiently wide to prevent metacarpophalangeal flexion and to allow and encourage interphalangeal flexion for grasp. **(I)**

The range of active motion continued to increase over 8 to 10 and even to 12 months after tendon grafting.

If the need for re-exploration or tendolysis is being considered, it should be delayed until at least six months after grafting, and then only when no progress is being made by nonoperative methods to gain increased motion.

Avoidance of Sheath Constriction by Insertion of Silicone Rod

To avoid constriction of the fibrous flexor sheath at the site of injury, it is logical to consider insertion of a silicone spacer at the time of initial injury. **(J)** Silicone rods have proved to be well tolerated in a finger. One may insert lengths of appropriate sized silicone rods which will extend proximally and distally to the sheath injury site to fill the empty sheath over the area left by spontaneous retraction of the tendons. **(K)** Nerve repair as necessary and skin closure may then be done. **(L)**

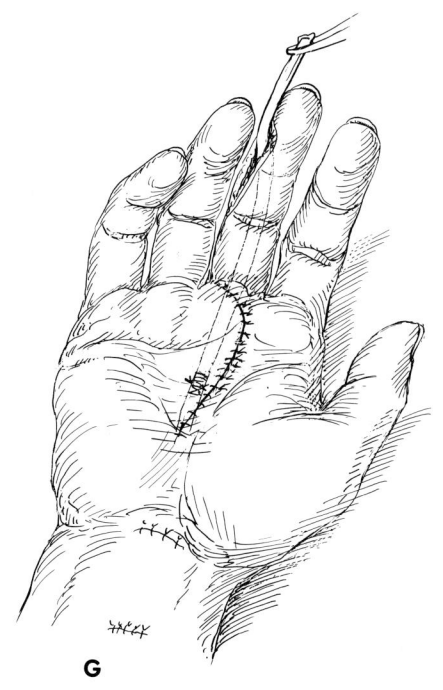

G

Tendons, Fascia and Muscles

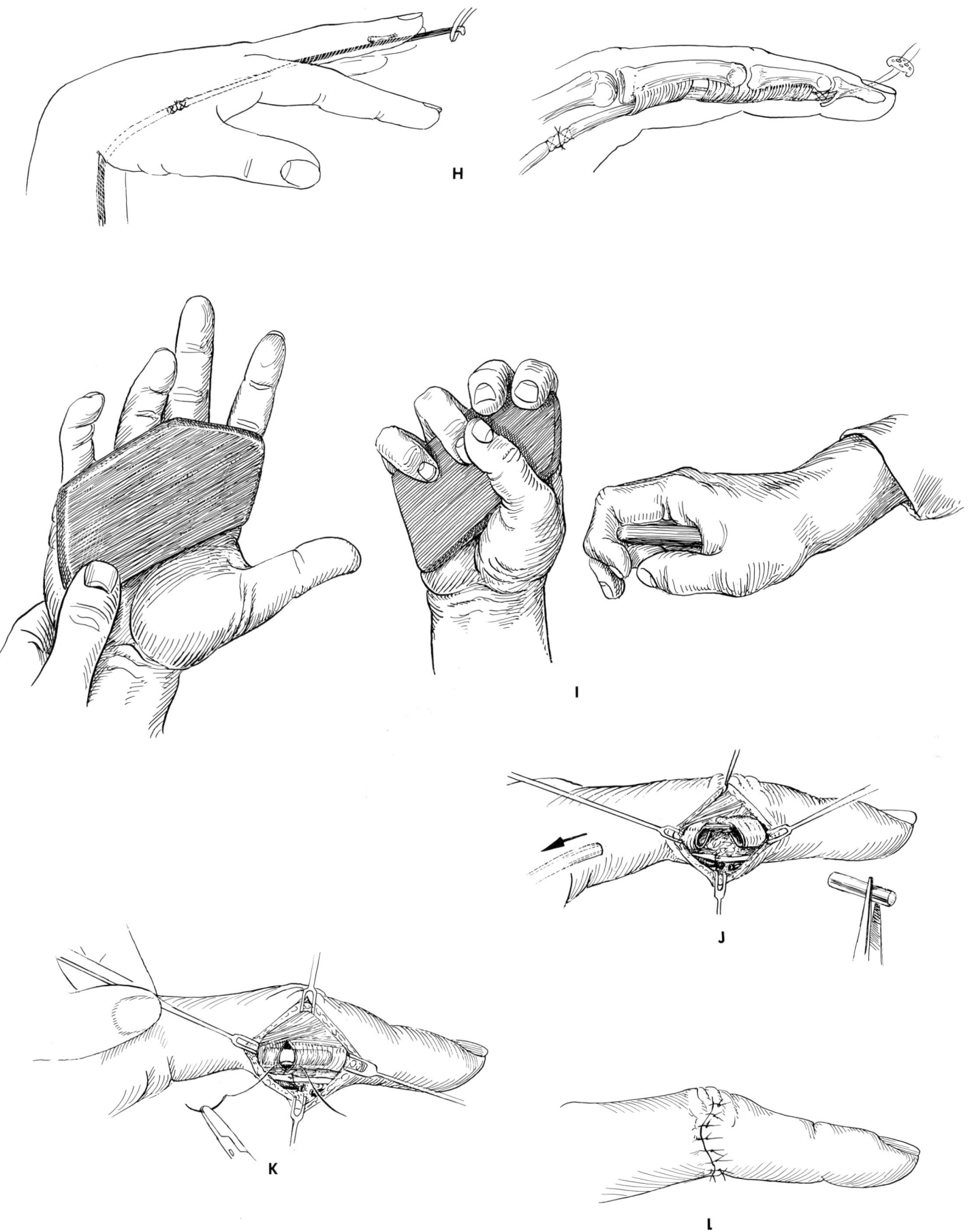

359

79 — Flexor Tendon Grafting

After healing of the skin wounds, the full length tendon graft as a secondary procedure may be done without the need for excision of the area of sheath constriction described above.

It seems logical to consider the same maneuver when flexor profundus repair is planned, using the delayed primary technique. In this instance, the silicone rod is placed across the site of sheath injury and the flexor tendons are left unrepaired. Later, an incision distal in the finger retrieves the silicone rod and distal end of the profundus. (**M**)

At the secondary procedure the flexor profundus may be retrieved in the palm. (**N**)

With the wrist and digit flexed, one may pull the proximal profundus tendon distal to the old injury site, where an end-to-end juncture is created to the distal cut tendon end. The repair may then be dropped back into the intact sheath, where it is less likely to become adherent. (**O**)

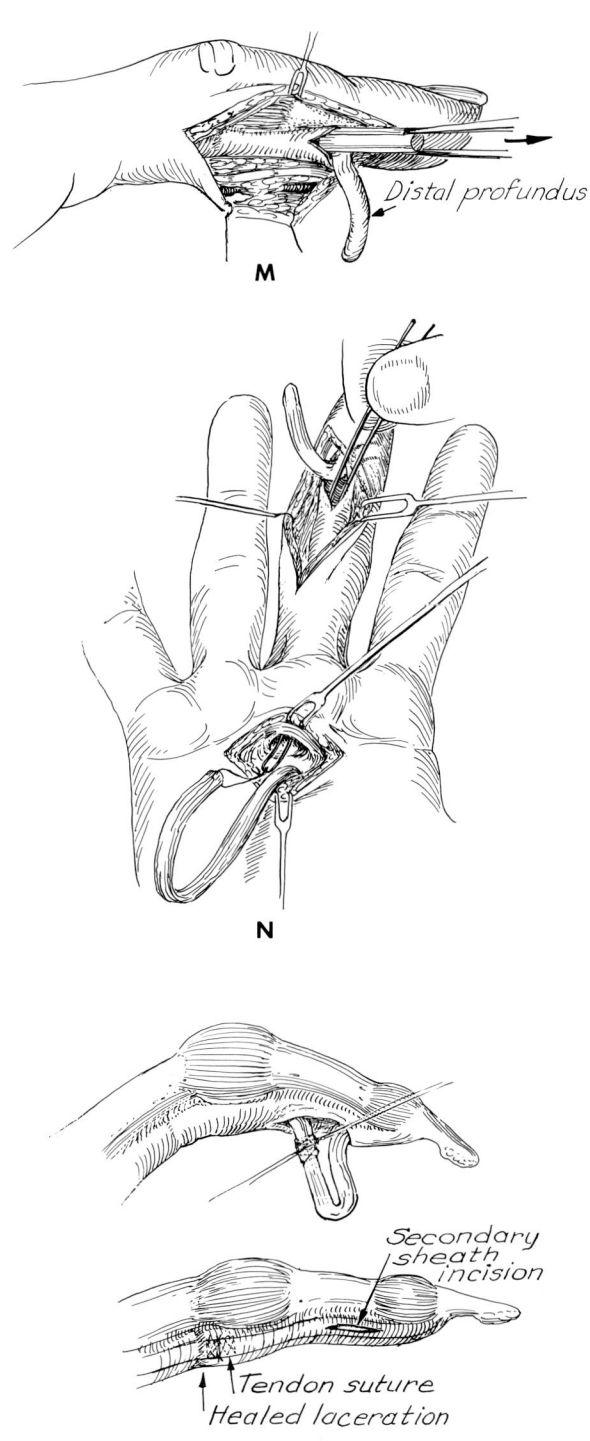

80

Tendon Graft Donor Sites

The palmaris longus tendon is a readily available, non-essential tendon which is commonly used as a free graft where an autogenous tendon graft is appropriate. It is absent in 15 to 20 per cent of the population. If it is absent or is unusable for any reason the plantaris tendon is an excellent second choice. The plantaris is absent in about the same percentage of people. The toe extensors may be removed as free grafts without serious loss of function because of the extensor brevis muscles which exist in the foot.

In a hand with multiple injuries it is possible that a tendon which will not be repaired or used may be removed to use as a free tendon graft. If no true tendon is available to use as a free graft, one may use a strip of fascia lata. As it becomes functional as a tendon, it remodels into a structure grossly indistinguishable from normal tendon.

The palmaris longus tendon may be removed for use as a tendon graft by a variety of techniques. One may expose the tendon just above the wrist and pass a smooth instrument beneath it. (**A**) By tenting the tendon on the instrument, and thus causing traction on it, it may be palpated over its entire length in the forearm. Tiny incisions over the tendon along its length will allow passage of an instrument beneath it. The tendon is sectioned proximal to its termination in the palmar fascia and reflected out through the proximal wounds. It is cut at its musculotendinous area for use as a graft.

One alternate method for securing the palmaris longus is to use a special tendon stripping instrument (Brand Tendon Stripper). (**B**) The palmaris is exposed just proximal to the wrist, where it is grasped with a hemostat and sectioned. The free proximal cut end is passed through the tubular blade of the stripper which is then advanced proximally into the subcutaneous forearm. The stripper is guided proximally by the palmaris longus, which is held taut by the hemostat. The tubular blade engages the muscle belly, which fills its leading cutting edge. As the instrument advances into muscle against the pull on the distal hemostat, the muscle gives way and the palmaris tendon is free to be drawn out at the wrist wound. (See technique for plantaris, page 362.)

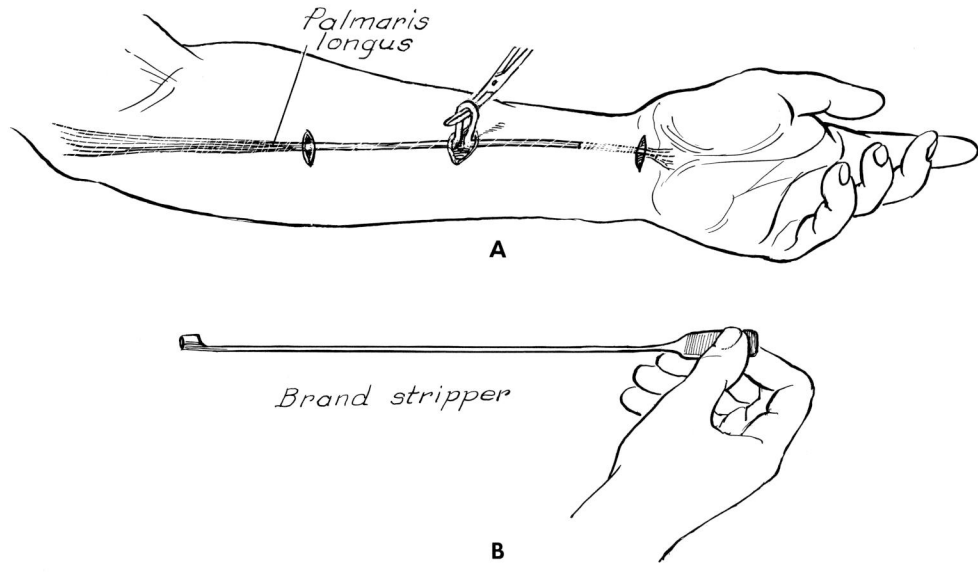

80 – Tendon Graft Donor Sites

The plantaris tendon may be removed by the same techniques, using a longer tendon stripper (Brand Tendon Stripper). The plantaris tendon is exposed through a small incision just in front of the medial side of the palpable Achilles tendon at the ankle level. (**C**) The tendon is sectioned and passed through the tubular blade of the tendon stripper, and the stripper is advanced up the leg with the knee extended. As the stripper passes around the gastrocnemius, penetrating the gastrocnemius fascia, there is a bit of resistance felt. As the stripper becomes filled with the plantaris muscle belly, the combined pull on the tendon distally and push on the instrument results in cutting into the muscle until the natural weakness of nonaponeurotic muscle gives way and the plantaris tendon slides out at the ankle wound. (**D**) It is important that the knee be kept in extension to avoid any possibility of having the stripper injure nerves and vessels in the popliteal area.

The plantaris, palmaris longus, and flat extensor tendons have a unique and useful characteristic not found in round flexor tendons. The collagen bundles are aligned parallel and the tendons may readily be split longitudinally for use as two or more separate grafts. (**E**)

If one grasps the opposite sides of the tendon, it may be stretched out like bubble gum into a flat, thin sheet. (**F**) This is useful in creating certain types of tendon junctures (see pages 412 and 413). If one attempts to spread a flexor tendon, the tendon will divide out into a lattice of fibrils by virute of its plexus of internal fibers.

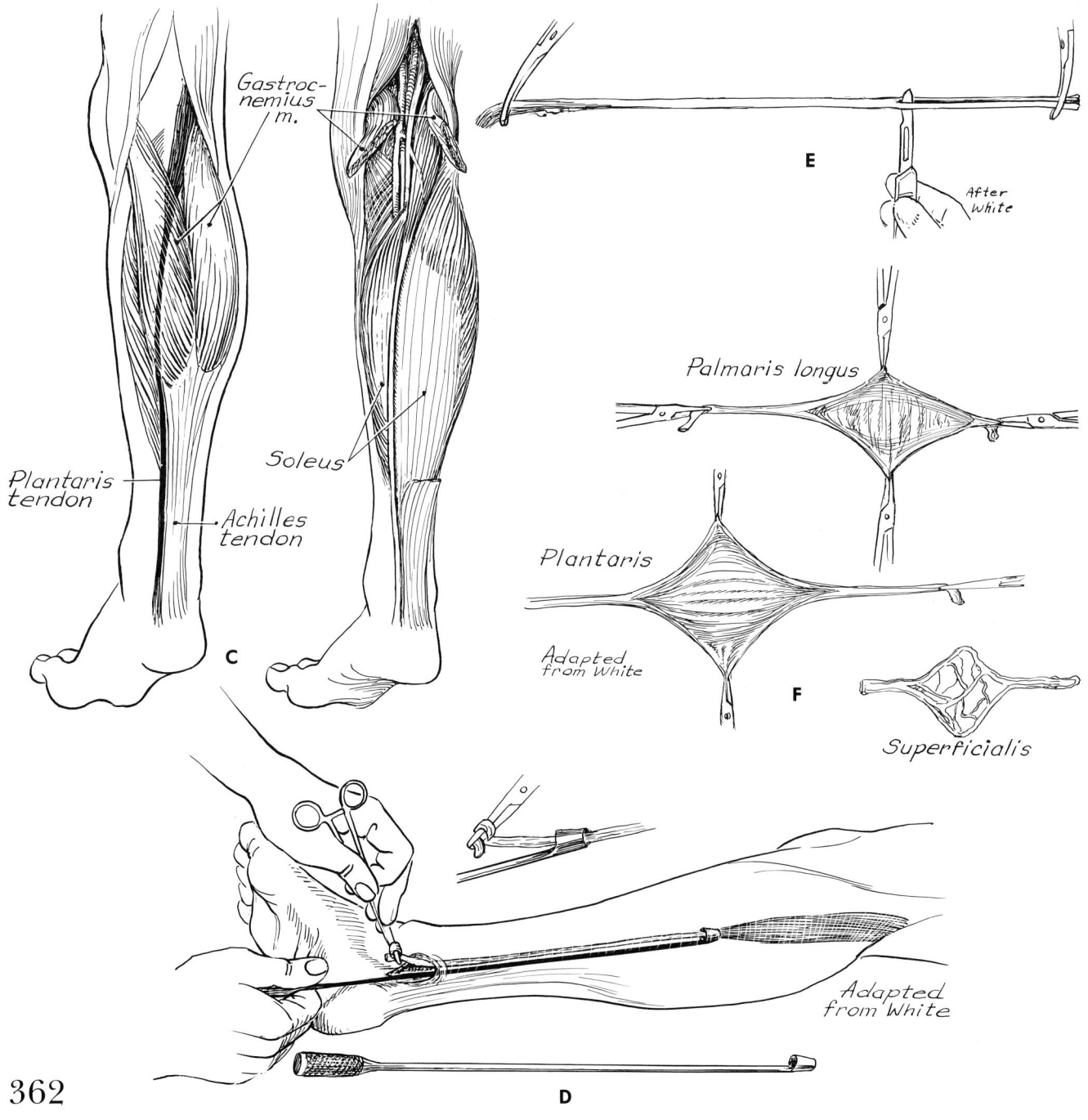

362

81
Laceration of the Flexor Pollicis Longus

Laceration of the flexor pollicis longus poses problems in repair that are different from those of the profundus tendons of the fingers. Anatomically there is no second extrinsic flexor of the thumb equivalent to the flexor digitorum superficialis of the fingers. There is no lumbrical taking origin from the flexor pollicis longus, and the muscle acts independently of the other distal phalangeal flexors. (**A**)

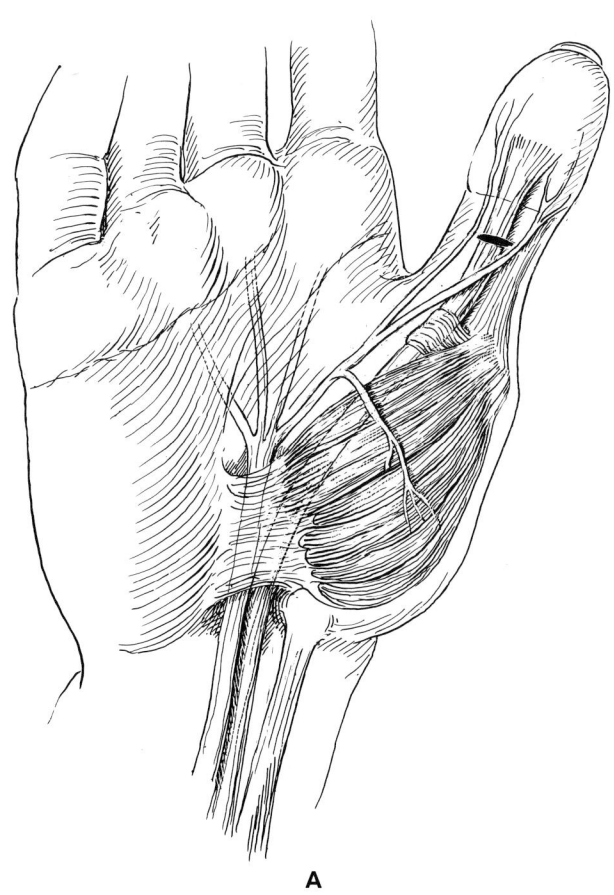

A

81 — Laceration of the Flexor Pollicis Longus

When the flexor pollicis longus is lacerated at the level of the proximal phalanx, the proximal end is not held distally by a lumbrical, and it frequently retracts deep into the thenar area or to the wrist. (**B**)

The proper digital nerve to the radial side of the thumb and the recurrent motor branch of the median nerve to the thenar muscles both cross superficial and close to the flexor pollicis longus.

The concavity of the palmar side of the thumb in full flexion is not as acute as it is in the fingers and, therefore, bow-stringing of the flexor pollicis longus is less likely to be a problem. Therefore, the fibrous flexor sheath may be removed with relative impunity.

The results from primary repair of this independent solitary long flexor of the thumb are good at every level, but care must be exercised in the technical aspects of surgical care.

Attempts to retrieve the proximal tendon end by reaching or grasping with instruments from the wound site endanger the nerves crossing the flexor pollicis longus. (**C**) The recurrent motor branch of the median nerve particularly must be kept in mind since inadvertent injury to it may create severe disability.

The safest and best method to retrieve the proximal tendon end is to withdraw it at the wrist. After placing the proximal tendon suture in the cut end, the tendon is redirected through its original course by passing a probe from the distal wound proximally and threading the sutures through the sheath by withdrawing the probe. (**D**)

The tendon may be sutured end-to-end or it may be reinserted into the distal phalanx using the pull-out wire technique. (See reinsertion pull-out wire technique, pages 352 and 353.)

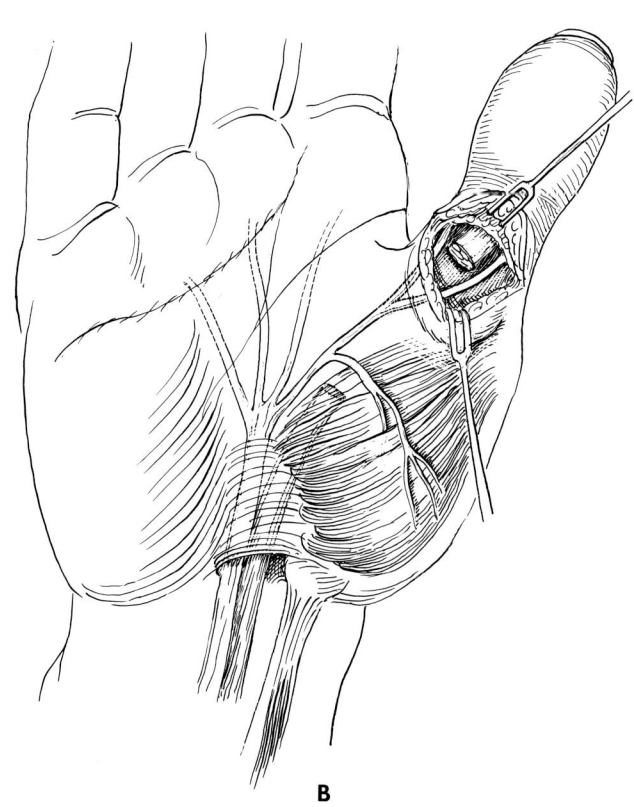

B

Tendons, Fascia and Muscles

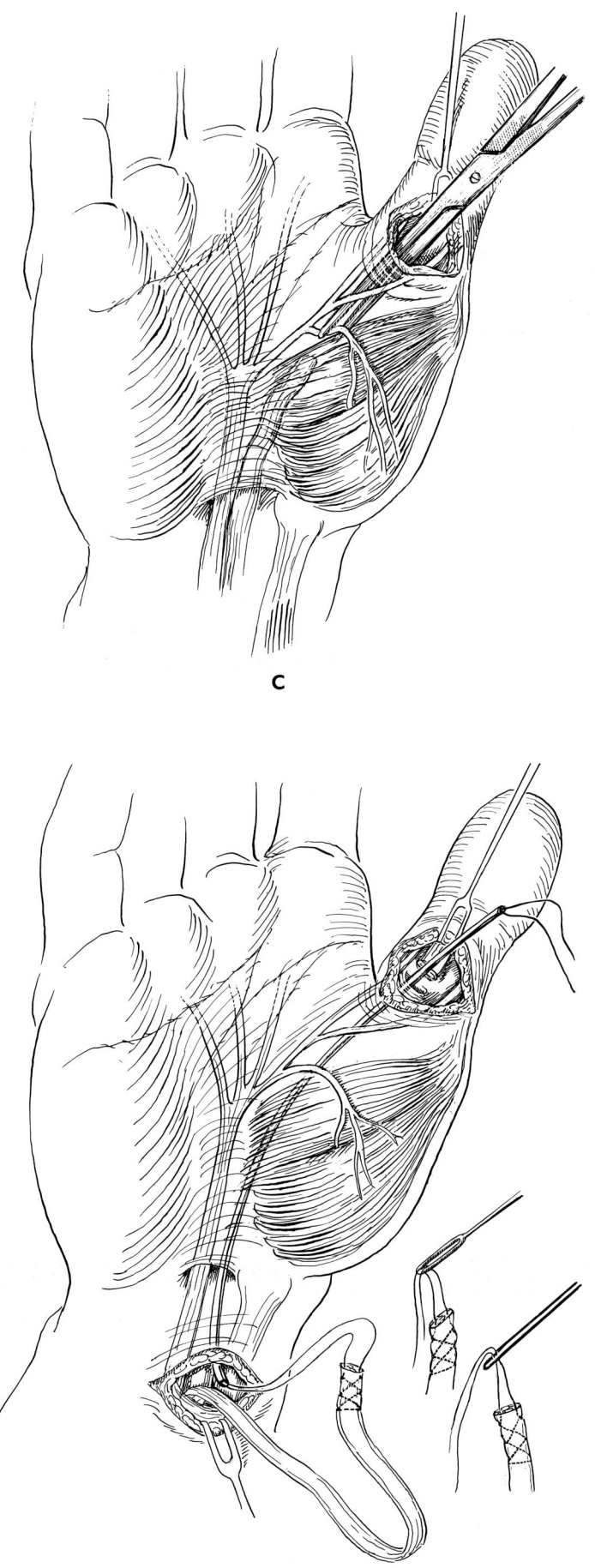

C

D

365

Palmar Wrist Laceration

Severe wrist laceration with transection of all structures on the palmar aspect is not uncommon. The surgeon responsible for initial care of such an injury must set priorities on structures to be repaired and must be prepared to leave some structures unrepaired to achieve the best possible result. (**A**)

The profundus tendons and flexor pollicis longus retract and are very difficult to manage secondarily if they are left unrepaired for several weeks. These distal phalangeal flexors deserve top priority as structures to be repaired if the wound is clean enough and recent enough to warrant primary closure.

The median and ulnar nerves should also be repaired primarily although they may be more easily and successfully repaired after a delay than the profundus tendons and the flexor pollicis longus.

Although blood supply to the hand is adequate for survival when both radial and ulnar arteries are cut, an attempt should be made to repair them to avoid late problems caused by less than full blood supply to the hand.

The flexor carpi ulnaris need not be repaired. To repair it adjacent to the ulnar nerve repair may, in fact, incorporate the ulnar nerve repair in tendon callus, diminishing the likelihood of nerve repair success. The flexor carpi radialis need not be repaired for restoration of adequate wrist flexion but if it can be done without adding significantly to the procedure, it should be.

The superficialis tendons should not be repaired if all structures are cut since repair of both superficialis and profundus tendons crowds the carpal tunnel, and all tendons heal in a common scar mass, ruining all long flexor function. The palmaris longus is essentially superfluous and should not be repaired.

Injury to the superficialis tendons without concomitant injury of the profundi warrants repair of the superficialis tendons. This is particularly important in children.

Tendons, Fascia and Muscles

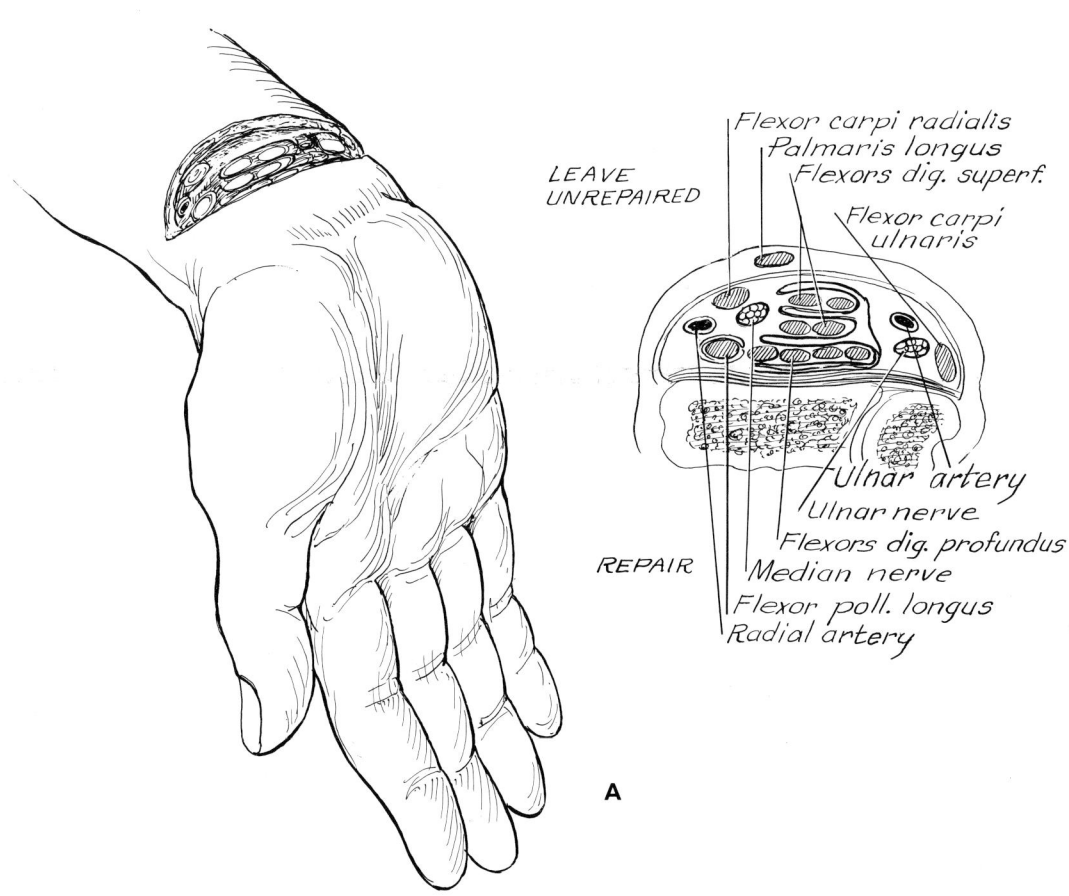

83

Extensor Tendon Lacerations

Principles

An injury which transects a digital long extensor over the knuckle area is common.

Adhesions between overlying skin and the tendon repair do not interfere with function. The short excursion of the extensor coupled with the mobile dorsal skin with its loose areolar fascia means that the skin will move enough to allow full excursion of the tendon even if the two are adherent.

The skin, in fact, acts as good backing for the tendon repair. This is helpful since sutures in the flat extensor tendons, with their longitudinally oriented collagen bundles, hold sutures poorly. There is a tendency for sutures to pull through the tendon as a comb pulls through hair.

Experience with repair of such tendon injuries with permanently buried non-absorbable sutures has resulted in a substantial percentage of foreign body inflammatory and rejection episodes. Repair with removable sutures has proved a more reliable and satisfactory method of reconstitution.

Example

A glass cut occurred over the extensor aspect of the index finger extensors just proximal to the metacarpophalangeal joint. Both long extensors to the finger were divided and the patient was unable to extend the finger at the metacarpophalangeal joint. The figure-of-eight suture repair of long extensor tendons at this level was satisfactory. The technique for each tendon consisted of passing a wire suture through skin-tendon-tendon-skin in figure-of-eight fashion. The wire was tied outside the skin. The dermis acted as a stabilizing backing for the repair. (**A**)

The hand was immobilized with the wrist extended and the metacarpophalangeal joint extended. The interphalangeal joints were immobilized in comfortable position just short of full extension. (**B**)

The finger and wrist were immobilized for four weeks, after which gentle motion was started with the pull-out wire still in place. The figure-of-eight sutures were removed five weeks after repair.

After function was fully restored and healing was solid, the surgeon and patient decided that revision of the small scar and separation of the tendons from the adherent skin was appropriate.

ALTERNATE TECHNIQUE

An alternate method of repair for an extensor tendon injury just proximal to the metacarpophalangeal joint utilizes the Bunnell pull-out principle. The extensor tendon is repaired, using the standard criss-cross method with a pull-out suture at one end and a button over dental cotton at the other. (**C**)

The pull-out suture is left in place for five weeks, during the last week of which gentle motion may be started.

FIGURE OF EIGHT — Tendons, Fascia and Muscles

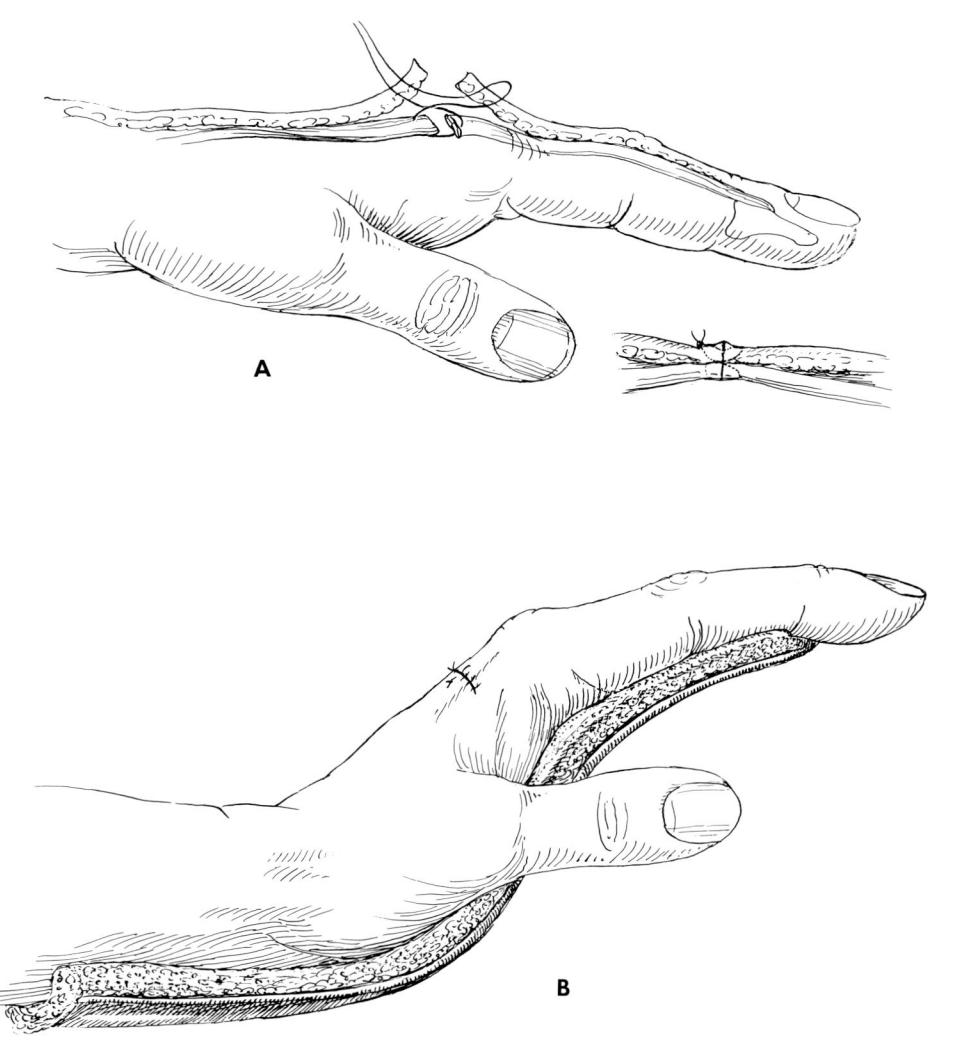

ALTERNATE TECHNIQUE

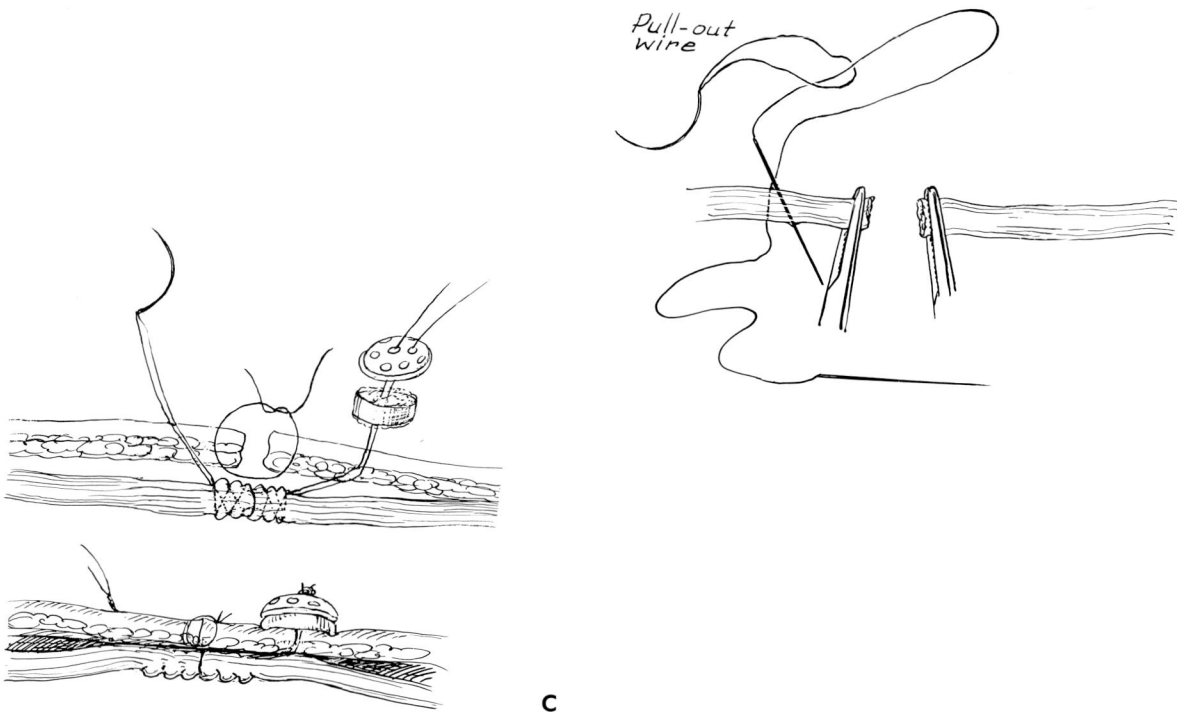

84

Digital Extensor Tendon Injuries

Principles

Rupture of the extensor tendon insertion into the distal phalanx may occur with or without a break in the overlying skin. When the injury occurs, the finger tip drops and it cannot be actively extended. This creates the deformity popularly referred to as "baseball finger." With rupture of the extensor at this site not only does the tip drop but, in addition, the entire extensor mechanism retracts in a proximal direction. All extension effort exerted by the long extensors and intrinsic muscles beyond the metacarpophalangeal joint acts to extend the *proximal* interphalangeal joint. If the rupture is left unrepaired, the patient's attempts to extend the distal joint commonly result in development of recurvatum deformity of the proximal interphalangeal joint. (**A**)

In closed injuries, immobilization of the distal joint in extension may be sufficient therapy. The finger should be positioned in exaggerated extension at the distal interphalangeal joint and moderate flexion at the proximal interphalangeal joint. The metacarpophalangeal joint should be held in comfortable neutral position. (**B**) Five or six weeks of immobilization, then gradual reintroduction of motion, first at the metacarpophalangeal joint, then at the proximal interphalangeal joint, and, finally, at the distal joint is frequently successful in treating a distal extensor rupture. Immobilization may be extended for several more weeks if the tip is still dropped when the splint is removed. External immobilization may be difficult in short fat fingers, and sometimes one is justified in threading a small Kirschner wire across the extended distal joint. The wire should cross *only* the distal joint and should be left for about six weeks.

An open wound over the site of rupture of the extensor may be an indication for surgical repair of the extensor. Secondary repair of the extensor mechanism is indicated when nonsurgical measures for more than four months have failed and the residual disability is significant.

Technique of Surgical Repair

The incision may be either transverse (**C**) or axial (**D**).

Sometimes direct repair is possible where there is a usable distal segment of the tendon. (**E**) The tendon ends are freshened and repaired with nonabsorbable suture material and the distal interphalangeal joint is immobilized for five or six weeks either with an external splint or transarticular Kirschner wire. (**F**)

More frequently, the extensor slip is better reinserted into the distal phalanx in a manner similar to flexor profundus tendon reinsertion (see technique, pages 352 and 353), using a pull-out suture. Violent rupture of the extensor insertion commonly occurs at the site of insertion. Sometimes a chip of the distal phalanx is pulled off with the extensor. (**G**)

An x-ray of the finger may show this and confirm the diagnosis of avulsion at the insertion site. The holding suture is passed through the tendon after looping a pull-out suture around it. The sutures are passed through the distal phalanx by using a straight (Keith) needle in a drill chuck. (**H**)

The tendon end is pulled snugly down into a freshened area on the dorsum of the distal phalanx, and the suture is tied over a bit of dental cotton and a button over the palmar digital pulp. (**I**)

The pull-out suture is passed through dorsal skin away from the wound if possible. (**J**) After five weeks of immobilization with the distal joint in extension and the proximal joints in comfortable flexion, the pull-out suture is removed and graded motion is allowed.

Tendons, Fascia and Muscles

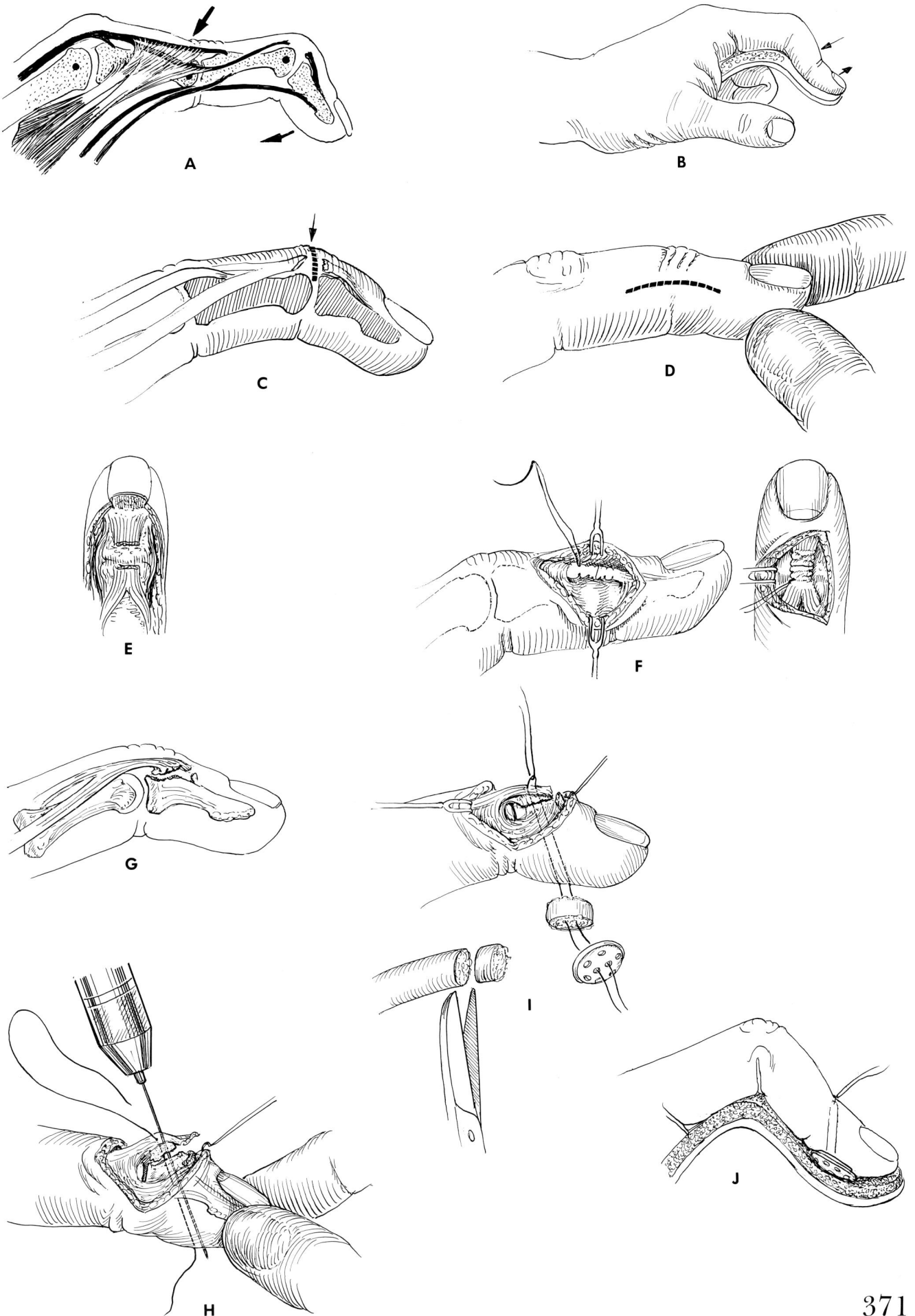

371

The Extensor Pollicis Longus

Principle

The extensor pollicis longus tendon is subject to injury because of its vulnerable superficial location on the radiodorsal surface of the hand and wrist. When it is divided in a clean wound, immediate end-to-end repair is indicated. The tendon may retract above the extensor retinaculum at the wrist. It should then be retrieved by an incision just proximal to the retinaculum. It may then be passed subcutaneously to the cut distal end to avoid a repair that will impinge itself upon the tight extensor tunnel at the wrist.

If the patient has sustained a traumatic division of the extensor pollicis longus which has gone unrepaired for several months, under most circumstances one would choose to transfer the extensor indicis tendon to the distal extensor pollicis longus. The extensor pollicis longus has a small muscle belly which is hidden beneath the ulnar border of the distal radius, and the shortening that occurs in the weeks after injury makes it technically difficult to locate the proximal tendon and very difficult to regain enough length for a secure repair. The extensor indicis transfer is simple and very effective and should be used in all but exceptional circumstances where independent extension of the index metacarpophalangeal joint is crucial as in a concert pianist.

The same general principle applies to the commonly occurring spontaneous rupture of the extensor pollicis longus in rheumatoid arthritis.

Example

A 63-year-old housewife with rheumatoid arthritis noted progressive inability to extend her right thumb tip and then the sudden total loss of ability to extend the thumb tip. (**A**) All function was intact in other finger extensor tendons.

Decision was made to restore function to the ruptured extensor pollicis longus by transfer of the extensor indicis tendon. The extensor pollicis longus distal to the wrist was exposed through a small curved incision. The site of rupture was evident and tension on the extensor resulted in extension of the thumb tip.

Through a small separate incision the extensor indicis tendon was isolated at the insertion into the dorsal hood just proximal to the metacarpophalangeal joint. The independent indicis tendon lies ulnar to the extensor digitorum to the index finger. Through the proximal incision, the extensor indicis tendon was located distal to the extensor retinaculum at the wrist. The tendon was divided at the distal site and was withdrawn to the proximal incision.

The thumb metacarpophalangeal joint and interphalangeal joint were extended, and traction was placed on the cut end of the extensor pollicis longus. The tendon and adjacent skin were transfixed with a straight needle to hold the tendon in position for juncture with the extensor indicis. The extensor indicis was routed to the extensor pollicis longus and a juncture was performed, passing the indicis extensor through the extensor pollicis longus, splitting the extensor indicis and suturing it to itself and the extensor pollicis longus by looping the two tails around it. (**B**)

The thumb and wrist were immobilized in moderate extension with a plaster splint for five weeks.

The patient regained good function in the thumb, without significant sacrifice of function in the index finger.

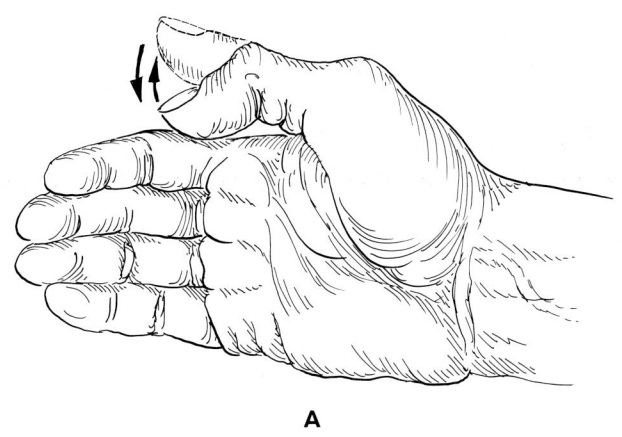

A

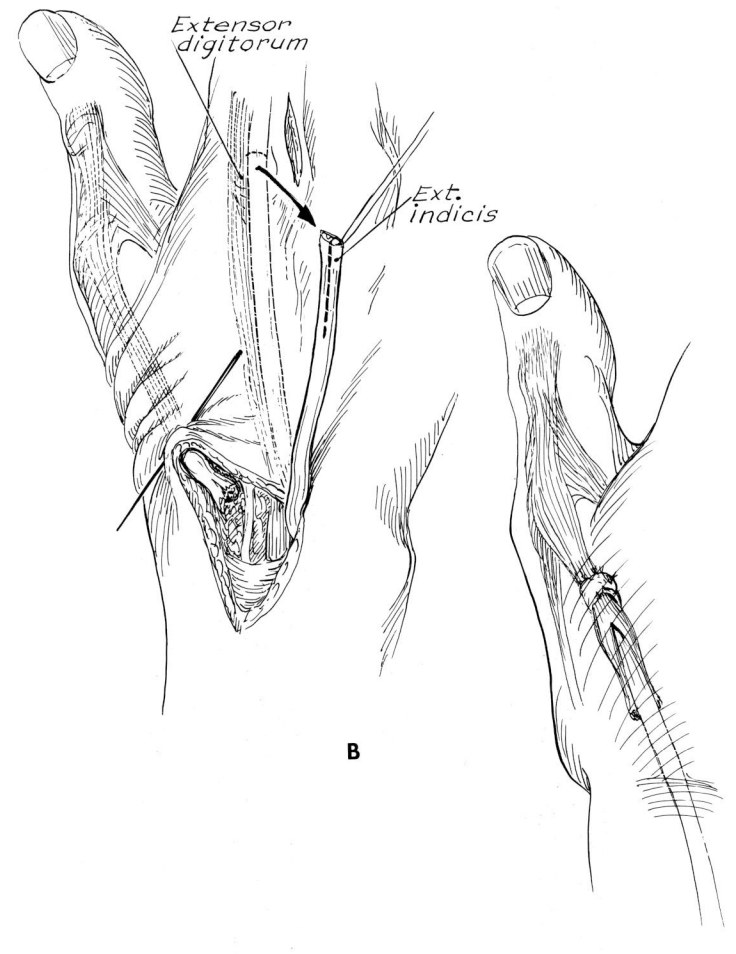

B

86
Deformities of the Fingers from Tendon Imbalance

Imbalance of forces which influence the three joints in each finger create standard deformities. Recurvatum deformity at the proximal interphalangeal joint may result from a variety of etiologies but fundamentally it occurs when the primary extensor forces at this joint overbalance the primary flexor force. **(A)** The primary flexor is the flexor digitorum superficialis, while extensor force originates in the long extensor or the intrinsic muscles depending upon the position of the metacarpophalangeal joints. Hyperextension of the proximal interphalangeal joint is limited by the palmar capsule (volar plate) of the joint.

In the presence of a loose palmar capsule recurvatum may occur because of absence of the flexor digitorum superficialis or excessive pull or tightness of the intrinsic muscles or long extensor.

Testing for differentiation of tight long extensor versus tight intrinsic muscles is performed by checking the extent of recurvatum or degree of extension of the proximal interphalangeal joint. If there is passive increased extension of the proximal interphalangeal joint on passive flexion of the metacarpophalangeal joint, the problem is tightness of the long extensor. **(B)**

If the proximal joint extends on passive extension of the metacarpophalangeal joint, then the diagnosis is tightness of the intrinsic muscles. **(C)** When recurvatum deformity is a result of tight intrinsic muscles a simple release of the tightness by excision of a triangle from the side of the dorsal hood to include the lateral band may correct the imbalance. **(D)**

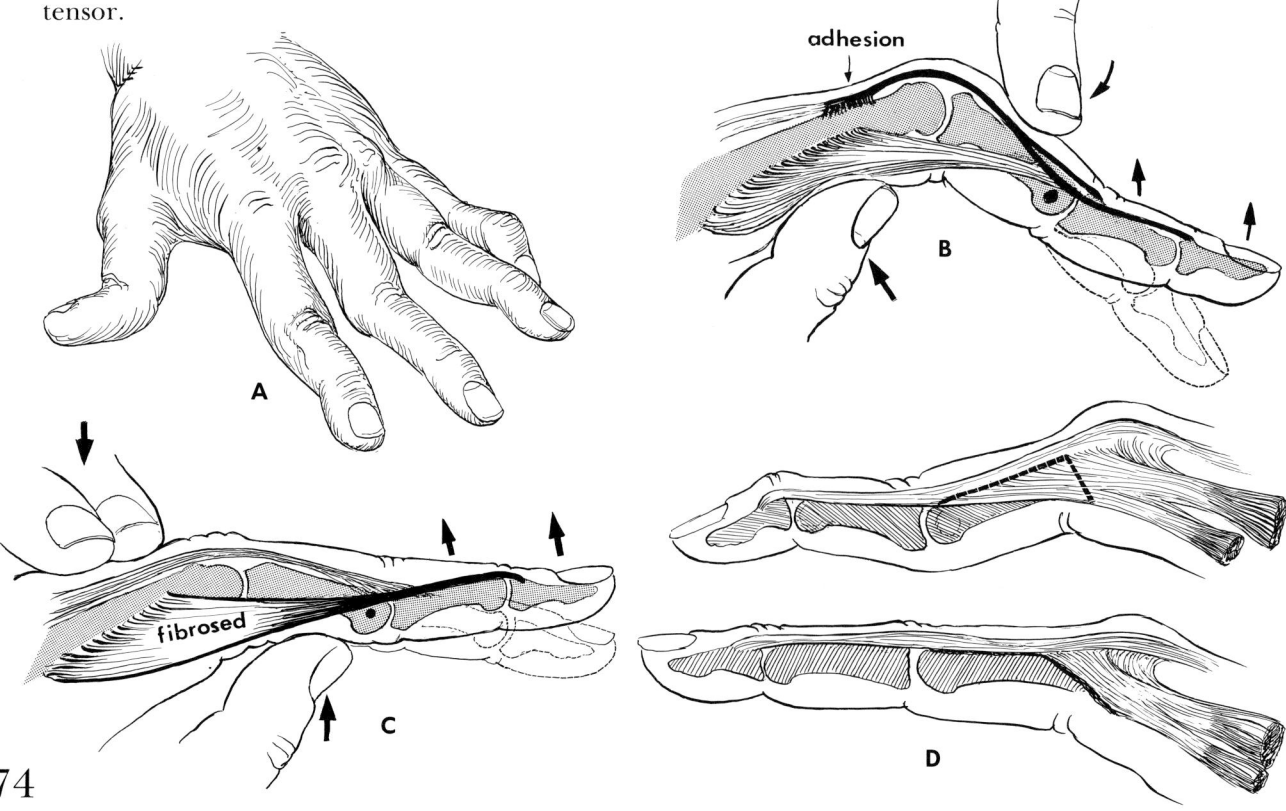

SWAN NECK DEFORMITY

Recurvatum deformity of the proximal interphalangeal joint coupled with dropped finger tip is present when a rupture or attenuation of the extensor insertion on the distal phalanx occurs in combination with overpull of either the long extensor or intrinsic muscles. It also is present with an intact distal insertion when the profundus flexor pull overpowers the extensor. This pull of the profundus coupled with tightness of the long extensor or intrinsic collapses the three-joint linkage into a zig-zag, with flexion of the metacarpophalangeal joint, hyperextension of the proximal interphalangeal joint and flexion of the distal interphalangeal joint. The most effective way to overcome the imbalance surgically is to redistribute the forces after Littler's technique. Instead of simply resecting the tight lateral bands, Littler advocates section of the lateral band proximally at the root of the finger and dissection of the lateral band from its attachments to the dorsal hood mechanism. It is dissected as a strip all the way to the distal interphalangeal joint just proximal to its insertion. This free lateral band is rerouted palmar to Cleland's ligament at the level of the mid-middle phalanx, to the side of the fibrous flexor sheath on the palmar aspect of the midproximal phalanx. This changes its vector relationship to the proximal interphalangeal joint by passing palmar to its joint axis. It becomes aligned anatomically with the oblique retinacular ligament of Landsmeer.

The cut end of the tendon is fixed to the fibrous flexor sheath with the proximal interphalangeal joint in 10 degrees of flexion and the distal interphalangeal joint in extension. This procedure separates the forces acting at the proximal interphalangeal joint from those acting at the distal interphalangeal joint. All motor power through the long extensor and residual intrinsic to the dorsal hood acts to extend the proximal interphalangeal joint. The distal interphalangeal joint automatically extends as the proximal interphalangeal joint is extended. By adjustment of tension in the transferred tendon it prevents hyperextension of the proximal interphalangeal joint.

Example

A 45-year-old patient with rheumatoid arthritis developed swan neck deformity in several fingers. (**A**) Passive extension of the metacarpophalangeal joints increased the recurvatum deformity at the proximal interphalangeal joints in each finger.

Release of tight intrinsic muscles by section of a lateral band and rerouting it was chosen as appropriate treatment. Through a longitudinal, gently curved, **S**-shaped incision in the dorsum of the finger, the entire extensor apparatus was exposed. The lateral band on the ulnar side of the finger was sectioned at the base of the finger and was dissected from the dorsal hood and from the central slip at the proximal interphalangeal joint all the way to the distal joint. (**B**) Traction on the tendon resulted in extension of the distal interphalangeal joint.

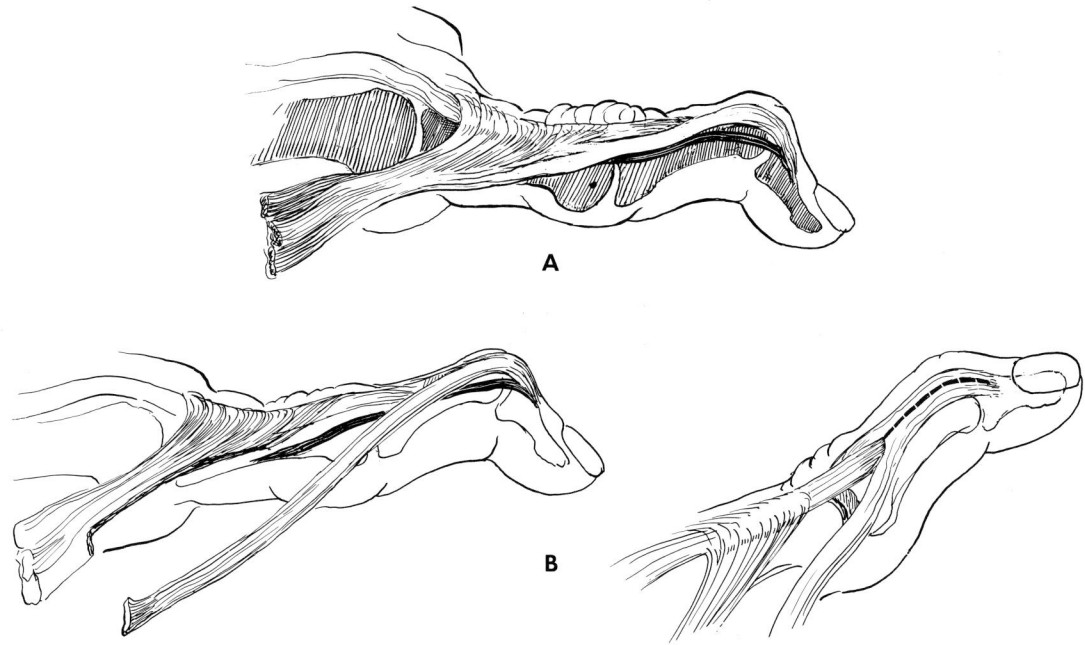

Cleland's ligament, which was readily visible, was left intact 1 cm. distal and 1 cm. proximal to the proximal interphalangeal joint. A probe was passed palmar to Cleland's ligament from mid-middle phalanx to mid-proximal phalanx and the freed lateral band was routed through the resulting tunnel. **(C)**

The tendon end was passed through the ulnar edge of the fibrous flexor sheath and its tension was adjusted to hold the proximal interphalangeal joint in flexion at about 10 degrees with the distal interphalangeal joint fully extended. **(D)**

Passive extension of the proximal interphalangeal joint resulted in tenodesis extension of the distal interphalangeal joint; hyperextension of the proximal interphalangeal joint was not possible.

The finger was immobilized on a splint in moderate flexion (30 degrees) at the metacarpophalangeal joint, the same at the proximal interphalangeal joint, with extension of the distal interphalangeal joint.

After five weeks of immobilization, the patient was allowed graded active exercise. Four months after the procedure the patient had nearly full range of digital flexion and extension without recurvatum deformity. In fact, the proximal interphalangeal joint failed to fully extend by 10 degrees.

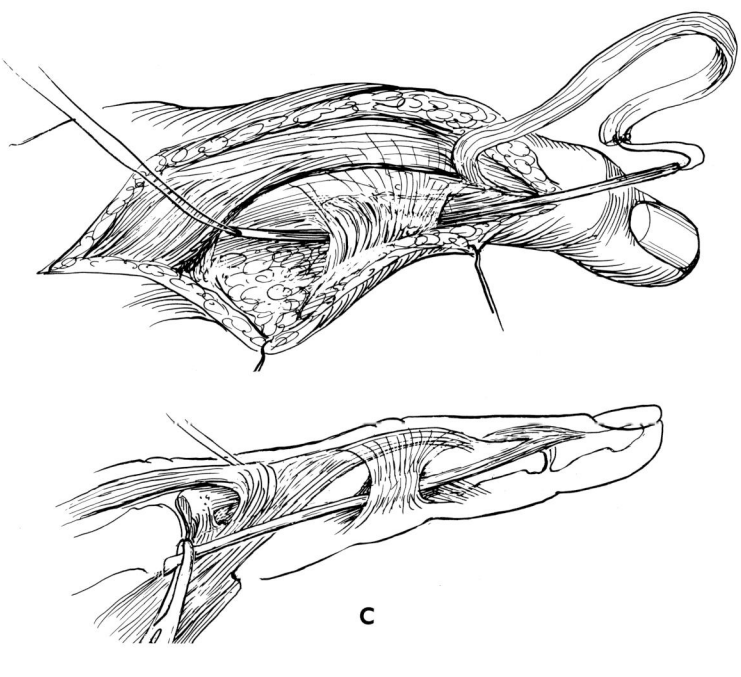

C

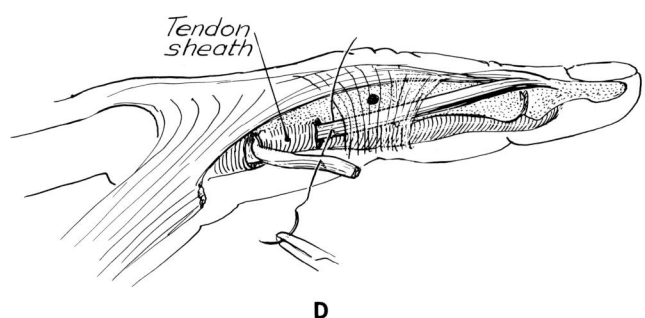

D

BOUTONNIERE DEFORMITY

Rupture or transection of the central slip of the long extensor tendon near or at its insertion into the middle phalanx left unrepaired frequently results in uncontrolled flexion of the proximal interphalangeal joint and hyperextension of the distal interphalangeal joint. Loss of the prime extensor of the proximal interphalangeal joint and palmar migration of the lateral bands to a point below the axis of the proximal interphalangeal joint has developed. Every effort on the part of the patient to extend his proximal interphalangeal joint using the long extensor or the intrinsic muscles not only fails to extend the joint but, in fact, flexes it. The same forces act to extend and finally hyperextend the distal interphalangeal joint. (**A**)

Correction is best managed by repair or reconstruction of the central slip by direct repair or tendon graft. As an alternative, the surgeon may choose to redistribute all interphalangeal extension power to the proximal interphalangeal joint. The distal interphalangeal joint may be extended by tenodesis, using the following redistribution technique:

The lateral bands of the finger are split longitudinally into two parts and cut in such a way that the dorsal half is sectioned distally over the middle phalanx and the palmar half is sectioned proximally at the root of the finger. (**B**)

The dorsal half of the lateral band remains the distal extension of the long extensor and the intrinsic muscles. The palmar half remains attached to the distal phalanx but is detached from the extensor and intrinsic muscles. (**C**) Traction on this band causes extension of the distal interphalangeal joint.

The dorsal band is sutured to the insertion site of the central slip of the extensor or may be passed through a small drill hole in the dorsum of the middle phalanx. This transfers all interphalangeal motor power to the task of extending the proximal interphalangeal joint. The palmar band is passed through Cleland's ligament at a point which diverts its course palmar to the proximal interphalangeal joint axis. It is sutured to the fibrous flexor sheath to act as a tenodesis extensor of the distal interphalangeal joint when the proximal interphalangeal joint is extended. (**D**)

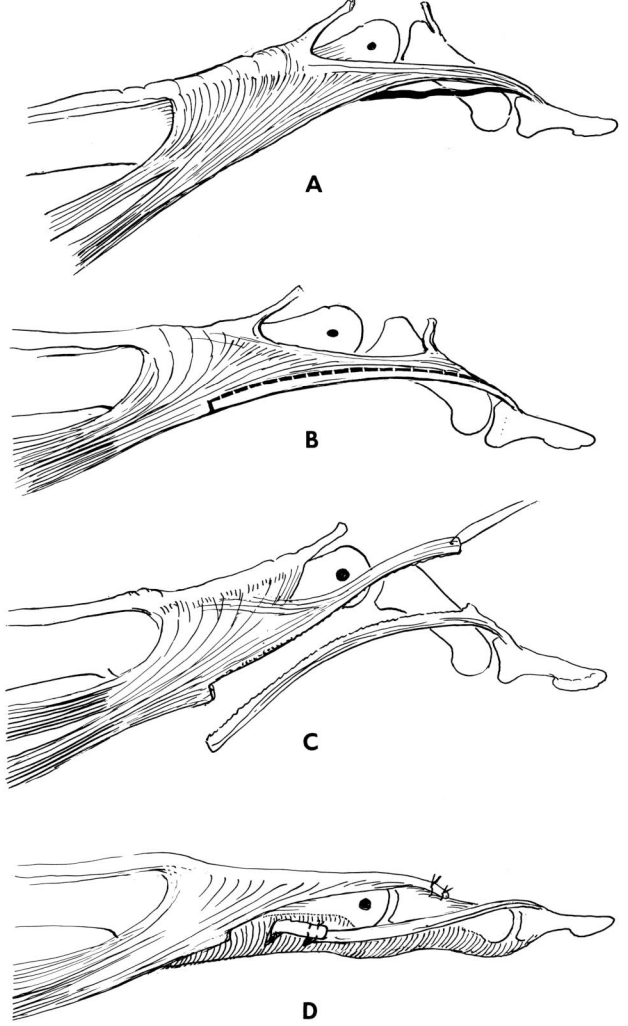

87

Dupuytren's Contracture

"It is a disease confined to Caucasian races, increasing with age, with little sex difference but more severe deformity in men and an association with epilepsy, chronic invalids, pulmonary tuberculosis and alcoholism but without relation to occupation."

HUESTON

Baron Dupuytren sought to elucidate the cause of the disease which now bears his name, and he tried desperately to find a means of treating it. His description of the findings in this disease recorded by his students have not been surpassed. Once contraction of the diseased palmar fascia is sufficient to cause disability, the most reliable therapy is surgery. The diagnosis is easily made when one sees thickening of the palmar fascia and inability to extend fully the metacarpophalangeal joint, proximal interphalangeal joint, or both. (**A**) The distal interphalangeal joint is never involved and, therefore, may be flexed and extended fully. (**B**)

Other findings commonly present are:

1. Lumpy tumefactions in the palmar fascia; (**C**)
2. Knuckle pads, the common term for thickening of subcutaneous fibrous tissue over the dorsum of the proximal interphalangeal joints; (**D**)
3. Fixation of plaques of palm skin over the palmar fascia, particularly at the distal joint crease proximal to an involved finger; (**E**)
4. Tumefactions and, rarely, contracture in *plantar* fascia; (**F** and **G**)
5. Peyronie's disease, characterized by a thick band of fibrosis in the investing fascia of the penis which causes angulation of the penis during erection.

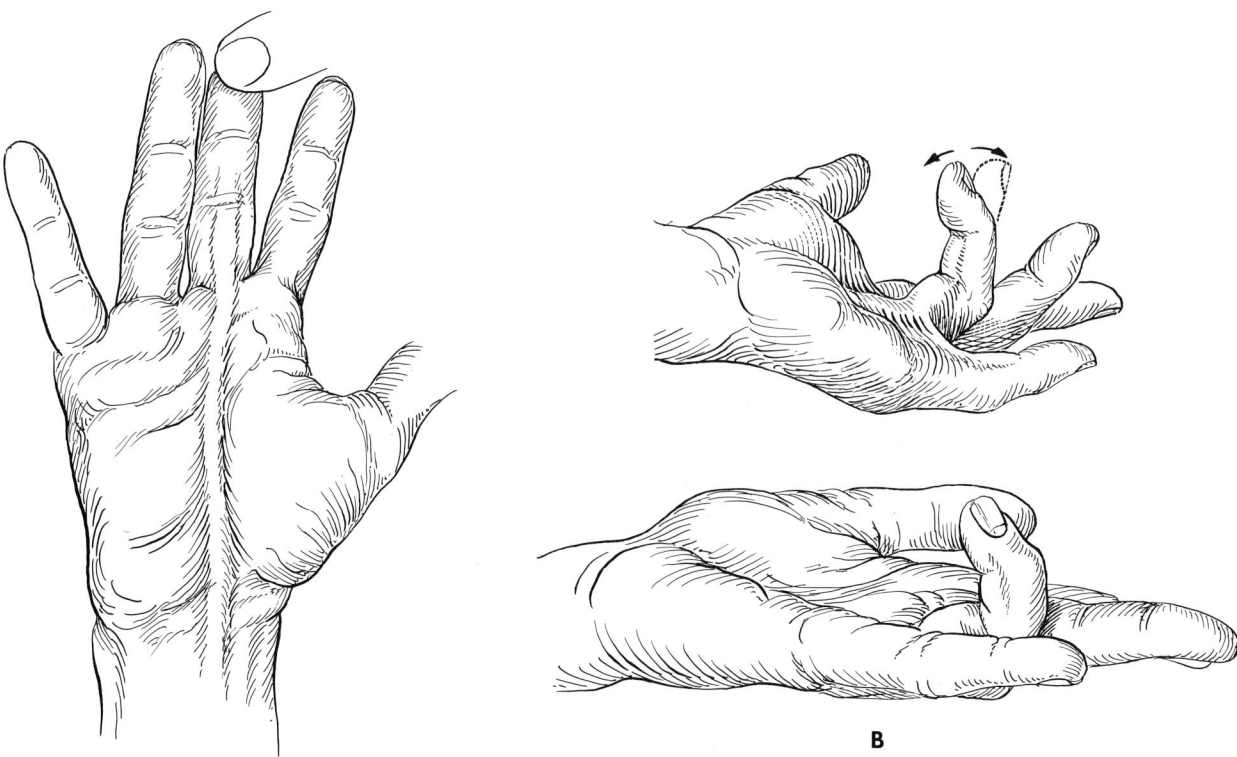

A

B

378

Tendons, Fascia and Muscles

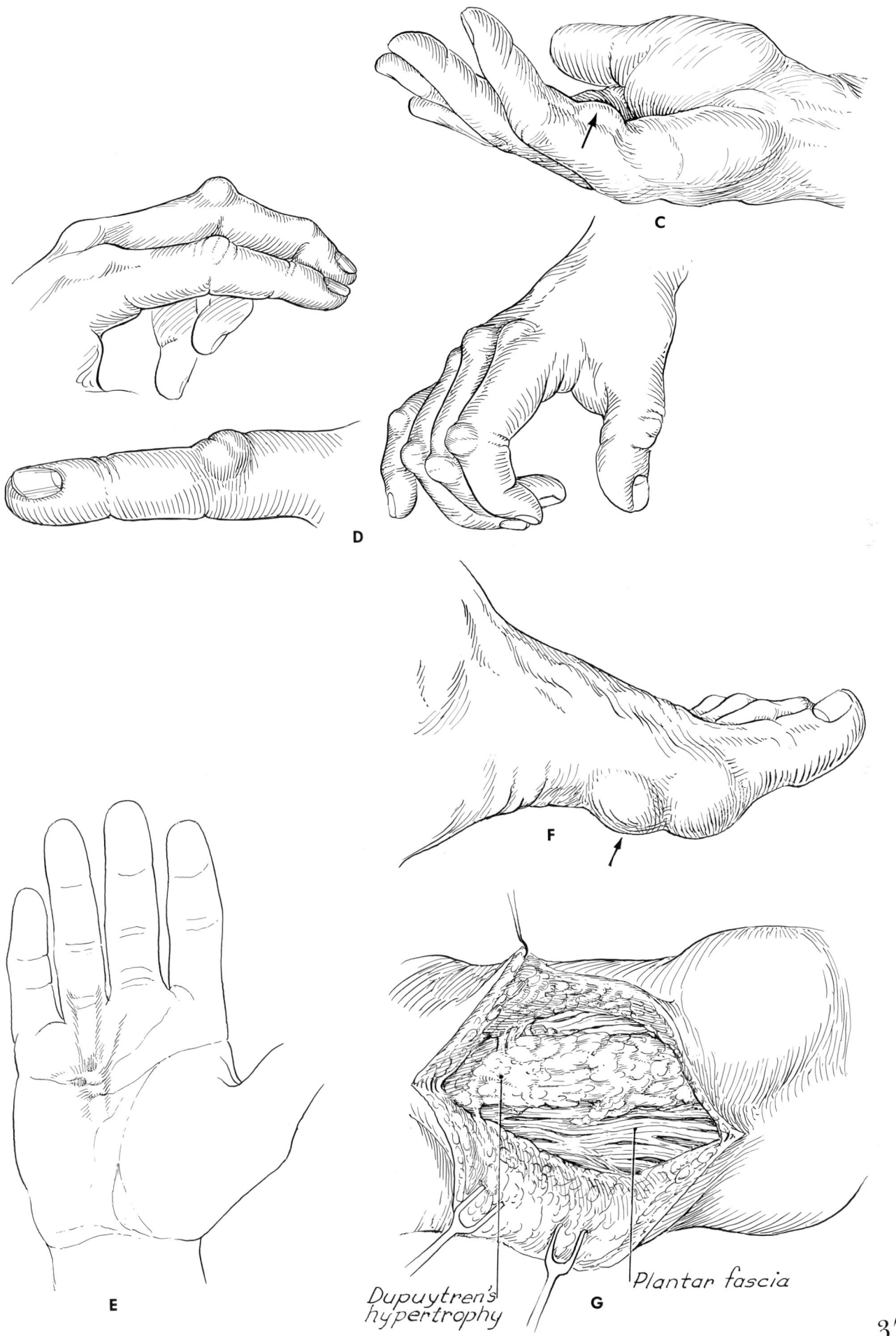

379

87 — Dupuytren's Contracture

PALMAR FASCIECTOMY

Principle

If Dupuytren's contracture involves the longitudinal fibers to a single finger, a limited fasciectomy for release is indicated. The incision preferred is a zig-zag, **W**-shaped incision, with its long axis along the thickened band of fascia in the palm and proximal phalanx of the finger. Alternatively, one may choose to make a longitudinal incision along the thickened contracted fibers to be followed by a multiple Z-plasty closure. Z-plasty is mandatory to avoid a disastrous midline flexion scar contracture.

Example: Z-Plasty Incision

A 60-year-old man with Dupuytren's contracture involving the longitudinal fibers of the palmar fascia to the left long finger asked for treatment because his inability to extend his metacarpophalangeal joint and proximal interphalangeal joint interfered with his activities.

The skin was lightly adherent to the thick strand of fascia, particularly in the distal palm. A longitudinal incision directly over the diseased fascia was planned. Two sets of parallel side cuts were designed for Z-plasty closure to avoid leaving a mid-palmar incision which would violate principles noted on page 37. (**A**)

The skin was cautiously dissected from the palmar fascial band and from the palmar fascia on both sides for adequate mobilization of the Z-plasty flaps. This may best be done by sweeping the scalpel blade beneath the skin with the blade held flat against the longitudinal fibers of the palmar fascia. (**B**) The transverse fascial fibers in the web spaces on each side of the base of the long finger were incised at the extremes of the dissection. (**C**)

The diseased longitudinal band of fascia was transected and removed, preserving the transverse fibers in the mid-palm. (**D**) When this portion of palmar fascia called the transverse palmar ligament can safely be preserved, the postoperative morbidity is diminished.

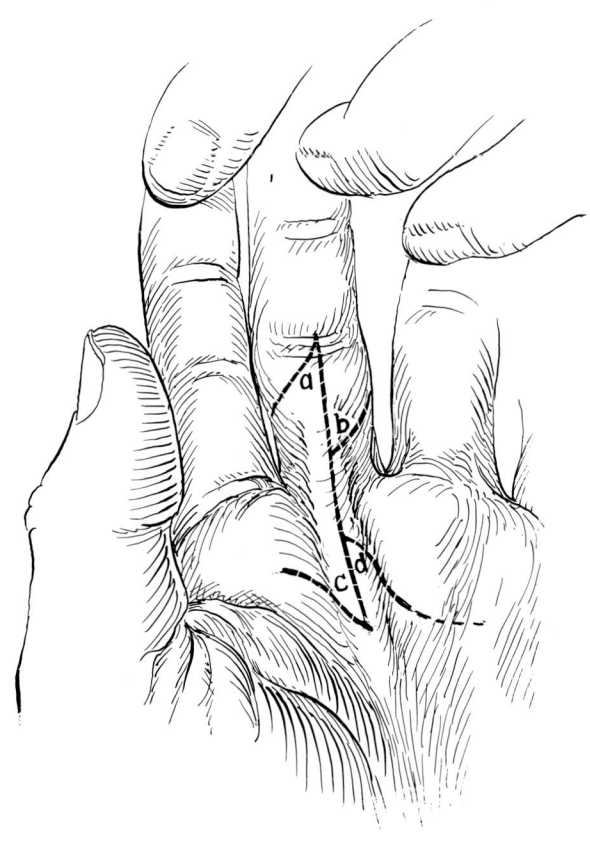

A

Tendons, Fascia and Muscles

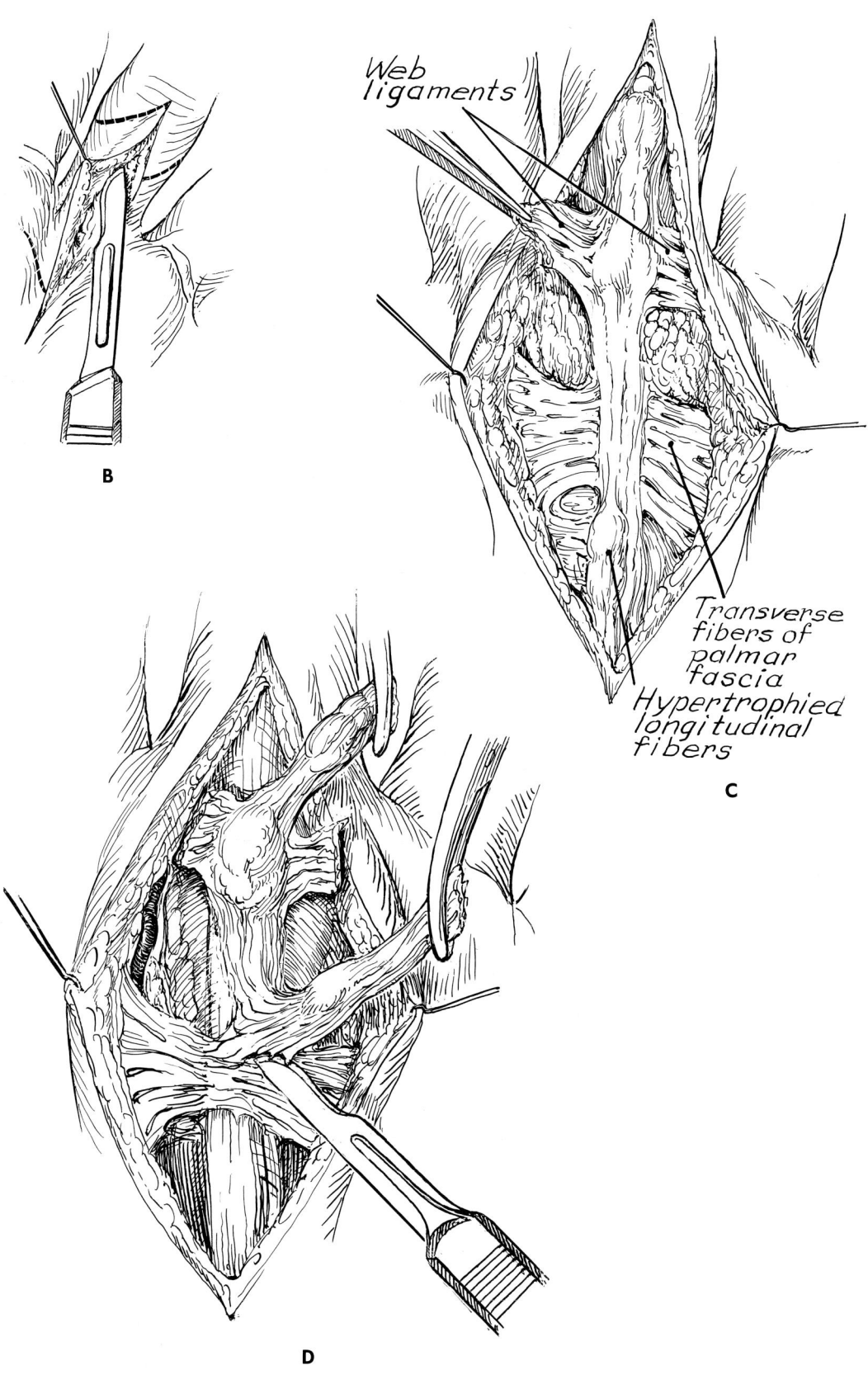

381

87 – Dupuytren's Contracture

Some of the penetrating vertical blood vessels to the skin flaps were spared to assure adequate skin blood supply.

When the longitudinal diseased band of fascia was removed, full passive extension was readily achieved.

The side cuts were made in preparation for Z-plasty shifts and, with the finger pulled into extension, the exchange flaps fell into place for closure. **(E)**

The tourniquet was released and removed from the arm at this time to check for adequacy of hemostasis. A few bleeding points required ligation. The skin wounds were sutured closed. **(F)**

The residual closed incision was a zig-zag one without the potential for scar contracture in flexor as is the case with a palmar straight longitudinal scar. The Z-plasty flaps added longitudinal skin length to overcome the deficit created when the finger, long held in flexion, was released to full extension.

A smoothly applied bulky dressing of fluffed gauze, a springy gauze roll and a plaster splint with the hand in a comfortable position were applied.

It was left undisturbed for 10 days, with the patient instructed to keep the arm elevated in a sling at all times.

Progressive active motion was initiated two weeks after operation. Healing was prompt and full range of motion had been restored six months after surgery.

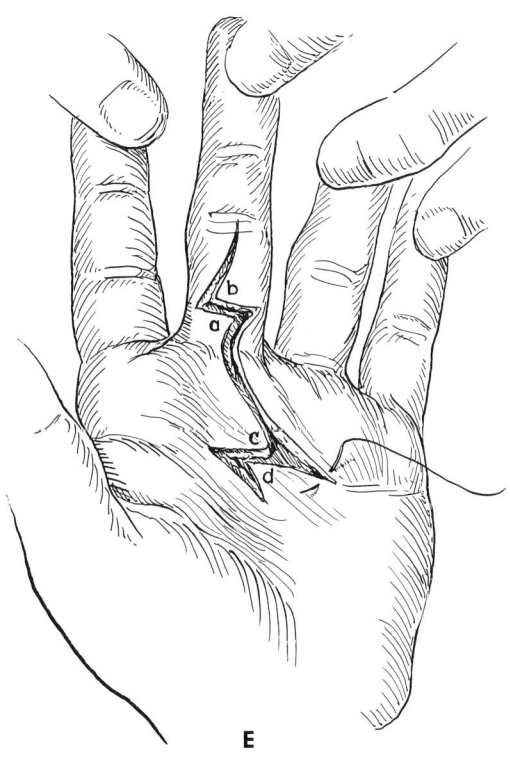

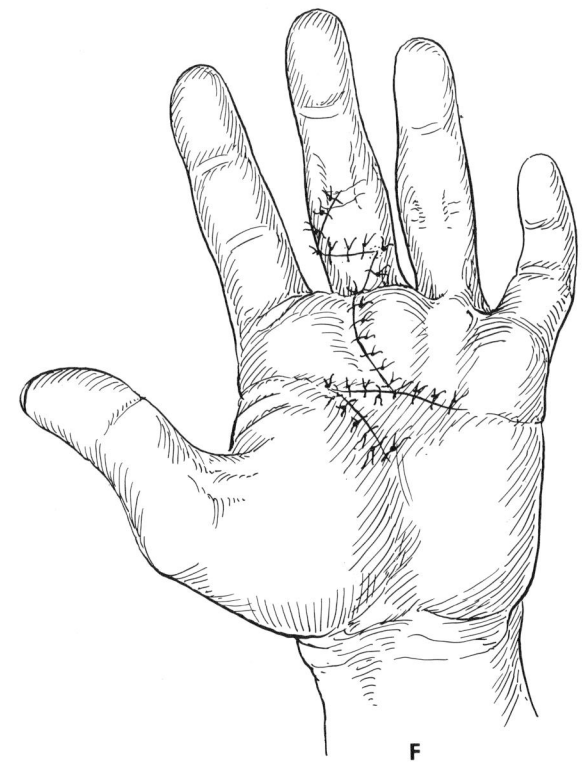

Tendons, Fascia and Muscles

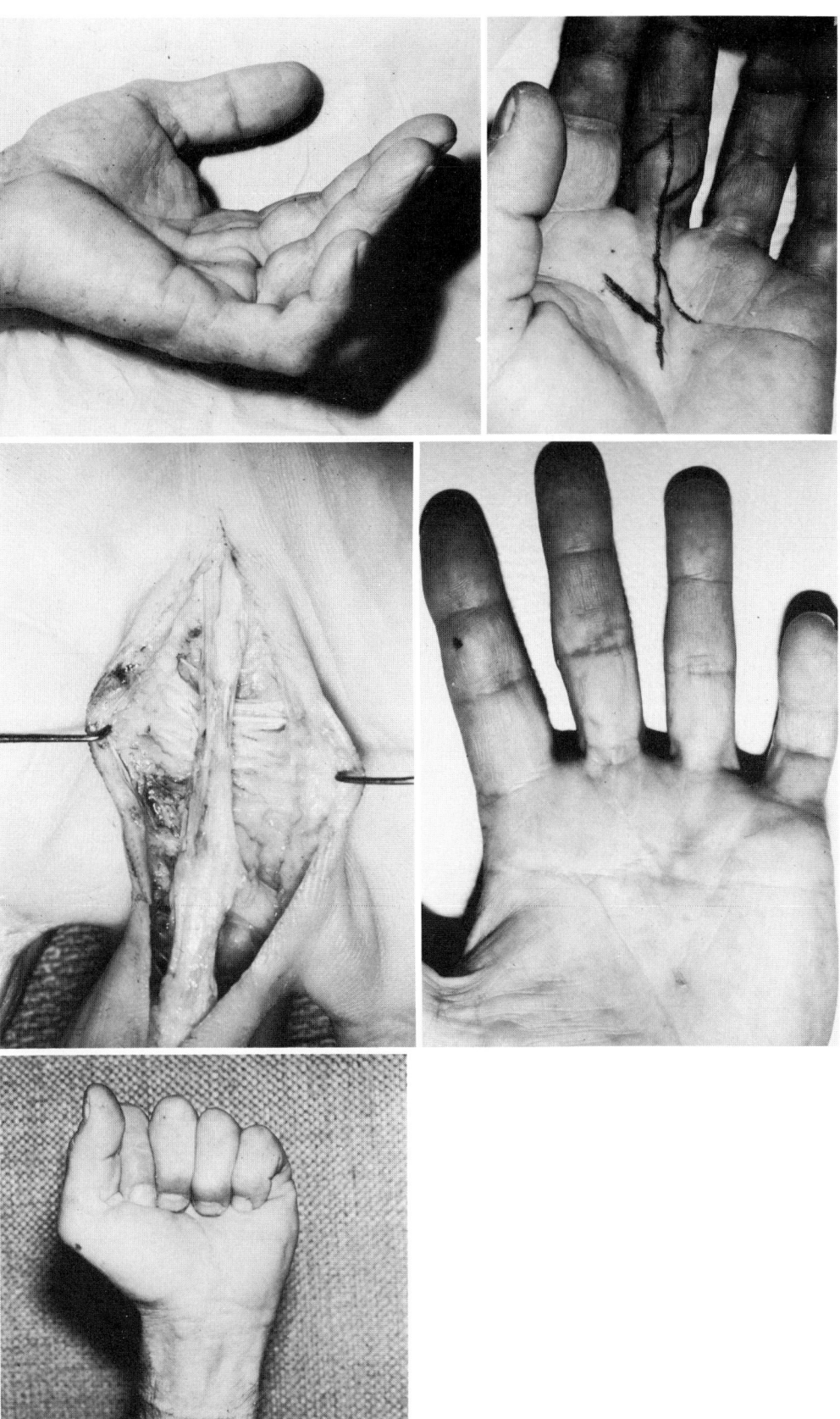

383

87 – Dupuytren's Contracture

Example: W-Incision

A 56-year-old patient with Dupuytren's contracture involving the ring finger of his right hand sought help for the disability caused by his inability to fully extend his ring finger at the metacarpophalangeal joint and proximal interphalangeal joint.

The palpable thickened band of palmar fascia seemed to involve only the ring finger. The flexion contracture, having been present for several years, had resulted in shortening of the skin along the line of the ring finger. The skin was tightly adherent to the diseased palmar fascia at one point at the distal palmar crease.

Selective excision of the diseased fascia was decided upon and a **W**-shaped incision was planned in such a way that one of the incision lines crossed the point of skin adherence. (**A**) This avoided placement of the thin plaque of adherent skin in the middle of one of the triangular flaps where it could compromise blood supply to the flap tip.

The skin was sharply dissected from the palmar fascia, being particularly careful where the skin flaps crossed the diseased palmar fascia to the ring finger. Removal of the diseased longitudinal fibrous palmar fascia allowed full extension of the finger. By progressively undermining the skin until the **W**-shaped flaps could be overlapped from side to side, it was possible to gain longitudinal skin length. (**B**)

To achieve this, the **V**-shaped triangular flaps were advanced into one another and incisions were made on the YV principle to release longitudinal tension and to insert the triangular wedges of skin, sacrificing unneeded transverse length for longitudinal length of skin. (**C**)

The skin wounds were closed after the tourniquet was released and hemostasis checked. (**D**) With the skin length gained by the procedure, it was possible to immobilize the finger in comfortable extension during the postoperative period.

Tendons, Fascia and Muscles

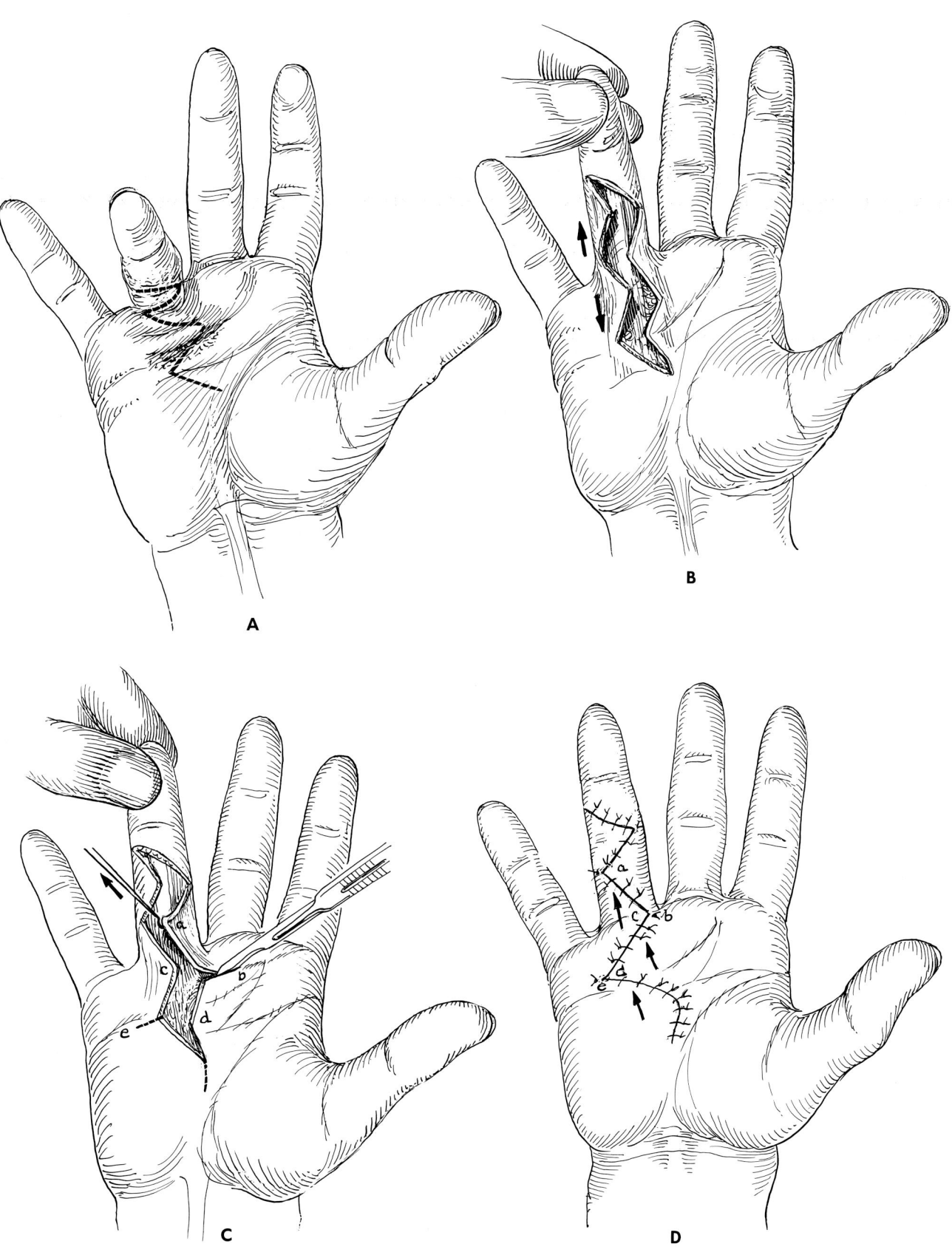

385

PITFALLS OF PALMAR FASCIECTOMY

Principle

The relationship of digital nerves to the palmar fascia may become distorted in advancing Dupuytren's contracture. This is most particularly true in the distal palm and at the base of the finger. Great care must be exercised during dissection of the fascia, particularly at this critical level.

Example: Distortion of Digital Nerve Anatomy in the Distal Palm

A patient with moderately advanced Dupuytren's contracture involving the ring and little fingers was operated upon using a **W**-shaped incision extending down the ring finger. **(A)** As the longitudinal fibrous band approached the finger at its base, it passed beneath the proper digital nerve to the ulnar side. The removal of this diseased fascia required careful release of the nerve from its surface. Once the nerve could be identified proximally and distally and free at this critical site, the diseased fascia could be safely excised. **(B)**

Tendons, Fascia and Muscles

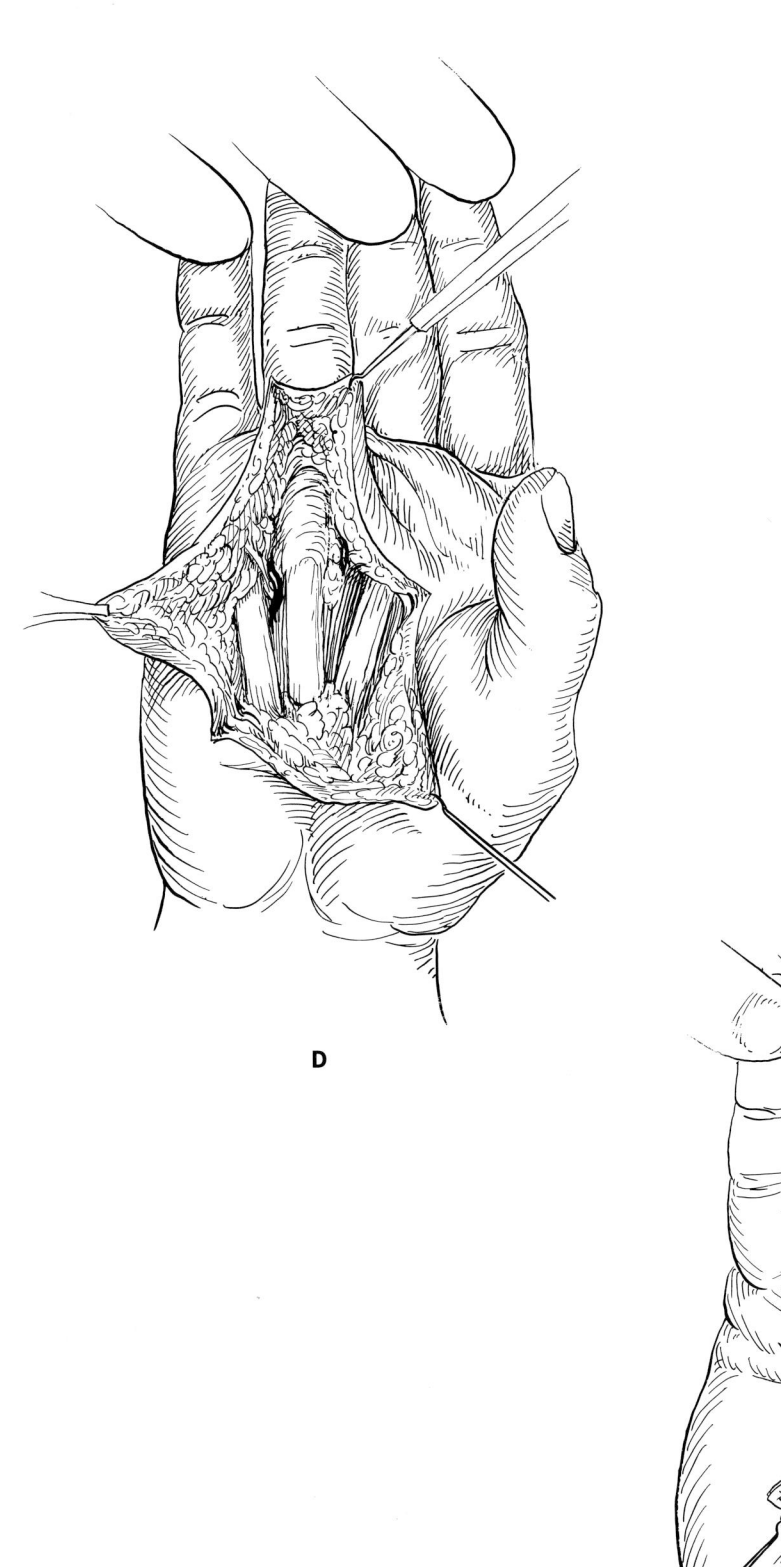

D

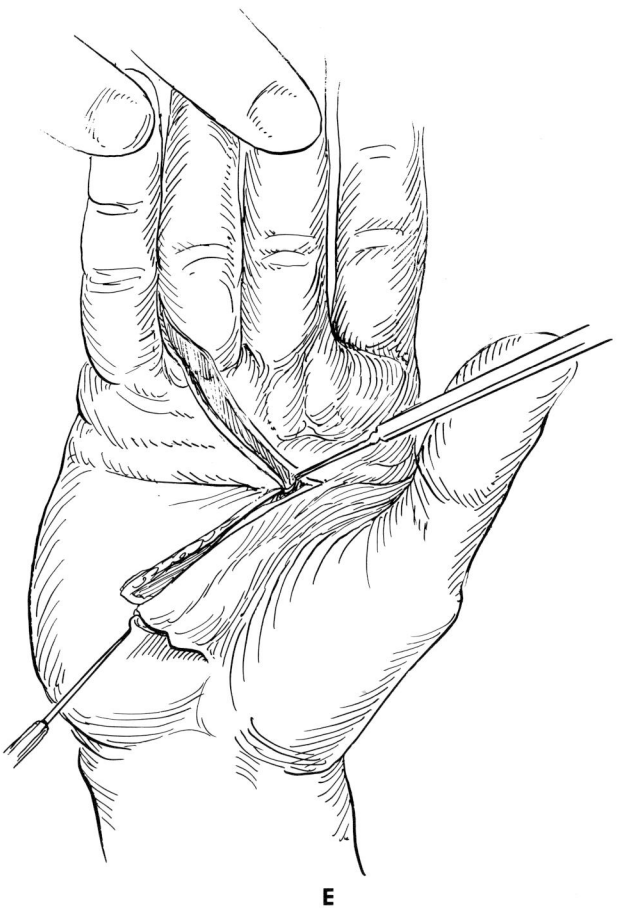

E

PALMAR FASCIOTOMY

Principle: Open Section

Flexion contracture of the proximal interphalangeal joint as a result of Dupuytren's contracture may be released without extensive dissection by transection of the skin and fascia and application of a free full thickness graft.

Example

An elderly man with marked flexion contracture of the proximal interphalangeal joint of the little finger was disturbed by its interference with his daily activities. (**A**)

Under local block anesthesia a transverse incision was made across the finger just proximal to the proximal interphalangeal joint. (**B**) While the finger was held in maximum extension, the incision was deepened into and through the diseased palmar fascia. (**C**) The digital neurovascular bundles were carefully preserved. The flexion contracture gave way as the diseased palmar fascia was cut across. With the release without skin undermining, a diamond-shaped skin deficit resulted.

A full thickness free skin graft was taken from the flank under local anesthesia. It was draped over the residual defect and sutured in place. (**D**)

The finger was immobilized in extension for 10 days. The graft took well and release has been effective in the two years subsequent to the operation.

Tendons, Fascia and Muscles

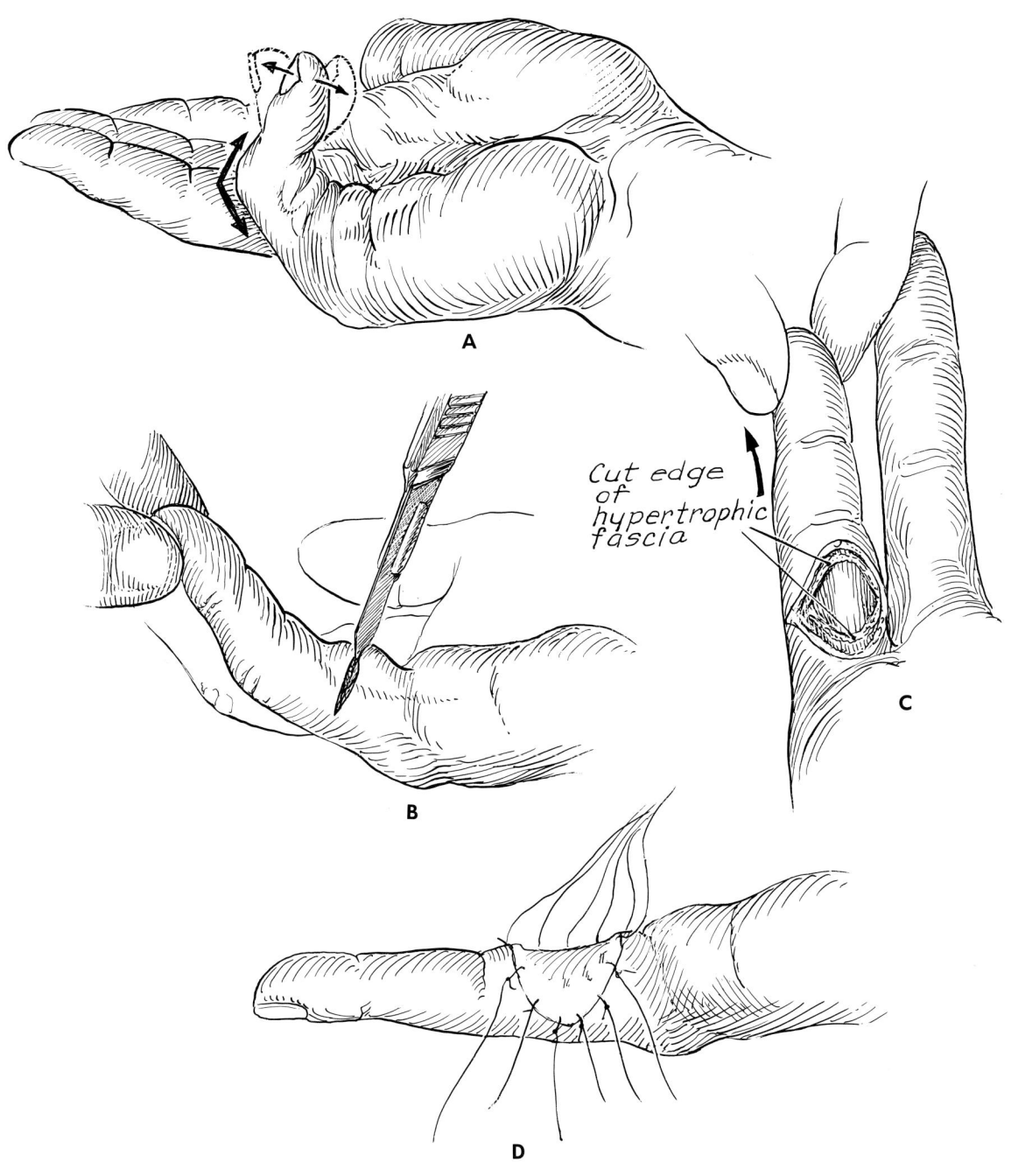

391

87 – Dupuytren's Contracture

Principle: Closed Section

In an elderly patient disabled by solitary digital involvement by Dupuytren's contracture, a subcutaneous fasciotomy may be useful. It is particularly practical when a more substantial procedure requiring more extensive anesthesia would not be well tolerated by the patient. The procedure may also be used for release of a tightly contracted metacarpophalangeal joint where folded palmar skin surfaces are subject to maceration and epidermophytosis. After release by subcutaneous fasciotomy the skin may improve to allow safe surgical incision for fascial excision. When closed fasciotomy is used, the transection should be done with tension pulling the finger into maximum extension. The taut fascia can then be cut like a tight string, whereas the loose digital nerves will fall away from the knife. The section is done at only one point. The point usually selected is at the distal palmar crease not closer to the base of the finger where the digital nerves become more superficial.

Example

A 75-year-old cigar maker was disabled by a bilateral progressive Dupuytren's contracture. It was confined to the ring finger and involved the metacarpophalangeal joints most severely. A subcutaneous closed fasciotomy was chosen because of his age and general condition.

Local anesthetic was injected from the hypothenar area to the mid-palm, just proximal to the distal palmar crease. (**E**)

A myringotomy knife was inserted into the subcutaneous tissues over the hypothenar area. It was advanced subcutaneously across the palm parallel to the distal palmar crease. As it reached the thick diseased band of palmar fascia, it was maneuvered between it and the overlying skin. The band of fascia was held taut by extension pull on the finger and the myringotomy knife was swept proximally and distally between the band and skin for about a centimeter proximally and a centimeter distally. (**F**)

With extension tension at a minimum, the knife was advanced and retracted in saw fashion, to cut the band of fascia transversely. The contracture gave way as the fascia was being transected. (**G**)

The knife was removed and a bulky pressure dressing was applied with the finger in release extension. The release was adequate to allow the patient to return to his trade without further surgery.

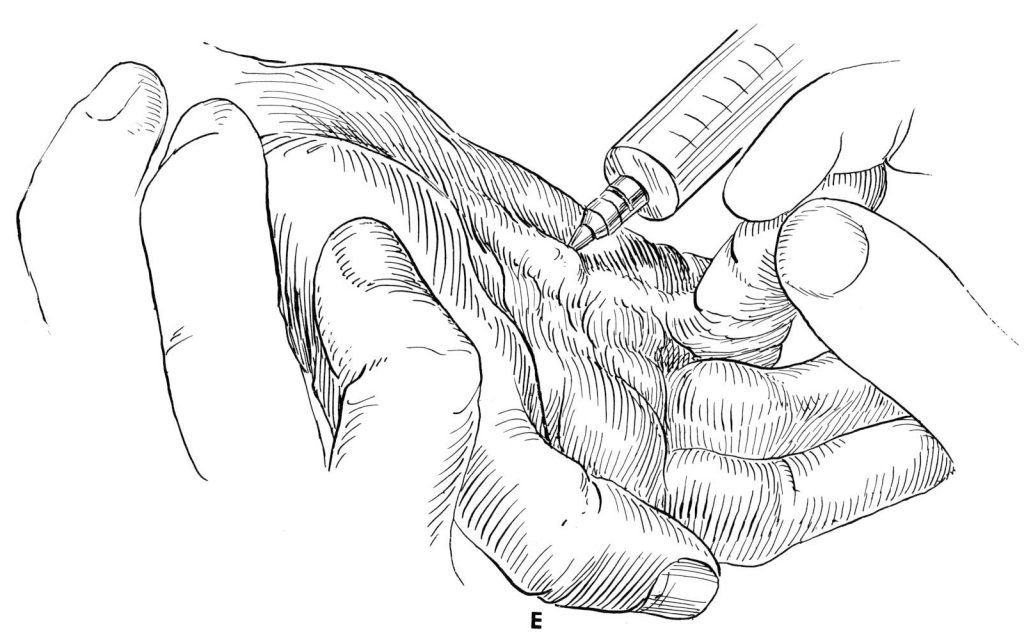

E

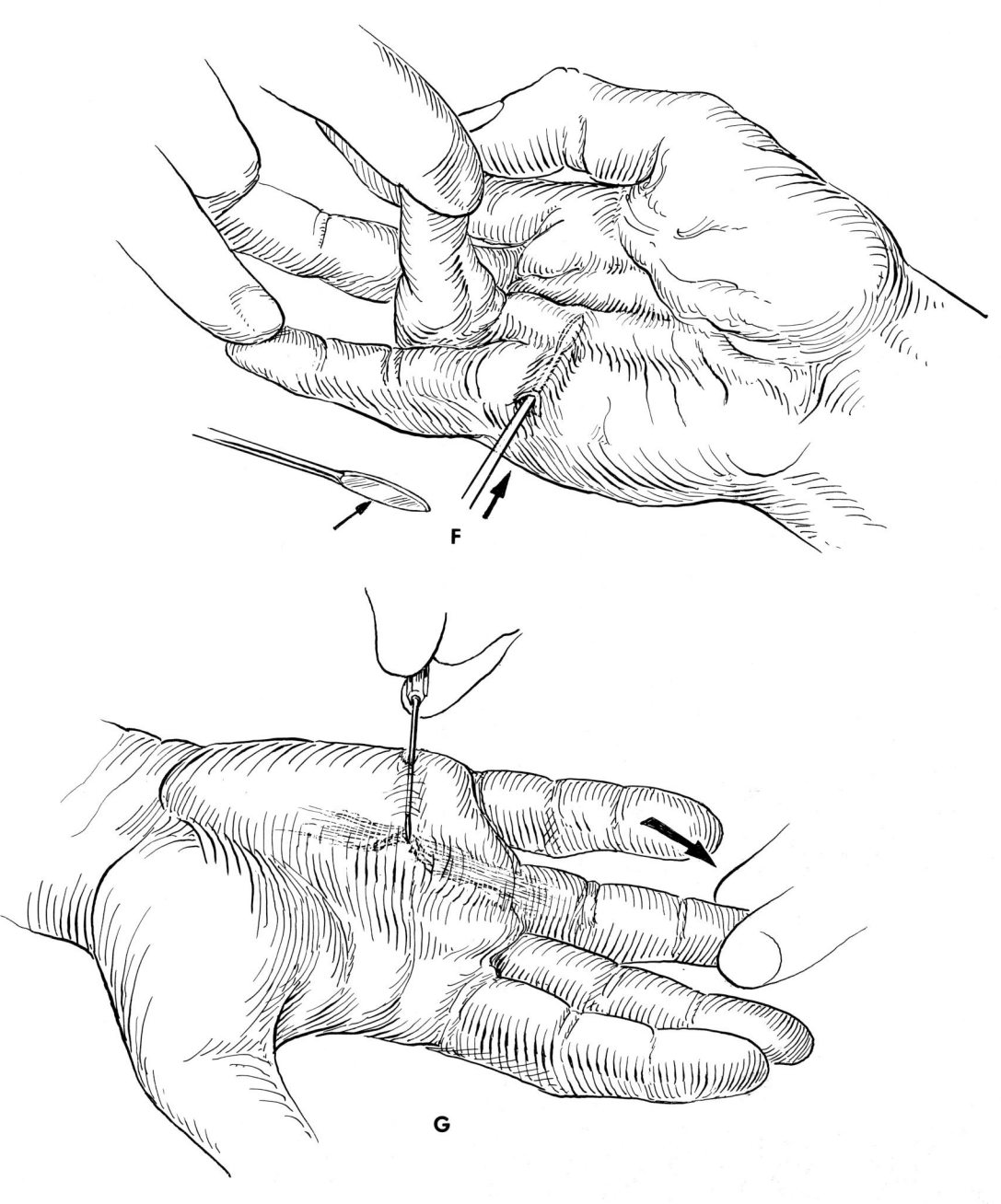

87 – Dupuytren's Contracture

RAY AMPUTATION FOR SEVERE DUPUYTREN'S CONTRACTURE OF THE LITTLE FINGER

Principle

The results of surgical excision of palmar fascia for Dupuytren's contracture of the little finger are poorer than those of any of the other fingers. Irreversible joint fixation is more frequent after long term contracture of the little finger from any cause. Recurrence of Dupuytren's contracture after surgery is more common in the little finger than in the others.

When treatment of Dupuytren's contracture in the little finger fails, and irreversible joint fixation results, a ray amputation is one appropriate means of diminishing disability. Such a ray amputation may liberate the dorsal undiseased skin and soft tissue as a pedicle flap to overcome the common skin deficiency in the palm.

Example

A 55 year-old-lawyer who had undergone repeated surgical procedures for treatment of his Dupuytren's contracture had disabling residual deformity of both little fingers. The finger on each hand was fixed in sharp flexion at the proximal interphalangeal joint. (**A**) There, skin deficiency on the palmar surface over the proximal phalanx of the digit and the palm skin distal to the distal palmar crease was scarred and deficient. Bilateral ray amputation (see Section 34) combined with digital fillet (see Section 23) to procure additional palm skin was decided upon. In each case, a mid-palmar digital incision and incision circumscribing the severely scarred distal palmar skin was planned. The ray amputation was carried out through the palmar incision, and the dorsal skin of the finger was draped into the palm defect and trimmed to size. (**B**) The wounds were closed, leaving the patient with smooth symmetrical three fingered hands. (**C, D,** and **E**)

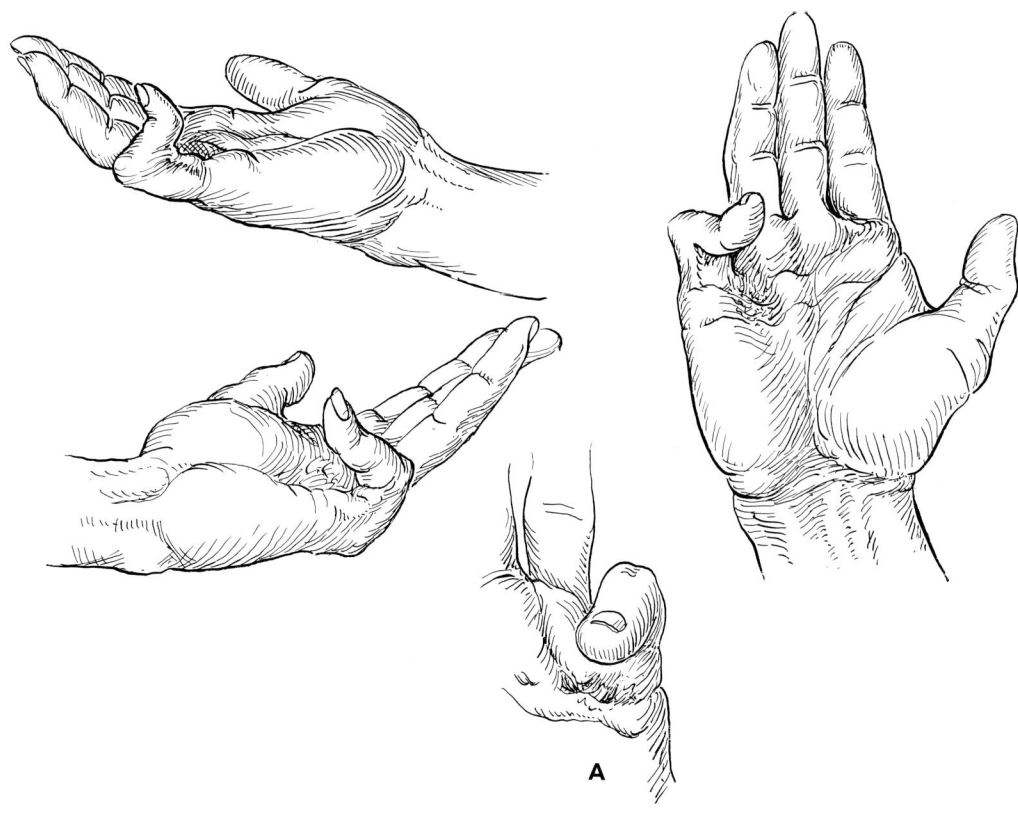

Tendons, Fascia and Muscles

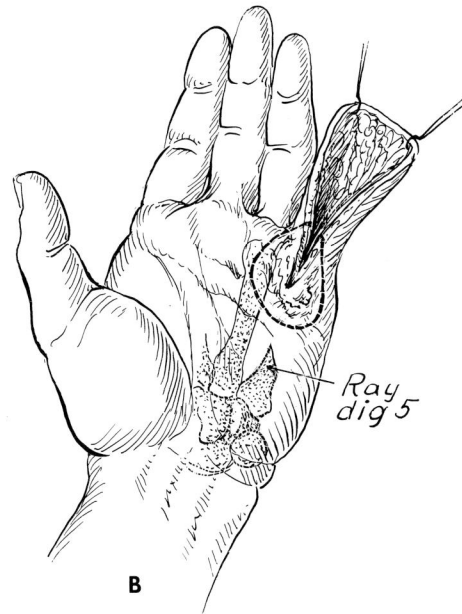
B

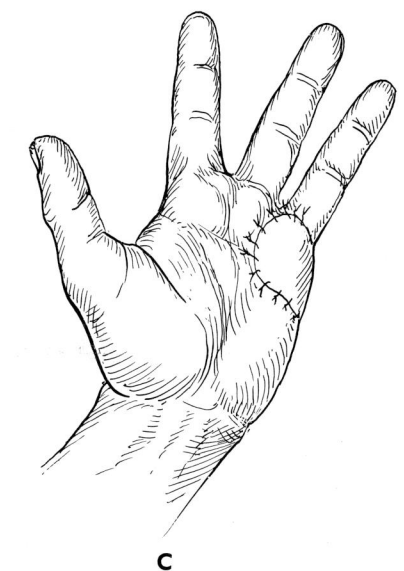
C

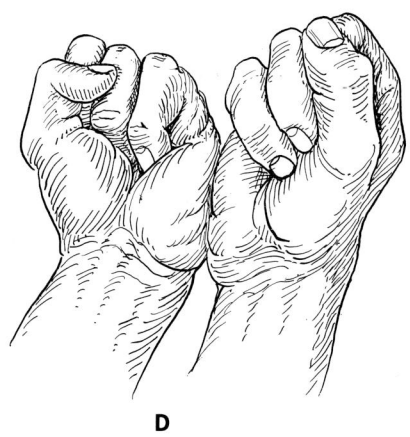
D

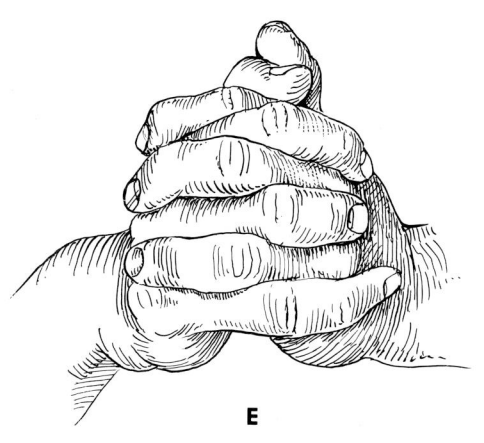
E

88

Tendon Transfers

Anatomy

The neurophysiology of muscle groups is such that there is central control of each muscle belly, which may be separated out centrally to function as a solitary unit. With education of that muscle unit through proper feedback information, it is possible to utilize its functional capability for a purpose entirely foreign to its original prime functional duty. Thus, whole muscle units and to some extent even portions of a muscle may be directed to take on new functions after transfer of its tendon. The period of reeducation of the neuromuscular unit is shorter to the point of being automatic, if one transfers a musculotendinous unit to assume a function which is normally synergistic with the primary function of the transferred muscle.

For example, finger flexion is normally coupled with wrist extension. The transfer of a wrist extensor to assume the function of paralyzed finger flexors sets the stage for natural assumption of finger flexion. The reverse—that is, finger flexor transfer to wrist extension function—is also quite natural. **(A)** To transfer a wrist flexor to assume the function of finger flexion is non-synergistic and unnatural. In time, cerebral reorientation occurs, and function may be transferred but the period necessary and the reeducation needed are longer and more extensive. In principle, however, any muscle-tendon unit may assume any new function assigned to it within the limitations imposed by its range of motion from full contraction to full relaxation.

A knowledge of which musculotendinous units are available for transfer in each case of paralysis requires a knowledge of relationships of muscles and tendons to one another and the usual innervation of each.

On the palmar aspect of the forearm the muscles are found in three layers—superficial, middle, and deep. The superficial group consists of muscles frequently used in musculotendinous transfers for radial nerve paralysis. The superficial layer may be readily remembered by placing one's hand on the opposite forearm with the heel of the thenar eminence at the elbow and dropping the little finger off the forearm on its ulnar side. **(B)** The thumb and fingers project precisely as the muscles in the superficial group do. The thumb falls over the pronator teres, the index finger over the flexor carpi radialis, the *long* finger over the palmaris *longus* and ring finger over the flexor carpi ulnaris.

The deep layer is easily recalled, since it consists of distal phalangeal flexors, the flexor digitorum profundi and the equivalent to the thumb, the flexor pollicis longus. **(C)** The residual muscle group making up the middle layer is the flexor digitorum superficialis. All of the muscles on the palmar aspect of the forearm are median nerve innervated except the flexor carpi *ulnaris* and the *ulnar* two or three profundi. They are *ulnar* nerve innervated.

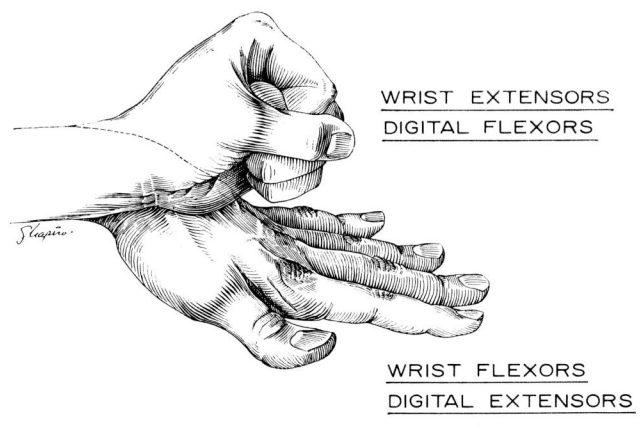

A

From White

Tendons, Fascia and Muscles

SUPERFICIAL LAYER

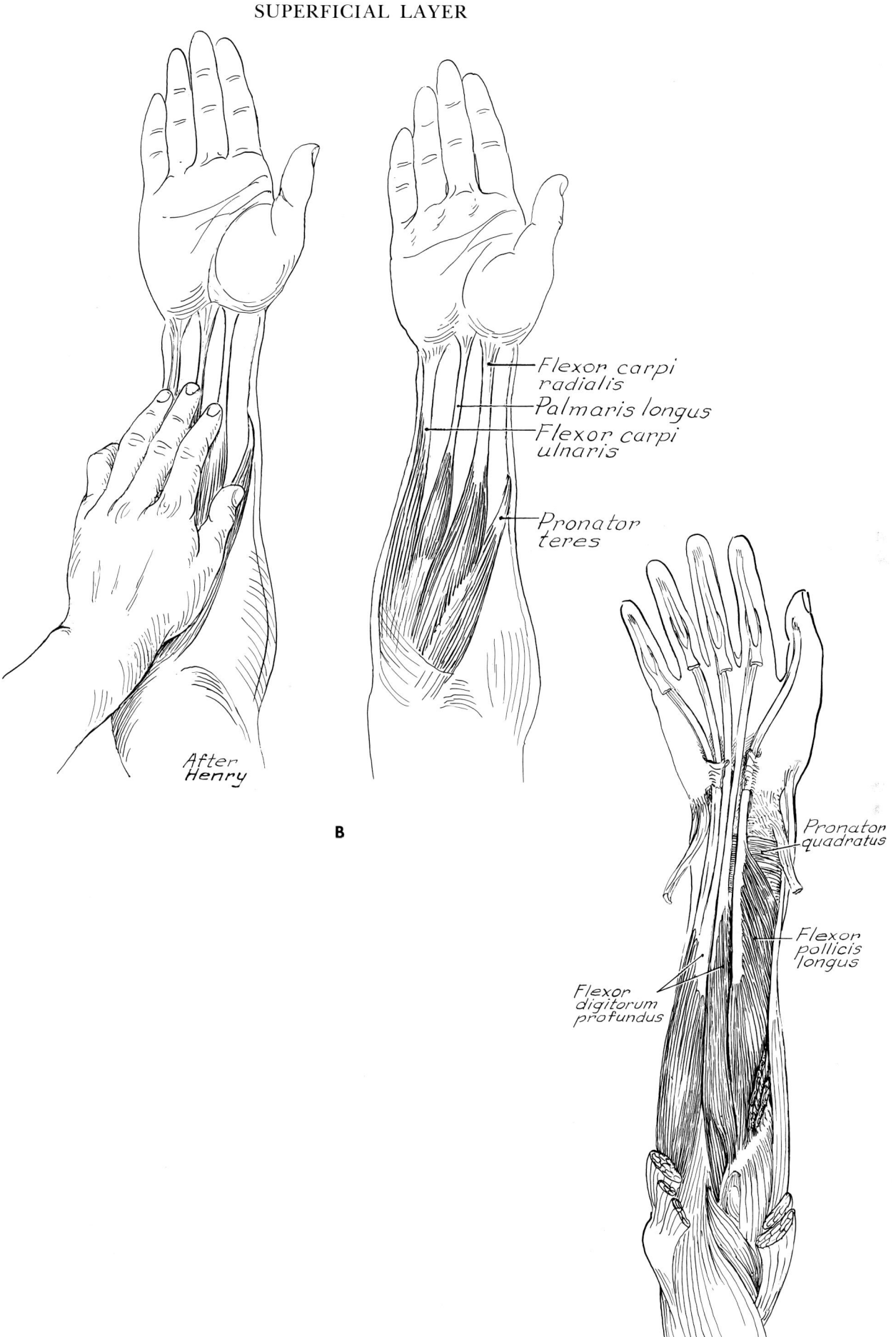

88 – Tendon Transfers

The muscles on the dorsal aspect of the forearm consist of digital extensors, wrist extensors, the oblique muscles to the thumb, and the supinator. The brachioradialis and the radial wrist extensors (extensor carpi radialis longus and brevis) make up the "mobile wad" of muscles of the radiodorsal aspect of the forearm below the elbow. This group of muscles may be picked up between the contralateral thumb and index finger as a group. (**D**, **E**, and **F**)

All of the muscles on the dorsal aspect of the forearm are innervated by the radial nerve.

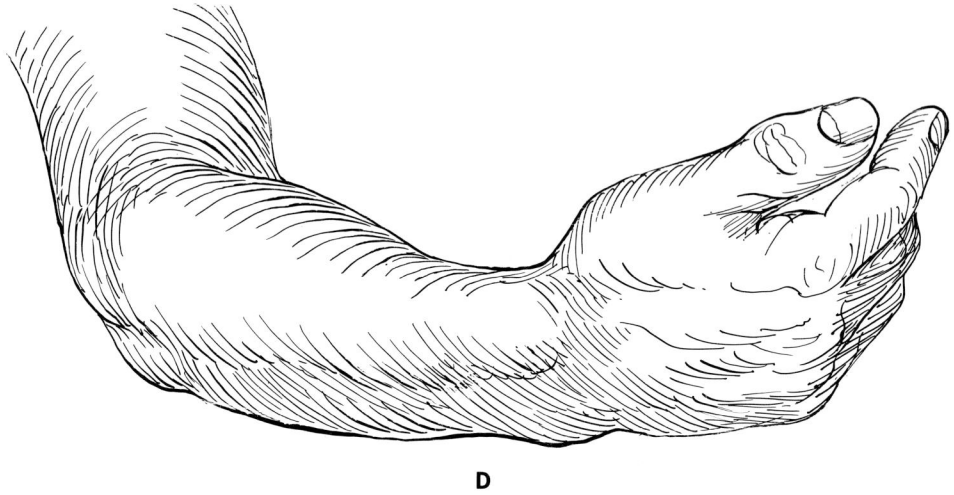

D

Tendons, Fascia and Muscles

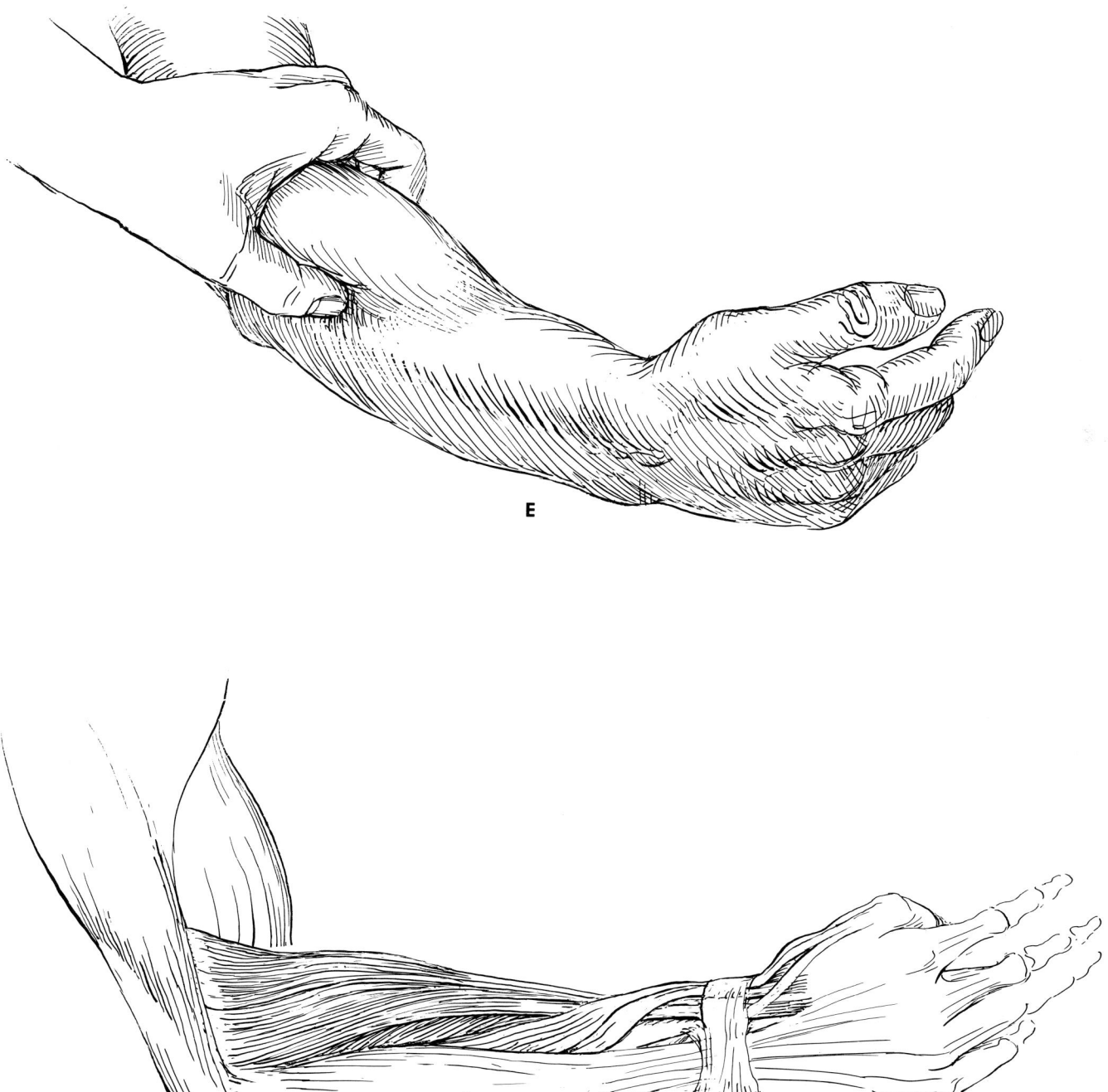

E

F

89
Tendon Transfers for Ulnar Nerve Paralysis

If an ulnar nerve injury at the wrist has resulted in intrinsic paralysis in the hand for more than a year, a repair or re-repair of the nerve to restore sensibility may justifiably be coupled with specific procedures to overcome the motor disability.

If the ulnar nerve lesion is at the elbow or above, the procedures might be done at the time of or shortly after the initial nerve repair. This requires an understanding patient who does not need to experience the disability implicit in ulnar nerve paralysis to understand the need to sacrifice some less important function for overall improved hand action. If there is any question in the surgeon's mind, the corrective procedure should be delayed, but not for a period long enough to evaluate whether or not intrinsic muscle function will return as a result of nerve repair. The prognosis for such return in high ulnar nerve palsy is so slim in adults that the risk of development of fixed deformity prompts a recommendation for early corrective intervention.

Two major functional problems are created by classical paralysis of ulnar innervated intrinsic muscles. They are: (1) thumb adduction weakness, and (2) clawing of the fingers—particularly the ring and little.

Ulnar Claw Hand

When intrinsic muscles to the fingers are paralyzed, they have lost the prime flexors of the metacarpophalangeal joints and they have also lost the ability to extend the interphalangeal joints when the metacarpophalangeal joints are in hyperextension. The combination of intact long flexors of the fingers with long extensors results in discoordination and a classical clawing posture. The long extensors, attempting to extend the fingers in the absence of balanced flexion of the metacarpophalangeal joints, hyperextend the metacarpophalangeal joints. In this position, the long extensor has lost its ability to extend the interphalangeal joints. The inability of the long extensors to extend the interphalangeal joints, combined with paralysis of the intrinsic extensors of these joints, leaves the joints influenced entirely by the long extensors and thus in a flexed position. Before the long flexors, the flexor digitorum superficialis and profundus, can effectively flex the metacarpophalangeal joint, they fully flex the interphalangeal joints, where opposing active extension is absent. The fingers roll up sequentially, first at the proximal interphalangeal joints and finally at the distal interphalangeal joints. The normal, coordinated sweep of the fingers into the palm is lost and the roll up of the fingers may actually push large objects out of attempted grasp. (**A**)

If one passively blocks hyperextension of the metacarpophalangeal joint in ulnar nerve paralysis, the patient may actively extend the interphalangeal joints using the unparalyzed long extensors. One means of correcting claw deformity of a finger or fingers is to block hyperextension of the metacarpophalangeal joint by surgical bone block of the joint or by metacarpophalangeal joint capsulodesis as recommended by Zancolli.

Tendons, Fascia and Muscles

NORMAL   INTRINSIC PARALYSIS

A

401

ULNAR CLAW HAND CORRECTION

Principles

The variety of procedures available and used to correct ulnar palsy clawing of the hand is not attributable to the fact that none is very good but to the variable functional deficits that appear from one patient to the next with ulnar palsy. A person whose normal range of extension in the finger metacarpophalangeal joints is limited as a variation of normal may not develop significant claw deformity. Individuals with loose capsular structures and an excessive range of metacarpophalangeal joint extension may develop severe clawing to the point of dorsal subluxation of the metacarpophalangeal joints.

Corrective procedures are numerous but they fall generally into the categories of tendon transfers, tenodeses, capsulodeses, osteotomy, or fusion. Frequently, clawing sufficient to require surgical correction occurs only in the ring and little fingers in isolated ulnar palsy. The median-nerve supplied lumbricals to the index and long fingers are often sufficient to prevent claw deformity in those fingers.

A few of the common successful procedures have been chosen as examples. None of the procedures should be done on a stiff hand. Maximum mobility of finger joints must be acquired by physical therapy, splinting, and casting prior to surgery.

Example: Metacarpophalangeal Joint Capsulodesis

A patient with ulnar nerve paralysis demonstrated clawing of the fingers on extension. (**A**) Function appeared nearly normal when hyperextension of the metacarpophalangeal joints was passively blocked. Treatment by palmar metacarpophalangeal joint capsulodesis (Zancolli) was decided upon. The principle is to shorten the palmar joint capsule or to fix it to the metacarpal head in such a way that metacarpophalangeal joint extension is limited. There are a number of techniques used to achieve this. In each method the approach to the palmar capsule is through a transverse incision just distal to the distal palmar crease. (**B**) The flexor tendons are retracted after incising the flexor retinaculum. (**C**)

1. One may carry out a simple transverse elliptical excision of the palmar glenoid capsule of the metacarpophalangeal joint with careful suture closure. (**D, E,** and **F**) Sufficient capsule is removed to hold the metacarpophalangeal joint to 10 to 30 degrees of flexion when extension is attempted. (**G** and **H**) Strong patients with powerful extensor tendons may in time stretch this simple capsular repair with resulting recurrence of clawing.

2. Capsular fixation to the metacarpal may be accomplished by incising the glenoid capsule and then suturing it to the metacarpal to limit extension of the metacarpophalangeal joint to 10 to 30 degrees of flexion. This procedure requires drilling holes in the metacarpal for secure fixation (**I** through **O**).

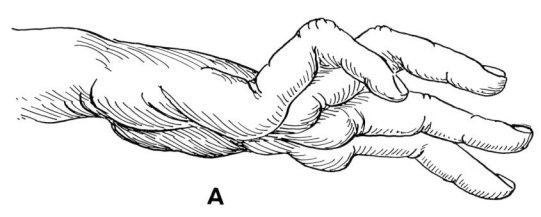

A

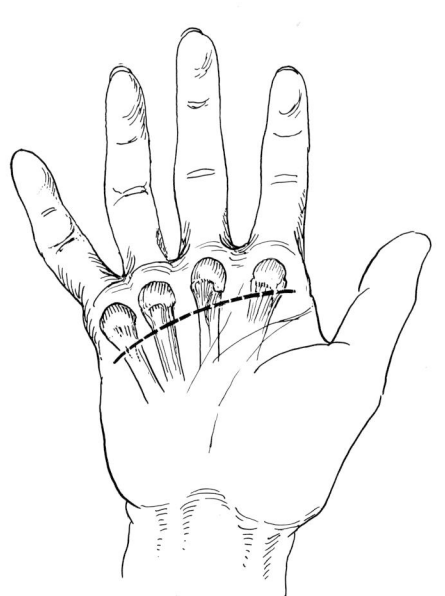

B

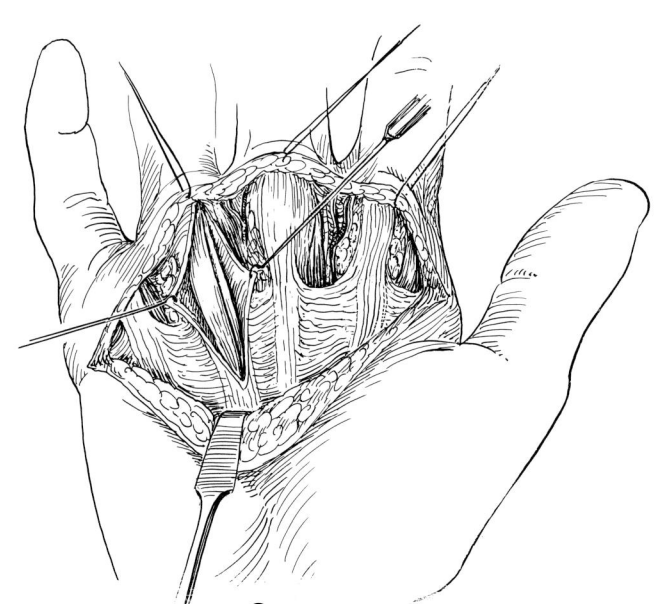

C

Tendons, Fascia and Muscles

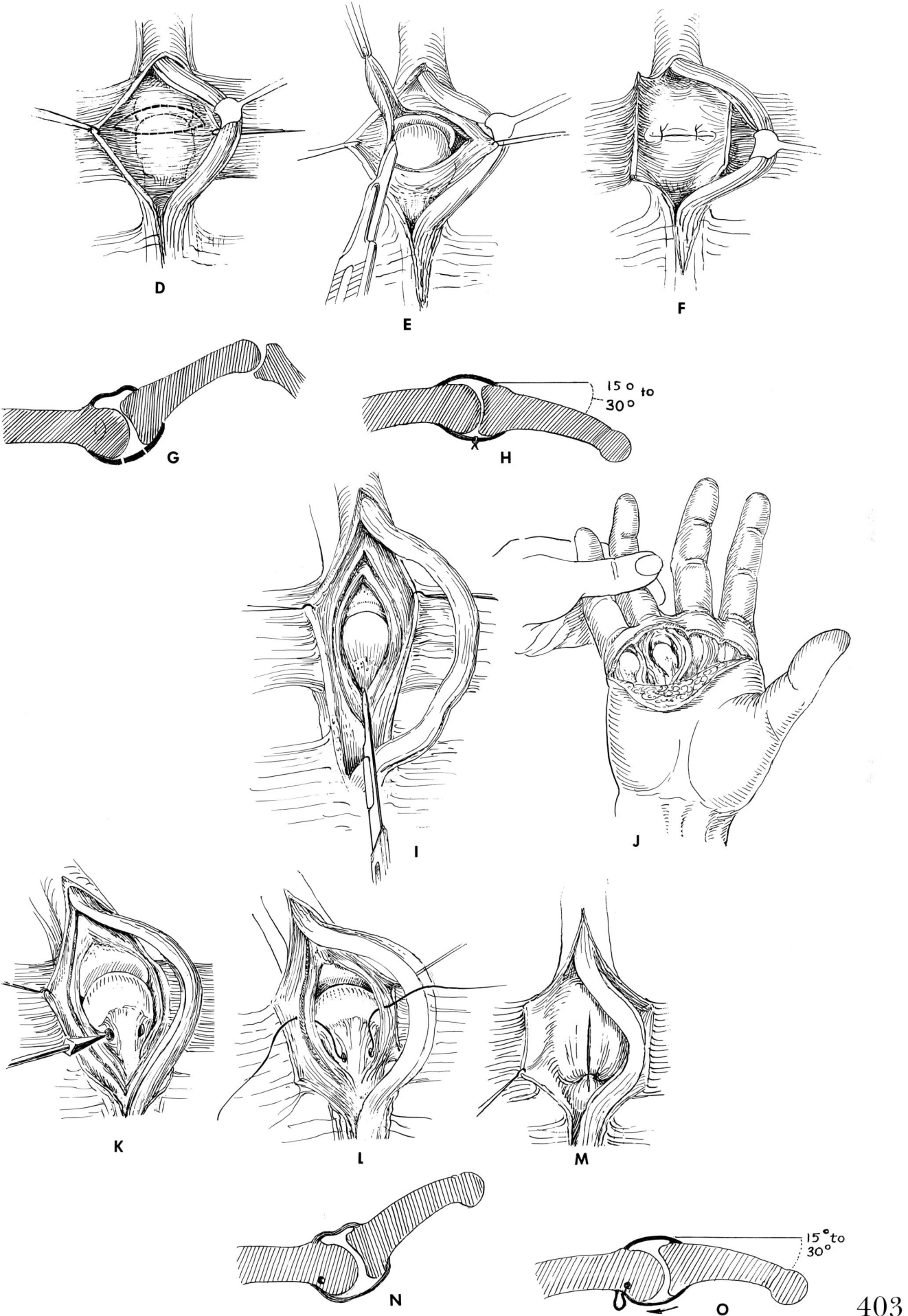

403

3. A combination of capsular shortening and fixation to bone may be chosen and was selected in this case.

The glenoid capsule was incised to create a distally based tongue, which was to be fixed to the metacarpal. (**P**) Excision of triangular capsular components to shorten the residual lateral capsule prevented folding of the capsule and further secured the limitation of metacarpophalangeal joint extension.

The tongue of glenoid capsule was fixed to the metacarpal by drilling through the metacarpal, passing a nonabsorbable suture through the tongue and bone, and tying it dorsally. (**Q**) The holes were placed in such a way that the suture would not interfere with long extensor tendon function. The metacarpophalangeal joint was held in 15 to 30 degrees of flexion. (**R**)

The metacarpophalangeal joints were immobilized in flexion for three weeks after the operation. If immobilization is difficult, a Kirschner wire may be run across the joint for three or four weeks. (**S**) The patient was allowed gradually to reassume full activity. Function, the equivalent of that demonstrated preoperatively by passive limitation of metacarpophalangeal joint extension, resulted after two months.

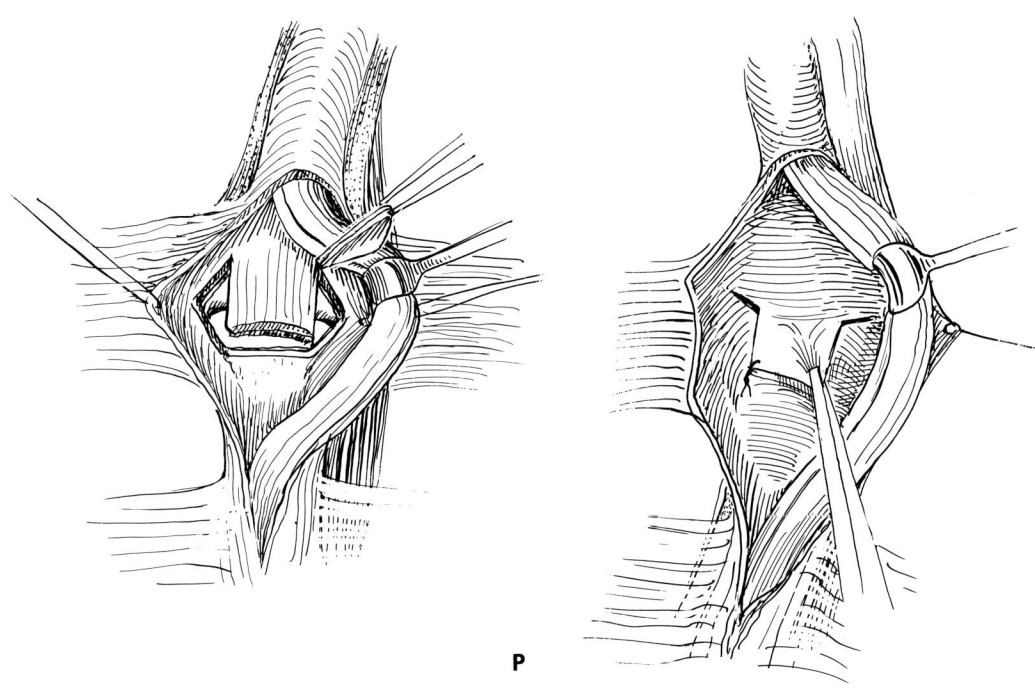

P

Tendons, Fascia and Muscles

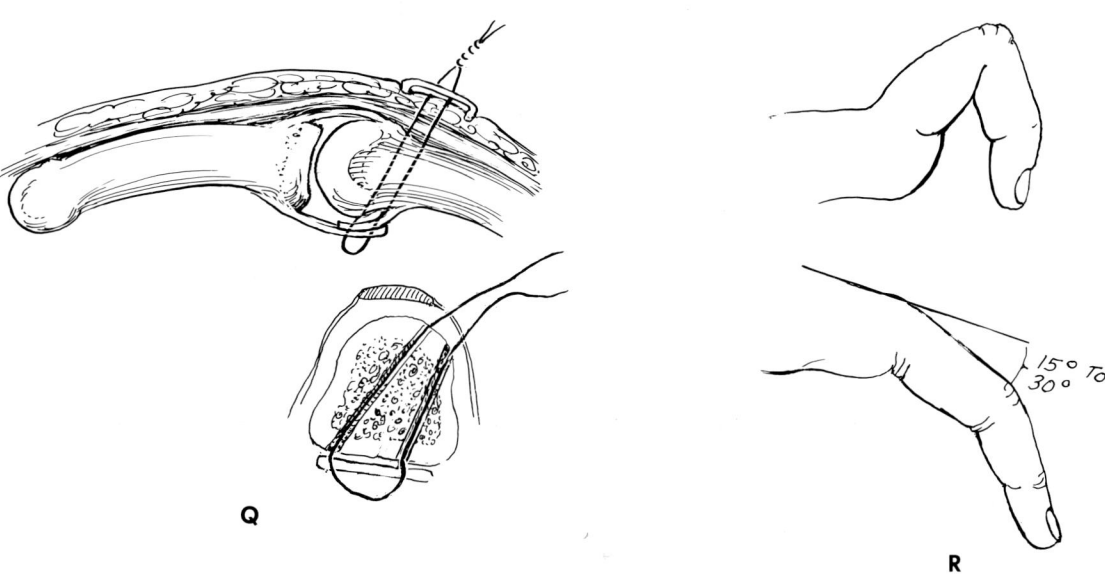

Q

R

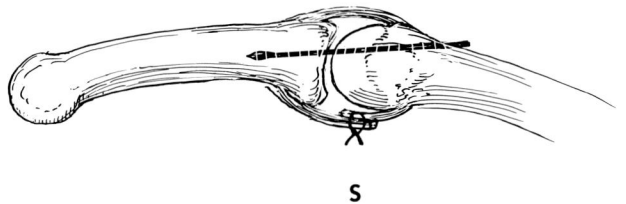

S

405

Example: Tenodesis

Prevention of hyperextension of the metacarpophalangeal joints may be achieved in combination with augmentation of interphalangeal joint function if a tenodesis rather than a capsulodesis is used.

The tenodesis crosses the metacarpophalangeal joint to insert into the lateral band of the extensor mechanism; thus, it acts to extend the interphalangeal joints as the metacarpophalangeal joint is extended; or, conversely, as the interphalangeal joints are actually flexed, the metacarpophalangeal joint is automatically flexed. If the tenodesis is carried above the wrist on the dorsal aspect, flexion of the wrist will cause flexion of the metacarpophalangeal joints and extension of the interphalangeal joints, depending on the tension in the primary flexors and extensors of those joints. Bits of tendon available locally, or a tendon graft from another site, may be used to perform a tenodesis for finger clawing. The palmaris longus tendon may be used as a free tendon graft for tenodesis of the ring and little finger. (**T**)

Tendons, Fascia and Muscles

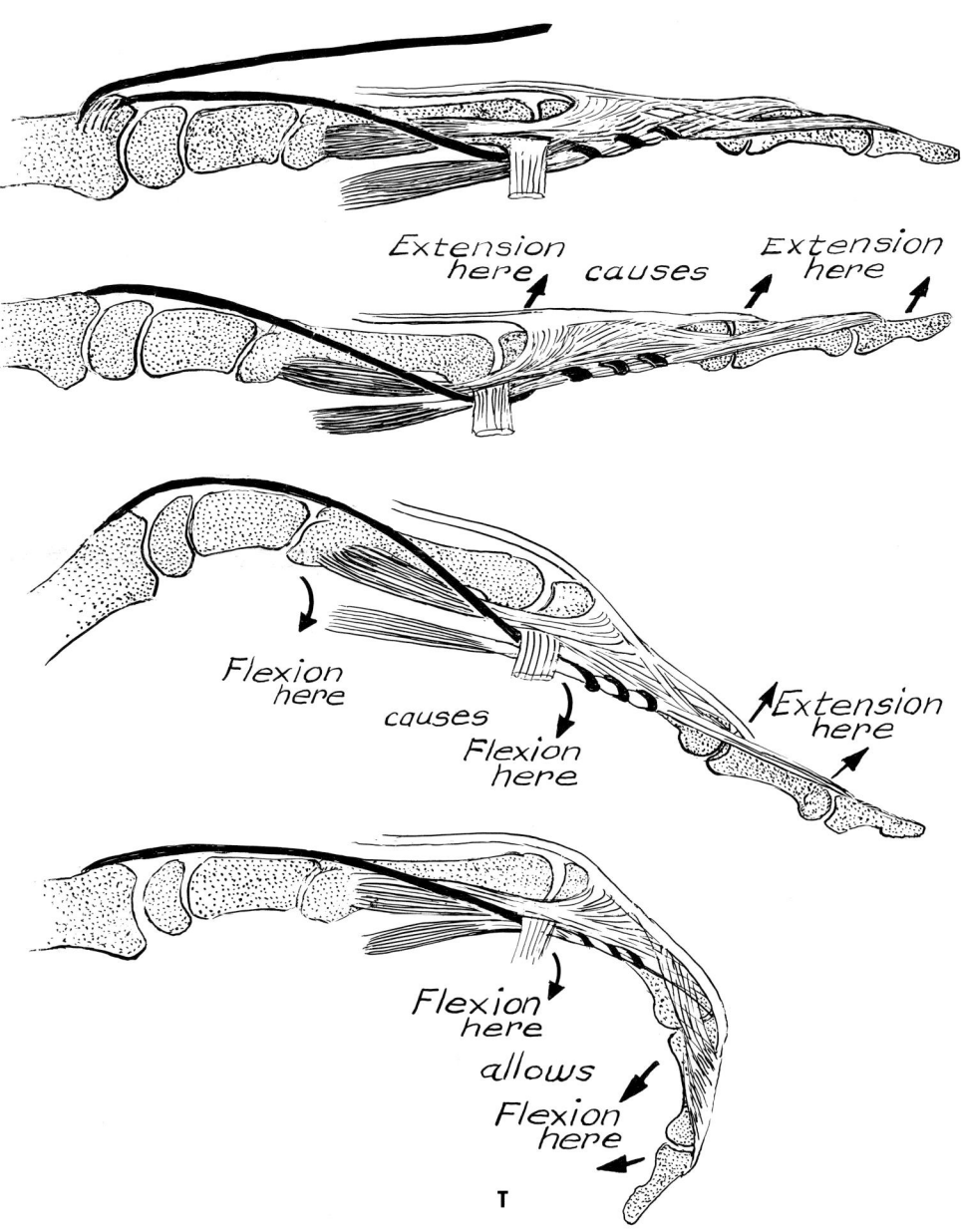

89 – Tendon Transfers for Ulnar Nerve Paralysis

A longitudinal incision on the radiodorsal aspect of the fingers readily exposes the lateral band and dorsal aponeurosis of the finger. A small transverse incision at the wrist will expose the distal edge of the extensor retinaculum. (**U**)

A blunt-nosed tendon passer laid on the lateral band in the finger with the metacarpophalangeal joint flexed can be passed proximally through the lumbrical canal palmar to the intermetacarpal ligament. (**V**) The instrument can then be directed dorsally and it will pass through the intermetacarpal space with little resistance. (**W**) It should be directed subcutaneously to emerge through the dorsal skin wound. One end of the tendon graft may then be grasped and pulled through the tunnel to the finger.

The other end of the graft may be passed through a hole made in the extensor retinaculum midway between the projection of the proximal ends of the little finger and ring finger metacarpals. The tendon passer is eased through the lumbrical canal of the other finger and passed through the intermetacarpal space to the dorsal incision. The end of the tendon is pulled through the canal to the finger. (**X**) The tendon graft ends are sutured to the radial lateral bands of the ring and little fingers. (**Y**)

Tension is adjusted by fixing the tendon graft with sutures, retaining the metacarpophalangeal joints in full flexion and the interphalangeal joints in extension with wrist flexed. Alternatively, the tension may be fixed, with the interphalangeal joints extended and the metacarpophalangeal joints of the ring and little fingers flexed 10 and 20 degrees, respectively, with the wrist in extension. (**Z**)

Passive flexion of the wrist should disallow hyperextension of the metacarpophalangeal joints at the end of the procedure. Reversed segments of the brachioradialis left attached above the wrist have been used in a manner similar to the technique described.

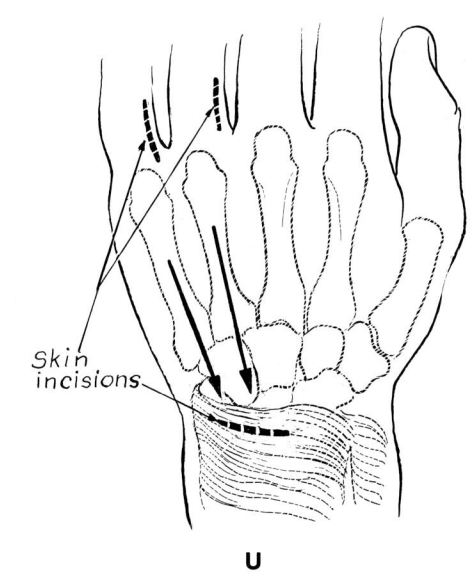

U

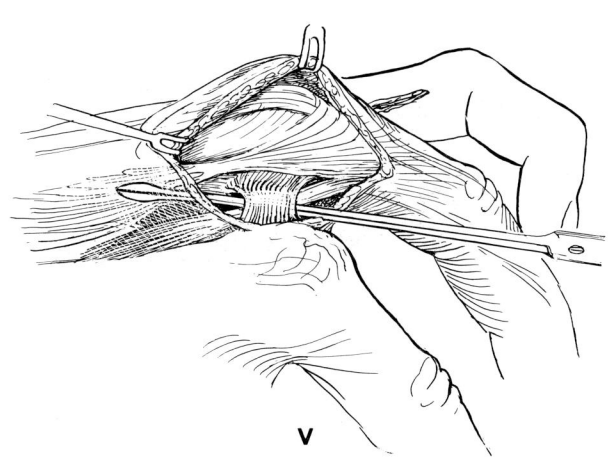

V

Tendons, Fascia and Muscles

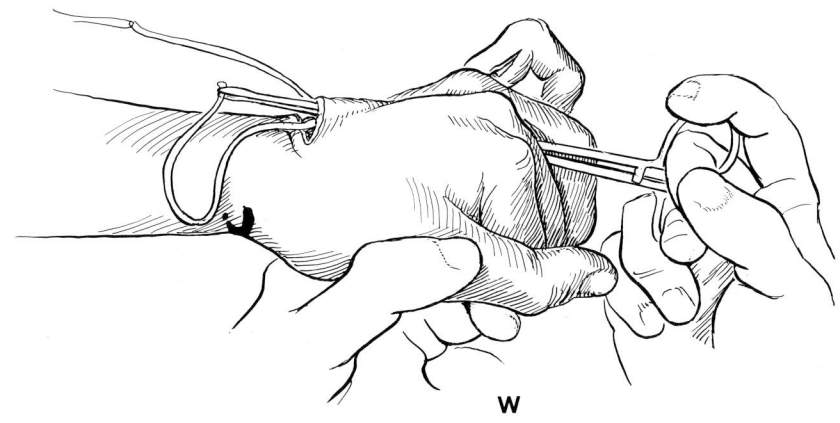
W

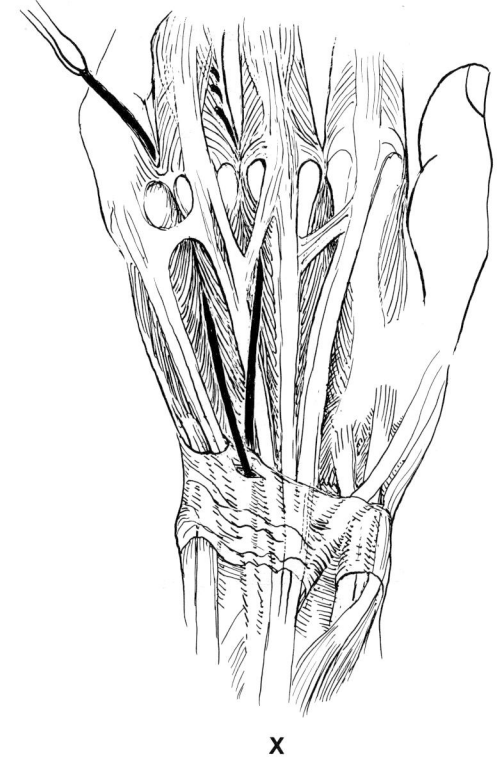
X

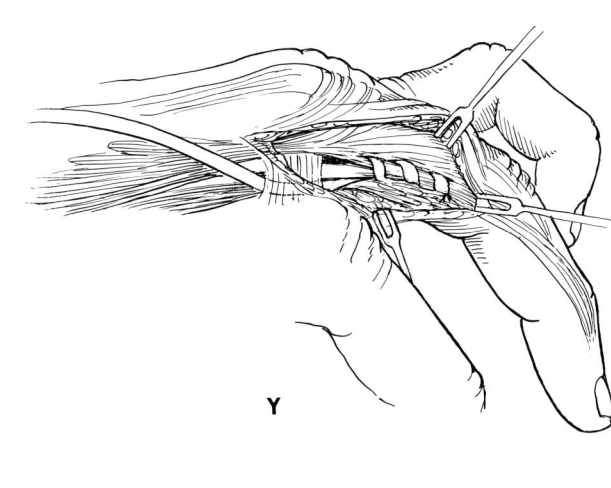
Y

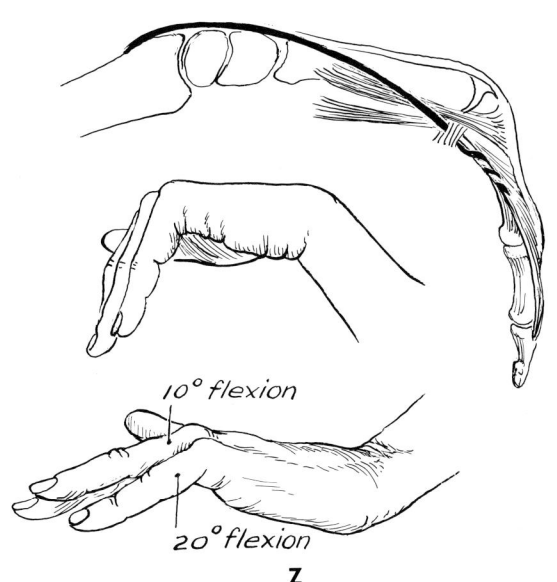
10° flexion
20° flexion
Z

MOTORIZED TENDON TRANSFERS

Fowler Procedure (Riordan Modification)

This operation utilizes the extensor indicis muscle tendon unit as the motor. The extensor indicis tendon is sectioned at the dorsal aponeurosis of the index finger and split into two parts. (**A**) These two tendons are passed through the intermetacarpal spaces to insert on the radial lateral bands of the ring and little fingers. The technique for passage of the tendon is precisely that described for the tenodesis.

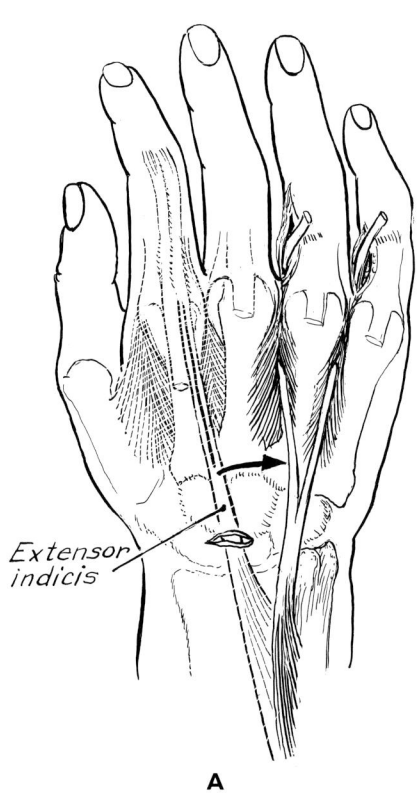

Tendons, Fascia and Muscles

Brand Procedures I and II

The motor unit for this operation is the extensor carpi radialis longus. (**A**) The tendon must be extended by a tendon graft which can be divided into two or four tails (depending on the number of fingers being corrected). The procedure consists of identification and release of the extensor carpi radialis longus from its insertion on the base of the index metacarpal. (**B**) This wrist extensor is reflected out proximal to the oblique muscles to the thumb through a small separate incision. (**C**)

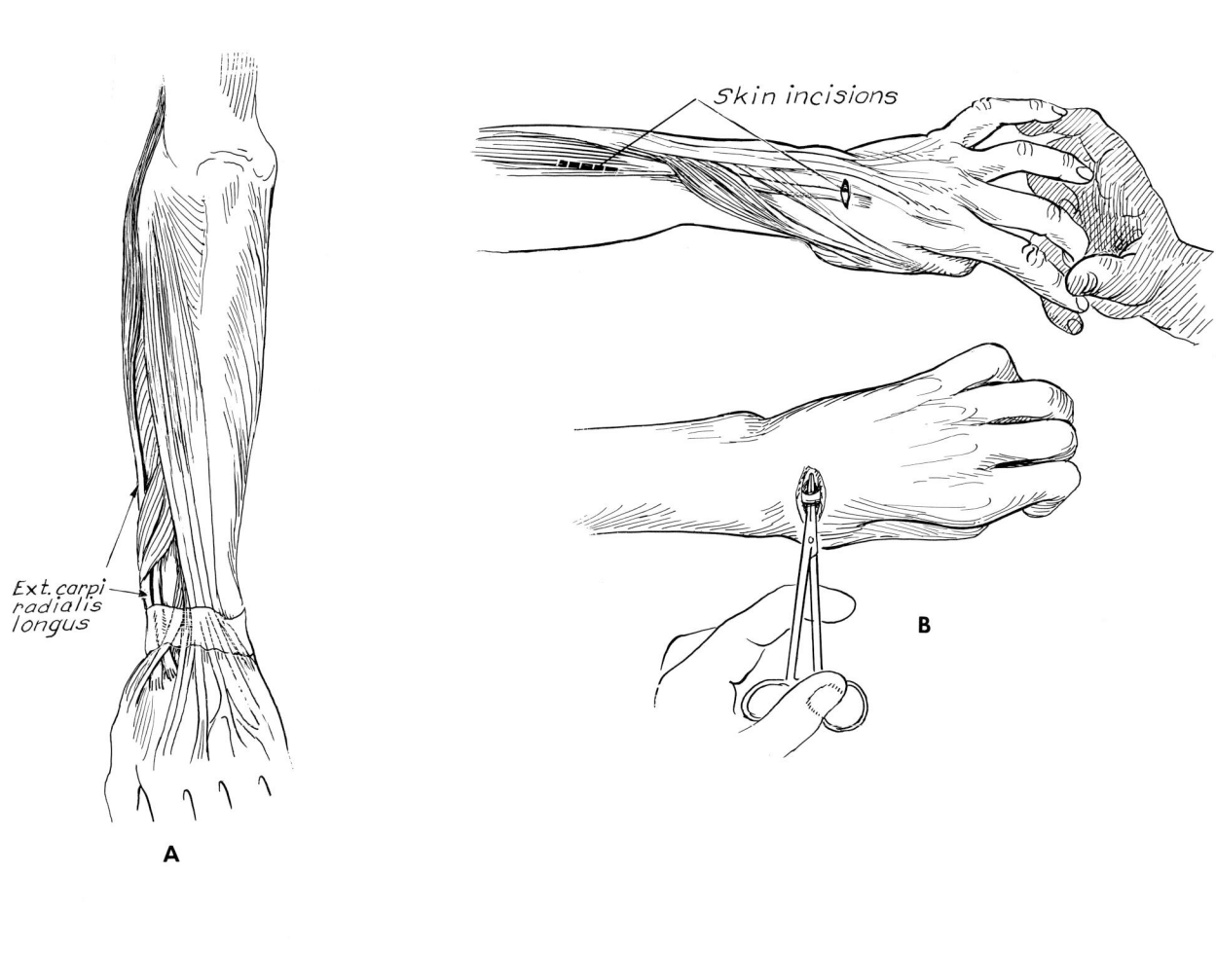

89 – Tendon Transfers for Ulnar Nerve Paralysis

A tendon graft, consisting of the plantaris tendon folded upon itself or even fascia lata if the plantaris is unavailable, is attached to the cut end of the extensor carpi radialis longus. The technique recommended by Brand is preferred. The extensor carpi radialis is laid open longitudinally, forming a flat sheet of tendon by splitting it along one side and working it flat. (**D**)

A small opening is made in the flattened tendon, and the point at which the plantaris is folded upon itself at its midpoint is pulled through the hole. (**E**)

It is sutured in place with several nonabsorbable sutures and the extensor carpi radialis tendon is rolled back to its original shape and closed over the inserted graft using a fine running suture of monofilament steel or plastic. (**F**)

One limb of the plantaris is picked up by fine hemostats at the edges of the flat tendon just beyond its site of emergence from the wrist extensor. (**G**) Gentle, repeated traction on the hemostats will pull the flat tendon into a sheet, which is then used to wrap the free cut end of the extensor carpi radialis. It is sutured closed over the tendon end, using the same running sutures as that used to close the wrist extensor tendon itself. (**H**)

The two tails of the plantaris are split to create one tendon for each of the four fingers.

Brand I

The tendon graft ends are then passed to the radial lateral bands of the long, ring, and little fingers and the ulnar lateral band of the index. (**I**) The technique for this is exactly that described above for the tenodesis. Tension is adjusted with the wrist extended and the metacarpophalangeal joints flexed with increasing tension from the index to the little finger, and all interphalangeal joints are extended. (**J**)

Flat dorsal and palmar plaster slabs are applied over the dressings to hold the hand in this position. (**K**)

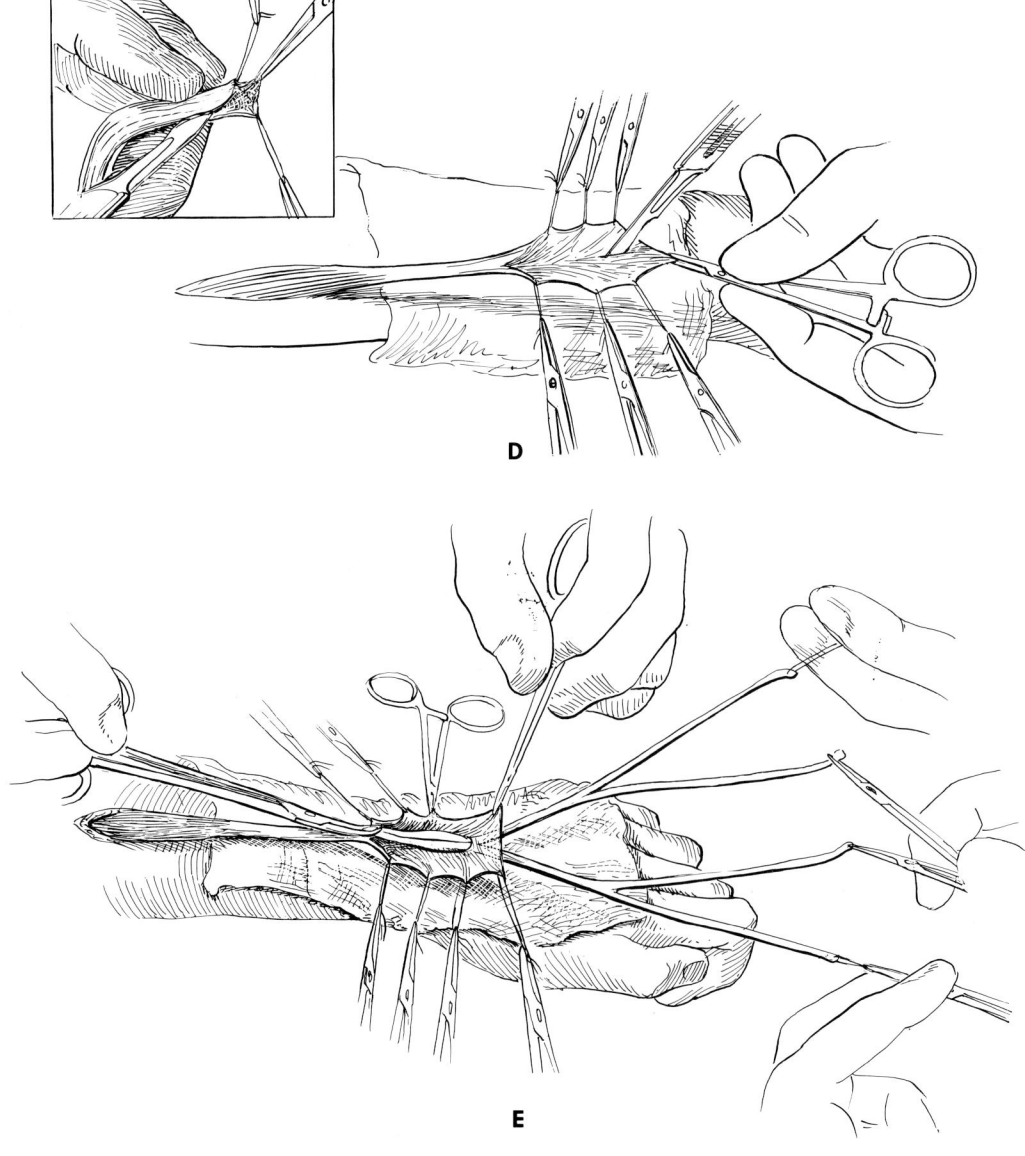

Tendons, Fascia and Muscles

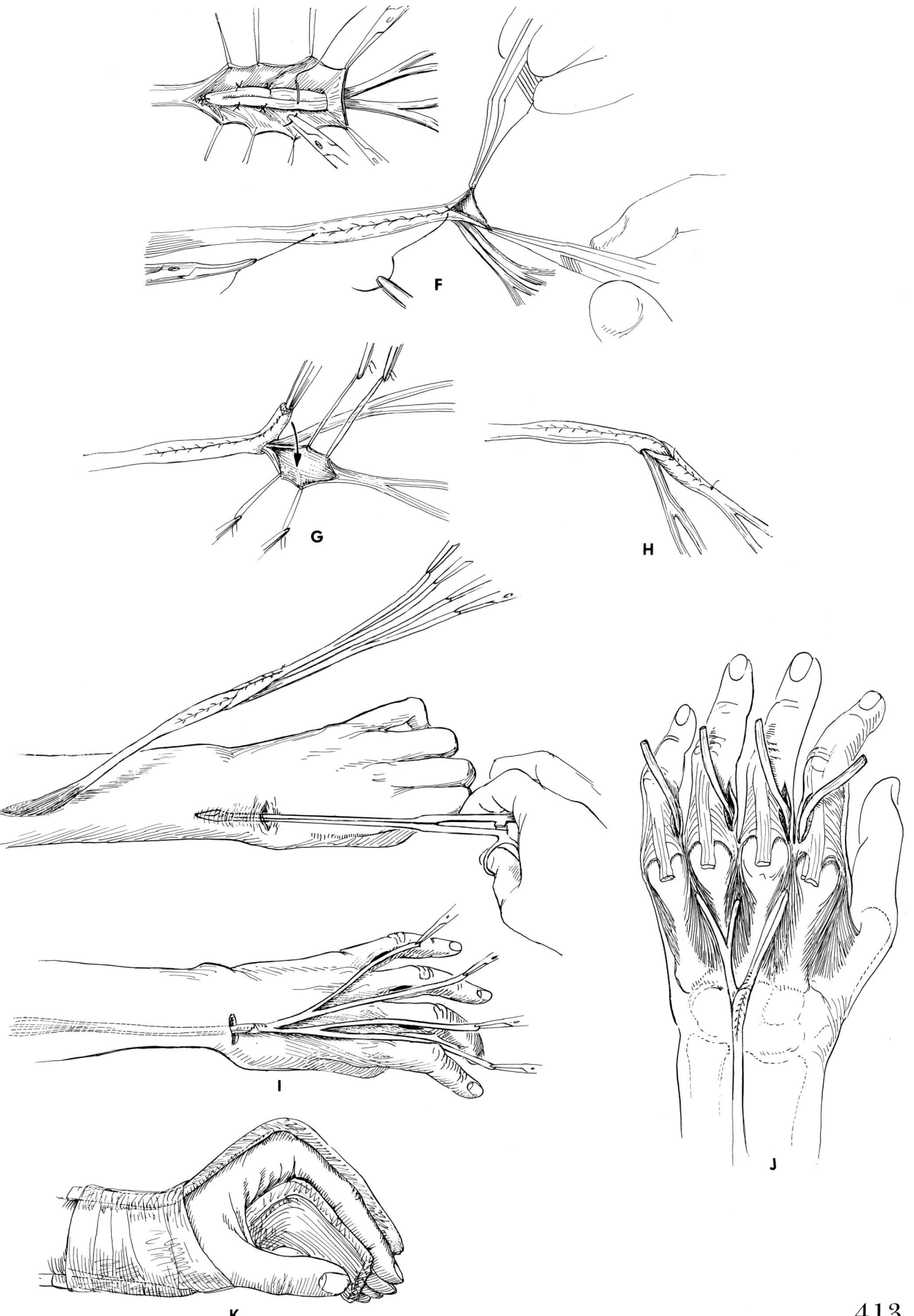

413

89 – Tendon Transfers for Ulnar Nerve Paralysis

Brand II

The alternate route for passage of the four tendon tails is generally preferable. It routes the tendon transfer beneath the brachioradialis to the palmar aspect of the forearm and through the carpal tunnel to the lumbrical canals. A mid-palmar incision is made, and the blunt nosed tendon tunneller is passed retrograde to the depths of the palm between the long flexors of the long and ring fingers. It passes without resistance through the carpal tunnel. (**L**)

By gentle positioning of the wrist, the tunneller can be directed radiodorsally to a nonresistant plane beneath the brachioradialis and to the dorsal forearm wound. The tendon graft ends are grasped and pulled through to the palm. (**M**)

The longitudinal incisions in the radiodorsal aspect of the skin over the proximal phalanges of the long, ring, and little fingers and the ulnar dorsal aspect of the index finger exposes the lateral bands of each finger. (**N**) The tendon tunneller is passed along the lateral band of each finger, through the lumbrical canal and out the palmar incision. Thus, each tendon graft is pulled through a tunnel of its own for suture insertion into the lateral band. (**O**)

Tension is adjusted to hold the fingers in flexion at the metacarpophalangeal joint, with the interphalangeal joints in extension with the wrist in neutral position. (**P**)

It is important that the tension be tighter for each finger, progressing from index to little.

The hand is held in a plaster splint with the wrist in neutral position, the metacarpophalangeal joints flexed progressively more sharply from index to little, and the interphalangeal joints in extension. This position is maintained for three to four weeks, after which progressive active motion is at first allowed, then encouraged. A good program of reeducation by an understanding, knowledgeable physical therapist is very important. (**Q**)

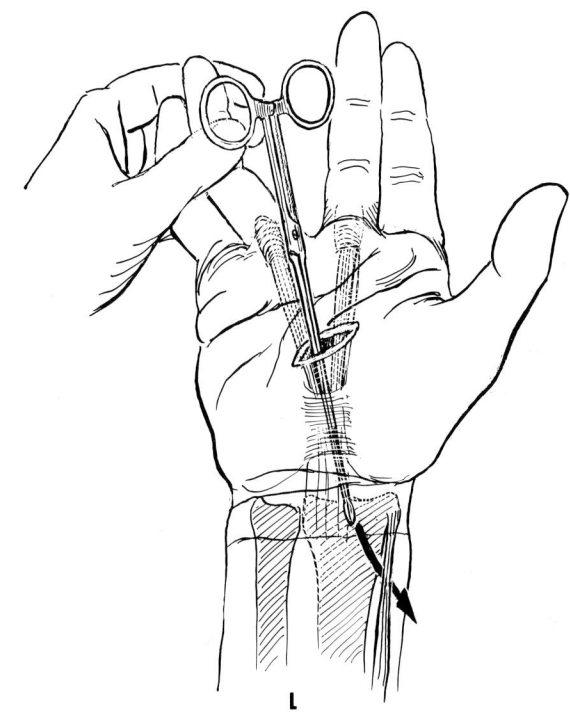

L

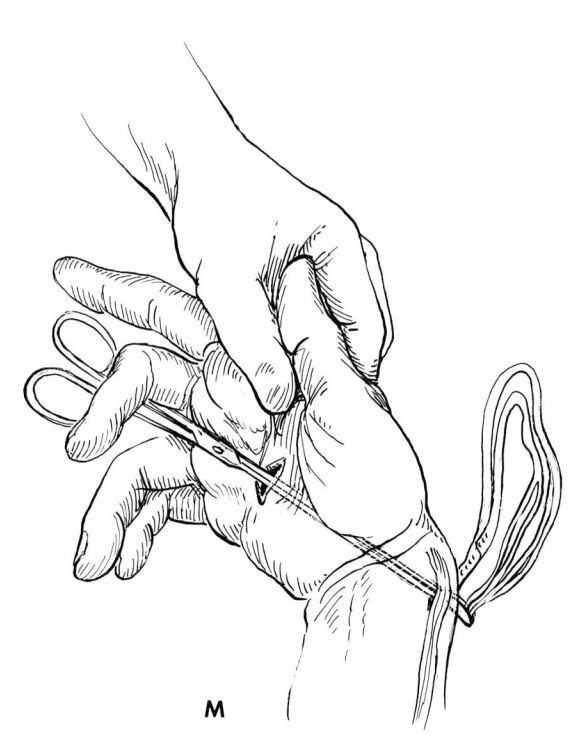

M

Tendons, Fascia and Muscles

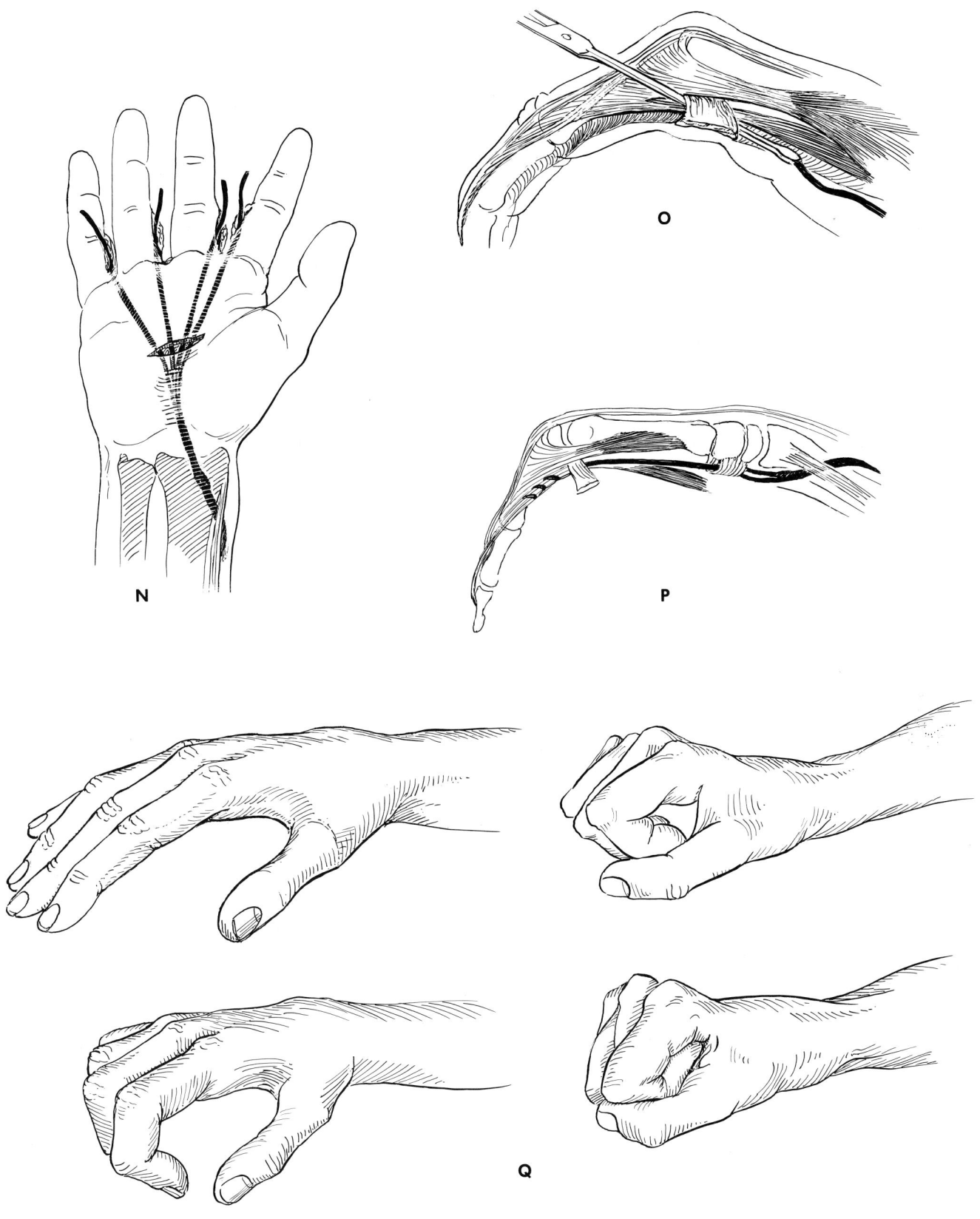

415

89 – Tendon Transfers for Ulnar Nerve Paralysis

The Stiles Bunnell Procedure

This operation makes use of superficialis motor power taken from fingers where the profundus is unparalyzed. High ulnar palsy results in profundus palsy in the ring and little fingers, and should a superficialis flexor be robbed from such a finger, it would lose all extrinsic flexor power. If one chooses to use one of these superficialis tendons, surgical adhesion of the profundus of the donor finger to the index and long finger profundus must be done.

There is a variety of combinations, including (1) use of the long finger superficialis (**R**) split into two (**S**) or four (**T**) tails; (2) use of each superficialis sutured to its own digit's lateral band (**U**); or (3) use of the central two superficialis tendons to all four fingers by splitting each tendon into two.

The passage and insertion into the lateral bands is done exactly as described for the Brand II procedure. Not uncommonly, the great power of the superficialis, coupled with removal of the prime flexor of the proximal interphalangeal joints, may result in recurvatum of the proximal interphalangeal joints. Intrinsic plus deformity has developed in many patients after this procedure. This procedure, therefore, is reserved for patients who have stiffness of the proximal interphalangeal joints.

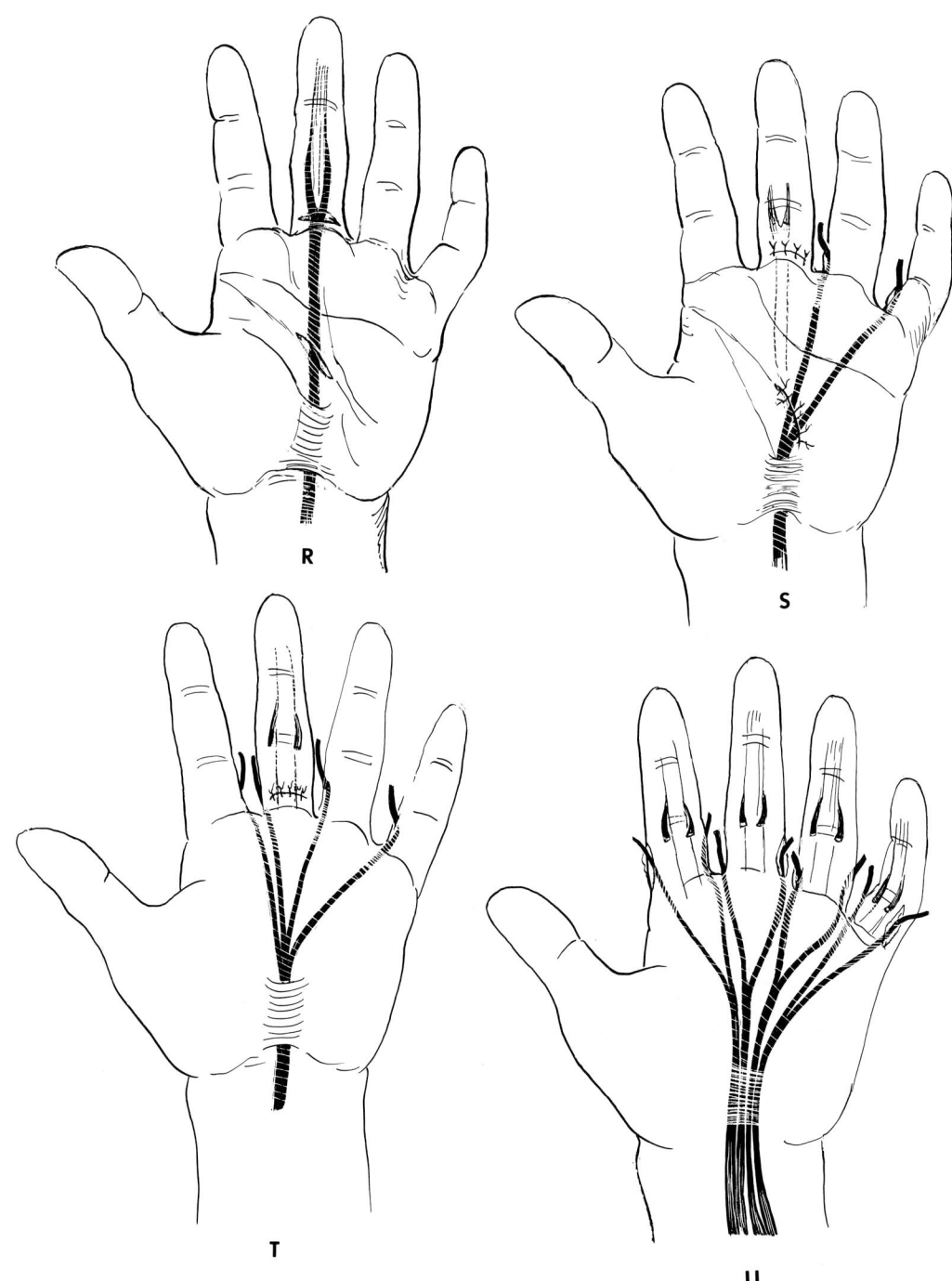

THUMB ADDUCTOR PARALYSIS CORRECTION

Although the greatest improvement in appearance of the hand is achieved by correcting the claw deformity of the fingers, successful substitution for paralysis of the thumb adductor is most appreciated by the patient where function is concerned.

In Low Ulnar Palsy

All the extrinsic muscles are intact and, if function in all of them is normal, one has a wide choice of donor muscles for transfer to substitute for the paralyzed thumb adductor. The ring finger superficialis is most frequently chosen because of its superficial position, independent functional ability, tendon size, and position in the hand. The long finger superficialis serves well if the ring finger superficialis has been injured with the ulnar nerve.

The long finger superficialis is exposed through a small transverse incision just distal to the palmar metacarpophalangeal joint crease. The two flat extensions of the superficialis may be seen through the thin synovial window just distal to the thickened proximal pulley. Through a small palmar incision the tendon can be indentified and picked up, using a smooth, dull probe.

A small incision on the ulnar side of the thumb close to the metacarpophalangeal joint will expose the normal insertion of the adductor pollicis muscle.

A blunt-nosed tendon passer is inserted over the adductor insertion and gently advanced across the palm toward the proximal end of the ulnar side of the palm. The instrument is directed upward to emerge behind the flexor tendons into the palm wound over the ring finger superficialis. The tendon tails are cut in the finger and the tendon is reflected into the palm. (**A**)

The cut ends of the superficialis tails are grasped by the tendon passer and the tendon is pulled through the tunnel to the insertion of the adductor pollicis. (**B**)

The tendon is inserted into the aponeurotic position of the adductor and sutured after adjustment of tension to allow full passive abduction, with the wrist in acute flexion and assumption of thumb adduction by passive extension of the wrist. (**C**)

This transfer is very much appreciated by the patient since it restores stable pinch.

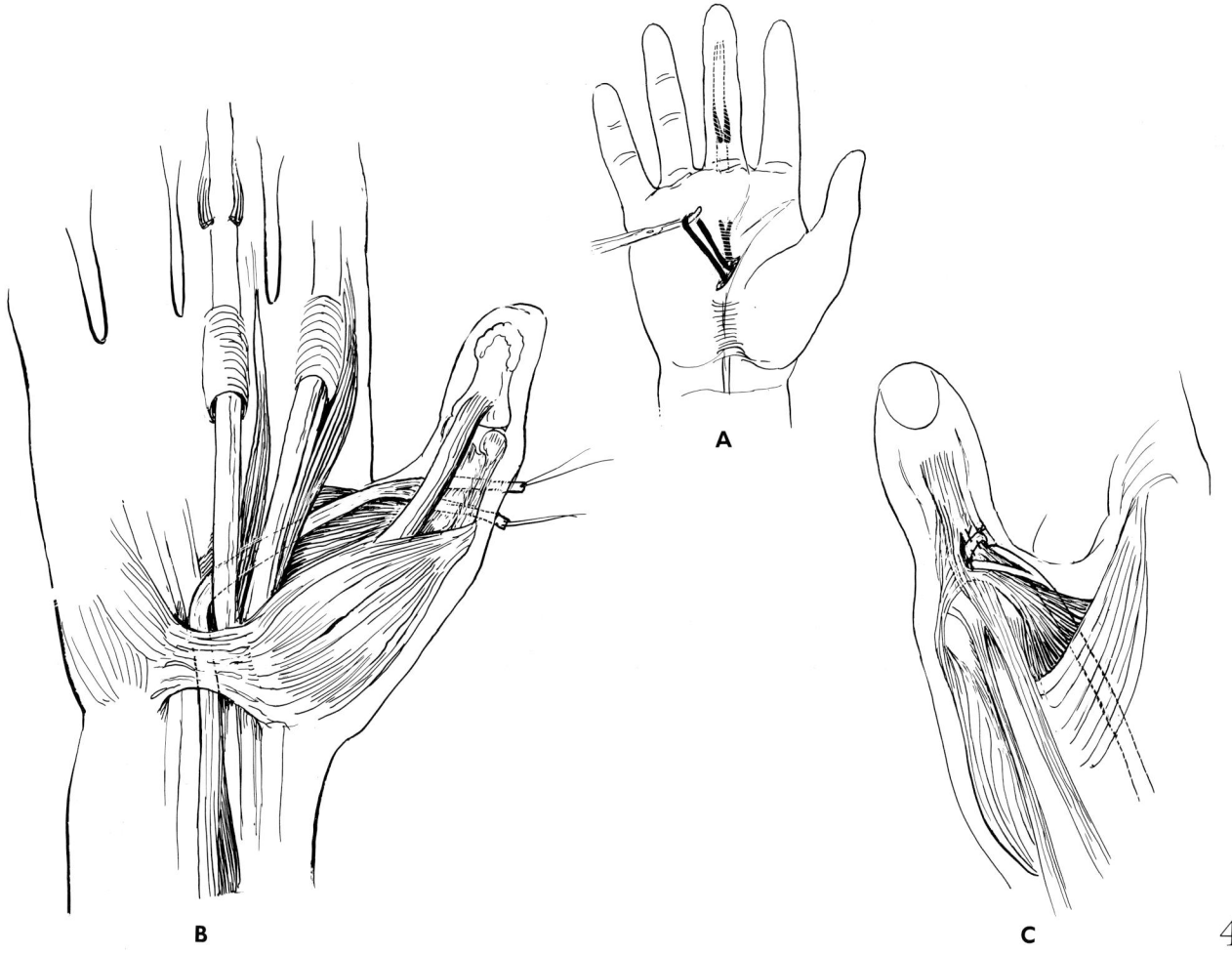

90
Tendon Transfers for Median Nerve Paralysis

When median nerve motor function is irreversibly lost, substitution by redistribution of muscle power is designed on the basis of available unparalyzed muscles. Median nerve paralysis from injury at the wrist, therefore, is treated differently than median paralysis from injury at the elbow or above.

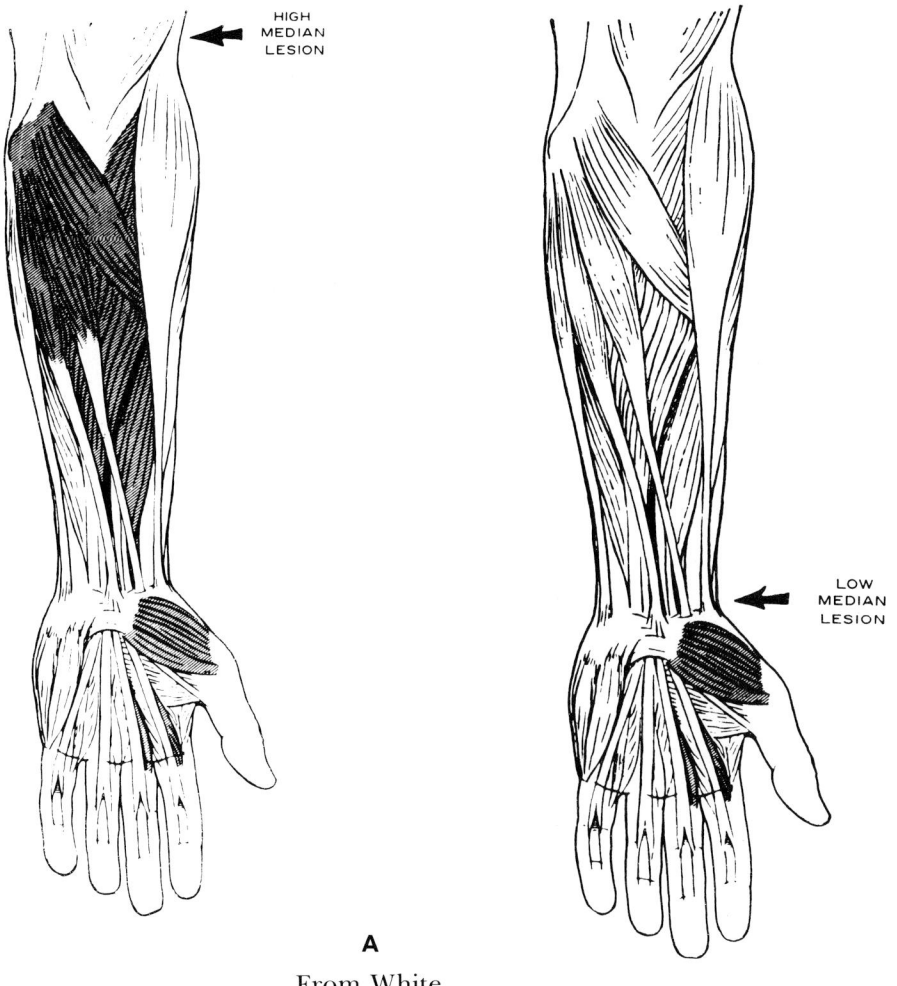

A

From White

LOW MEDIAN NERVE PARALYSIS

Median nerve interruption at the wrist level leaves the patient unable effectively to position his thumb for pulp-to-pulp opposition with the fingers. The specific muscles usually paralyzed are the two and one-half thenar muscles radial to the flexor pollicis longus. These are the abductor pollicis brevis, the opponens pollicis, and the superficial head of the flexor pollicis brevis. The lumbricals to the index and long fingers also are paralyzed but no substitution for their loss is necessary. (**A**)

Such a distal injury leaves all the median innervated extrinsic flexors intact and available for tendon transfer to substitute for the thumb positioning opponens muscles.

The most commonly used substitution is the transfer of a superficialis tendon routed subcutaneously over the thenar eminence and inserted into the thumb by any of a number of techniques.

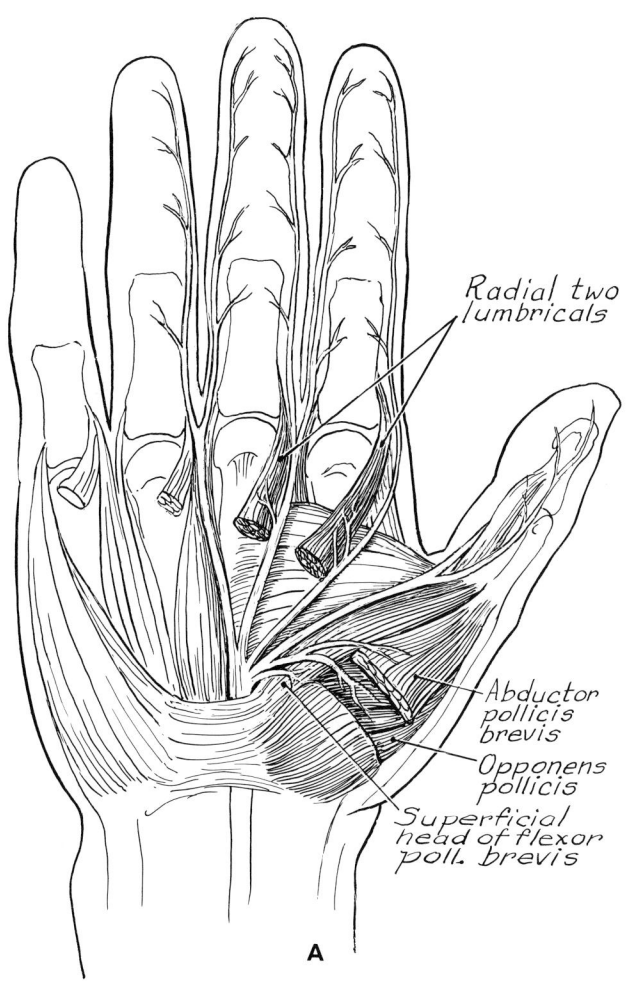

90 — Tendon Transfers for Median Nerve Paralysis

Example

A 60-year-old man with median nerve paralysis from an injury sustained three years prior to the consultation had recovered protective sensibility in his thumb and fingers but had persistent total paralysis of his thenar positioning muscles. All profundus and superficialis finger flexors were functionally intact. An opponens transfer using the ring finger superficialis was chosen as appropriate. The procedure was initiated by identifying the insertion of the abductor pollicis brevis, through a small curved incision over the radial side of the thumb at the level of the metacarpophalangeal joint of the thumb. A second small incision was made above the wrist on the ulnar side of the forearm just radial to the flexor carpi ulnaris. Through this incision the distal tendinous flexor carpi ulnaris was split for a distance of 4 centimeters proximal to its insertion. The radial one half of the tendon was sectioned proximally and left attached at its insertion. (**B**) The far proximal end of the tendon was sutured to the insertion site to create a pulley loop for passage of the superficialis to be transferred. Through the wrist incision, the superficialis to the ring finger was identified in preparation for its withdrawal. A small transverse incision was made over the proximal phalanx of the ring finger. (**C**)

The fibrous flexor sheath was perforated in the thin portion proximal to the middle pulley and the two tails of the superficialis were seen. (**D**) One tail was reflected out of the wound with the finger and wrist flexed. It was cut across after a clamp was applied proximal to the site chosen for section. (**E**) The tendon was pulled distally by the clamp with the wrist flexed. This brought the other tail of the superficialis into view and its was sectioned. (**F**)

The tendon was then withdrawn at the wrist (**G**) and passed through the pulley constructed of flexor carpi ulnaris.

The tendon was then passed subcutaneously over the thenar eminence to the exposed insertion of the abductor pollicis brevis. This subcutaneous passage was precisely defined to place the tendon line palmar to the axis of the metacarpophalangeal joint.

The natural split in the superficialis tendon was deepened and the tendon was passed around and through the tendinous insertion of the abductor pollicis brevis and sutured to itself and the insertion under moderate tension with the thumb palmar abducted and the wrist in comfortable flexion. (**H**)

The wrist and the thumb were immobilized in this position for three weeks, after which splinting was removed and graded active exercise was started. Attempts to pinch the thumb pulp against the ring finger in flexion exercised the transferred superficialis and demonstrated to the patient his new ability to position the thumb for opposition.

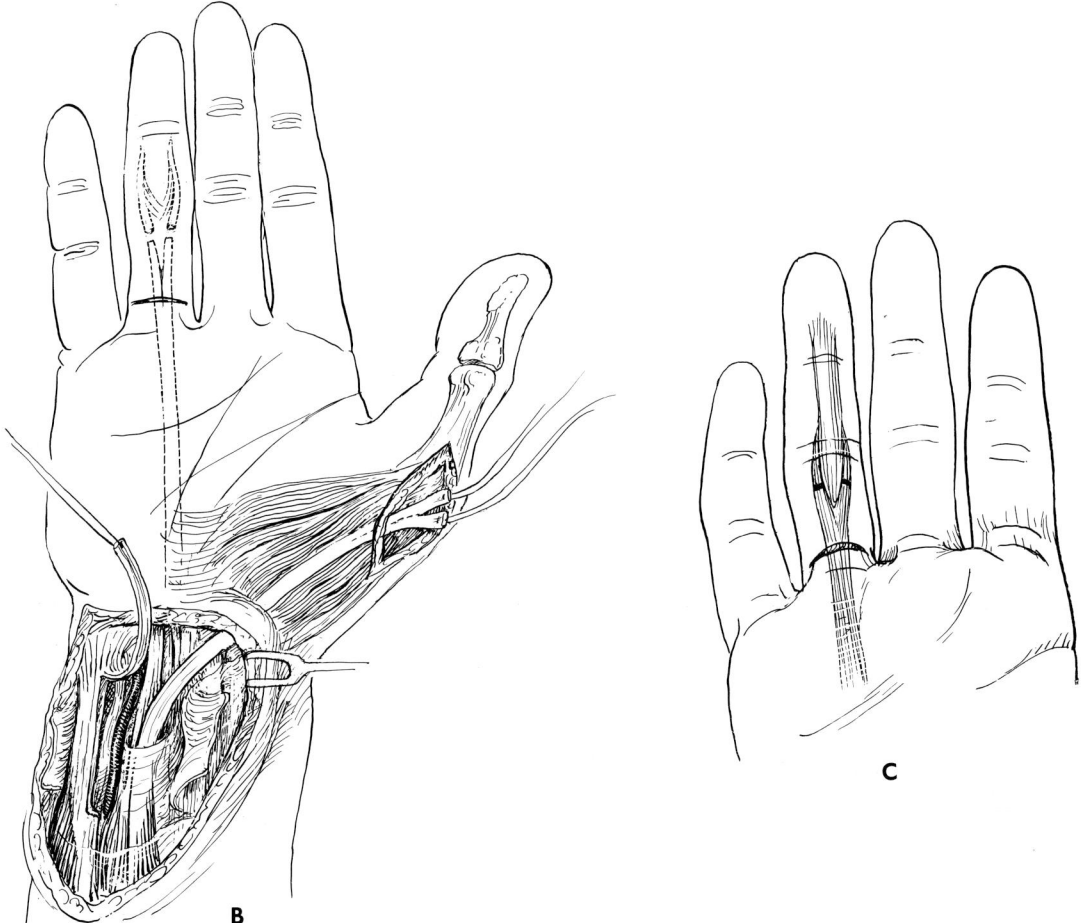

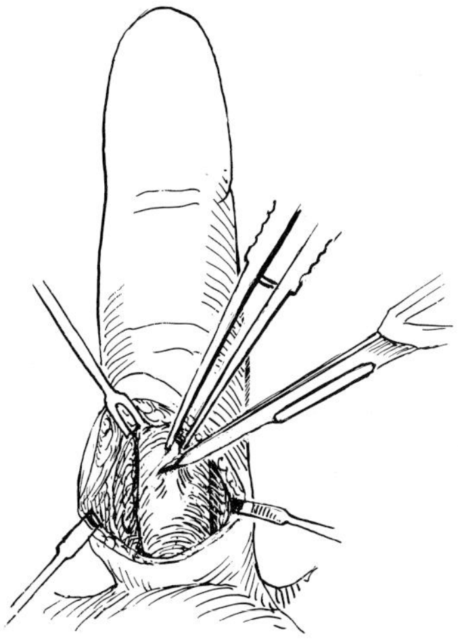

Tendons, Fascia and Muscles

D

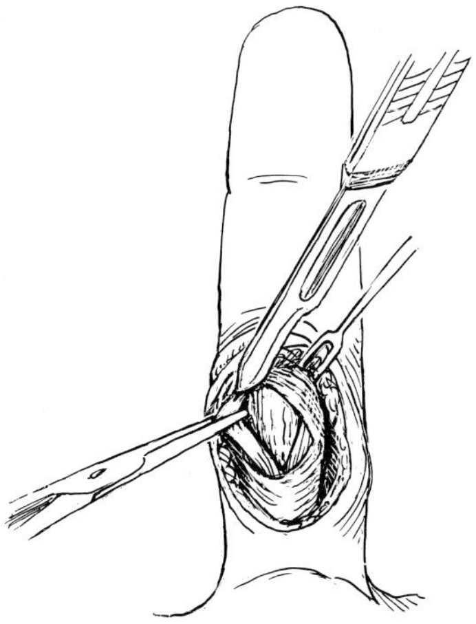

E

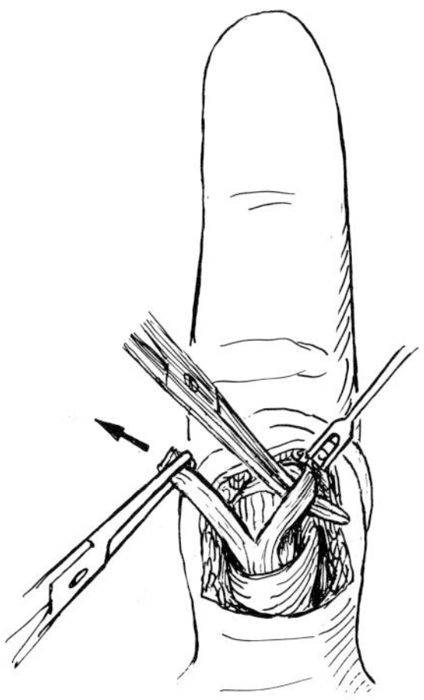

F

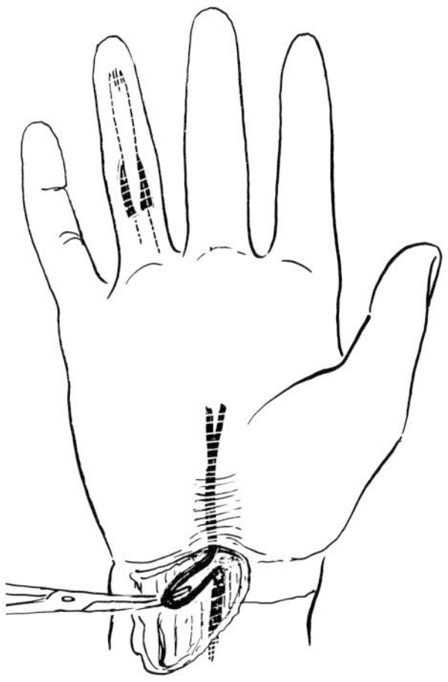

G

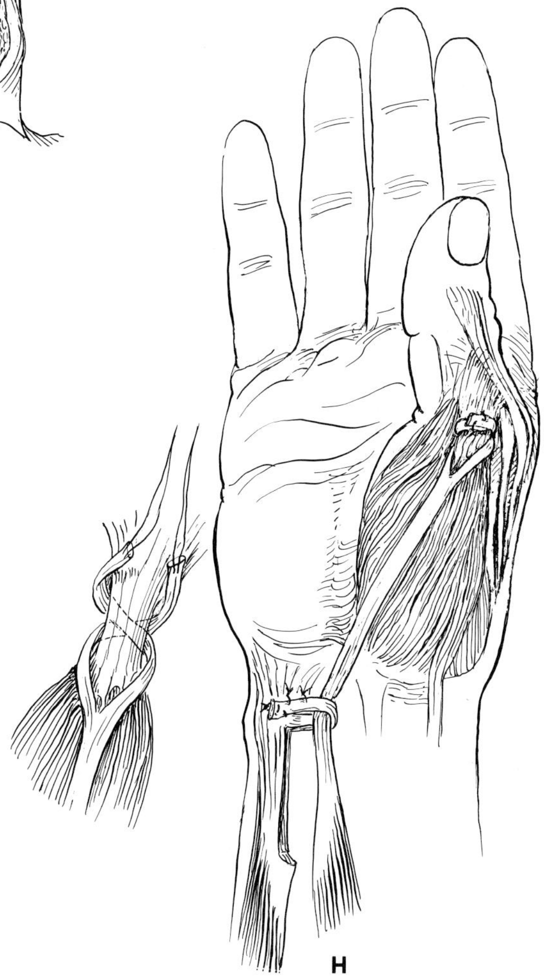

H

PREOPERATIVE

POSTOPERATIVE

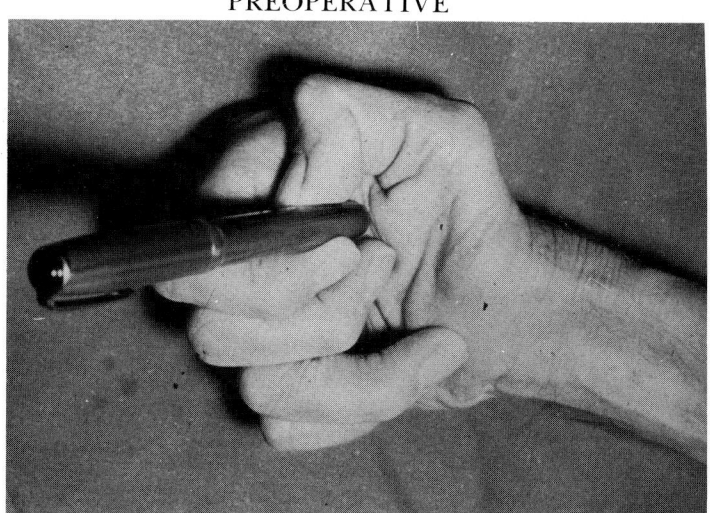
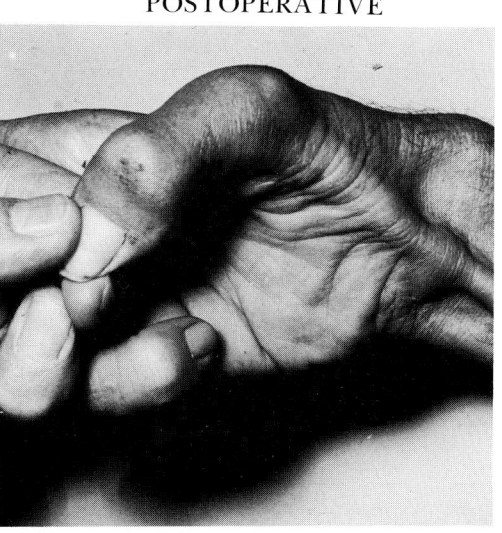

421

90 — Tendon Transfers for Median Nerve Paralysis

HIGH MEDIAN NERVE PARALYSIS

Interruption of the median nerve above the elbow results in paralysis of the palmar forearm structures as well as the thenar thumb positioning group. The pronator teres and digital flexors, except for the flexor carpi ulnaris and the profundus muscles to the long, ring and little fingers, are all paralyzed. Opponens substitution remains important in the rehabilitation of such a hand but the possible muscle tendon available for transfer is not limited. One may use the unparalyzed flexor carpi ulnaris, a wrist extensor, the brachioradialis, or the abductor digiti minimi.

Flexor Carpi Ulnaris Transfer

The flexor carpi ulnaris may be used as the motor but, since it will not reach the thumb, the extensor pollicis brevis may be sectioned proximally close to its muscle belly; then it may be rerouted across the thenar eminence to suture to the flexor carpi ulnaris. The extensor pollicis brevis must be split off the extensor mechanism to a point distal to the metacarpophalangeal joint so it will pass below the joint axis to the thenar areas over the abductor pollicis brevis. (**A**, **B**, and **C**)

Extensor Carpi Radialis Longus Transfer to Opponens

Another alternative is to use a wrist extensor or the brachioradialis rerouted all the way across the dorsum of the hand around the ulnar side of the forearm to the thenar area. This requires the interposition of a tendon graft. (**D**, **E**, and **F**)

If high median nerve palsy remains uncorrected, substitution of motor power is necessary to reactivate the flexor pollicis longus and flexor digitorum profundus to the index finger. The ulnar profundi are intact and functional since they are innervated by the ulnar nerve. The profundus to the index finger may be sutured side to side to the other profundi to provide interphalangeal joint flexion to the index finger. (**G**)

The flexor pollicis longus may be remotored by direct transfer of the brachioradialis to it. (**H**)

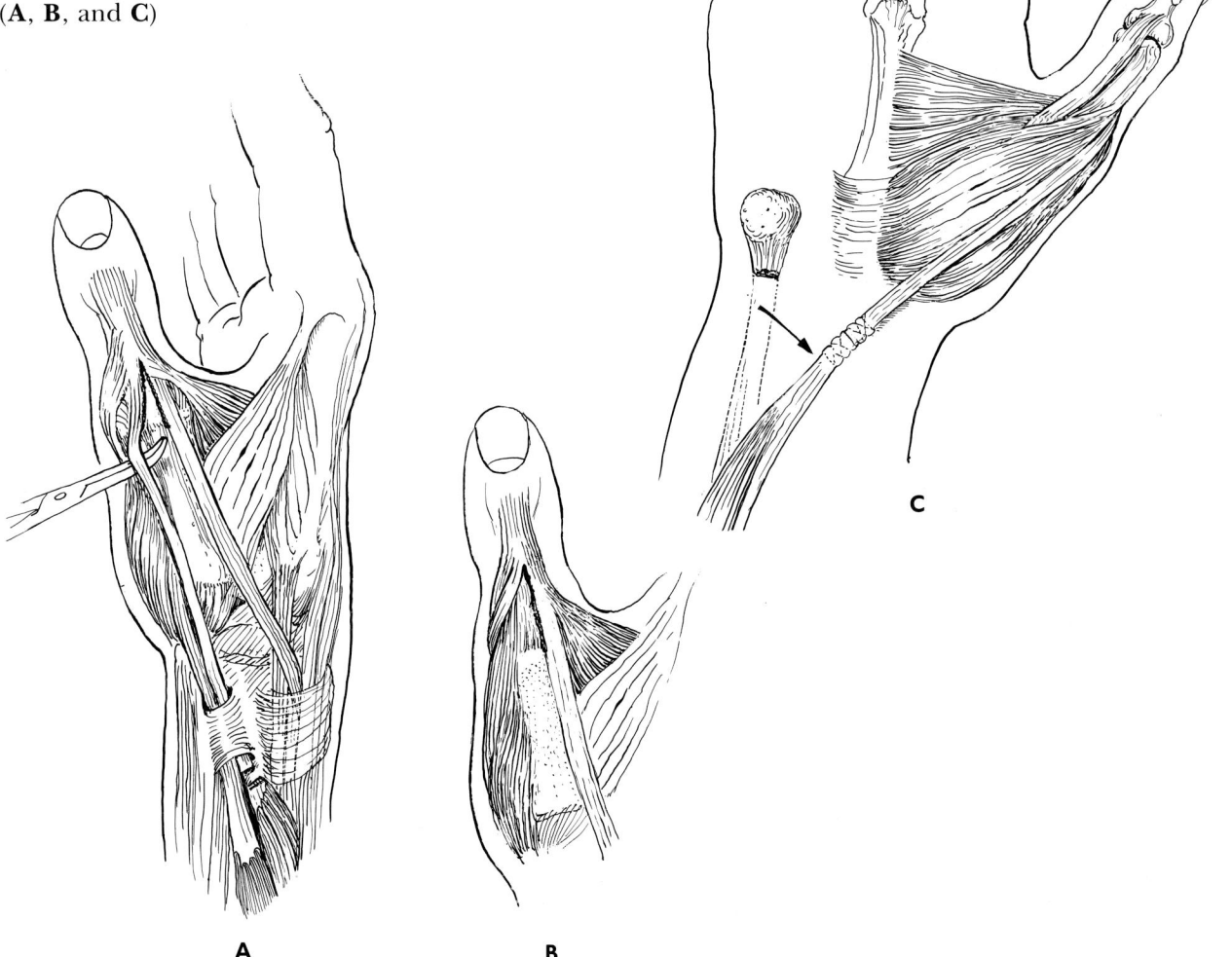

Tendons, Fascia and Muscles

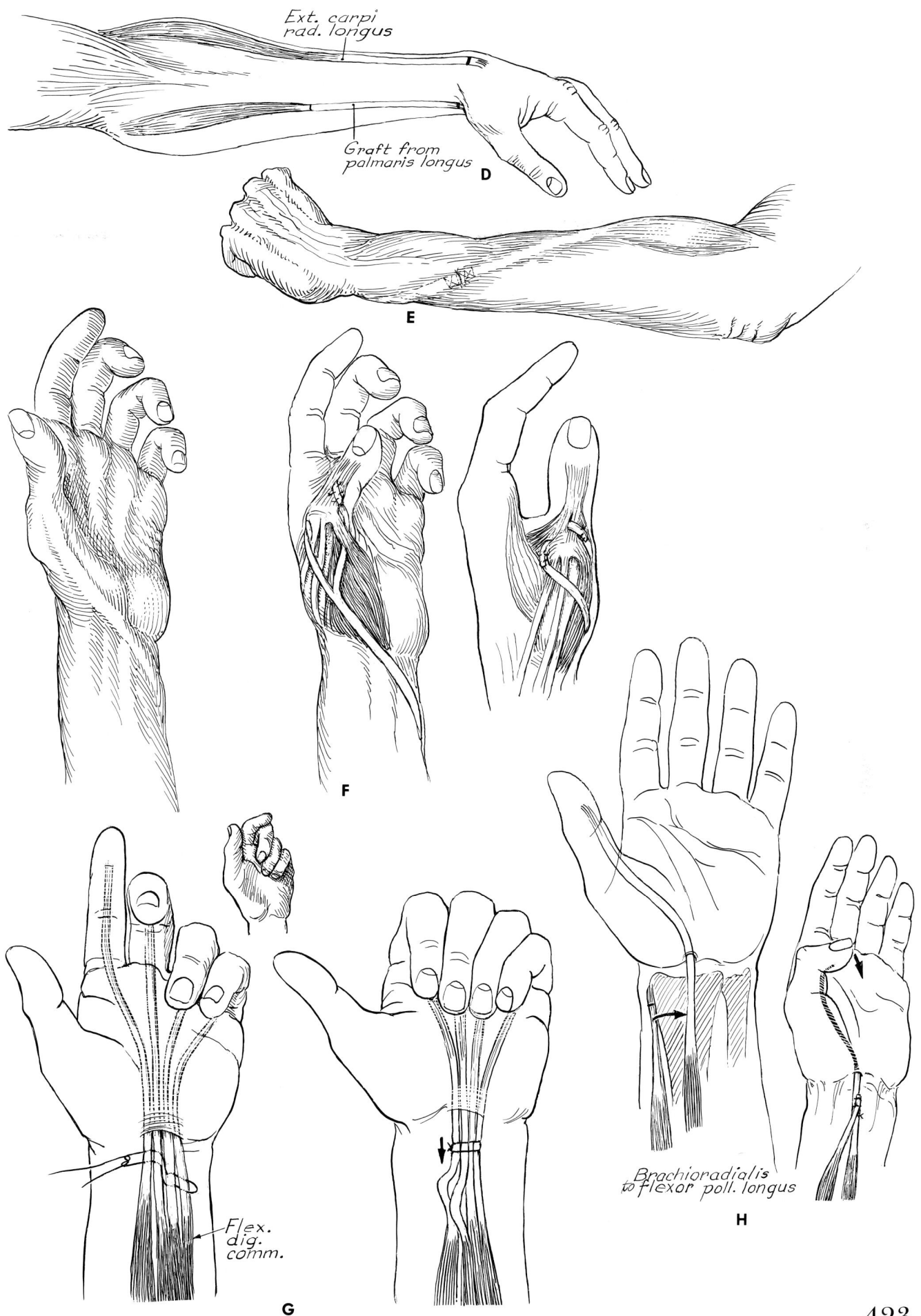

INTRINSIC TRANSFER FOR OPPONENS PARALYSIS

Opponens transfer using the abductor digiti minimi is excellent for the patient suffering from high level median nerve paralysis. In high median palsy, the patient has lost not only his thumb positioning intrinsic muscles for opposition but also the pronators and long flexors, except for the flexor carpi ulnaris and ulnar two or three profundi. (**A**)

Since superficialis flexors are weak or paralyzed the available muscles for opponens transfer are limited. Some of the alternate extrinsic muscles for opponens transfer have been described. The surgeon may choose to use the ulnar innervated intrinsic muscle, the abductor digiti minimi, to transfer to the paralyzed abductor pollicis brevis.

A combination of three procedures — (1) flexor profundus side-to-side juncture; (2) brachioradialis transfer to the flexor pollicis longus; and (3) abductor digiti minimi to the abductor pollicis brevis — is an appropriate approach to high median nerve paralysis. (**B**)

Example

A 30-year-old male patient sustained a severe laceration below the elbow which severed his median nerve. The nerve was repaired and, after 10 months, he was starting to regain sensibility and some function in the median innervated extrinsic muscles. The thenar muscles were paralyzed and atrophic. Transfer of the abductor digiti minimi to the abductor pollicis brevis was elected.

Transfer of the abductor digiti minimi was carried out using a mid-lateral ulnar incision at the metacarpal level. The abductor digiti minimi was exposed and sectioned far enough distal on the lateral band of the little finger to preserve its tendinous insertion. It was easily dissected from the other hypothenar muscles. The nerve and blood supply at its base were carefully preserved. Dissection at the proximal end was carried far enough to allow the surgeon to reflect the muscle to the thenar area without undue tension. This required release of the muscle from the underlying hamate bone.

A small incision was made over the radial side of the thumb at the level of the metacarpal phalangeal joint to expose the tendinous insertion of the abductor pollicis brevis. A subcutaneous tunnel was dissected across the proximal palm between the two incisions and widened sufficiently to allow easy passage of the muscle across the thenar area. (**C**) The tendinous part of the abductor digiti minimi was sutured to the abductor pollicis brevis insertion with the thumb in oppositional position. (**D**)

After wound closure, the thumb was splinted in opposition (palmar abduction). The wounds healed without event and all immobilization was removed in three weeks. The patient quickly learned to use the transferred muscle to achieve thumb positioning for opposition.

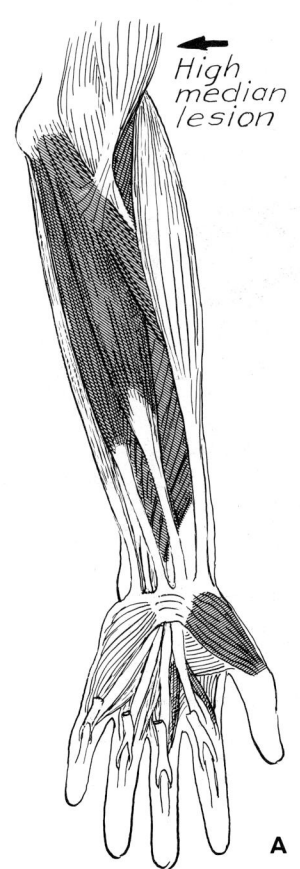

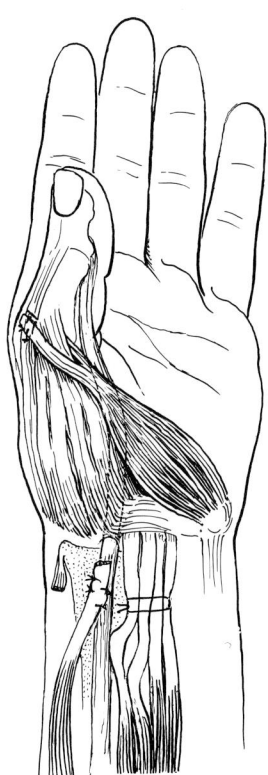

Combined transfers for high median nerve paralysis.

Tendons, Fascia and Muscles

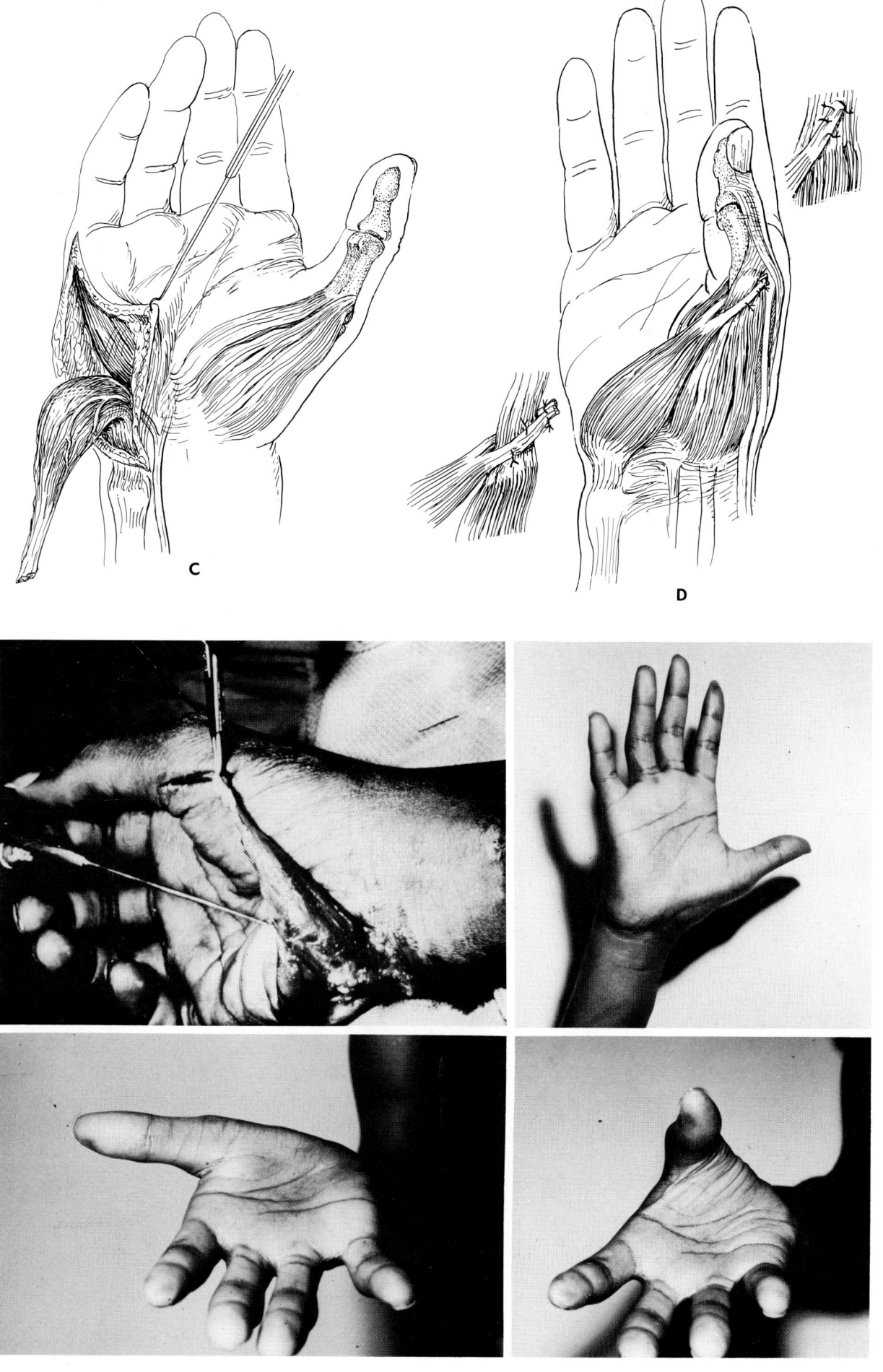

90 — Tendon Transfers for Median Nerve Paralysis

Complications of Opponens Transfer

Removal of the superficialis from a finger must be done with caution. *First,* one must determine that the patient has a functioning profundus flexor in the donor finger, otherwise he will be robbed of all interphalangeal joint flexors. *Second,* one should check the hypertensibility and, therefore, the integrity and tightness of the palmar capsule of the proximal interphalangeal joint of the donor finger. Where the capsule is lax one must remove the superficialis, leaving adequate length for the distal superficialis tails to attach proximal to the joint to prevent occurrence of recurvatum deformity of the joint. (**E**)

The finger should be splinted in ten degrees of flexion for two weeks postoperatively to avoid this complication. It may be corrected if it does occur by tenodesis of the distal tails of the superficialis across the proximal interphalangeal joint. (**F**)

Third, one must place the transferred superficialis tendon on the surface of the thenar muscles along a line which places its pull palmar to the joint axis of the metacarpophalangeal joint. If it falls dorsal to the joint axis, it may pull the joint into hyperextension, creating a collapse recurvatum of the metacarpophalangeal joint. (**G** and **H**)

If the tendon transfer is functional except for this complication, it is best corrected by fusion of the metacarpophalangeal joint. (**I**)

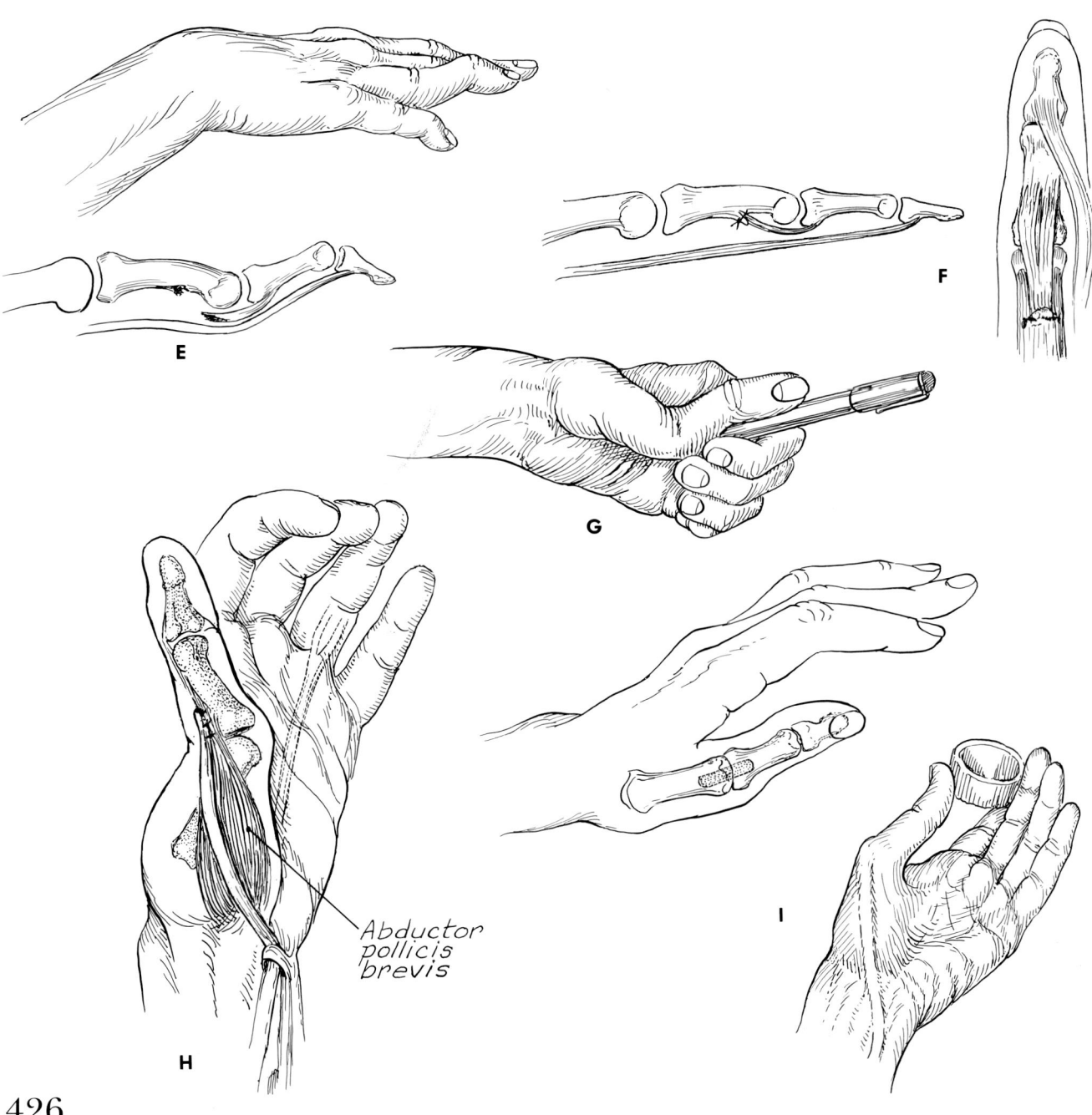

91

Tendon Transfers For Radial Nerve Paralysis

Paralysis of the muscles innervated by the radial nerve may successfully be substituted for by a variety of tendon transfers. Commonly the radial nerve is injured at the mid-humeral level where it lies superficial in the spiral groove. Fracture of the humerus may result in radial nerve paralysis at this susceptible level, but in a large percentage of closed fractures the nerve will recover spontaneously.

The key function attributable to the radial-innervated muscles is wrist extension. Power grip is critically dependent upon fixation of the wrist in extension. Extension and abduction of the thumb through the oblique muscles to the thumb (abductor pollicis longus, extensor pollicis longus, and extensor pollicis brevis) is next in the priority of functions requiring substitution in radial paralysis. Extension of the fingers, particularly at the metacarpophalangeal joints, also requires motor substitution. Supination is weakened but not lost in most positions since the secondary function of the innervated biceps is supination.

The uncorrected paralytic position in radial nerve palsy, therefore, consists of wrist drop, finger drop at the metacarpophalangeal joints, thumb adduction, and thumb flexion. To avoid fixed deformity, the full range of motion in all joints must be maintained. This is best done by a combination of passive range of motion exercises and splinting. A dynamic splint should be designed to hold the wrist in "cock-up" extension position, the metacarpophalangeal joints in extension, and the thumb in radial abduction and extension. Splinting and range of motion exercises keep the limb in proper condition to regain maximum function if paralysis is reversed or if tendon transfers are done.

The extensor-supinator group of muscles on the dorsal aspect of the forearm paralyzed in radial palsy are substituted for by transfer from a variety of muscles in the pronator flexor group innervated by the median and ulnar nerves.

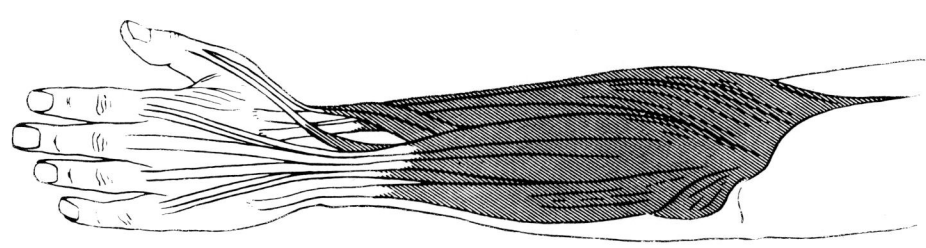

From White.

91 – Tendon Transfers for Radial Nerve Paralysis

In pure radial nerve palsy all of the muscles of the superficial layer on the palmar aspect of the forearm are fully innervated and available for transfer. (See page 397.) In addition, the superficialis and flexors of the fingers, each with individual functional capability, are also intact and innervated. The pronator teres crosses beneath the brachioradialis and extensor carpi radialis longus and brevis to insert on the mid-radius. (**A**) By releasing its insertion around the radius, it may be transferred to the extensor carpi radialis brevis and, with little change in direction of pull, it becomes a motor replacement for this prime wrist extensor. The fleshy muscle is best rerouted superficial to the brachioradialis to insert into the extensor carpi radialis brevis or into both brevis and longus. The juncture is made with the wrist held passively in full extension and with substantial tension on the pronator teres. (**B**) After transfer the pronator teres still acts as a pronator, though it is somewhat less effective.

Loss of active extension of the fingers at the metacarpophalangeal joint and weakness of interphalangeal joint extension, particularly with the metacarpophalangeal joints in flexion, is a hallmark of radial palsy. It may be overcome best by using a naturally synergistic wrist flexor as a substitute source of power. The flexor carpi ulnaris and part of its distal origin in the distal forearm, released from its insertion at the wrist, may be rerouted subcutaneously to the extensor digitorum to all fingers. (**C**) The extensor digitorum should be extensively unroofed by removal of the deep fascia over the musculotendinous units proximal to the extensor retinaculum at the wrist. The end of the flexor carpi ulnaris may be sutured to the extensor pollicis longus as well.

Tendons, Fascia and Muscles

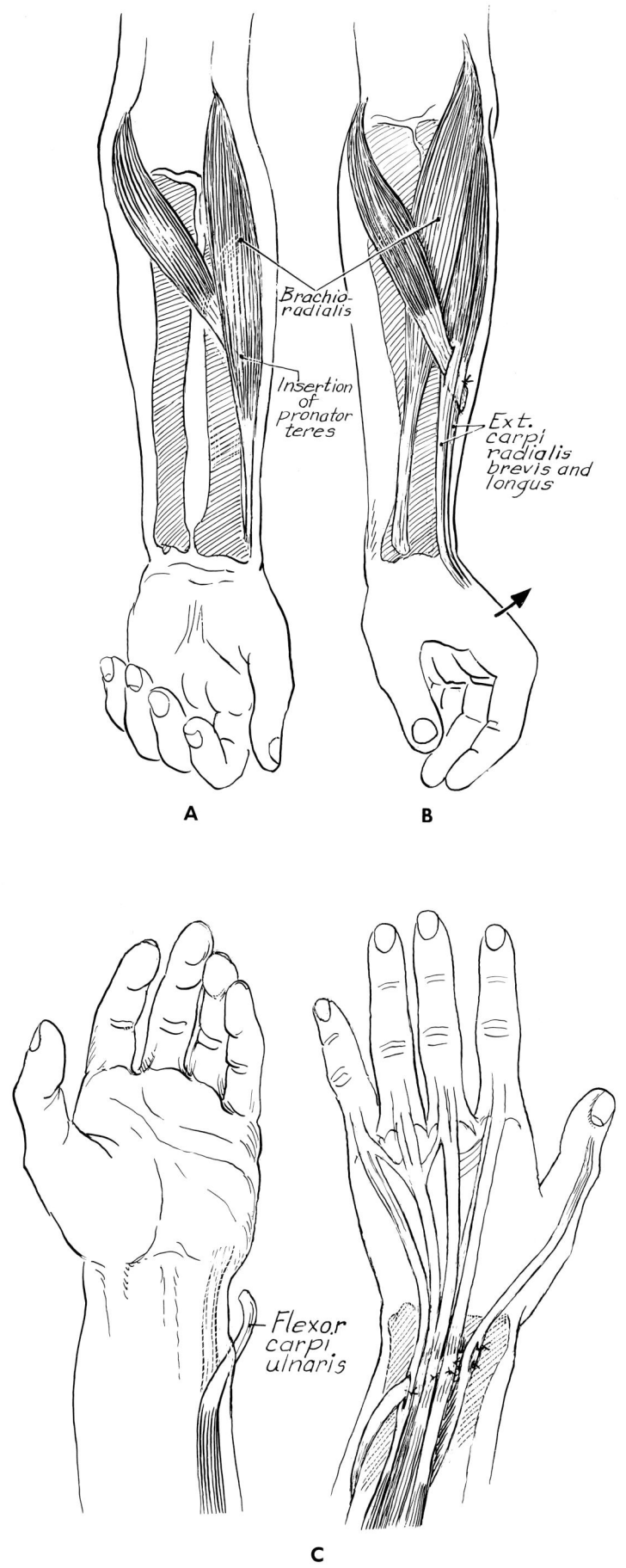

91 – Tendon Transfers for Radial Nerve Paralysis

Alternatively, the flexor carpi radialis is cut near its insertion and passed around the radial side of the forearm for insertion into the extensor pollicis longus and extensor indicis. (**D**, **E**, **F**, and **G**)

Further thumb stability may be achieved by transfer of the palmaris longus into the extensor pollicis brevis. If all other primary wrist flexors have been used, the palmaris longus should be left *in situ*. Even then it is possible to release the extensor pollicis brevis from its wrist tunnel and to reroute it for side-to-side suture with an uninterrupted palmaris longus. (**H**)

After the transfers are complete the hand is put up in a dressing with a splint fashioned to hold the wrist and metacarpophalangeal joints of the fingers in extension and the thumb in radial abduction and extension. This position is held for four weeks, after which progressive activity is first allowed then urged over several months.

A variety of other transfers may be successful and even more useful in specific cases. For example, all of the superficialis tendons are available for use, since in isolated radial nerve paralysis, all fingers have intact profundi. The palmaris longus is available to aid in thumb stabilization in abduction if the flexor carpi radialis is left intact as an active wrist flexor.

Thoughtful ingenuity on the part of the surgeon assessing the disability and functioning muscles available for transfer will result in use of a proper combination of transfers in an individual case.

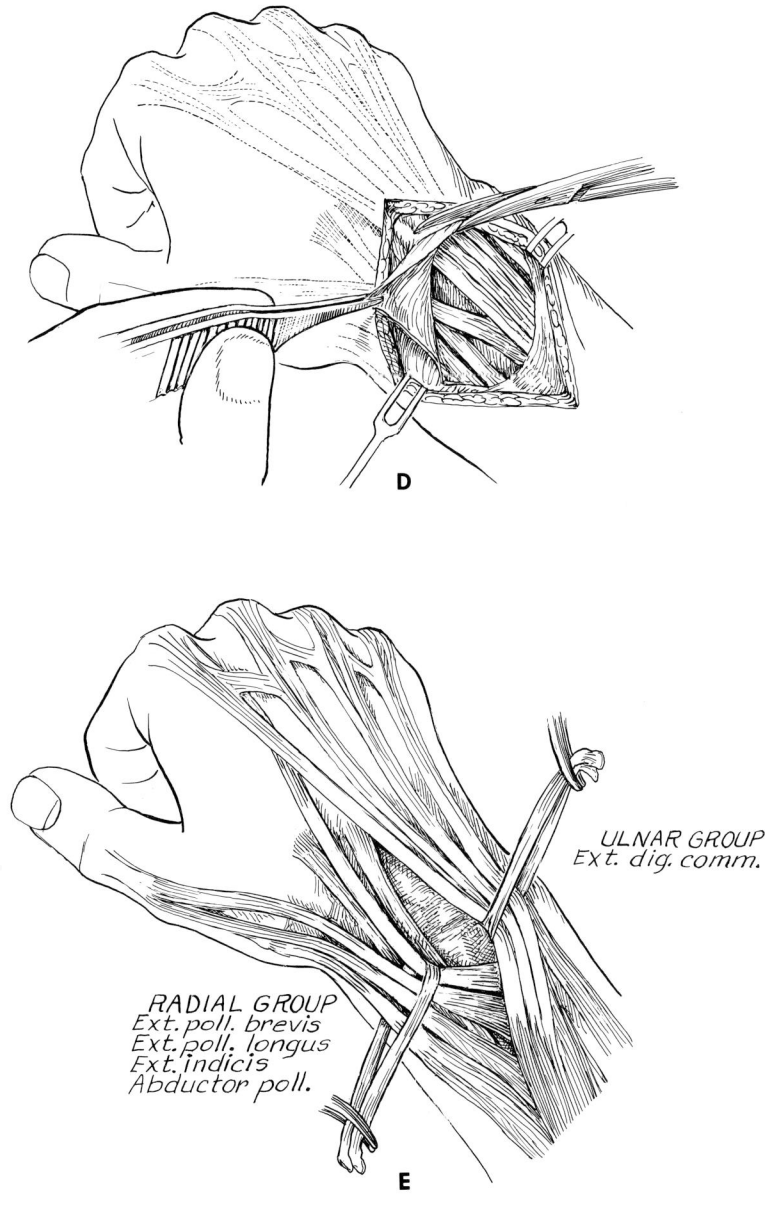

Tendons, Fascia and Muscles

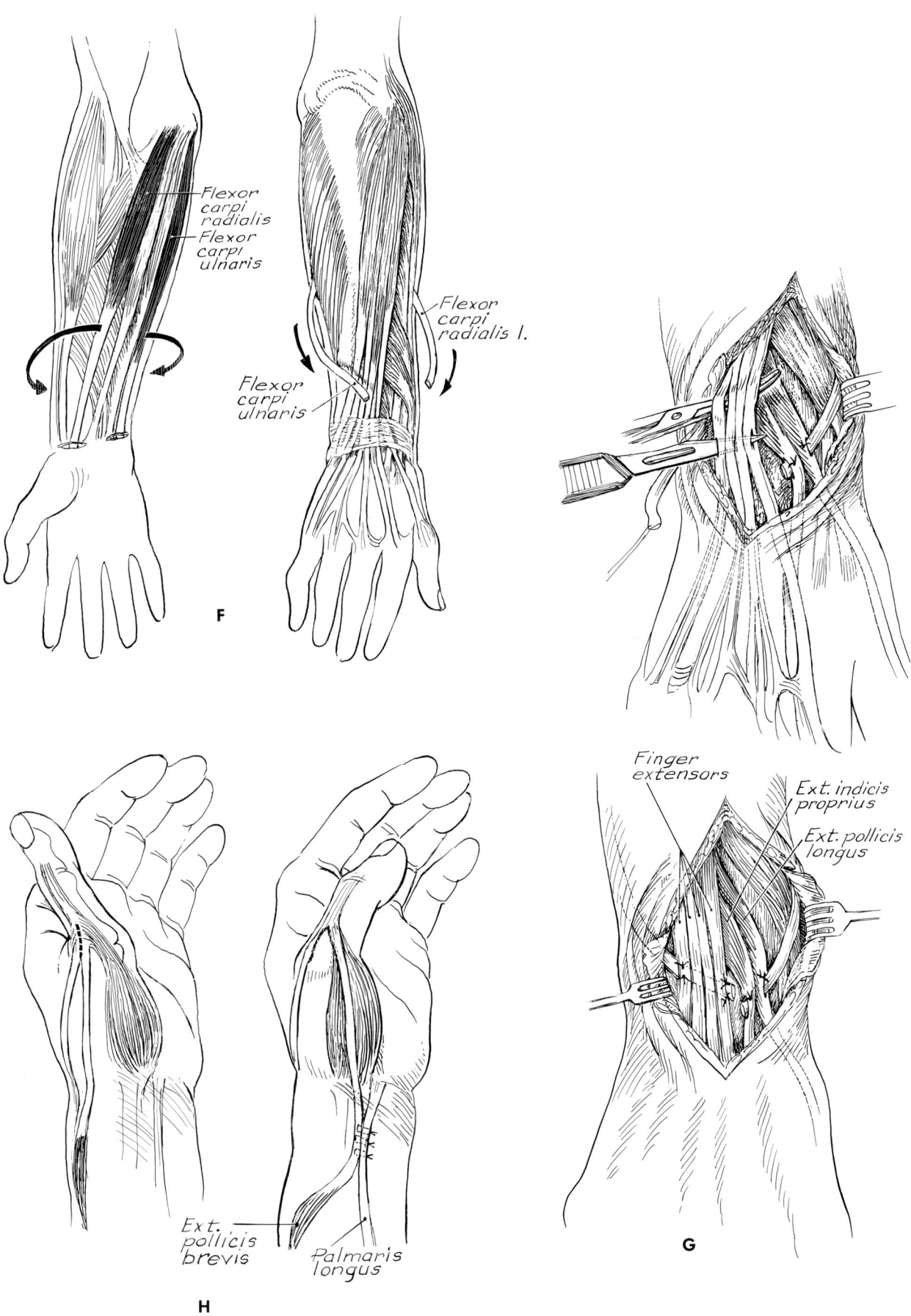

431

Index

Abrasion, avulsion, of hand, with loss of skin and tendons, 121–125
Abscess, collar button, 60
Advancement flap, in fingertip amputation, 82–84
Allen's test, in vascular reconstruction, 195–197
Amputated parts, as a source of free skin and nerve grafts, 166
Amputation(s), 147–193
   avulsion, of fingertip, 66
   of fingertip, replantation of fingertip after, 66
   of fifth ray, 158
   of index finger, 150
   of index ray, 151
   of little finger ray, in severe Dupuytren's contracture, 394–395
   of long finger ray,
      rotation of ring and little fingers in, 184
   of ring finger metacarpal, 188
   of thumb, subtotal, 295
         pollicization for, 301–304
   ray, for severe Dupuytren's contracture, 394–395
   replantation after, 68–69, 198
   single digit, 148–150
   two-stage, with cross-finger flap, 116–119
Anesthesia, of finger tips, after ulnar nerve injury at wrist, 212
   nerve block. See *Nerve block anesthesia.*
Arthritis, rheumatoid, surgery of, 319–345. See also *Rheumatoid arthritis.*
Arthroplasty, finger, 332–339
   implant, 334–339
      in metacarpophalangeal joint destruction, 334
      in proximal interphalangeal joint destruction, 336
      joint prostheses for, Niebauer vs. Swanson, 338
   wrist, in rheumatoid arthritis, 321–345
Arthroplasty implant, preparation of, 336
Atrophy, of denervated muscles, after nerve transection, 208
   of skin over finger tips, after ulnar nerve injury at wrist, 212
   of ulnar innervated muscles, after ulnar nerve injury at wrist, 212
Autogenous nerve grafts, to overcome nerve gaps, 236
Avulsion, of finger skin by ring, 130–133
   of ring finger, island pedicle flap in, 174
Avulsion abrasion of hand, with loss of skin and tendons, 121–125
Avulsion amputation, of fingertip, 66
Avulsion injuries, severe, of index finger, 172
   of thumb, 176
Axillary brachial plexus block, 30

Base pedicle, importance of, 144
Bennett's fracture, 253
Blade, Weck, 40
Bone, cortical vs. cancellous, for bone grafts, 258
   donor, iliac, 260
      of hand, 264
      rib, 262
      tibial, 258
      ulnar, 262
   salvage of, in severe hand injuries, 162

Bone and joint reconstruction, 245–291
Bone blocks, in stabilization of first metacarpal, 275
Bone grafting, 258–265
   metacarpal, 270–275
   phalangeal, 266–269
Bone graft(s), donor sites for, 258
   in thumb reconstruction, 68
   phalangeal, 266
Bony ankylosis, in stiff proximal interphalangeal joints, 254
Boutonniere deformity, in proximal interphalangeal joint, 377
Brand procedures I and II, in motorized tendon transfers, 411–415
Brand tendon stripper, 361
Brown-Padget dermatome, 44
Bunnell pull-out technique, in extensor tendon repair, 368–369

Capsulodesis, at metacarpophalangeal joint, in correction of ulnar claw hand, 402
Carpometacarpal joint, of thumb, fusion of, 280–282
   implant arthroplasty to, 338
Closed section palmar fasciotomy, 392–393
Collar button abscess, 60
Combined island pedicle and nerve transfer techniques, 242–244
Composite transfer, of joint, 190–193
Contracture, Dupuytren's, 378–395. See also *Dupuytren's contracture.*
   flexion, 35
   hyperextension, in burn or avulsion injuries, 92
   in stiff proximal interphalangeal joints, 254
Cross-finger flap, 71–73
   two-stage amputation with, 116

Deep sensibility, test of, late after nerve injury, 229
Deficits, sensory, in acute nerve injury at wrist, 202–204
Deformity(ies), boutonniere, 377
   of fingers, from tendon imbalance, 374–377
      recurvatum, 374
      swan neck, 375–376
Degeneration, Wallerian, following nerve transection, 208
Degloving injury, total, 134
Denervated muscles, atrophy of after nerve transection, 208
Dermatome, air, Hall, 44
   Brown-Padget, 44
   Davol/Simon, 40
   drum, 46–53. See also *Drum dermatome.*
   electric, 44
   mesh graft, Tanner-Vandeput, 54
   Silver, 40
   special, 44–53
Diagnostic tests, late after nerve injury, 229–233
Digital extensor tendon, technique of surgical repair of, 370
Digital fillet, secondary, 104–109
Digital joints, surgical fusion of, 283–288
Digital nerve repair, 216
   Tinel's sign in, 217

Index

Digits, damaged, use of as composite transfers, 164
Direct nerve stimulation, as diagnostic tool, late after nerve injury, 230
Discrimination, two point, 230
Distal phalanx, fractures of, 251–252
Distant pedicle flap(s), 120
    combined with secondary local island pedicle flap, 178
Dorsal skin, characteristics of, 32
Dorsum, of hand, skin grafting on, 92–95
Drainage, surgical. See *Surgical drainage.*
Dressing, stent, 55
Drum dermatome, method of operation, 46–53
    Padgett, 46
    Reese, 46
Dupuytren's contracture, 378–395
    dissection of palm skin in, 34
    in stiff proximal interphalangeal joints, 254
    knuckle pads in, 378
    palmar fasciectomy in, 380
    Peyronie's disease in, 378
    ray amputation for, 394–395
Dystrophy, sympathetic, after ulnar nerve injury at wrist, 212

Elbow, median nerve injury at, 228
    repair of ulnar nerve at, 222
    ulnar nerve injury at, 222
Elective skin incisions, 35–39
Electric dermatome, 44
Electromyography, late after nerve injury, 230
Elevator, Joseph, 152
Extension, dynamics of, 10
Extensor carpi radialis longus, transfer of to opponens, in high median nerve paralysis, 422
Extensor muscles, extrinsic, 14
Extensor pollicis longus tendon, injuries to, 372–373
Extensor tendon(s), digital, injuries to, 370
    lacerations of, 368–369
    rupture of, 342–343
    synovectomy of at wrist, 340–341
Extremity, shortening of, to overcome nerve gaps, 234

Fascia, palmar, 32–34
Fasciectomy, palmar. See *Palmar Fasciectomy.*
Fasciotomy, palmar, closed section, 392–393
    open section, 390–391
Felon, incision and drainage of, 57
Fifth ray amputation, 158
Fillet principle, in acute injury, 112–115
Finger(s), avulsion of skin of by ring, 130–133
    deformities of from tendon imbalance, 374–377
    immobilization of, in fracture in hand, 246
    index. See *Index finger.*
    individual, nerve block anesthesia for, 30
    interphalangeal joints of, fusion of, 284
    little, amputation of, 148
        ray amputation of, for severe Dupuytren's contracture, 394–395
    long, amputation of, 148, 184
    long flexors of, and interphalangeal joints, 14
    multiple use of parts of after amputation, 168–171
    ring, avulsion of, 174
    third, fourth and fifth, action of, 4
Finger arthroplasty, 332–339
Finger drop, in radial nerve palsy, 227
Finger fillet, to resurface thumb, 110
Fingernail, injuries to, 70
    salvage of, in severe hand injuries, 162
Fingertip, avulsion amputation of, 66
    injuries to, 61–84
        minor soft tissue loss in, 63–65
    loss of, advancement flap for, 82–84
    replantation of after amputation, 68–69

Finger to thumb pedicle flap, 74–77
First web space, contracture in, 138
    distant pedicle flap in cleft of, 140
    loss of skin and soft tissue in, 136
    Z-plasty in contracture in, 138
Flap(s), cross finger, 71–73, 97–99
    infraclavicular, 126–133
    pedicle, finger to thumb, 74–77
    island. See *Island pedicle flap.*
    vascularized, 71
Flexion, dynamics of, 10
Flexion contracture, 35
Flexor carpi ulnaris, detection of paralysis of, 222
    transfer of, in high median nerve paralysis, 422
Flexor digitorum profundus, detection of paralysis of, 222
Flexor muscles, extrinsic, 16
Flexor pollicis brevis, heads of, table of innervation of, 221
Flexor pollicis longus, lacerations of, 363–366
Flexor sheath, avoidance of constriction of by insertion of silicone rod, 358
Flexor tendon(s), grafting of, 356–360
    lacerations of, 348–355
        primary management of, 352
Foot, plantar surface, as source of skin graft, 90
Fowler procedure (Riordan modification), in motorized tendon transfer, 410–411
Fracture(s), Bennett's, 253
    immobilization of hand in, 246
    in hand, 246–253
    of distal phalanx, 251–252
    open metacarpal, 250
    unstable closed metacarpal, 248
Freehand grafts, 40–43
Free skin grafts, 86–95
Froment's sign, after ulnar nerve injury at wrist, 212
Fusion, surgical. See *Surgical fusion.*

Graft(s). See also specific types; e.g., *Bone grafts, Skin grafts.*
    bone, cortical vs. cancellous, 258
        donor sites for, 258
        in thumb reconstruction, 68
    free, full thickness, in avulsion amputation of fingertip, 66
    freehand, 40–43
    free skin, in finger injuries, 36
        in minor soft tissue loss in fingertip, 63
    tendon, donor sites for, 361–362
Grafting. See also specific types; e.g., *Bone grafting, Skin grafting.*
    bone, 258–265
    mesh, 54
    of flexor tendons, 356–360
    nerve, to overcome nerve gaps, 236
    skin, 40–55. See also under *Skin grafting.*

Hall air dermatome, 44
Hand, adaptive elements of, 4
    anatomy of, 3–20
    as bone graft source, 264
    avulsion abrasion of dorsum of, with loss of skin and tendons, 121–125
    bone from, as bone graft source, 264
    dorsum of, skin grafting on, 92–95
    elective incisions of, planning of, 35
    flexion and extension of, 10
    fractures in, 246–253
    functionally important areas of sensibility of, 221
    immobilization of, in fracture, 246
    skeleton and neuromuscular apparatus of, 4–9
    skeleton of, architecture of, 4
        fixed unit of, 4
    skin grafting of palm of, 86–89
    total degloving injury of, 134–135
    ulnar nerve motor innervation in, 210

Index

Hand degloving injury, 134
Hand function, dynamics of, 10–19
Hand injuries, severe, salvage of usable parts in, 162
High median nerve paralysis, 422–423
Humby knife, in freehand skin grafting, 42
Hyperextension contracture, in burn or avulsion injuries, 92

Iliac bone, as bone graft source, 260
Immobilization, of hand, in fracture, 246
 of joint, in hand fracture, 246
Implant arthroplasty, 334–339
 in metacarpophalangeal joint destruction, 334
 in proximal interphalangeal joint destruction, 336
 in thumb carpometacarpal joint, 338
 joint prostheses for Niebauer vs. Swanson, 338
Implant, arthroplasty, preparation of, 336
Incision, W-shaped, in repair of Dupuytren's contracture, 384
 Z-plasty. See *Z-plasty incision.*
Index finger, action of, 4
 amputation of, 149, 150
 avulsion injury to, 172
 blast injury to, 172
 metacarpal transfer in, 184–187
Index ray, amputation of, 151
 osteotomy of, 152
Infections, 56–60. See also specific types; e.g., *Paronychia, Synovial infections.*
Infraclavicular flap, advantages and disadvantages of, 126
Injury(ies), acute, fillet principle in, 112–115
 of motor branch of ulnar nerve, 213–215
 avulsion, to index finger, 172
 fingernail, 70
 median nerve, 202, 208, 228
 nerve. See *Nerve injury.*
 severe, of hand, salvage of usable parts in, 162
 severe avulsion, of index finger, 172
  of thumb, 176
  ring, 174
 tendon, 346–347
 to digital extensor tendon, 370
 to fingernail, 70
 to fingertip, 61–84
 to median nerve, at elbow, 228
  at wrist, 202
 to thumb tip, 74
 total hand degloving, 134
 to ulnar nerve, at elbow, 222
Intermetacarpal ligaments, insertion of, 8
Interphalangeal joints, action and architecture of, 8
 boutonniere deformity in, 377
 collateral ligaments of, 6
 long flexors of fingers and, 14
 proximal, flexor digitorum profundus muscle and, 16
 of thumb, implant arthroplasty to, 336
 stiff, 254–257
 surgical fusion of, 284
 swan neck deformity in, 375–376
Intrinsic muscle(s), salvage of, in severe hand injuries, 162
 transfer of, for opponens paralysis, 424
Island pedicle flap, for fingertip loss, 78–81
 in avulsion or blast injury to index finger, 172
 in ring avulsion injury, 174
 in thumb avulsion injury, 176
 in thumb reconstruction, 310
 primary, for salvage after trauma, 172–182
Island pedicle technique, 238–241
 neurovascular, in thumb reconstruction, 310

Joint(s), carpometacarpal, of thumb, 280–282, 338
 digital, surgical fusion of, 283–288

Joint(s) (*Continued*)
 immobilization of, in fracture in hand, 246
 interphalangeal. See *Interphalangeal joints.*
 metacarpophalangeal. See *Metacarpophalangeal joint(s).*
 positioning of, to overcome nerve gaps, 234
 relation of skin creases to, 8
 salvage of, in severe hand injuries, 162
 skin creases and, 8
 surgical fusion of, principles of, 276
 thumb carpometacarpal, fusion of, 280–282
 thumb metacarpophalangeal, fusion of, 276–279
 wrist, action and architecture of, 8
  fusion of, 288–291
Joint prostheses, for implant arthroplasty, Niebauer vs. Swanson, 338

Kirschner wire(s), in Bennett's fracture of metacarpal, 253
 in composite transfer of metacarpophalangeal joint, 192
 in fractures of distal phalanx, 251–252
 in fractures of hand, 246, 248
 in fusion of thumb carpometacarpal joint, 282
 in metacarpal transfer, 184
 in open metacarpal fracture, 250
 in thumb avulsion injury, 176
 in thumb pollicization, 308
 in unstable closed metacarpal fracture, 248
Knuckle pads, in Dupuytren's contracture, 378

Laceration(s), of extensor tendon, 368–369
 of flexor pollicis longus, 363–366
 of flexor tendons, 348–355
 of wrist, palmar, 366–367
Ligaments, intermetacarpal, insertion of, 8
Light touch, evaluation of late after nerve injury, 229
Little finger, amputation of, 148
 metacarpal transfer in, 188
 ray amputation for severe Dupuytren's contracture, 394–395
Littler, technique of, in thumb reconstruction, 310
Local pedicle shift, 100–103
Long finger, amputation of, 148, 184
Low median nerve paralysis, 419–421
Lumbrical muscles, action of, 18

Manometer, and pneumatic tourniquet, 22
Median nerve, motor innervation in hand, 202
 tests of, 202–204
 palmar cutaneous branch of, 219
 sensory pattern of, 202
 transection of, at elbow, 228
  at wrist, 205
Median nerve injury, at elbow, 228
 at wrist, 202
 findings and treatment late after, 208
 simultaneous nerve repair and opponens transfer late after, 208
Median nerve paralysis, high, 422–423
 findings in, 228
 low, 419–421
 tendon transfers for, 418–426
Mesh grafting, 54
Metacarpal, Bennett's fracture of, 253
 first, stabilization of, 275
 of thumb, bone grafting in, 274
 open fracture of, 250
 unstable closed fracture of, 248
Metacarpal bone grafting, 270–275
 technical variations, 273
Metacarpal transfer, 182–189
 index finger, 184–187
 little finger, 188
 principle of, 182

435

Index

Metacarpophalangeal joint(s), action of, 6
  capsulodesis at, in correction of ulnar claw hand, 402
  collateral ligaments of, 6
  composite transfer of, 190
  hyperextension contracture in after burn or avulsion injuries, 92
  of fingers, fusion of, 283
  of thumb, implant arthroplasty to, 334
    fusion of, 276–279
  synovectomy at, in rheumatoid arthritis, 326–333
  tenodesis at, in correction of ulnar claw hand, 406
  volar plates of, 8
Mitten hand, 134
Moberg, technique of, in thumb reconstruction, 310
Moberg ninhydrin test, 202–204
Motor deficits, in acute nerve injury at wrist, 202–204
Motorized tendon transfers, Brand procedures I and II in, 411–415
  Fowler procedure (Riordan modification) in, 410–411
  Stiles-Bunnell procedure, 416
Muscles, extrinsic, extensor, 14
  flexor, 16
  intrinsic, positioning, 12
    salvage of, in severe hand injuries, 162
  of forearm, anatomy of, 396–399

Nail bed, infections around, 56
Nerve, digital, repair of, 216
  Tinel's sign in, 217
  median. See *Median nerve.*
  radial. See *Radial nerve.*
  salvage of, in severe hand injuries, 162
  ulnar. See *Ulnar nerve.*
Nerve block anesthesia, 24–31
  as diagnostic tool, late after nerve injury, 230
  axillary brachial plexus block, 30
  combined wrist and elbow block, 28
  elbow block: median nerve, 28
  elbow block: ulnar nerve, 28
  for individual fingers, 30
  in diagnosis late after nerve injury, 230
  wrist block: dorsal nerve, 26–27
  wrist block: median nerve, 24–25
  wrist block: ulnar nerve, 26–27
Nerve conduction time, measurement of, late after nerve injury, 230
Nerve crossover, to overcome nerve gaps, 234
Nerve gap(s), 234–237
  island pedicle technique to treat, 238–241
Nerve graft(s), autogenous, to overcome nerve gaps, 236
  free, amputated parts as source of, 166
Nerve grafting, to overcome nerve gaps, 236
Nerve injury(ies), at wrist, facts influencing care of, 221
  sensory and motor deficits after, 202–204
  diagnostic tests late after, 229–233
  partial, repair of by secondary surgery, 232
Nerve repair, digital, 216–217
  primary, 205–207
Nerve stimulation, at nerve exploration, 230
Nerve surgery, 201–244
Nerve transection, atrophy of denervated muscles after, 208
  Wallerian degeneration following, 208
Neuroma, painful, after transection of palmar cutaneous branch of median nerve, 219
  at wrist, after ulnar nerve injury, 212
Neurovascular island pedicle technique, in thumb reconstruction, 310
Nicoladoni, technique of, in thumb reconstruction, 310

Open metacarpal fracture, 250
Open section palmar fasciotomy, 390–391
Opponens paralysis, transfer of intrinsic muscle for, 424
Opponens transfer, in high median nerve paralysis, 424
  complications of, 426
Osteotomy, oblique, of fifth ray, 158
  of index ray, 152

Palm, free plantar skin graft to, 90
  skin grafting of, 86–89
Palmar fascia, characteristics of, 32–34
Palmar fasciectomy, distortion of digital nerve anatomy in distal palm in, 386
  in Dupuytren's contracture, 380
  pitfalls of, 386
  preservation of synovial sheaths in, 388
Palmar fasciotomy, closed section, 392–393
  open section, 390–391
Palmar skin, characteristics of, 32
Palmar wrist laceration, 366–367
Palsy, low ulnar, thumb adductor paralysis in, 417
Paralysis, of flexor carpi ulnaris, detection of, 222
  of flexor digitorum profundus, detection of, 222
  of radial nerve, 226–227
  of thumb adductor, correction of, 417
  of ulnar nerve, tendon transfers for, 400–417
  opponens, transfer of intrinsic muscle for, 424
Paronychia, 56
Paronychial abscess, surgical drainage of, 56
Pedicle(s), base, importance of, 144
  vascularized, soft tissue replacement using, 96
Pedicle flap(s), 96–103
  anatomical placement of, 145
  delay in procedure, advantages and disadvantages of, 146
  distant, combined with secondary local island pedicle flap, 178
  finger to thumb, 74–77
  indication for, 142
  infraclavicular, advantages of, 128
  in thumb reconstruction, 310
  island. See *Island pedicle flap.*
  local, 97–103
  misuse of, 142
  proper use and care of, 142–146
  transfer from distant sites, 120–125
  tubed, in thumb reconstruction, 310
  vascularized, 71
Pedicle nerve grafts, 236
Pedicle shift, local, 100–103
Pedicle soft tissue from distant sites, 120–125
Peyronie's disease, in Dupuytren's contracture, 378
Phalangeal bone grafts, 266
Phalanges, use of bone grafts in, 266–269
Plates, volar, of metacarpophalangeal joints, 8
Pollicization, for congenital absence of thumb, 306–309
  for subtotal thumb loss, 301–304
  thumb reconstruction by, 300–309
  principle of, 300
Primary island pedicle flap, for salvage after trauma, 172–182
Primary nerve repair, 205–207
  principle of, 205
Primary surgery, in nerve repair, 205–207
Prostheses, joint, for implant arthroplasty, Niebauer vs. Swanson, 338

Radial nerve, dorsal branch of, 218
  repair of, 219
  paralysis of, 226–227
    tendon transfers for, 427–431
Radial nerve palsy, wrist drop and finger drop in, 227

Index

Ray, index, amputation of, 151
   osteotomy of, 152
  little finger, amputation of, for severe Dupuytren's contracture, 394–395
Records, of physical findings, keeping of, 21
Recurvatum, after ulnar nerve injury at wrist, 212
  in proximal interphalangeal joint, 375–376
Reese drum dermatome, 46
Reinsertion pull-out wire technique, in tendon repair, 352–353
Replantation, of amputated fingers, 198
  of fingertip after amputation, 68–69
Resection, of ulnar head, 344–345
Rheumatoid arthritis, surgery of, 319–345
  synovectomy at metacarpophalangeal joint in, 326–333
  synovectomy of extensor tendons at wrist in, 340
  wrist arthroplasty in, 321–325
Rheumatoid synovitis, 342
Rib, as bone graft source, 262
Ring avulsion, island pedicle flap in, 174
Ring finger, amputation of, 148
Ring finger metacarpal, amputation of, 188

Salvage of usable parts in severe hand injuries, 162–163
Scar contracture, in stiff proximal interphalangeal joints, 254
Secondary digital fillet, 104–109
Secondary surgery, repair of partial nerve injury by, 232
Sense of touch, 20
Sensibility, of hand, functionally important areas of, 221
  tests of, 229–230
Sensory deficits, in acute median nerve injury at wrist, 202–204
Sensory nerve branches, small, 218–220
Severe hand injuries, salvage of usable parts in, 162–163
Sheaths, synovial, preservation of, in palmar fasciectomy, 388
Sheath constriction, avoidance of, 358–360
Shortening of extremity, in repair of nerve gaps, 234
Single digit amputation, 148–150
Skin, and subcutaneous tissue, 32–34
  dorsal, 32
  elective incisions of, 35–39
  palmar, 32
    dissection of in Dupuytren's contracture, 34
  ring avulsion of from finger, 130–133
  salvage of, in severe hand injuries, 162
  sensibility of to pain, 20
Skin and soft tissue losses, 85
Skin creases, relation of to joints, 8
Skin grafting, 40–55
  freehand graft, 40–43
  on dorsum of hand, 92–95
  on palm of hand, 86–89
Skin grafts, free, amputated parts as source of, 166
  free plantar to palm, 90–91
    plantar surface of foot as source of, 90
Skin incisions, elective, 35–39
Soft tissue, of fingertip, extensive loss of, 66
  minor loss of, 63–65
Space infections, 58
Special dermatomes, 44–53
Square transection of peripheral nerve ends, 205
Stabilization of first metacarpal, 275
Staphylococcus, in nail bed infections, 56
Steinmann pins, in wrist arthroplasty, 322
Stent dressing, 55
Stiff proximal interphalangeal joints, 254–257
Stiles-Bunnell procedure, in motorized tendon transfer, 416
Strange-Seddon nerve graft procedure, 236

Subcutaneous tissue, 32–34
Subtotal amputation of thumb, 295–296
  pollicization for, 301–305
Sudomotor function, evaluation of, late after nerve injury, 229
  testing of, 204
Surgery, nerve, 201–244
  of rheumatoid arthritis, 319–345
  primary, in nerve repair, 205–207
  secondary, repair of partial nerve injury by, 232
Surgical drainage, of collar button abscess, 60
  of paronychial abscess, 56
  of synovial sheath infections, 58
Surgical fusion, of digital joints, 283–288
  of finger metacarpophalangeal joints, 283
  of interphalangeal joints, 284
  of joints, principles of, 276
  of thumb carpometacarpal joint, 280–282
  of thumb metacarpophalangeal joint, 276–279
  of wrist joint, 288–291
Swan neck deformity, 375–376
Syndactylism, surgical, in cross-finger flaps, 98
Synovectomy, at metacarpophalangeal joint, 326–333
  of extensor tendons at wrist, 340–341
Synovial infections, 58
Synovial sheaths, preservation of in palmar fasciectomy, 388
Synovitis, destructive, of wrist, in rheumatoid arthritis, 321
  rheumatoid, 342

Tanner-Vandeput Meshgraft Dermatome, 54
Tendon(s), anatomy of, 396–399
  extensor, lacerations of, 368–369
    rupture of, 342–343
    synovectomy of at wrist, 340–341
  extensor pollicis longus, injuries to, 372–373
  flexor, grafting of, 356–360
    lacerations of, 348–355
      primary management of, 352
  salvage of, in severe hand injuries, 162
  transected, end-to-end repair of, 346
Tendon graft(s), donor sites for, 361–362
  in avulsion abrasion, 124
Tendon imbalance, deformities of fingers from, 374–377
Tendon injuries, 346–347
Tendon transfers, 396–399
  for median nerve paralysis, 418–431
  for radial nerve paralysis, 427–431
  for ulnar nerve paralysis, 400–417
Tendon tunneler, in tendon graft, 124
Tendons, fascia and muscles, 346–431
Tenodesis, at metacarpophalangeal joint, in correction of ulnar claw hand, 406
Test, Allen's, in vascular reconstruction, 195–197
  diagnostic, after nerve injury, 229–233
  Moberg ninhydrin, 202–204
  of sensibility,
    late after nerve injury, 229–230
      deep, 229
      light touch, 229
      sudomotor function, 229
      Tinel's sign, 230
      two-point discrimination, 230
  of motor function, late after nerve injury, 230
Thumb, amputation of, 148
  avulsion, with loss of skin in excess of bone, 127–129
  subtotal, pollicization for, 301–304
  carpometacarpal joint of, fusion of, 280–282
    implant arthroplasty to, 338
  congenital absence of, pollicization for, 306–309
  finger fillet to resurface, 110
  interphalangeal joints of, fusion of, 284
  metacarpal of, bone grafting in, 274
  metacarpophalangeal joint of, fusion of, 276–279

Thumb (Continued)
  range of motion of, 4
  reconstruction of, 293–317
    after pulp loss, finger to thumb pedicle flap in, 74
      island pedicle flap in, 78
    by pollicization, 300–309
    local soft tissue advancement and bone graft in, 68
    pedicle flap, bone graft, island flap method in, 310–317
    technique of Nicoladoni in, 310
  subtotal amputation of, 295
    pollicization for, 301–304
  surgical fusion of joints of, 276
Thumb adductor, paralysis of, correction of, 417
Thumb avulsion, island pedicle flap in, 176
Tibia, as bone graft source, 258
Tinel's sign, evaluation of, late after nerve injury, 230
  in digital nerve repair, 217
Total hand degloving injury, 134–135
Touch, sense of, 20
Tourniquet, Esmarch, in nerve block anesthesia, 28
  pneumatic, 22–23
    technique and rules in use of, 22
Transection, of median nerve at wrist, 205
  square, of peripheral nerve ends, 205
Transfer(s), composite, use of damaged digits as, 164
  metacarpal, 182–189
Trauma, primary island pedicle flap for salvage after, 172–182
Two-point discrimination, evaluation of, late after nerve injury, 230
Two-stage amputation, with cross-finger flap, 116–119

Ulcers, on skin over fingertips, after ulnar nerve injury at wrist, 212
Ulna, as bone graft source, 262
  head of, resection of, 344–345
Ulnar claw hand, 400
  after ulnar nerve injury at wrist, 212
  correction of, 402
Ulnar nerve, acute injury of motor branch, 213–215
  dorsal branch of, 219
  paralysis of, tendon transfers for, 400–417
  repair of at elbow, 222
  sensory pattern of, 210
  transection of, at elbow, 222
    at wrist, acute, 210–212
  transposition of, 224
    to overcome nerve gaps, 234

Ulnar nerve injury, at elbow, 222
  at wrist, findings immediately after, 210
    progressive changes after, 212
Upper extremity, sensibility in, 20

Vascular reconstruction, 195–200
  after replantation, 198
  Allen's test in, 195–197
  principles of, 198
Vascularized pedicle flap, 71
Vascularized pedicles, as soft tissue replacement, 96
Vi-drape, in median nerve transection, 205
Volar plates, of metacarpophalangeal joints, 8

Wallerian degeneration, following nerve transection, 208
Web space, deepening of, in thumb reconstruction, 68
  first. See *First web space.*
Weck blade, for small split thickness skin grafts, 40
Weinstein-Semmes Pressure Aesthesiometer, in light touch evaluation, 229
Wounds, deep, pain in, 20
Wrist, acute nerve injury at, motor and sensory deficits in, 202–204
  acute ulnar nerve transection at, 210–212
  functionally important areas of sensibility of, 221
  median nerve injury at, 202, 208
  nerve injuries at, facts influencing care of, 221
  palmar, laceration of, 366–367
  synovectomy of extensor tendons at, 340–341
  ulnar nerve injury at, 210
    findings immediately after, 210
    progressive changes after, 212
  variations in intrinsic muscle innervation patterns of, 221
Wrist arthroplasty, in rheumatoid arthritis, 321–325
Wrist block anesthesia, 24–27
Wrist drop, in radial nerve palsy, 227
Wrist joint, action and architecture of, 8
  fusion of, 288–291
W-shaped incision, in repair of Dupuytren's contracture, 384

Z-plasty incision, in finger injuries, 36
  in first web space contracture, 138
  in repair of Dupuytren's contracture, 380
  in skin grafting of dorsum of hand, 92